CRITICAL CARE INFECTIOUS DISEASES TEXTBOOK

CRITICAL CARE INFECTIOUS DISEASES TEXTBOOK

Edited by

Jordi Rello, M.D., Ph.D.
HOSPITAL UNIVERSITARI JOAN XXIII.
AND
UNIVERSITY ROVIRA & VIRGILI
TARRAGONA, SPAIN

Jordi Valles, M.D., Ph.D.
CORPORACIO SANITARIA PARC TAULI,
SABADELL, BARCELONA, SPAIN

Marin H. Kollef, M.D.
WASHINGTON UNIVERSITY SCHOOL OF MEDICINE
AND
BARNES-JEWISH HOSPITAL
ST. LOUIS, MISSOURI, USA

Springer-Science+Business Media, B.V.

Library of Congress Cataloging-in-Publication Data
Critical care infectious diseases textbook / edited by Jordi Rello, Jordi Valles, Marin H. Kollef.
p. ; cm.
Includes bibliographical references and index.
ISBN 978-1-4613-5674-5 ISBN 978-1-4615-1679-8 (eBook)
DOI 10.1007/978-1-4615-1679-8
1. Communicable diseases. 2. Critical care medicine. 3. Intensive care units. 4. Nosocomial infections. 5. Opportunistic infections. I. Rello, Jordi. II. Valles, Jordi, 1953– III. Kollef, Marin H.
[DNLM: 1. Cross Infection – therapy. 2. Anti-Infective Agents – therapeutic use. 3. Community-Acquired Infections – therapy. 4. Critical Care – methods. 5. Infection Control – methods. 6. Intensive Care Units. WX 167 C934 2001]
RC112 .C75 2001
616.9 – dc21

00-066407

Printed on acid-free paper.

CONTENTS

PREFACE

Infections and their complications are a very important clinical area in the intensive care unit setting. Community-acquired infections and nosocomial infections both contribute to the high level of disease acquity common among critically ill patients. The importance of accurately diagnosing nosocomial infections and providing appropriate therapies, to include antimicrobial therapy effective against the identified agents of infection, have been shown to be important determinants of patient outcome. Critical care practitioners are in a unique position in dealing with infectious diseases. They are often the initial providers of care to seriously ill patients with infections. Additionally, they have a responsibility to ensure that nosocomial infections are prevented and that antimicrobial resistance is minimized by prudently employing antibiotic agents. It is our hope that this textbook will provide clinicians practicing in the intensive care unit a reference to help guide their care of infected patients. To that end we have brought together a group of international authors to address important topics related to infectious diseases for the critical care practitioner.

Jordi Rello, M.D., Ph.D.
Jordi Valles, M.D., Ph.D
Marin H. Kollef, M.D

SECTION 1: GENERAL ASPECTS

J. Rello

1. OPPORTUNISTIC INFECTIONS: AN OVERVIEW

Guillem Prats and Ferran Sánchez

Introduction

Opportunistic infections occur in patients who have local or systemic factors favoring infection and are caused by non-pathogenic microorganisms, which form part of the normal flora of man or of the environment.

Patients admitted to hospital and in particular to Intensive Care Units (ICU) have different factors predisposing them to infection; some local factors such as intravascular catheters, indwelling urinary catheters, and tracheal intubation are very prevalent. Moreover, diseases such as granulocytopenia, AIDS or cirrhosis, among others, constitute systemic processes favoring infection (Table 1). This chapter focuses on infections due to local predisposing factors.

Opportunistic Microorganisms

Opportunistic microorganisms form part of the normal human flora or are telluric microorganisms, which are found in the inanimate environment or have temporarily colonized man.

The skin and the mucouse membranes of the respiratory, digestive and genital tract are normally coated with numerous different microorganisms, mainly bacteria. The concentration and diversity of these microorganisms depends on the territory assessed [1].

Gram-positive bacteria such as the coagulase-negative staphylococci (*Staphylococcus epidermidis* and others) and the corynebacteria, are predominant on the skin.

The nasal cavity is the natural habitat of *Staphylococcus aureus*, and various species of commensal neisseries, *viridans* streptococci, pneumococci and some anaerobic bacteria can be found in the oropharynx.

The number of bacteria is progressively higher in the small intestine and in the colon reaches 10^{9-10} bacteria per gram of faeces. The main components of the intestinal flora are the anaerobic bacteria, the enterobacteria (such as *Escherichia coli* and others) and the enterococci. Yeasts of the genus *Candida* are also occasionally found.

Under normal conditions a slightly varied flora, but with a marked preponderance of lactobacilli (Döderlein bacilli) is found in the vagina of the woman of fertile age. Table 2 indicates the main microorganisms of the normal human flora.

Some Gram-negative rods, such as *Pseudomonas aeruginosa*, *Acinetobacter baumannii* and others are widely distributed in nature, in water, earth and plants (Table 2). When they become established in a ward or ICU, they can be found on the floor, on the surfaces, in recipients with water and even in antiseptics. These microorganisms, in addition to being resistant to some antiseptics, also tend to be resistant to numerous antimicrobials commonly used in therapy.

Their widespread distribution and persistence in the environment makes their eradication difficult. Although most of them do not form part of the normal stable human flora, they can colo-

TABLE 1. Factors predisposing to infection

I **Local factors**
- A *Damaged integument*
  - 1 Traumatic
  - 2 Surgical
  - 3 Intravascular devices
  - 4 Indwelling urinary catheters
  - 5 Endotracheal intubation
  - 6 Central nervous system shunts
  - 7 Peritoneal dyalisis and hemodialysis
- B *Foreign bodies*
  - 1 Prosthetic joint / heart valves
  - 2 Pacemaker
- C *Contaminated surgery*

II **General factors**
- A Granulocytopenia
- B Transplantation
- C AIDS
- D Liver cirrhosis
- E Chronic renal failure
- F Diabetes mellitus (?)

nize man for long periods of time, adhering to foreign matter such as tracheal and other catheters, but also occur in the skin and the digestive tract, in particular in people in which their normal flora has been eradicated by the administration of antibiotics.

MAIN OPPORTUNISTIC MICROORGANISMS

Staphylococcus epidermidis, *Escherichia coli*, *Enterococcus faecalis* and *Pseudomonas aeruginosa* cause the great majority of opportunistic infections in patients with catheters, drainages, tracheostomy or subject to dialysis. However, in specific areas of the hospital, such as urology and neurology wards, ICU or operating theatres, other microorganisms may appear alongside these, such as the methicillin-resistant strains of *Staphylococcus aureus* (MRSA), *Enterococcus faecium*, multiresistant *Pseudomonas aeruginosa*, *Acinetobacter baumannii* or other endogenous or telluric bacteria causing sporadic infections or epidemics (Table 2).

After surgical operations carried out on the oropharynx or the digestive tract, polymicrobial infections can occur caused by bacteria of the oropharyngeal or intestinal flora, including anaerobes such as *Peptostreptococcus*, *Bacteroides*, *Prevotella*, *Fusobacterium*, *Eubacterium*, *Bifidobacterium* and *Clostridium*, among others.

STAPHYLOCOCCI

The staphylococci are non-fastidious, facultative aerobic and anaerobic Gram-positive cocci which are usually classified into two groups: coagulase-positive and coagulase-negative (CoN).

The coagulase-negative staphylococci form a group which includes some 30 species, of which a dozen have been described as colonizing the skin and mucouse membranes of man [2].

Unlike *Staphylococcus aureus*, which is coagulase-positive and has a great pathogenic capacity, the coagulase-negative staphylococci are non-pathogenic human commensals. However, over recent decades it has been possible to document the fact that these microorganisms very frequently cause opportunistic infections related to the use of in dwelling catheters and prosthetic devices.

The most frequent species from this group which cause device-related infections to are *S. epidermidis*, *S. haemolyticus*, *S. capitis*, *S. lugdunensis*, *S. schleiferi* and *S. warneri*, with a marked prevalence of *S. epidermidis* which, in our experience, is responsible for 42% of all venous catheter-associated infections and 29% of all clinically significant sepsis. *S. lugdunensis* has been correlated to a greater pathogenic capacity within the group [3].

There is a subgroup of coagulase-negative staphylococci characterized by being novobiocin-resistant which rarely cause disease except for *S. saprophyticus*, which causes urinary infections in women. However, over recent years, *S. hominis* subsp. *novobiosepticus* has been associated with septicaemia.

The coagulase-negative staphylococci, and in particular *S. epidermidis*, have a great capacity of adherence to polyethylene, polyvinyl chloride or silicone catheters, as they form an exopolysaccharide which behaves as a glicocalix or slime which ends up surrounding the bacteria and

TABLE 2. Most common opportunistic microorganisms

NORMAL INDIGENOUS MICROBIAL FLORA

Skin
- Coagulase-negative staphylococci:
  Staphylococcus epidermidis and others
- Coryneform bacteria:
  Corynebacterium spp
- Propionibacteria[1]

Nose
  Staphylococcus aureus

Oro- and nasopharyngeal cavity
- Commensal neisseria
- Streptococcci "*viridans* group"
- Anaerobic bacteria
  Peptostreptococcus, *Prevotella*, *Porphyromonas*, *Actinomyces* and others

Intestine
- Anaerobic bacteria
  Peptostreptococcus, *Prevotella*, *Porphyromonas*, *Fusobacterium*, *Eubacterium*, *Bifidobacterium*, *Actinomyces*, *Clostridium* and others
- *Enterobacteriaceae*
  Escherichia coli, *Proteus mirabilis*, *Klebsiella pneumoniae*, *Citrobacter freundii*
  Enterobacter cloacae, *Enterobacter aerogenes* and others
- Enterococci
  Enterococcus faecalis, *E. faecium* and others
- Yeast
  Candida albicans

Urethra
- Coagulase-negative staphylococci
- *Enterobacteriaceae*
- Enterococci

Vagina
- Lactobacilli
  Döderlein bacilli
- Anaerobic bacteria

TELLURIC BACTERIA[2]
- Non-fermentative Gram-negative rods
  Pseudomonas: P. aeruginosa, *P. fluorescens*, *P. putida*, *P. stutzeri* and others
  Burkholderia: B. cepacia
  Stenotrophomonas: S. maltophilia
  Acinetobacter: A. baumannii
  Alcaligenes
  Flavobacteriaceae: *Flavobacterium*, *Chryseobacterium* and others
- Telluric enterobacteria
  Some species of: *Klebsiella*, *Enterobacter*, *Serratia*, *Pantoea* and others

[1] Anaerobic.
[2] Many other telluric bacteria may be established in a ICU's on the floor, surfaces, materials and solutions. They can temporally colonize medical instruments and also the skin, trachea or gut of the patients, particularly if the normal flora has been eradicated by the administration of antibiotics.

adhering it to the foreign body [4]. This exopolysaccharide also hinders the penetration and action of antibiotics.

The identification of the staphylococci at species level is not easy, but there are some simple tests which allow the identification of the main species causing infections in man with an acceptable specificity. Commercial and automated methods for identification have variable reproducibility and accuracy of 70 to >90%. The standardization of identification tests is very important when collaborative and long-term studies are developed in order to obtain comparable results [5].

Conventional diffusion tests are adequate to assess the susceptibility of staphylococci. *S. epidermidis* and other CoN staphylococci are multi-resistant. Roughly 90% of *S. epidermidis* strains are resistant to penicillin and 70% to methicillin. Those methicillin-resistant strains should also be considered clinically resistant to all penicillins, cephalosporins and carbapenems, and usually have an associate resistance to other antimicrobials (macrolides, aminoglycosides, quinolones); they thus raise a serious treatment problem, with vancomycin sometimes being the only active therapeutic agent.

The coagulase-positive pathogenic species *S. aureus* can also produce infections in patients with catheters and who are intubated. Moreover, MRSA can establish itself endemically or epidemically in an ICU or other areas of the hospital. These strains have the same virulence as the methicillin-sensitive strains.

Typical strains of *S. aureus* are not difficult to identify, but in some MRSA strains it is difficult to interpret the slide coagulase test and the heteroresistance to methicillin is also difficult to reveal. These strains can be identified correctly by means of adequate techniques or genetic tests.

CORYNEFORM BACTERIA

The coryneform bacteria include a very extensive group of club-shaped Gram-positive rods characteristically arranged in V forms, in palisade or Chinese letter, both aerobic and facultative anaerobic. Over 20 genera with numerous species have been included in this informal group, the genus *Corynebacterium* being the one which includes the species detected with the greatest frequency as causing opportunistic infection in man, such as *C. amycolatum*, *C. jeikeium*, *C. riegelii*, *C. striatum* and *C. urealyticum*. However, other related genera, such as *Arthrobacter*, *Dermabacter*, *Brevibacterium*, *Oerskovia* or *Microbacterium* also include species which can cause opportunistic infections [6].

The commensal species of the genus *Corynebacterium* form part of the normal human flora, being located in the mucouse membranes (pharyngeal and urethral) and the skin, occupying specific niches. Some species, such as *C. urealyticum* or *C. jeikeium* can also be detected in the inanimate environment of hospitals. The natural habitat of the other genera of coryneform bacteria is mainly the environment.

A large number of these microorganisms cause infections in catheters, urinary infections and sepsis in a similar way as the coagulase-negative staphylococci [7].

It is not easy to identify this species, either using home-made or commercial methods. When for epidemiological studies or other reasons the identification at species level and/or the typing of the corynebacteria is necessary, it is recommended to resort to a reference laboratory in which, together with the metabolic tests, chromatographic and genetic studies are carried out.

In the species which grow slowly, are fastidious, capnophilic or rough, it is very difficult to study the sensitivity to the antimicrobials, both by diffusion and by dilution methods, and the National Committee for Clinical Laboratory Standards has not published rules to perform these tests. Various proposals have been made to overcome these difficulties. *Propionibacterium acnes* is an anaerobic coryneform bacteria located in the skin, that can cause catheter infections.

ENTEROCOCCI

The enterococci has its natural habitat in the digestive tract of animals, including man, but their ability to survive in the environment makes them ubicuitary [8]. Two species, *Enterococcus faecalis* and *E. faecium*, are frequently found in the digestive tract of man and are those which cause opportunistic infection with the greatest frequency, in particular *E. faecalis*. The molecular mechanisms which facilitate these infections are not entirely known [9].

The enterococci are facultative aerobic and anaerobic Gram-positive cocci which grow well in the usual media. They can easily be cultured in conventional, enriched or selective media and their identification is carried out, with a high specificity, by means of simple home-tests or using commercialized systems. The susceptibility to antibiotics can also be determined by means of conventional techniques (diffusion, E-test or microdilution).

The recent appearance of multi-resistant strains of enterococci, particularly in *E. faecium*, some of which are also resistant to vancomycin, has made them even more difficult to treat [10].

ENTEROBACTERIACEAE

This family is made up of non-fastidious, aerobic and facultative anaerobic Gram-negative rods. Over 30 genera and 100 species have been described, with a very heterogenous habitat and pathogenicity, but they are included in the same family in view of the similarity of their biochemical characteristics and their genomic homology [11].

Together with species which inhabit the digestive tract of warm-blooded animals, including man, such as *Escherichia coli* and to a lesser extent *Proteus mirabilis*, *Klebsiella pneumoniae* or *Citrobacter freundii*, there are others which inhabit plants or the inanimate environment, such as *Klebsiella oxytoca*, *Enterobacter aerogenes*, *Serratia marcescens* or an exclusively telluric habitat, such as *Pantoea agglomerans*, *Serratia rubidaea* or *Budvicia aquatica* [12].

In relation to pathogenicity, it can be said that together with non-pathogenic species, for which neither colonization nor infection of man have been described, such as *Budvicia aquatica*, and others which only cause opportunistic infections, such as *E. aerogenes*, there are highly pathogenic genus for man, such as *Salmonella*, *Shigella* or *Yersinia*. However, *E. coli* is the enterobacteria which causes sepsis with the greatest frequency, in general from urinary, respiratory or abdominal foci and, together with *Staphylococcus epidermidis*, they are probably the bacteria which cause opportunistic infection with the greatest prevalence.

In fact enterobacteria, such as *E. coli*, *P. mirabilis*, *K. pneumoniae* or *C. freundii* and other species with a human habitat, cause urinary infections both in healthy and with in dwelling-urinary–catheter people, they likewise colonize the respiratory tract of intubated patients and can cause pulmonary infection and also regularly form part of the polymicrobial flora which causes post-surgical abdominal infection [13].

In patients with urinary catheters or tracheostomy subjected to previous antibiotic treatment, these infections are caused by multi-resistant strains of enterobacteria, such as *K. oxytoca*, *Morganella morganii*, *E. aerogenes*, *E. cloacae* and *S. marcescens* or non-fermentative Gram-negative rods like *Pseudomonas* and others (see page 8).

The telluric enterobacteria, such as *Pantoea* (*Enterobacter*) *agglomerans* or *Klebsiella oxytoca*, and also non-fermentative rods can contaminate bottles with fluids for perfusion or connections of the catheters, producing sepsis [14].

Some molecular virulence factors responsible for the pathogenicity of the enteropathogenic enterobacteria (*Salmonella*, *Shigella* and *Yersinia*) are known, but it is not known with precision if factors such as haemolysin, aerobactin, capsular type, resistance to serum and others present in opportunistic bacteria have any importance in those infections.

The enterobacteria grow well in usual culture media and in general it is easy to identify them and to study their sensitivity, numerous systems having been commercialized.

Diffusion tests are useful to detect the susceptibility of these bacteria and the antibiotic treatment should be guided by the results of those tests, as the susceptibility of the enterobacteria to antibiotics is highly variable. The resistance to beta-lactam antibiotics, including the third generation cephalosporins, depends on both chromosomal and plasmidic beta-lactamases, and the latter can diffuse among the different species [15]. The resistance to quinolones is also significant for many species, but most conserve their sensitivity to carbapenems and aminoglycosides.

ANAEROBIC BACTERIA

The strict anaerobic bacteria form a very widespread and varied group of microorganisms which are found in the digestive tract, from the mouth to the rectum, together with the enterobacteria and enterococci, and constitute, quantitatively and qualitatively, the most abundant bacterial group of the intestine [16]. It should not be forgotten that some anaerobic bacteria and enterobacteria colonize the vagina in a more or less transitory manner.

In practical terms, the numerous and extremely varied contingent of anaerobic bacteria can be distributed into two groups. 1) The non-pathogenic group, which includes Gram-positive cocci, such as *Peptostreptococcus*, Gram-negative rods, such as *Bacteroides*, *Fusobacterium*, *Porphyromonas* and *Prevotella*, and coryneform Gram-positive rods, such as *Eubacterium*, *Actinomyces* and others (Table 2). These bacteria only produce post-surgical oropharyngeal, abdominal and pelvic infections associated with aerobic bacteria of these territories. 2) The primary pathogenic clostridia, such as *Clostridium tetani* (tetanus), *C. perfringens* (gas gangrene), *C. difficile* (pseudomembranous colitis, see below) and *C. botulinum* (botulism) which cause disease in specific circumstances.

The isolation of these bacteria require an appropiate collection and transport of specimens, in order to avoid contact with the air. Therefore, before taking a clinical sample which may contain anaerobic bacteria, it is necessary to contact the laboratory to specify the collection method. In any case, the culture must be carried out promptly, on enriched media incubated in anaerobiosis [17]. These bacteria tend to grow for between three and seven days or more. The specific drugs for the treatment of infections due to anaerobic bacteria are penicillin, cephamycins (cefoxitin and others), carbapenems (imipenem and others), tetracyclines, chloramphenicol, clindamycin and metronidazole. The susceptibility of the anaerobic bacteria to the anaerobicide drugs is variable, although in general is high. *Bacteroides fragilis* is resistant to penicillin. Some species are resistant to the clindamycin and to a greater extent to the tetracyclines, but the susceptibility to metronidazole is very conserved [18]. The susceptibility of the bacteria isolated in mixed infections does not tend to be studied, the treatment being established with empirical bases. Surgical debridement is essential.

CLOSTRIDIUM DIFFICILE

This is a strict anaerobic endospore former Gram-positive rod, fastidious from the nutritional point of view and very sensitive to oxygen.

C. difficile can be considered as a primary enteropathogenic bacteria which causes enteritis due to the production of two exotoxins, A and B, producing clinical symptoms which vary from self-limited benign diarrhoea to serious symptoms of pseudomembranous colitis [19].

However, it has been observed that there are around 5–10% of healthy carriers, a figure which may be higher in infants. Moreover, symptomatic infections occur with a certain opportunistic character and severe cases are more frequent in elderly patients with debilitating diseases and after surgery, particularly if they have been treated with antibiotics and/or antiacids. Epidemics have also been described in hospitals as a result of the diffusion of spores into the environment and from contact with the hands of the healthcare staff [20].

The diagnosis is carried out through the detection of toxins in the faeces or by culture; in this case the samples must be transferred urgently to the laboratory and processed immediately. All strains are sensitive to vancomycin and metronidazole which constitute the specific treatment for this infection.

NON-FERMENTATIVE GRAM-NEGATIVE RODS

There is a group of species of generally non-fastidious strict aerobic Gram-negative rods, which are found in water, soil and plants and which conceptually, from the pathogenic point of view, can be considered as practically identical to the telluric enterobacteria [21]. As with the latter, naturally multi-resistant strains are easily selected and can be established in an endemic or epidemic manner in a specific setting (ward, ICU) their treatment and eradication being extraordinarily difficult.

The non-fermentative Gram-negative rods include various families and very numerous genera and species, some of which are primarily pathogenic for plants, but the vast majority are innocuous for man. From this enormous variety of species a few account for the majority of human infections, such as *Pseudomonas aeruginosa*, *Pseudomonas* from the "*fluorescens-putida* group" and *A. baumannii*, and also *Burkholderia cepacia* and *Stenotrophomonas maltophilia* are isolated with some frequency. In fact, the relative frequency of these microorganisms varies from time to time, ward to ward and hospital to hospital.

These microorganisms cause urinary infections in patients with in dwelling catheters, respiratory infection in intubated patients and colonization of the catheters hubs and blood stream intections.

The molecular virulence factors, if any, of these microorganisms which facilitate their infection are not known in detail. In the case of *P. aeruginosa*, the strains which cause pulmonary infection in patients with cystic fibrosis are mucoid due to the overproduction of alginate.

The culture of these organisms is not difficult, as the majority are non-fastidious. The identification of some species, such as *P. aeruginosa* or *A. baumannii*, using home-made techniques is very simple to the expert microbiologist, but other species are very difficult to identify without the study of many biochemical characters. Many strains are multi-resistant, but the study of the susceptibility to antibiotics can be carried out by diffusion and dilution techniques and the treatment should be guided by these data.

CANDIDA

The genus *Candida* includes over 150 species which are widely distributed in nature. Some, such as *Candida albicans*, can colonize, scarcely, the mouth, the digestive tract and the vagina of healthy people in a proportion which ranges from 30% to 70% of the population, therefore being considered as forming part of the normal human flora. To a lesser extent, other species can be found in the digestive tract or in the vulva, such as *Candida glabrata* (10%), *C. parapsilosis* (5%), *C. krusei* (2%) or *C. tropicalis* (2%) [22].

C. albicans is the species which causes opportunistic infections with the greatest frequency. In persistent and multi-treated opportunistic infections, a progressive change of etiologic agents is usually seen, and more to more resistant microorganisms have been involucrated. *Candida*, which are naturally resistant to all antibacterial agents, are usually found at the end of this process.

The use of imidazoles and triazoles for the treatment of these processes can eradicate *C. albicans*, but allows a reinfection from species naturally resistant to these drugs, such as *C. glabrata* or *C. krusei*, or even from strains of *C. albicans* which have become resistant to these antifungal agents [23].

The candida are yeast, and therefore single-cells, which present an oval morphology and a size of between 5 and 7 μm. These microorganisms grow for 1 to 3 days in most conventional bacteriological and mycological culture media. Their correct identification, although requiring a certain experience, does not tend to be difficult.

The standardization and interpretation of results of susceptibility tests for fungi are in progress, but may be indicated in some severe candida infections.

Opportunistic Infections Associated With Local Predisposing Factors

INFECTIONS ASSOCIATED WITH INTRAVASCULAR CATHETERS

Infections and sepsis originating in the perfusion systems can be due to 1) colonization of the cannula 2) colonization of the junctions or 3) contamination of the infusate [24]. Infection at the insertion site occurs in the tunnelized area and can progress, causing a phlebitis around the catheter. In these cases the infections are caused by *S. epidermidis*, coryneform bacteria which reside in the skin, including the anaerobe specie *Propionibacterium acnes* and *S. aureus*. The colonization of the hubs can be caused by these bacteria, but more frequently by telluric *Enterobacteriaceae* and non-fermentative Gram-negative rods, such as *Enterobacter*, *Pantoea*, *Serratia*, *Pseudomonas* and *Acinetobacter*.

Telluric bacteria are found in contaminated perfusion fluids, such as *Pantoea agglomerans* and *Stenotrophomonas maltophilia*, in addition to *Candida* (*C. tropicalis* and others) and more exceptionally *Malassezia*, which is a lypophilic yeast. These contaminations can be intrinsic if they occur during manufacture of the infusate, or extrinsic if they take place during the preparation for the perfusion. The catheter can also be contaminated by a haematogenous route with a microorganism originating in another source.

In catheter related bacteremic, for approximately every 100 infections of cutaneous origin, 10 occur starting from the hub and much less due to contamination of the infusion which fortunately are unusual; the haematogenous colonization of the catheter not being rare [25]. In the absence of local symptoms, the diagnosis of catheter infection is intended to establish the involvement of the latter as a port of entry for a bacteraemia or source of febrile symptoms of unknown origin. Some microbiological techniques have been developed for this purpose, and can be divided into those which require the removal of the catheter and those which try to diagnose catheter infection avoiding its removal.

In relation to the studies which involve the removal of the catheter, in 1977 Maki *et al.* developed a semi-quantitative culture technique and introduced a new concept in the diagnosis of the catheter-related infection, that of quantification, and the possibility of differentiating between colonization and infection. This method only assesses the colonization of the external surface of the catheter and does not consider the intraluminal progression of the colonization, which would justify an overall sensitivity of 85% [26].

The first techniques which assessed and quantified the colonization of the intraluminal surface of the catheter were performed by Cleri and collaborators in 1980.

In addition to these culture techniques, several rapid diagnosis procedures have been developed [27] consisting of the application of Gram's staining method or acridine orange at the catheter tip. These staining procedures have a sensitivity and specificity greater than 80%, but are technically difficult, require a lot of time and also need the culture to isolate the causal agent.

The negativity of the cultures in case of suspected infection by catheter is common, and especially frequent in the ICU, in which it is considered that the study of febrile episodes finally attributable to other causes makes it unnecessary to remove between 75% and 85% of catheters. This high percentage of unnecessarily removed catheters and the importance of maintaining them in place determined the appearance of conservative diagnostic processes. These diagnostic techniques, although less sensitive and specific, can, on certain occasions, be very useful. The culture or Gram's staining with a smear taken from the periphery, either on the skin surrounding the catheter insertion site or at the level of the hubs, is a simple, cheap and practical method which has a high effectiveness and a negative predictive value estimated at around 95%. It should, however, be taken into account that the peripheral, especially cutaneous, colonization is a dynamic process and that the same microorganisms which have been isolated on the smear are not necessarily going to be found on the catheter [28]. Another approximation to the conservative diagnosis of catheter-associated bacteraemia is the comparative quantitative blood cultures, as has been demonstrated that the colony counts on blood samples removed through the catheter are significantly higher than the counts from the blood obtained by puncture of a peripheral vein [29]. More recent introductions to the arsenal of conservative diagnostic techniques are the staining of the pellet obtained after centrifugation of the blood obtained through the catheter, or the calculation of the differential positivity time values (>2 hours) between the blood removed through the catheter and peripheral blood samples [30].

INFECTIONS ASSOCIATED WITH CSF DERIVATIONS OR OTHER DRAINAGE SYSTEMS

The central nervous prosthetic devices usually inserted in the ventricles can be closed or open systems. The closed systems tend to be ventriculoperitoneal or ventriculojugular (atrial) shunts, which are generally used when it is necessary to decompress a hydrocephalus for a prolonged period of time. The open systems tend to be maintained for a short period of time, and are generally used for temporary drainage or decompression, in order to monitor the intraventricular pressure or for the administration of therapeutic agents.

Infection constitutes the foremost complication of CSF shunt implantation, with an infection rate of between 1% and 10% with closed shunts and around 10% with the open systems [31]. These rates vary in accordance with the drainage system used (subarachnoid screw, subdural cup catheter or intraventricular catheter) and various other factors, such as age, surgeon's experience and time, which is one of the factors best correlated to the infection, as occurs with other drainage systems or catheters. The highest risk of infection, however, occurs with the reinsertion of the system after a prior infection.

Infections are caused by bacteria of the skin flora (*S. epidermidis*, *P. acnes*, *S. aureus*), such as in the infections of venous catheters. The colonization in the open systems probably occurs as a result of handling the same, while with the closed systems (shunts) this tends to occur during the surgical operation or through the incisions, but the exact pathogenic mechanism is not known.

INFECTIONS ASSOCIATED WITH URINARY INDWELLING CATHETERS

Infections of the urinary tract are the most frequent nosocomial infections and are generally due to the presence of an indwelling catheter [32]. These infections occur even when using closed systems. Their frequency can diminish on taking extreme care with the catheter, but in general if the catheterization is prolonged the infection ends up occurring. Indeed, it is very difficult to maintain the urine sterile after two weeks, although it is not infrequent to observe bacteriuria without pyuria.

The infection tends to begin due to colonization of the area located between the catheter and the urethra, where a magma of mucus occurs with microorganisms which ascend up to the bladder [33]. This area constitutes a protected area for microbial multiplication. Inoculation at the time of placing the catheter or intraluminal, and in particular the latter, is less frequent than the periluminal. Likewise, in catheterized patients, it would appear that the resistance of the vesical mucosa to infection is reduced.

Urinary infections in catheterized patients for short periods tend to be caused by *E. coli*, *P. mirabilis* and enterococci, being relatively sensitive strains. If the catheterization is prolonged and the patient is treated with antibiotics, these species tend to be replaced by others more resistant from the genera *Enterobacter*, *Morganella*, *Providencia*, *Pseudomonas* or *Acinetobacter* and also by *Candida*. Moreover, polymicrobial infections are common in these patients.

In relation to microbiological diagnosis, it is generally accepted that in the catheterized patient, any bacterial count should be reported when a maximum of two different microorganisms are isolated in the urine sample, and that the isolation of three or more bacterial species should be assessed in accordance with the results of previous cultures, the bacterial count and the presence or absence of pyuria, it being not infrequent in prolonged catheterizations to isolate more than two microorganisms. The presence of yeasts should also be reported, although rarely correspond to a true infection, tending to be vesical colonizations which will disappear with catheter removal. However, true *Candida* infections and bladder fungus ball can occur.

It is important to cultivate a sample representative of the vesical urine, and therefore should be collected by aseptic puncture and aspiration through the catheter zone created for this purpose. The urine stored in the bag should never be cultivated. The practice of suprapubic punctures is unusual, but in certain circumstances can be used to ensure the vesical origin of the microorganisms [34].

Some authors recommend the culture of urethral smears to position the extraluminal colonization of the urinary catheters, but although it has been demonstrated that urethral colonization precedes the isolation of the microorganisms in the urine, the practical value of these cultures is not clear.

INFECTIONS ASSOCIATED WITH ENDOTRACHEAL INTUBATION

Nosocomial pneumonia, which generally appears in intubated patients, although is not the most frequent hospital infection, is associated with attributable mortality. It is accepted that 60% of the cases are caused by Gram-negative rods and the crude mortality rate may be 50% [35].

Although the lung is in communication with the outside through the respiratory tract, there are a series of defence mechanisms which prevent its colonization by microorganisms. The inhaled particles are trapped by the nasal or tracheobroncheal mucus and eliminated to the outside by the mucociliary system. The non-pathogenic microorganisms which reach the alveolus are phagocyted and destroyed without a noticeable inflammatory reaction. Various factors affect these defence mechanisms, such as diabetes, alveolar oedema, which affect the migration of the macrophages; acidosis and hypoxia, which affect their bactericidal capacity. Moreover, tracheal intubation prevents coughing and the action of the mucociliary system, damages the epithelium and increases the secretion of the mucus to which some bacteria adhere.

The infections would appear to be more frequent in tracheotomized than in intubated patients. The pulmonary infections which appear soon after the intubation in patients with cerebral trauma and coma tend to be caused by *S. aureus*, *H. influenzae* or streptococci [36]; on the contrary, late infections, which represent the majority, are mainly caused by Gram-negative rods, particularly *Pseudomonas* and enterobacteria. These microorganisms, which do not form part of the oropharyngeal flora, colonize this region and subsequently the airways. This occurs due to a change in the receptors of the epithelium of these regions which allows the adherence of the Gram-negative rods. The origin of this flora is telluric, the humidifiers and taps constituting one of the most frequent reservoirs. It remains controversial if the colonization of the stomach of patients with anti-acid treatment constitutes a prior colonization before reaching the respiratory tract [37].

The diagnosis of pneumonia should be made on the basis of clinical and radiological signs but, in the intubated patient subjected to mechanical ventilation, the appearance of fever, leucocytosis or pulmonary infiltrates can be due to non-infectious causes or have an extrapulmonary origin (see Chapter 2). The sensitivity of the different diagnostic techniques to establish or to rule out the diagnosis of pneumonia will depend on their capacity to differentiate between colonization and a true parenchymatous infection.

The qualitative samples obtained by non-invasive techniques present little risk for the patient, but are not very useful in the diagnosis of bacterial pneumonias.

The lack of specificity of the microbiological study of the qualitative samples has led to the search for more sensitive and specific diagnostic methods, such as pulmonary biopsy by thoracotomy, percutaneous pulmonary biopsy and transthoracic puncture, but although these are techniques with great diagnostic effectiveness, they can present serious complications and are not used to diagnose VAP.

Various technical variants are based on the bronchoscopy, which allows direct access to the lower respiratory tract and the possibility to access the respiratory secretions of a specific bronchoalveolar area, avoiding as far as possible contamination with flora from the upper respiratory tract.

However, the value of these diagnostic techniques will be determined by the possibility of using a quantitative technique, which should involve protected methods which prevent the entry of secretions from the upper tracts into the canal of the fibrobronchoscopy, such as protected brushing or double telescoped catheter and protected bronchoalveolar washing to obtain the highest specilicity.

With the protected bronchoalveolar lavage, 120 ml of saline solution are instilled which will be subsequently recovered and processed. In theory, the sample represents the secretions present in approximately 1% of the pulmonary surface, it being estimated that 1 ml of secretions can be found diluted in the recovered liquid. This technique is suitable to detect microorganisms that are not usually found in the airways, like *Mycobacterium tuberculosis*, *Legionella*, *Pneumocystis carinii*, *Histoplasma capsulatum* or citomegalovirus. With protected brushing, once the area required has been reached with the catheter, the brush is advanced to collect the sample. Using this method the brush collects from 0.001 to 0.01 ml of the secretions present in a single bronchiolus, which, to be transported, will be diluted in 1 ml of saline solution.

On the basis of quantitative criteria, it has been established that concentrations of $\geq 10^3$ UFC/ml in the protected brush samples indicate infection rather than colonization [38].

INFECTIONS ASSOCIATED WITH PROSTHESES OR OTHER FOREIGN BODIES

Valvular prostheses, vascular grafts, joint, ocular and other prostheses, constitute closed systems, some of which when infected can produce local pathology (articular, ocular prostheses) or general complications which can require general or specialized ICU admission (endocarditis, graft infection, etc) [39].

These infections could be classified as early or late. This temporal characteristic is related to the time of the infection (during surgery or lately by hematogenous route) being in the former *S. epidermidis* the most frequent causative agent.

Pacemakers are formed by a pulse generator and conductivity system and an electrode. The former is subcutaneous and the latter two endovascular. Pacemakers become infected during implantation (in the pulse-generator pocket), from a skin injury or by hematogenous route. *S. epidermidis* and *S. aureus* cause 75% [40] of the infections, followed by members of *Enterobacteriaceae* and *Candida*.

INFECTIONS ASSOCIATED WITH CONTAMINATED SURGERY

Any surgical operation on a contaminated area, in particular the oropharynx, the intestine, colon, rectum and vagina, can cause an infection in its contiguity in the mediastinum or abdomen (peritoneal cavity) and/or at the surgical wound [41].

The risk of infection depends on the preparation of the patient, including the use of a suitable prophylaxis, on the duration and complexity of the operation and on the experience of the surgeon.

The etiology of these infections reflects their topography (pharynx, oesophagus, stomach, colon or vagina), but they all tend to be mixed aerobic and anaerobic polymicrobial infections. The pharyngeal infections tend to be caused by *viridans* streptococci and bacteroids. Infections from the colonic area are caused by a mixed flora, with enterobacteria, enterococci, bacteroids, fusobacterium, eubacterium and clostridia.

A microscopic examination (Gram stain) reveals the existing flora and allows initiation of an empiric antibiotic treatment. In most cases, surgical drainage is usually the most effective therapeutic action (see Chapter 49 and Section 8).

BLOODSTREAM INFECTIONS

Bacteraemia can occur from any of the previous locations, in particular catheter-related infections, and worsens the prognosis of the patient. Blood culture is the most practical and effective method for the diagnosis of bacteraemias and fungemia [42].

Most laboratories currently have automated systems capable of detecting, rapidly and with high sensitivity, the bacterial growth in blood culture bottles. The processing has been simplified and the handling of the samples has been reduced. Using automated systems with continuous agitation around 40% of the bacteria are recovered in the first 12 hours of incubation, at

24 hours 75% of the microorganisms have been recovered, and 90% at 48 hours, blind cultures in the negative flasks thus being unnecessary [43].

The volume of blood cultivated is the parameter which can most influence the recovery of the bacteria, and it has been well demonstrated that the volume extracted for blood culture should not be less than 10 ml (nor more than 30 ml) [44]. Moreover, carrying out several extractions increases the recovery index and facilitates the interpretation of the results, helping to differentiate the significant isolations from those possibly due to contamination. The recommendation to carry out two or three independent blood cultures per septic episode should be generalized, endeavoring to inoculate 20 ml of blood for sample (between 1 and 5 ml with small or newborn children).

If the volume of the sample is the greatest determinant of sensitivity, the specificity basically depends on the number of falsely positive blood cultures [45]. To succeed in minimizing the false positives is only possible with a meticulous extraction technique, which is moreover essential in order to determine the value of an isolation, as it should be remembered that many of the bacteria which cause true sepsis are the same as those which colonize the skin.

The skin surface should be carefully prepared before the extraction, cleaning it first with 70° alcohol and then with an antiseptic, such as iodine or some other iodofor, which should be left to act for at least two minutes. Venopuncture material and sterile gloves will be used for the extraction, the puncture area should not be touched and any contact of the needle with lints or other dressings will be avoided. The blood culture bottles should be inoculated at the bed-side.

Epidemiology of the Infection

Endemic or epidemic outbreaks due to some microorganisms, the majority of which are multi-resistant, frequently occur in the ICU, and other areas where seriously ill patients are admitted (Chapter 22).

The control of the diffusion of epidemic strains should be carried out taking into account certain simple but essential guidelines: 1) early detection in the laboratory of the bacteria with epidemic ability, and 2) rapid passing of information to the clinician responsible for the patient, so that the suitable isolation measures for each case can be taken immediately [46].

The main objective in these situations is to prevent the diffusion of the bacteria. It is not a question of carrying out complex academic studies in order to unequivocally determine the identity of apparently similar strains, but rather of taking universal precautions and adequate isolation measures immediately after detecting any bacteria with an epidemic ability, such as methicillin resistant *S. aureus*, *Enterococcus faecium*, *Pseudomonas aeruginosa*, *Klebsiella oxytoca*, klebsiellae producing wide spectrum beta-lactamases, *Enterobacter*, *Serratia marcescens* and *Acinetobacter baumannii*, among others.

This does not mean that it is of no interest to confirm the identity of the strains involved in an intra-hospital outbreak for epidemiological and also control purposes.

There are phenotypical and genotypical methods to determine the identity of bacteria. The phenotypical methods tend to be useful, each for a single bacterial group or species and some are not very reproducible [47]. The most frequently used are biotyping, which makes it possible to differentiate two strains in accordance with metabolic differences, serotyping, which is based on anti-genic differences, phagotyping, based on the difference in sensitivity (lysis) to a set of bacteriophages, and anti-biotyping. There are also more complex techniques which are routinely used less frequently, such as the profile of membrane proteins or multilocus enzyme electrophoresis.

The genetic methods include some based on the restriction of the DNA (PFGE), occasionally with subsequent hydridation (for example ribotyping), or on the polymorphism of amplification of repeated sequences in the chromosome [48]. The selection of the tests for these studies should be based on cost, simplicity and speed of completion, which are as important as their discriminatory power and their reproducibility.

References

1. Tannock GW. Normal microflora. London: Chapman & Hall, 1995.
2. Kloos WE, Bannerman TL. *Staphylococcus* and *Micrococcus*. In Murray PR, Baron EJ, Pfaller MA, Tenover FC, Yolken RH (eds). Manual of clinical microbiology. 7th edn, Washington DC: American Society for Microbiology, 1999:264.
3. Huebner J, Goldmann DA. Coagulase-negative staphylococci: role as pathogens. Annu Rev Med 50:223, 1999.
4. Foster TJ, McDevitt D. Molecular basis of adherence of staphylococci to biomaterials. In Bisno AL, Waldvogel FA (eds). Infections associated with indwelling medical devices, 2nd edn, Washington DC: American Society for Microbiology, 1994:31.
5. Weinstein MP, Mirrett S, Van Pelt L, McKinnon M, Zimmer BL, *et al*. Clinical importance of identifying coagulase-negative staphylococci isolated from blood cultures: evaluation of microscan rapid and dried overnight gram-positive panels versus a conventional reference method. J Clin Microbiol 36:2089, 1998.
6. Funke G, Bernard KA. Coryneform gram-positive rods. In Murray PR, Baron EJ, Pfaller MA, Tenover FC, Yolken RH (eds). Manual of Clinical Microbiology, 7th edn, Washington DC: American Society for Microbiology, 1999:319.
7. Funke G, von Graevenitz A, Clarridge III JE, Bernard KA. Clinical microbiology of coryneform bacteria. Clin Microbiol Rev 10:125, 1997.
8. Facklam RR, Sahm DF, Teixeira LM. *Enterococcus*. In Murray PR, Baron EJ, Pfaller MA, Tenover FC, Yolken RH (eds). Manual of Clinical Microbiology, 7th edn, Washington DC: American Society for Microbiology, 1999:297.
9. Jett BD, Huycke MM, Gilmore MS. Virulence of enterococci. Clin Microbiol Rev 7:462, 1994.
10. Huycke MM, Sahm DF, Gilmore MS. Multiple-drug resistant enterococci: the nature of the problem and an agenda for the future. Emerg Infect Dis 4:239, 1998.
11. Farmer III JJ, Davis BR, Hickman-Brenner FW, McWhorter A, Huntley-Carter GP, *et al*. Biochemical identification of new species and biogroups of *Enterobacteriaceae* isolated from clinical specimens. J Clin Microbiol 21:46, 1985.
12. Farmer III JJ. *Enterobacteriaceae*: introduction and identification. In Murray PR, Baron EJ, Pfaller MA, Tenover FC, Yolken RH (eds). Manual of Clinical Microbiology, 7th edn, Washington DC: American Society for Microbiology, 1999: 442.
13. Eisentein BI, Zaleznik DF. *Enterobacteriaceae*. In Mandell GL, Bennett JE, Dolin R (eds). Mandell, Douglas and Bennett's principles and practice of infectious diseases, 5th edn, Philadelphia: Churchill Livingstone, 2000:2294.
14. Maki DG. Nosocomial bacteremia. Am J Med 70:183, 1981.
15. Livermore DM. β-lactamases in laboratory and clinical resistance. Clin Microbiol Rev 8:557, 1995.
16. Duerden BI, Drasar BB (eds). Anaerobes in human disease. London: Edward Arnold, 1991.
17. Rodloff AC, Appelbaum PC, Zabransky RJ (eds). Practical anaerobic bacteriology. Cumitech 5A. Washington DC: American Society for Microbiology, 1991.
18. Hecht DW. Susceptibility testing of anaerobic bacteria. In Murray PR, Baron EJ, Pfaller MA, Tenover FC, Yolken RH (eds). Manual of Clinical Microbiology, 7th edn, Washington DC: American Society for Microbiology, 1999:1555.
19. Spencer RC. Clinical impact and associated costs of *Clostridium difficile*-associated disease. J Antimicrob Chemother 41 Suppl C:5, 1998.
20. Samore MH, Venkataraman L, DeGirolami PC, Arbeit RD, Karchmer AW. Clinical and molecular epidemiology of sporadic and clustered cases of nosocomial *Clostridium difficile* diarrhea. Am J Med 100:32, 1996.
21. Richard C, Kiredjian M. Méthodes de laboratoire pour l'identification des bacilles à gram-négatif aérobies stricts (*Pseudomonas*, *Alcaligenes*,

Flavobacterium, *Acinetobacter*, *Brucella*, *Bordetella*). 2 edn, Paris: Institut Pasteur, 1995.

22. Kwon-Chung KJ, Bennett JE. Medical Mycology. Philadelphia: Lea & Febiger, 1992.
23. Denning DW, Baily GG, Hood SV. Azole resistance in *Candida*. Eur J Clin Microbiol Infect Dis 16:261, 1997.
24. Rello J, Vallès J. Infecciones por catéter. In Net A, Quintana E (eds). Infecciones en el paciente crítico. Barcelona: Springer-Verlag Ibérica, 1997:22.
25. Maki DG, Cobb L, Garman JK, Shapiro J, Ringer M, Helgerson RB. An attachable silver-impregnated cuff for prevention of infection with central venous catheters. A prospective randomized multi-centre trial. Am J Med 85:307, 1988.
26. Siegman-Igra Y, Anglim AM, Shapiro DE, Adal KA, Strain BA, Farr BM. Diagnosis of vascular catheter-related bloodstream infection: a meta-analysis. J Clin Microbiol 35:928, 1997.
27. Farr BM. Accuracy and cost-effectiveness of new tests for diagnosis of catheter-related bloodstream infections. Lancet 354:1587, 1999.
28. Atela I, Coll P, Rello J, Quintana E, Barrio J, *et al.* Serial surveillance cultures of skin and catheter hub specimens from critically ill patients with central venous catheters: molecular epidemiology of infection and implications for clinical management and research. J Clin Microbiol 35:1784, 1997.
29. Capdevila JA, Planes AM, Palomar M, Gasser I, Almirante B, *et al.* Value of differential quantitative blood cultures in the diagnosis of catheter-related sepsis. Eur J Clin Microbiol Infect Dis 11:403, 1992.
30. Blot F, Nitenberg G, Chachaty E, Raynard B, Germann N, *et al.* Diagnosis of catheter-related bacteraemia: a prospective comparison of the time to positivity of hub-blood versus peripheral-blood cultures. Lancet 354: 1071, 1999.
31. Bisno AL, Sternau L. Infections of central nervous system shunts. In Bisno AL, Waldvogel FA (eds). Infections associated with indwelling medical devices, 2nd edn, Washington DC: American Society for Microbiology, 1994: 91.
32. Stamm WE. Catheter-associated urinary tract infections: epidemiology, pathogenesis and prevention. Am J Med 91(Suppl 3B):65S, 1991.
33. Brau J, Pericas R, Lopez L, Virto JL, Prats G, Verger G. Estudio de la infección urinaria en pacientes con sondaje vesical de corta duración. Med Clin (Barc) 96:161, 1991.
34. Shea YR. Specimen collection and transport. Section 1. Aerobic bacteriology. In Isenberg HD (ed). Clinical Microbiology Procedures Handbook. Washington DC: American Society for Microbiology, 1992:1.1.1.
35. Gross PA, Neu HC, Aswapokee P, Van Antwerpen C, Aswapokee N. Deaths from nosocomial infections: experience in a community hospital. Am J Med 68:219, 1980.
36. Rello J, Quintana E, Ausina V, Puzo C, Net A, Prats G. Risk factors for *Staphylococcus aureus* nosocosmial pneumonia in critically ill patients. Am Rev Respir Dis 142:1320, 1990.
37. Driks MR, Craven DE, Celli BR, Manning M, Burke RA, *et al.* Nosocomial pneumonia in intubated patients given sucralfate as compared with antacids or histamine type 2 blockers. N Engl J Med 317:1376, 1987.
38. Baselski VS, Wunderink RG. Bronchoscopic diagnosis of pneumonia. Clin Microbiol Rev 7:533, 1994.
39. Bisno AL, Waldvogel FA (eds). Infections associated with indwelling medical devices. 2nd edn, Washington DC: American Society for Microbiology, 1994.
40. Phibbs B, Marriott HJL. Complications of permanent transvenous pacing. N Engl J Med 312: 1428, 1985.
41. Douglas SK, Kaiser AB. Postoperative infections and antimicrobial prophylaxis. In Mandell GL, Bennett JE, Dolin R (eds). Mandell, Douglas and Bennett's principles and practice of infectious diseases, 5th edn, Philadelphia: Churchill Livingstone, 2000:3177.
42. Prats G, Sánchez F. El hemocultivo en los tiempos de la reacción en cadena de la polimerasa [editorial]. Med Clin (Barc) 108:534, 1997.
43. Alonso C, Rello J, Mirelis B, Pericas R, Navarro F, Prats G. Comparación del sistema automatizado de incubación y lectura de hemocultivos BacT/ALERT® con un sistema convencional. Enferm Infecc Microbiol Clin 13:17, 1995.
44. Reller LB, Murray PR, MacLowry JD. Blood cultures II. In Washington JA II (ed). Cumitech 1A. Washington DC: American Society for Microbiology; 1982.
45. Mirelis B, Ausina V, Coll P. *et al.* Sepsis en un Hospital General Universitario (1976–1986). II Congreso SEIMC. Granada. Mayo 1988.
46. Wenzel RP (ed). Prevention and control of nosocomial infections, 3rd edn, Baltimore: Williams & Wilkins; 1997.

47. Arbeit RD. Laboratory procedures for the epidemiologic analysis of microorganisms. In Murray PR, Baron EJ, Pfaller MA, Tenover FC, Yolken RH (eds). Manual of Clinical Microbiology, 6th edn, Washington DC: American Society for Microbiology, 1995:190.

48. Arbeit RD. Laboratory procedures for the epidemiologic analysis of microorganisms. In Murray PR, Baron EJ, Pfaller MA, Tenover FC, Yolken RH (eds). Manual of Clinical Microbiology, 7th edn, Washington DC: American Society for Microbiology, 1999:116.

2. PATHOGENESIS AND DIFFERENTIAL DIAGNOSIS OF FEVER AND APPROACH TO THE FEBRILE PATIENT IN THE INTENSIVE CARE UNIT

Bekele Afessa and G. Umberto Meduri

Introduction

Normal body temperature is considered to be 37°C or 98.6°F. This temperature varies by 0.5–1.0°C in healthy individuals, depending on the circadian rhythm and menstrual cycle [1]. With heavy exercise, body temperature can rise 2–3°C [2]. Temperature is usually measured orally, rectally, or in the axilla. Electronic probes are used to measure tympanic membrane temperature. In critically ill patient, the thermistor of a pulmonary artery catheter is used as the gold standard device for measuring temperature [3]. Thermistors in indwelling bladder catheters provide temperature readings that are identical to those provided by thermistors in pulmonary artery catheters [3]. In addition to many biological processes, environmental factors, such as specialized mattresses, hot lights, air conditioning, cardiopulmonary bypass, peritoneal lavage, dialysis, and continuous hemofiltration, can alter patient body temperature in an intensive care unit (ICU) [2]. Thermoregulation can be disrupted by drugs or by damage to the central or autonomic nervous system [2]. In many ICUs, all patients with temperature ≥38.3°C (100.9°F) are considered to be febrile and warrant special attention [2].

A wide range of biological processes can cause fever. Although we consider infection to be the main cause of fever, noninfectious processes can also cause fever. Sepsis, a systemic inflammatory response to infection, is a frequent cause of fever in ICU patients. Patients admitted to the ICU for respiratory failure, hemodynamic instability, or central nervous dysfunction caused by the systemic inflammatory response syndrome (SIRS) resulting from infection are considered to have primary sepsis. Sepsis that develops in patients after admission to the ICU for noninfectious conditions is defined as secondary sepsis. Some patients may have normal or low temperature, despite having infection (Table 1). In this chapter, we will review the pathogenesis, differential diagnosis, and investigation of fever in critically ill, immunocompetent adults.

Pathogenesis

Endogenous and exogenous pyrogens cause fever [1]. Exogenous pyrogens come from outside the host, whereas endogenous pyrogens are produced by the host. The majority of exogenous pyrogens are microbes, their toxins, and other products. Endotoxins produced by Gram-negative bacteria and exotoxins and enterotoxins produced by streptococci and staphylococci are examples of exogenous pyrogens. Many exogenous pyrogens act by inducing the formation of endogenous

TABLE 1. Conditions associated with the absence of fever despite the presence of sepsis

Old age
Severe sepsis
Open abdominal wounds
Large burns
Extracorporeal membrane oxygenation
Antiinflammatory medications
Antipyretic medications

TABLE 2. The mechanisms of actions of some medications and substances impairing the febrile response to infection

Affect prostaglandin synthesis
Block brain cyclooxygenase, e.g., aspirin, nonsteroidal antiinflammatory drugs, corticosteroids
Alter the ability of endogenous pyrogens to stimulate prostaglandin production, e.g., somatostatin, arginine vasopressin, α-melanocyte stimulating factor, adrenocorticotropin and corticotropin-releasing hormone
Interfere with neural transmission, e.g., acetaminophen

pyrogens via stimulation of the host's cells. However, lipopolysaccharide, an exogenous pyrogen produced by Gram-negative organisms, can act directly on endothelial cells of the brain to generate fever. Fever occurs when an inflammatory process of infectious or noninfectious origin stimulates primarily monocyte/macrophages, but also lymphocytes, endothelial cells, hepatocytes, epithelial cells, keratinocytes, and fibroblasts, to synthesize and release endogenous pyrogens: e.g., tumor necrosis factor (TNF), interferon, interleukin-1 (IL-1), and interleukin-6 (IL-6). Upon reaching the hypothalamic thermoregulatory center these inflammatory cytokines induce an abrupt release of prostaglandins that increase the thermostatic set point and produce heat [1]. To produce fever two conditions must be met: the hypothalamic thermostat needs to be raised to a higher setting and the peripheral mechanisms regulating peripheral heat loss (peripheral vasoconstriction) and/or internal heat production (shivering) must be intact [1].

Medications and other substances impair the febrile response to infection by different mechanisms (Table 2).

In many situations, elevating body temperature increases chances for survival. The growth and virulence of several bacteria are impaired at high temperatures. Fever improves host defense responses by enhancing neutrophil migration, increasing production of antibacterial substances, increasing production of interferon, increasing the antiviral and antitumor activity of interferon, increasing T cell proliferation, and decreasing the growth of microorganisms in an iron-poor environment [4]. Fever may also protect against pathogen-induced disturbances in homeostasis [4]. High temperature increases the phagocytic and bactericidal activity of neutrophils and enhances the cytotoxic effects of lymphocytes. However, fever can increase the metabolic demand and lead to cardiac decompensation, weight loss, negative nitrogen balance, muscle wasting, decreased mental status and seizure.

Differential Diagnosis

The cause of fever in the ICU varies according to the patient population and type of ICU. Both infectious and noninfectious conditions can cause fever in critically ill patients [5, 6]. The diagnostic approach to fever in critically ill patients is based on the magnitude of the fever, fever pattern, and presence of localizing signs. Temperatures above 41.1°C (106°F) are rarely caused by an infection [5]. Temperature elevations ≤38.9°C (102°F) may or may not result from an infection [5]. Although ICU patients with a temperature between 38.9°C (102°F) and 41.1°C (106°F) may have noninfectious causes of fever, most temperature elevations >38.9°C (102°F) in critically ill patients result from infection, except for drug fever and acute adrenal insufficiency [5]. Single fever spikes with temperature between 38.9°C (102.°F) and 41.1°C (106°F) that terminate spontaneously are unlikely to result from an infection [5]. Infection is the most common cause of prolonged fever (> five days) in critically ill patients [6].

Sepsis is a major threat to the recovery of critically ill patients and represents a diagnostic challenge to physicians in charge of their care. Clinical criteria are insensitive in identifying causes of fever. Furthermore, several pathologic conditions may coexist in a single patient and make correct diagnosis and treatment even more difficult. The host response to noninfectious tissue injury of critically ill patients can lead to fever. Such causes include hematomas, traumatic injury to soft tissue, tissue ischemia without infection, pulmonary contusion, atelectasis, chemical pneumonitis, and acute respiratory distress syndrome (ARDS). Subarachnoid hemorrhage can produce a severe febrile response, usually a few days following the acute bleeding. Certain noninfectious conditions present with a sepsis-like picture. Neuroleptic malignant syndrome, systemic vasculitides, anaphylaxis, acute pancreatitis, extensive tissue injury due to crush, rhabdomyolysis, vascular occlusion, and heat stroke can mimic sepsis. The sympathomimetic and anticholinergic activity associated with cocaine and phenothiazine intoxication, the cholinesterase blockade from organophosphate poisoning, and withdrawal from alcohol, opiates, and barbiturates can also lead to fever. A thorough understanding of the epidemiology and the various causes of fever is necessary to avoid misdiagnosis and inappropriate treatment. This understanding then allows a systematic approach in the diagnosis of the causes of fever and use of the most appropriate tests. The infectious and noninfectious causes of fever in critically ill patients are listed in Table 3.

EPIDEMIOLOGY OF SEPSIS

The incidence of infection and the spectrum of causative organisms in the ICU change over time [7]. In a multicenter study of 12,001 patients in the United States, the incidence of sepsis was two per 100 hospital-admissions [8]. Fifty-five per cent of the episodes of sepsis originated in an ICU. The sources of infection were respiratory in 42%, bacteremia with undetermined site in 12%, genitourinary in 11%, abdominal in 10%, device-related in 6%, wound/soft tissue in 5%, central nervous system in 2%, endocarditis in 1%, others in 3%, and undetermined in 8%. The organisms identified to cause the septic episodes were Gram-negative in 39.8%, Gram-positive in 31%, fungi in 6.1%, intraabdominal anaerobes in 2%, unclassified organisms in 4.8%, and polymicrobial in 16.3%. The most common Gram-negative organisms were Enterobacteriaceae in 27.1%, *Pseudomonas* in 9.8%, and *Haemophilus* in 1.3%. The most common Gram-positive organisms were *Staphylococcus aureus* in 13.9%, Enterococcus in 6.1%, coagulase-negative Staphylococcus in 5.7%, and Pneumococcus in 2%. In a nationwide surveillance network of hospitals in the United States, 10,617 episodes of nosocomial blood stream infections were identified [9]: 64.4% due to Gram-positive organisms, 27% due to Gram-negative organisms, and 8.4% due to fungi. Coagulase-negative staphylococci and *Staphylococcus aureus* were the two most common organisms; 29% of the *S aureus* and 80% of the coagulase-negative staphylococci isolates were methicillin-resistant; 3% of the *Enterococcus fecalis* strains and 50% of *Enterococcus faecium* isolates displayed resistance to vancomycin.

The sources of infection in the ICU reported through the National Nosocomial Infections Surveillance System in the United States and European Prevalence of Infection in the Intensive Care are listed in Table 4. Analysis of surveillance data, collected through the National Nosocomial Infections Surveillance System on 181,993 patients from medical ICUs in the United States showed 87% of primary blood stream infections were associated with central lines, 86% of nosocomial pneumonias were associated with mechanical ventilation, and 95% of urinary tract infections were associated with urinary catheters [10]. Coagulase-negative

TABLE 3. Infectious and noninfectious causes of fever in critically ill patients

Infectious	Noninfectious
Central nervous system	Intracranial bleeding
Meningitis	Intracerebral
Encephalitis	Subarachnoid
Intracranial pressure monitor infection	Subdural
	Nonhemorrhagic infarction
	Seizures
Cardiovascular	Dissecting aortic aneurysm
Endocarditis	Dressler's syndrome
Intravascular catheter infection	Venous thrombophlebitis
Suppurative phlebitis	Myocardial infarction
	Pericarditis
Respiratory	Fibroproliferative phase of ARDS
Pneumonia	Pulmonary emboli/infarction
Tracheobronchitis	Atelectasis
Empyema	Chemical pneumonitis
Ear, nose and throat	
Suppurative parotitis	
Sinusitis	
Posterior pharyngeal space infection	
Otitis	
Renal	
Urinary tract infection	
Pyelonephritis	
Abdominal	Nonviral hepatitis
Viral hepatitis	Cholecystitis
Acalculous cholecystitis	Pancreatitis
Intraabdominal abscess	Ischemic colitis
Peritonitis	Inflammatory bowel disease
Spontaneous bacterial peritonitis	
Antibiotic-associated colitis	
Pseudomembranous colitis	
Diverticulitis	
Skin and soft tissue	
Wound infection	
Mediastinitis	
Burn infection	
Decubitus ulcer infection	
Musculoskeletal	
Osteomyelitis	
Septic arthritis	
Metabolic/endocrine	Adrenal insufficency
	Hyperthyroidism
	Alcohol or drug withdrawal
	Heat stroke
	Malignant hyperthermia

TABLE 3 (Continued)

Infectious	Noninfectious

Hematologic	Deep venous thrombosis
	Hemolysis
	Hemorrhage
	  Gastrointestinal
	  Occult hematoma
	  Retroperitoneal
	Sickle cell crisis
	Thrombotic thrombocytopenic purpura

Neoplastic	Lymphoreticular/hematopoietic
	Metastasis
	Solid tumors
	  Carcinoma of pancreas, lung, bone, colon
	  Hepatocellular carcinoma
	  Hypernephroma

Miscellaneous	Drugs
	Fat embolism
	Procedures
	  Bronchoscopy
	  Colonoscopy
	  Intravenous catheter placement
	  Urinary catheterization
	Surgery
	Toxic epidermal necrolysis
	Transfusion
	Collagen vascular disease
	Gout/pseudogout
	Vasculitis
	Reaction to intramuscular injection
	Intravenous contrast reaction

staphylococci (36%) were the most common bloodstream infection isolates, followed by Enterococci (16%), and *Staphylococcus aureus* (13%). Twelve per cent of bloodstream isolates were fungi. The most common isolates from pneumonia were Gram-negative aerobic organisms (64%). *Pseudomonas aeruginosa* (21%) and *Staphylococcus aureus* (20%) were the most frequently isolated organisms. *Candida albicans* was the most common single pathogen isolated from urine and constituted just over half of the fungal isolates. Certain pathogens were associated with device use: coagulase-negative staphylococci with central lines, *Pseudomonas aeruginosa* and *Acinetobacter* species with ventilators, and fungal infections with urinary catheters.

In a multicenter survey of 10,038 patients from ICUs of 17 West European countries, 44.8% had infection [11]. The most frequently isolated organisms were Enterobacteriaceae (34.4%), *Staphylococcus aureus* I (30.1%), *Pseudomonas aeruginosa* (28.7%), coagulase-negative staphylococcus (19.1%) and fungi (17.1%).

In another multicenter study of 1589 patients treated in ICUs in France, infections were

TABLE 4. The sources of nosocomial infection in the ICU in the United States and Europe

	NNIS[10] N = 181,993	*EPIC*[11] N = 10,038
Urinary tract	31%	14.6%
Pneumonia	27%	38.9%
Blood stream	19%	9.9%
Wound	NR	5.7%
Ear, nose, throat	4%	4.3%
Skin and soft tissue	NR	4.0%
Gastrointestinal	5%	3.7%
Cardiovascular	4%	2.4%
Other	10%	16.5%

NNIS = National Nosocomial Infections Surveillance System.
EPIC = European Prevalence of Infection in the Intensive Care.
NR = Not reported.

identified in 13.1% of patients [12]: the ventilator-associated pneumonia (VAP) rate was 9.6%; sinusitis, 1.5%; central venous catheter-associated infection, 3.5%; central venous catheter-associated bacteremia, 4.8%; catheter-associated urinary tract infection, 7.8%; and bacteremia 4.5%.

Pneumonia, nosocomial sinusitis, intravascular catheter-related infection, and urinary tract infection account for most of the infections seen in ICUs [13]. Most of these infections occur in the presence of a foreign object – a catheter or a tube [13]. Even when one source of infection is identified, other concomitant sources of infection with different pathogens are common in the ICU [13].

INFECTIOUS CAUSES OF FEVER IN THE ICU

Pneumonia. Pneumonia results when a particularly virulent organism or a very large inoculum reaches the lower airways and overwhelms lung defenses. A local inflammatory response follows, with accumulation of neutrophils and other effector cells in the peripheral bronchi and alveolar spaces. Locally, the inflammatory exudate produces purulent sputum and consolidation that can be detected by physical examination and chest radiography. Systemically, it causes, among others things, fever and leukocytosis.

Pneumonia is subdivided into community- and hospital-acquired. VAP is defined as pneumonia that develops in patients who have been endotracheally intubated for 48 hours or more. Risk factors for VAP include pack-years history of smoking, chronic obstructive pulmonary disease (COPD), low serum albumin level, the presence of intracranial pressure monitor, prior antibiotic use, absence of antibiotic therapy, multiple organ failure, large volume gastric aspirate, H_2 blockers and antacids, gastric colonization and high pH, colonization of upper respiratory tract with respiratory Gram-negative bacilli, supine head position, positive end-expiratory pressure (PEEP) level, reintubation, tracheostomy, duration of mechanical ventilation, failure of subglottic aspiration, and low intracuff pressure [14–16]. The cumulative incidence of pneumonia in ICU patients requiring mechanical ventilation is 12.1% compared to 0.74% in those who do not require mechanical ventilation [16]. For patients receiving mechanical ventilation for 48 h or more, the incidence of pneumonia is 20.5 cases per 1,000 mechanical-ventilation days [16].

The incidence of the organisms causing hospital-acquired pneumonia varies from hospital to hospital and within different units of the same hospital. Early-onset hospital-acquired pneumonia is likely to be caused by *Streptococcus pneumoniae*, nonpseudomonal Enterobacter species, *Escherichia coli*, *Hemophilus influenzae*, *Klebsiella* species, *Serratia marcescens*, and methicillin-sensitive *Staphylococcus aureus* [17]. Late-onset hospital-acquired pneumonia is likely to be caused by *Pseudomonas aeruginosa*, methicillin-resistant *Staphylococcus aureus*, and *Acinetobacter* species, in addition to the organisms causing early-onset pneumonia [17]. Certain risk factors are associated with specific pathogens: recent abdominal surgery and witnessed aspiration with anaerobes; coma, head trauma, diabetes mellitus, and renal failure with *Staphylococcus aureus*; high-dose corticosteroid therapy with *Legionella*; and prolonged ICU stay, steroid therapy, antibiotics, and structural lung disease with *Pseudomonas aeruginosa*. Uncommon pathogens can cause nosocomial pneumonia under certain conditions. Clusters of Legionellosis have been related to contaminated water and cooling towers, as well as to soil movement, in an area related to the hospital. *Candida* species can cause pneumonia in patients on broad spectrum antibiotics. *Aspergillus fumigatus* should be considered as a possible pathogen when there are construction activities and faulty ventilator systems around a hospital. *Staphylococcus aureus* and *Pseudomonas aeruginosa* are the two most common organisms causing VAP [16]. About 40% of VAP have polymicrobial etiology [16]. Anaerobes are uncommon causes of VAP in critically ill patients [18].

The diagnosis of pneumonia in noncritically ill patients is usually made on the basis of symptoms, signs, chest radiographs, and respiratory secretions. In ventilated patients, this combination of signs is shared by a variety of other conditions occurring either alone or in combination, making it difficult to distinguish VAP from other infectious or noninfectious processes, characterized by fever and pulmonary densities. In a study of 50 critically ill patients with fever and pulmonary densities, a comprehensive diagnostic approach led to definitive diagnosis in 90% of the patients [13]. Although infections were the most common causes of the fever and pulmonary densities, pneumonia was identified in 40% [13]. In six other studies [19–24] involving 317 patients on mechanical ventilation with suspected VAP, only 110 (35%) had pneumonia. An alternative diagnosis for pulmonary densities was described for 118. Chest radiographic findings are nonspecific for the diagnosis of pneumonial [21, 25–27]. Alternative diagnoses for radiographic densities in patients with suspected VAP include atelectasis, congestive heart failure, ARDS, pulmonary embolism, pulmonary fibrosis, pulmonary hemorrhage, neoplastic disorders, nonbacterial pneumonia, chemical aspiration, near-drowning, neurogenic pulmonary edema, smoke inhalation, fat embolism, drug reaction, pulmonary contusion, acute interstitial pneumonitis, occupational lung disease, bronchiolitis obliterans organizing pneumonia, connective tissue diseases and hypersensitivity pneumonia [13, 28]. Patients with atelectasis and congestive heart failure may have one or more extrapulmonary infectious sources of fever.

In selecting a diagnostic method, the following factors should be considered: cost effectiveness, availability, expertise, severity, and likelihood of changing empirical treatment. An attempt should be made to establish a correct etiologic diagnosis of pneumonia to permit optimal antibiotic selection and to identify pathogens of potential epidemiological significance. Using invasive methods to diagnose VAP is controversial [29, 30]. However, a recent, randomized, controlled, multicenter study showed reduced mortality and antibiotic use in patients who underwent bronchoscopy for the diagnosis of VAP [31].

Urinary Tract Infection. Urinary tract infection (UTI) is a common nosocomial infection in ICU patients [32]. Bacteremia occurs in up to 4% and usually results from pyelonephritis, perinephric abscesses, or obstructive uropathy, often in diabetic patients. Progression of UTI to sepsis results in a 14% excess mortality [33, 34]. Eighty per cent of these infections are related to using urinary catheters [35]. Placing a urinary catheter creates several avenues for bladder colonization: loss of the normal urethral washing mechanism, catheter contamination at the catheter-tubing junction, and retrograde flow of microbes from the collecting bag. Indwelling catheters may result in incomplete bladder emptying, providing a culture medium for unchecked proliferation of bacteria [36]. Bladder mucosal damage from catheter manipulation or overdistention from a blocked catheter may enhance bacterial invasion [37]. Rarely, UTI may arise by hematogenous seeding from a distant site.

Risk for UTI is highest in patients who require catheterization for more than a week [38]. Fifty per cent of UTIs occur within 10 days of ICU admission [32]. Aerobic Gram-negative rods are the predominant pathogens, with *Escherichia coli* being the most common. In hospitalized patients, a high frequency of *Pseudomonas* spp, *Enterococcus* spp, coagulase-negative staphylococci, and *Candida* spp are encountered. *Candida albicans* is the most common organism isolated from the urine of patients in United States ICUs [39]. Anaerobic UTI may occur in critically ill surgical patients and should be suspected when cultures are negative with a positive Gram stain [40]. Anaerobes multiply in the urinary tract when the oxygen tension is low, such as in scar tissue, tumors, and necrotic tissue. Persistent or relapsing *Proteus mirabilis* bacteriuria should prompt evaluation for staghorn calculus. *Corynebacterium urealyticum* is associated with an alkaline urine and renal stones [41]. Isolation of *Staphylococcus aureus* from the urine culture should raise the possibility of seeding from the bloodstream.

Signs and symptoms of local inflammation, such as suprapubic tenderness and dysuria, are rarely found in critically ill patients with UTI. UTI should be suspected in bladder-catheterized patients with fever and leukocytosis. Cultures of urine obtained by aspiration from a sampling port on the catheter itself are probably adequate to diagnose UTI. Studies show that cultures obtained by this method correlate with cultures from suprapubic aspiration in at least 90% of cases [42]. The usual threshold of 10^5 organisms used in noncatheterized patients may be inappropriate for patients with indwelling catheters. Although prospective studies to establish a specific quantitative level diagnostic of infection have not been done, some sources suggest that bacteriuria of 10^2 colony forming unit (CFU)/ml should be considered significant and treated as UTI [43]. The urinalysis should be consistent (presence of leukocytes, large numbers of bacteria, positive nitrite test, positive leukocyte esterase) to rule out a false-positive culture resulting from a delay in culturing the specimen.

Ultrasound is used to investigate patients with upper urinary tract infection and suspected obstruction. Complications such as cortical abscess, acute focal bacterial nephritis, and perinephric abscess are better defined by CT scan. Accurate placement of percutaneous drains into suppurative collections may require CT scan guidance. Intravenous urography is superior in demonstrating the collection system and thus confirming a diagnosis of papillary necrosis. Emphysematous pyelonephritis is characterized by gas formation in the renal parenchyma and surrounding tissues and is observed in patients with uncontrolled diabetes. The diagnosis can be made by plain radiograph, ultrasound or CT [44]. CT may show gas in the muscular layer of the bladder in patients with pyocystis [45].

Intravascular Catheter-Related Infections. Nosocomial infections related to intravascular lines continue to be an important and serious complication in critically ill patients. The microbial flora colonizing the skin at the insertion site are the primary source of exogenous contamination of the catheter [46–49]. Local trauma induced by introducing the catheter facilitates entry of microorganisms that proliferate on the surface of the catheter [50]. Bacteria either advance or multiply distally along the external catheter surface (within the subcutaneous tract) and ultimately gain access to the venous circulation. In the absence of any other externally provided nutrient, bacteria adhere to irregularities on the catheter surface within 30 minutes, and heavy colonization occurs within six to 12 hours. These colonies become covered by a slimy material (glycocalyx) that enhances bacterial adherence and serves as a barrier against the host defense mechanisms [51]. Additional but less common mechanisms of catheter-related infections include contamination of the catheter tip during episodes of bacteremia or fungemia and microbial contamination of the infusate.

A prospective multicenter cohort study reported that 9.3% of 623 central venous catheterizations were associated with infection [52]. The chance of a patient developing bacteremia from a central line has been estimated to be 0.3% to 0.5%/catheter/day [53]. Catheter-related sepsis is associated with substantial morbidity and an average added hospital cost of $4000 per episode [54]. Factors reported to increase the risk for catheter-related infections include age, loss of skin integrity, presence of neutropenia, chemotherapy, radiation therapy, thrombogenicity of catheter materials, not using antibiotic impregnated catheters, vascular cutdown, emergency catheter placement, transparent dressings, lack of aseptic technique at the time of placement, site of insertion (internal jugular > subclavian > peripheral), duration of catheterization, use of multilumen catheters, multiple attempts at vessel cannulation, excessive manipulation of the catheter, severity of underlying illness and infection at another site [55]. The type of skin disinfectant used prior to insertion may also be important. Ten per cent povidone-iodine and 70% isopropyl alcohol appear to be inferior to 2% aqueous chlorhexidine in preventing catheter-related infection and bacteremia [56]. The risk of bacteremia associated with peripheral venous catheters is less than 1% [57, 58]. The frequency of bacteremia related to peripheral arterial cannulation is about 1% [59, 60].

Because most episodes of catheter-related infection can be traced to bacteria that colonize the patient's skin at the insertion site, Staphylococcus species constitutue approximately two-thirds of all catheter-related infection [54]. *Coagulase-negative staphylococci* have a propensity to adhere to plastic catheters and result in catheter-related infections [61]. Enteric Gram-negative and fungal infections are more often related to hematogenous seeding from a distant site [62, 63].

Erythema, warmth, and purulence at the insertion site are often absent in patients with catheter-related infection. Fever and leukocytosis should alert the clinician that a central or arterial line may be the source of infection. Metastatic infection and endocarditis should heighten suspicion of a catheter source of infection. Signs of infection at the insertion site warrant removal of the catheter. Even in the absence of local signs of infection, fever in critically ill patients should prompt removal or exchange over a guide wire of any central venous catheter present for more than 48 hours. Catheters in place for less than two days rarely show significant growth [49]. Resolution of fever following catheter removal is consistent with a diagnosis of catheter-related infection.

Bacteriologic confirmation of catheter-related infection is based on isolating potential pathogens in significant numbers on semiquantitative cultures, according to guidelines established by the Centers for Disease Control and Prevention [64, 65]. When catheters <3 inches are removed, the entire catheter from just inside the skin surface to the tip should be cultured. When large central catheters are removed, both a 2-inch intracutaneous segment and the tip should be cultured. When pulmonary artery catheters are cultured, the introducer should be cultured as well. The culture is performed by rolling a 5-cm catheter segment (intracutaneous portion for long cathethers and tip for short catheters) across a blood agar plate in a reproducible manner. Growth of 15 or more colonies is considered diagnostic of catheter-related infection and is associated with a 16% incidence of bacteremia. In one study, no episodes of bacteremia or clinical infection occurred in cases with fewer than 15 colonies [50]. When catheter-related infection is suspected, at least two sets of blood cultures should be drawn. Comparison of blood cultures drawn through the catheter with those from a peripheral venipuncture has been suggested, but no clear advantage to this approach has been shown [66]. Differential quantitative blood cultures with a 10-fold or higher differential count from blood drawn from a catheter compared to blood drawn from a peripheral vein indicates catheter-related infection [67]. Multiple positive blood cultures are needed for organisms that may be disregarded as contaminants, such as coagulase-negative staphylococci, *Corynebacterium jeikeium*, *Bacillus* species, *Candida* species, or *Malassezia* species.

For patients with fever who are in stable condition, it is not necessary to remove or change all indwelling catheters. However, if there is evidence of tunnel infection, embolic phenomenon, vascular compromise, or sepsis, the catheter should be removed and cultured, and a new catheter should be inserted at a different site [2].

Nosocomial Sinusitis. Paranasal sinusitis is a frequently overlooked source of sepsis in critically ill patients. Sinusitis was first noted as a frequent problem in neurosurgical patients because of the frequent use of CT scan of the brain, which incidentally included the paranasal sinuses. The presence of a foreign object in the nasopharynx appears to be an important, but not essential, risk factor for the development of sinusitis. Foreign bodies in the nares can cause mucosal edema and inflammation, which may obstruct the sinus ostia, thereby impeding the drainage of the more than 500 ml of fluid produced by the paranasal sinuses each day [68, 69]. Stagnant secretions in a closed space contaminated by nosocomial pathogens may lead to sinusitis and systemic signs of sepsis. Once established in the maxillary sinuses, inflammation and infection can subsequently spread to the ethmoid and sphenoid sinuses [70]. Intracranial spread via diploic veins can have devastating consequences such as meningitis, brain abscess, osteomyelitis of the skull, and cavernous sinus thrombosis [71].

An epidemiological study of medical ICU patients with oral intubation found the incidence of sinusitis, diagnosed by cultures of maxillary aspirates, to be 7.7% [72]. In some critically ill patients, sinusitis may be the sole or contributing cause of fever. The incidence of sinusitis may exceed 15% in patients intubated longer than five days [73]. The incidence of sinusitis is higher in patients intubated nasotracheally than in those intubated orotracheally [74]. A randomized study assessing the systematic search for maxillary sinusitis demonstrated the presence of nosocomial sinusitis in 40% of nasotracheally intubated, mechanically ventilated patients [75]. In patients who are hospitalized in an ICU for at least 48 hours, the incidence rates of nosocomial sinusitis were 17.4 cases per 1000 patient-days and 19.8 cases per 1000 nasoenteric tube-days [72].

Risk factors for nosocomial sinusitis include nasal colonization with enteric Gram-negative bacilli, feeding via nasoenteric tube, sedative use, and low Glasgow coma score [72]. Additional factors also paly roles in the development of sinusitis in patients without nasal tubes. The recumbent position and limitation of head mobility prevent natural sinus drainage due to gravity [76, 77]. Recumbency also causes decreased venous blood return from the head and neck and results in increased nasal congestion and narrowing of maxillary sinus ostia [77]. Positive pressure ventilation, by raising central venous pressure, may compound this problem [78]. Impaired ability to cough or sneeze and the simple absence of airflow through the nares in mechanically ventilated patients may also predispose to sinus infection [78].

Localized symptoms of sinus infection are difficult to elicit in intubated patients, and the first manifestation of nosocomial sinusitis is often fever or even sepsis without an obvious source [79]. A purulent nasal discharge may be absent in up to 73% of cases [80]. Infected purulent secretions, when present, may appear in the proximal trachea due to aspiration, thus simulating tracheobrochitis and pneumonia. Sinusitis is a common alternate cause of fever in patients with suspected pneumonia and negative bronchoscopic cultures. Furthermore, pneumonia and sinusitis often coexist and are frequently caused by the same organism [13]. Sinusitis in ICU patients is most commonly due to Gram-negative bacilli, and *Staphylococcus aureus* [72, 76, 79, 81]. In a study using nasal disinfection with povidone-iodine solution prior to transnasal puncture to avoid contamination with colonizing organisms, Gram-negative bacilli accounted for 47% of infections with *Pseudomonas aeruginosa* being the most common; *Staphylococcus aureus* represented 20% and yeast were found in 18%

[74]. Nosocomial sinusitis is of polymicrobial etiology in 27–82% of the cases. Mucosal thickening, opacification, or air-fluid levels on sinus roentgenograms or CT scans suggest the diagnosis of sinusitis. A sinus puncture is helpful in patients with fever and positive findings on sinus films. If pus is obtained by maxillary puncture, a positive culture may be found in 80% of the cases. Antral puncture for drainage and specimen collection for Gram stain and culture can guide antibiotic selection. In the majority of patients with sinusitis, antibiotic therapy is changed as the result of antral puncture [82]. In the presence of purulence in the middle meatus on physical examination in conjuction with the presence of sinus disease on CT of the sinuses, antral lavage confirms purulence in 92% of the maxillary sinus [83].

The occurrence of VAP in patients undergoing prolonged mechanical ventilation via a nasotracheal intubation can be prevented by the systematic search and treatment of nosocomial sinusitis [75].

Intraabdominal Infection. Intraabdominal infections, although an infrequent cause of fever in a medical ICU, are a significant source of sepsis in patients with prior abdominal surgery or trauma. It is analyzed in detail in Section 7. Intraabdominal sepsis results when bacteria or fungi are introduced into the peritoneal cavity from penetrating trauma, surgery, instrumentation (e.g., peritoneal dialysis or paracentesis), perforated viscus, translocation through intact bowel (e.g., spontaneous bacterial peritonitis), ischemic bowel, and systemic bacteremia. The evolution of the infection depends upon the number of invading organisms and the immunologic response of the host. An effective inflammatory response causes localization of the infection with abscess formation. The progressively thicker fibrin deposit that surrounds the abscess, however, prevents host defenses from completely eradicating microbes, even when appropriate antibiotics are administered [84]. In patients without prior surgery, abscesses form most commonly in the lower quadrants of the abdomen or pelvis. Widespread contamination of the abdominal cavity results in peritonitis. In spontaneous bacterial peritonitis and peritonitis related to peritoneal dialysis catheters, chronic ascites becomes infected without overt loss of bowel mucosal integrity. Another cause of peritonitis in patients admitted to the ICU for nonsurgical problems is the development of ischemic enterocolitis from either a low cardiac output state or high-dose vasopressor therapy. Overgrowth of certain bacteria within the gut lumen, as occurs in antibiotic-associated colitis, can cause fever or can result in perforation.

Intraabdominal sources of fever are identified in 11% of patients with suspected VAP [13]. Intraabdominal infections represent a common infectious cause of fever in patients with ARDS and carry a poor prognosis. One prospective study found that the abdomen was a major site of infection in 13% of 129 ICU patients with ARDS [85]. In one autopsy study of ARDS patients, whose site of infection was undetermined antemortem, autopsy showed the lungs to be the source of infection in 8 of 10 patients with negative blood cultures and the peritoneum in 7 of 9 patients who had positive blood cultures [85].

Prompt diagnosis and treatment of intraabdominal infection results in decreased mortality [86]. Gastrointestinal bleeding, gastrointestinal malignancy, abdominal surgery, and pancreatitis are risk factors for intraabdominal infection.

Pain is a common manifestation of intraabdominal infection. The classical clinical findings suggesting an intraabdominal abscess are often absent in critically ill patients and are frequently masked by altered mental status and administration of sedatives, narcotics, neuromuscular blockers, or steroids. In one study of patients with intraabdominal abscess, only 36% had localized tenderness and 7% had a palpable mass [87]. Approximately one-third of patients with primary peritonitis have no signs or symptoms of sepsis referrable to the abdomen [88]. Because of these limitations, clinicians should suspect an intraabdominal source of infection in the presence of unexplained sepsis, hypovolemia, and abdominal distention. Abdominal distention with absence of bowel movements or diarrhea, derceased bowel sounds, and abdominal pain are nonspecific findings in intraabdominal infections. In the appropriate clinical setting, a febrile patient should have the abdomen evaluated even in the absence of localizing signs and symptoms.

Ultrasound examination will help in detecting biliary tract disease, and inflammatory processes or abscesses of the liver, perihepatic region, pancreas, retroperitoneum, and pelvis. CT scan is the examination of choice for suspected intraabdominal sepsis of unclear etiology, and it helps in detecting abscesses and inflammatory masses associated with the bowel [89].

PSEUDOMEMBRANOUS COLITIS. Pseudomembranous colitis usually presents with diarrhea and systemic symptoms following antimicrobial therapy. However, it will occasionally present with sepsis or an acute abdomen in the absence of diarrhea, blood per rectum, and tenderness over the descending colon. Repeated examination of the abdomen is needed, looking for persistent, localized pain, tenderness, or guarding. Consultation with a general surgeon is required. *Clostridium difficile* accounts for 10%–25% of all cases of antibiotic-associated diarrhea and 100% of antibiotic-associated pseudomembranous colitis [90]. When pseudomembranous colitis is suspected, a stool should be tested for *Clostridium difficile* toxin, and, if there is no diarrhea, sigmoidoscopy or colonoscopy may be diagnostic (see Chapter 44).

PERITONITIS. Primary peritonitis occurs in patients who have ascites secondary to cirrhosis of the liver, congestive heart failure, or end stage renal disease. Although most patients with peritonitis present with signs of peritoneal irritation, some have no symptoms or signs referrable to the abdomen. Gram stain and culture of peritoneal fluid usually yields aerobic enteric organisms. However, in about 35% of patients with bacterial peritonitis, the ascitic fluid cultures may be negative [91, 92]. Secondary bacterial peritonitis is caused by contamination from the gut lumen, and multiple organisms are usually found in the ascitic fluid. Patients with secondary bacterial peritonitis are unlikely to respond to antibiotics alone and usually require surgical treatment. Patients who develop peritonitis from an infected peritoneal dialysis catheter require removal of the catheter if the infection does not respond to antibiotic treatment (see Chapter 49).

CHOLECYSTITIS. Biliary tract infection should be considered when sepsis and hyperbilirubinemia coexist. Biliary tract infection results from calculous cholecystitis, acute cholangitis, and acalculous cholecystitis. Ultrasonography, CT, endoscopic retrograde cholangiography, and percutaneous hepatic cholangiography are used to detect dilated and obstructed biliary tree. Calculous cholecystitis results from obstruction of the cystic duct by a gallstone and is treated by cholecystectomy. Cholangitis, bacterial infection within the bile duct, presents with right upper quadrant abdominal pain, jaundice and fever. Treatment consists of biliary decompression and antibiotics. Biliary decompression can be achieved surgically, endoscopically, or percutaneously. Rapid clinical and biochemical improvement indicates the adequacy of the decompression. If a patient with acute cholangitis does not improve despite decompression, CT scan should be obtained to look for hepatic abscess induced by the cholangitis (see Chapter 47).

ACALCULOUS CHOLECYSTITIS. Acalculous cholecystitis may occur in a patient with no known biliary disease and require prolonged intensive care support. The cause is most likely multifactorial. Prolonged absence of enteral feeding results in decreased gallbladder emptying and progressive concentration of noxious bile acids within its lumen [93]. Prolonged spasm of the sphincter of Oddi caused by narcotic analgesics, especially morphine, promotes bile stasis [94]. Use of mechanical ventilation with PEEP produces decreased portal blood flow, biliary stasis, and elevated bilirubin [95, 96]. Hemodynamic instability and use of vasopressor agents may compromise circulation to the gallbladder epithelium. Taken together, these risk factors predispose to a combine ischemic-chemical injury and secondary infection by gut flora ascending the biliary tree [93].

Acalculous cholecystitis is diagnosed in less than 1% of long-term ICU patients [97]; however, at the time of surgery, 40% to 100% already have advanced disease with gangrene, empyema, or perforation [98]. The most common organisms cultured from bile are Gram-negative aerobes, such as *E coli*, *Klebsiella*, *Enterobacter* and *Proteus*. Streptococcus, Enterococcus, Staphylococcus, and anaerobes are also seen [93, 97, 99].

The onset of acalculous cholecystitis is insidious, its presenting symptoms are nonconstant, and its neglect can lead to necrosis of the gallbladder with sepsis and death [100]. Right upper quadrant pain and tenderness are absent in 50% to 75% of cases [93, 94]. Elevations of white blood cell count, alkaline phosphatase and bilirubin are neither sensitive nor specific for the diagnosis of cholecystitis. Elevated bilirubin may be seen as a manifestation of sepsis or multiorgan failure, where it is associated with the specific histologic finding of cholangiolar cholestasis [101]. The presence of fever without an obvious source should alert one to consider acalculous cholecystitis, especially in the presence of risk factors such as a prolonged critical illness, recent surgical procedure, use of narcotic analgesics, and prolonged absence of enteral nutrition [94, 97].

Filling of the gallbladder in a biliary radionuclide scan rules out cholecystitis [102]. Findings of pericholecystic fluid in the absence of ascites, intraluminal gas, or a sloughed mucosal membrane in ultrasonography or CT are diagnostic of acalculous cholecystitis [94]. A thick-walled gallbladder in a patient without generalized edema suggests acalculous cholecystitis. Percutaneous bile aspiration for culture has high false-positive and false-negative rates. If the clinical index of suspicion for acalculous cholecystitis in a deteriorating patient is high, surgical intervention will confirm the diagnosis and lead to improvement.

The traditional approach to treating acalculous cholecystitis has been urgent laparotomy and cholecystectomy. Recently, ultrasound-guided percutaneous placement of a cholecystostomy drainage catheter has become popular, especially in patients at high risk for surgery. One study reported an 87% long-term success rate and no mortality with this procedure [103]. Percutaneous transhepatic drainage can lead to significant clinical improvement in patients who are too sick to undergo laparotomy [104]. Postdrainage cholangiography can be done through the indwelling catheter and, if normal, may obviate the need for open cholecystectomy later [99]. Transpapillary endoscopic cholecystostomy has been reported to be another effective alternative for gallbladder drainage in patients at high risk for surgery [105]. Because one of the most consistent risk factors for acalculous cholecystitis is the absence of enteral nutrition, all attempts should be made to feed ventilated patients by this route. Mortality rates associated with acalculous cholecystitis range from 7% to 44% [94, 106].

INTRAABDOMINAL ABSCESS. Pyogenic liver abscess can result from trauma, perihepatic infection, systemic bacteremia, portal bacteremia and cholangitis. Patients with hepatic abscess usually present with right upper quadrant abdominal pain, and the diagnosis can be confirmed with ultrasound or CT. Percutaneous drainage is the preferred treatment of hepatic abscess.

Splenic abscess can result from trauma, direct extension, or bacteremia. The diagnosis can be established with ultrasound or CT of the abdomen, and the optimal treatment is splenectomy with percutaneous drainage as a temporizing measure.

Intraabdominal abscesses that are too small to be seen by CT or ultrasound examination and intraloop abscesses can lead to occult sepsis. At times, a short segment of ischemic or necrotic bowel may be difficult to detect. If such segment is in the left colon, colonoscopy may be needed.

Central Nervous System Infection. Although there are numerous noninfectious reasons for fever and change in mental status of a critically ill patient, intensivists should maintain a high index of suspicion for central nervous system (CNS) infection [107]. The diagnostic evaluation for suspected CNS infection includes CT of the brain and lumbar puncture. In patients with focal neurological findings suggesting disease above the foramen magnum, imaging of the brain is needed before lumbar puncture. In patients with suspected brain abscess, the bacteriologic yield of cerebrospinal fluid (CSF) analysis is too low to justify the risk of herniation associated with lumbar puncture [108]. Aspiration of the suspected brain abscess is the diagnostic procedure of choice [2]. When a patient with an intracranial device becomes febrile, CSF should be obtained for analysis. If the patient has a CSF reservoir, the reservoir should be aspirated [2]. If a patient with ventriculostomy or lumbar drain catheter develops signs of meningitis, the catheter should be removed and the tip cultured [2]. The CSF should be analyzed for cell count and white blood cell differential, glucose, protein, Gram stain, and bacterial culture. Additionally, tests for tuberculosis, fungal disease, and neoplasia should be performed if dictated by the clinical situation [2]. Lumbar puncture in surgical ICU patients without a recent history of head trauma or a neurosurgical operation has a low yield for the diagnosis of bacterial meningitis [109] (see Chapters 24, 29 and 30).

POSTOPERATIVE FEVER

Fever is seen in 9% of patients postoperatively [110]. Fever during the initial 48 hours after surgery is usually of noninfectious origin [111, 112]. Atelectasis is often considered to be a cause of postoperative fever. However, clinicians should be aware that aspiration during the perioperative period and community-acquired infection that has been incubating before surgery can cause fever postoperatively [2]. Persistence of fever > four days after surgery for intraabdominal infection should raise suspicion for persistent or new infection. The overall incidence of wound infection is 3%–6% in the United States. Wound infection, except from group A Streptococci and Clostridia, is uncommon during the first few days following surgery. Surgical wound sites should be examined for erythema, purulence and tenderness. If infection of the wound site is suspected, the wound should be opened and Gram-stain and cultures should be performed on pus or material obtained from deep within the wound site [2]. Postoperative fever can be caused by erysipelas, myonecrosis, and toxic shock syndrome from group A Streptococci or *Staphylococcus aureus*. Fever can also be caused by crush syndrome, hematoma and tetanus in a surgical patient. Other causes of postoperative fever include deep vein thrombosis, suppurative phlebitis, pulmonary embolism and catheter-related infection.

NONINFECTIOUS CAUSES OF FEVER

Many factors predispose critically ill patients to fever of noninfectious etiology. The common noninfectious causes of fever include neoplasia, central nervous system dieases, myocardial infarction, drug and transfusion reactions and alcohol withdrawal. In one study of critically ill patients, noninfectious sources of fever were more common in patients with ARDS, and most were caused by histologically proven pulmonary fibroproliferation [13]. The noninfectious causes of fever are listed in Table 3.

Pulmonary Fibroproliferation. ARDS is a clinical and physiopathological entity characterized by acute and diffuse injury to the endothelial and epithelial surface of the lung that leads to respiratory failure. Late ARDS refers to the clinical stage of ARDS when the lung attempts to repair the initial or persistent injury to the endothelial and epithelial lining of the respiratory units. Its histological correspondent is termed "fibroproliferative phase" which, if unhalted, can progress to extensive fibrosis. Histological and laboratory data indicate that an exaggerated and persistent inflammatory response in the lungs of patients with late ARDS results in recurrent injury to the alveolo-capillary barrier and amplification of intraalveolar fibroproliferation [113]. In addition to the inability to improve lung function, progressive fibroproliferation can manifest with fever and may be clinically indistinguishable from nosocomial pneumonia [114–116]. Fibroproliferation may be the sole cause of fever in up to 25% of the episodes of fever developing in patients with late ARDS [13]. Elevation in pulmonary and systemic inflammatory cytokines plays a pathogenic role in causing fever in the absence of infection [114]. A recent randomized trial has found prolonged methylprednisolone treatment to be highly effective in reducing inflammation and improving lung function in patients with unresolved ARDS [117].

Drug Fever. The diagnosis of drug fever requires that fever coincides with the administration of a drug and disappears after discontinuation of the drug and other causes are excluded. Clinicians need to look for evidence of allergy and inflammation in organs most commonly involved in adverse drug reactions: skin rashes, liver enzyme elevations, nephritis, hemolytic anemia, and thrombocytopenia. Drugs may not cause fever until one week into treatment. Clinical findings are nonspecific with relative bradycardia (10%), rash (18%) and eosinophilia (22%) occurring infrequently [118]. Withdrawal of the suspected drug is helpful. Antibiotics, particularly β-lactams, are the medications most commonly associated with drug fever [119, 120]. Quinidine, procainamide and phenytoin are also commonly implicated [119, 120]. However, any drug can cause fever. Some medications that cause fever, such as sedatives, analgesics, and sulfa-containing stool softeners, may be overlooked [121]. The mechanisms by which drugs induce fever have not been well delineated. The fact that drug fever occurs after days of exposure to the offending agent, are dose independent, recur immediately after a provocative dose of the offending agent, and are occasionally accompanied by eosinophilia may indicate an allergic mechanism. Other proposed mechanisms of drug fever include altered thermoregulation, pharmacologic action, idiosyncratic susceptibility from a hereditary biochemical defect, pyrogenic contaminants, and administration-related reaction [122, 123]. Some of the medications associated with drug fever are listed in Table 5.

TABLE 5. Medication associated with drug fever

Frequent	
Antimicrobials	β-lactam agents, sulfonamides, vancomycin, quinine, isoniazid, pyrazinamide, rifampin, amphotericin B
Inotropes/vasoactive	Methyldopa, hydralazine, amrinone, dobutamine
Antiarrhythmic	Quinidine, procainamide, amiodarone, atropine
Antiepileptic	Phenytoin, barbiturates, phenothiazines, carbamazepine
Others	Toxic level of salicylates, cytotoxic drugs, propylthiouracil, iodides, histamine type 2 blockers, ibuprofen
Infrequent	
Antimicrobials	Aminoglycosides, chloramphenicol, macrolides, tetracycline, clindamycin, metronidazole, vitamin preparations
Inotropes/vasoactive	Digoxin, nitroprusside, nitrates, intravenous adrenergic agents
Antiarrhythmic	Lidocaine, bretylium, β-blockers
Others	Benzodiazepines, acetaminophen, opiates, corticosteroids, theophylline, inhaled bronchodilators, insulin

Malignant hyperthermia and neuroleptic malignant syndrome can cause high fever. Malignant hyperthermia is caused by medications such as succinylcholine and inhalational anesthetics. Although malignant hyperthermia is often identified in the operating room, its onset can be delayed for 24 hours. Neuroleptic malignant syndrome is associated with antipsychotic drugs such as phenothiazines, thioxanthines and butyrophenones.

Acute Pancreatitis. Pancreatitis is an inflammatory disease of the pancreas. Acute pancreatitis is characterized by an inflammatory response caused by the release of pancreatic enzymes with resultant tissue destruction and septic complications and multiple organ failure [124]. The two most common conditions associated with acute pancreatitis are ethanol use and biliary tract stones. The etiology of pancreatitis in ICU patients may be multifactorial and include trauma [125]; upper abdominal surgery [126–128]; cardiopulmonary bypass [126–129]; heart, liver, and kidney transplantation [130–132]; endoscopic retrograde cholangiopancreatography [133]; abdominal aortic aneurysm repair [134]; and drugs including thiazides, ethacrynic acid, furosemide, azathioprine, dideoxyinosine and pentamidine [135].

Although it is difficult to evaluate the critically ill, patients with acute pancreatitis may complain of abdominal pain, nausea and vomiting. Fever, leukocytosis and unexplained hemodynamic instability may be seen. Serum and urine amylase are useful for diagnosing of pancreatitis. But serum lipase is more reliable. Routine chest and abdominal radiographs may show atelectasis, pleural effusion, ileus, pancreatic calcification, gallstones, and free intraperitoneal fluid. However, these findings are nonspecific, and ultrasound or CT is needed to better visualize the pancreas and other intraabdominal structures. The local complications of pancreatitis include necrosis, pancreatic abscess, and pseudocyst, which may be infected. These complications may require percutaneous drainage and surgical debridement, in addition to antibiotics (see Chapter 46).

Other Causes. Fever associated with transfusion of red blood cells and platelets most frequently occurs in patients who have received multiple transfusions. The fever may present alone or with intravascular hemolysis and ARDS.

The rapid lysis of a large burden of tumor cells in tumor lysis syndrome and the liberation of biologically active fragments of lysed organisms in the Jarisch-Herxheimer phenomenon can be associated with fever.

Infusion of IL-2, granulocyte-macrophage colony-stimulating factor, and granulocyte colony-stimulating factor an lead to cytokine-related fever.

Penicillins, erythromycin, vancomycin, amphotericin B, potassium chloride, and certain chemotherapeutic agents can cause phlebitis associated with fever when they are peripherally administered.

APPROACH TO PATIENTS WITH FEVER IN THE ICU

In most ICUs, VAP, nosocomial sinusitis, catheter-related infection, and urinary tract infection are the leading sources of fever, followed by intraabdominal infections and pulmonary fibroproliferation in patients with ARDS [5]. Because multiple infections are a common occurrence, identifying one source of fever cannot exclude the concomitant presence of another source. The work-up of a critically ill patient with fever should start with a search for a source of infection. Recognizing the complex differential diagnosis in critically ill patients, every ICU should develop a diagnostic protocol, taking into consideration the prevalence of specific conditions and the diagnostic yield of individual tests. Although most sources of infection can be detected with a systematic approach, a number of patients will have negative results of all tests. In stable patients, we prefer withholding new antibiotic therapy while the diagnostic evaluation is in progress. However, if the patient has

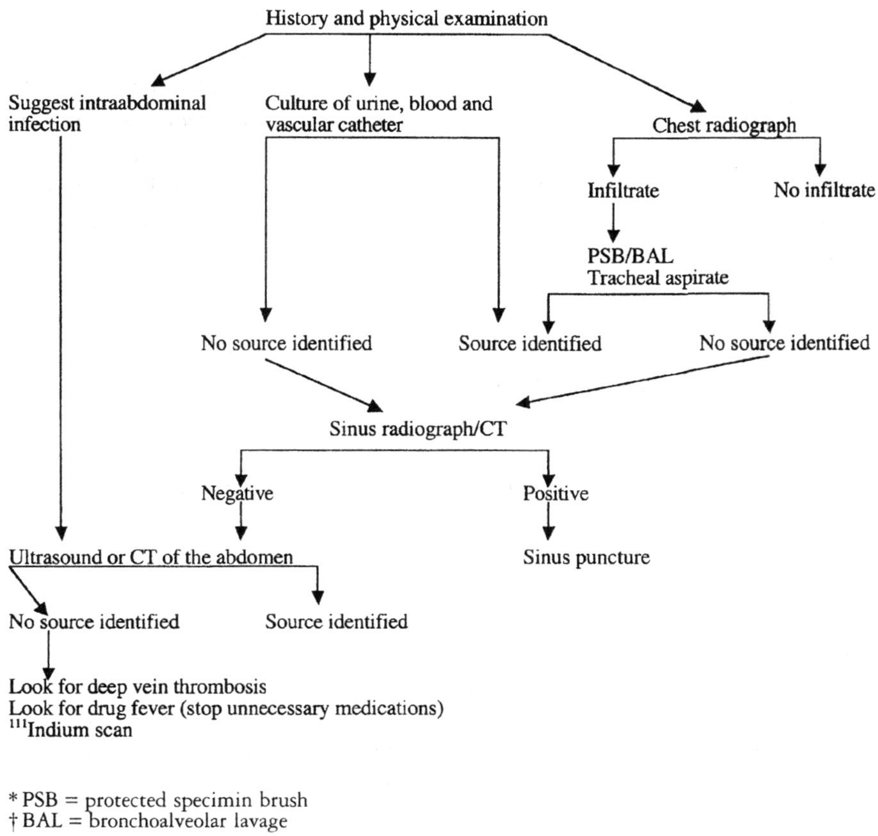

FIGURE 1. Diagnostic approach to fever in critically ill, endotracheally intubated patients.

clinical evidence of a severe infection with systemic involvement characterized by hypotension, metabolic acidosis, or worsening organ function, initiating broad-spectrum antibiotic therapy should not be delayed. Because antipyretics have the potential of decreasing host defense mechanisms and preventing the use of fever as a diagnostic aid, they should not be administered to patients unless the fever presents a threat [5].

The approach to critically ill, endotracheally intubated patients with fever is outlined in Figure 1. Investigation of a critically ill patient with fever should start with a thorough history and physical examination. During the physical examination, special attention should be paid to sites of catheter or tube insertion (i.e., chest tube, intracranial pressure monitor, central lines, urinary catheter, nasoenteric tube), and the abdomen [5]. However, physical findings are insensitive for identifying the source of infection in critically ill patients. Abdominal sources of fever and urinary tract infection are not correctly diagnosed in the majority of cases. Clinical assessment fails (most of the time) to correctly predict pulmonary fibroproliferation, empyema, catheter-related infection, or nosocomial sinusitis [13]. Pneumonia can present without the typical findings and without infiltrates on chest radiograph, especially in intravascularly volume-depleted patients. Central nervous system infection usually manifests as nuchal rigidity, headache, or impaired level of consciousness, but confusion may be the only manifestation, particularly in the elderly. Urinary tract infection can present without localizing symptoms, particularly in the elderly. Urinary tract infection presents without pyuria in diluted urine, ureteric obstruction, perinephric abscess, and prostatitis. Abnormal physical findings are almost nonexistent in mesenteric ischemia.

General

The diagnostic work-up of a critically ill patient with fever should include complete blood cell count, chest radiograph, urinalysis, urine culture and blood culture. Blood culture should be performed for ICU patients with new fever, even when clinical findings do not strongly suggest an infectious cause [2]. The site of venipuncture should be cleaned with either 10% povidone iodine or 1%–2% tincture of iodine. Because of needle-stick injury, the needle used for venipuncture need not be replaced by a sterile needle to inoculate blood into a culture tube [136]. At least 10–15 ml of blood should be drawn for each blood culture. The sensitivity of blood culture depends on the volume of blood drawn [137]. Blood culture collection systems for children should not be used for adults, because the concentration of organisms in children is higher than in adults [138].

The usefulness of antibiotic removal devices in blood culture systems is controversial. No more than three blood samples for culture need to be drawn during the initial 24 hours after onset of new fever, and in most situations two blood samples are sufficient. Each sample should be drawn by separate venipuncture [2]. Drawing two blood samples from separate venipuncture sites, 10 minutes apart, is recommended [2]. If venipuncture is difficult to perform and if there is an intravascular device in place, the second blood sample can be drawn from the device. However, in cases of discordant results, where blood drawn from the device is positive and blood drawn by venipuncture is negative, the isolate is usually considered contaminant. Additional investigation can be obtained as indicated (Table 6). Even in the absence of fever, the presence of leukocytosis, left shifted leukopenia,

TABLE 6. Suspected sites of infection and suggested diagnostic work-up

Suspected intracranial infection	CT scan of the head, lumbar puncture
Respiratory infection	Sputum or tracheal secretion for Gram stain and quantitative culture
	Bronchoscopy with PSB[1] and/or BAL[2] or (P)BAL[3]
	Ultrasound or CT scan of the chest
	Radiograph of nasal sinuses followed by needle aspiration
	Needle aspiration of pleural fluid
Wound infection	Gram stain and culture of wound drainage
Intraabdominal infection	Imaging of abdominal contents by ultrasound or CT scan
	HIDA[4] scan
	Needle aspirate of peritoneal fluid collection or abscess
Bone or joint infection	Radiograph and/or bone can, needle aspiration for Gram stain and culture of joint
Complicated urinary tract infection	Ultrasound or CT scan of kidney and perinephric space
Primary bacteremia	Semiquantitative culture of all indwelling vascular catheters
	Echocardiogram (preferably transesophageal)
General	^{67}Gallium scan, ^{111}Indium scan
	Surgical exploration

[1] PSB = protected specimen brush.
[2] BAL = bronchoalveolar lavage.
[3] (P)BAL = protected bronchoalveolar lavage.
[4] HIDA = hepatic iminodiacetic acid.

thrombocytopenia, respiratory alkalosis, hypoxemia, cholestasis, elevated transaminases, hyperglycemia and lactic acidosis calls for the work-up to identify a focus of infection.

PULMONARY

Diagnosing the cause of fever and pulmonary densities based on findings of the physical examination, laboratory tests and chest radiograph is not reliable [13, 139]. Although bedside chest radiographs are adequate in identifying clinically important abnormalities in critically ill patients, CT of the thorax may identify unsuspected sources of fever in selected patients [140]. If a patient is suspected of having lower respiratory tract infection, lower respiratory secretions should be obtained for direct examination and culture. Respiratory secretions can be obtained by expectoration, hypertonic saline induction, deep tracheal suctioning, bronchoscopic and nonbronchoscopic protected brush, or bronchoscopic or nonbronchoscopic alveolar lavage. Early microscopic identification of organisms within the alveolar cells (≥2% intracellular organisms) recovered by bronchoalveolar lavage is helpful in establishing the presence of pneumonia, and the Gram stain is helpful in selecting antimicrobial therapy. Pulmonary secretions should be transported to the laboratory and processed within two hours of collection so that any fastidious organisms, such as *Streptococcus pneumoniae* do not die. A Gram stain should be performed in most situations. In appropriate circumstances, direct tests such as potassium hydroxide wet mount for detecting fungi, enzyme immunoassay (EIA) for influenza A virus, an acid fast stain for mycobacteria, a fluorescent antibody stain for *Legionella*, or an immunofluorescent stain for *Pneumocystis carinii* should be performed. Pleural fluid should be obtained for Gram stain and routine culture if there is an adjacent infiltrate or another reason to suspect infection and the fluid can be safely aspirated. Blood should be obtained for culture in patients with suspected pneumonia. Although blood culture has low yield, the isolation of a respiratory pathogen is highly specific for diagnosing bacterial pneumonia. Pulmonary fibroproliferation as a cause of fever remains a diagnosis of exclusion, after ruling out pneumonia and extrapulmonary sources of infection. Methods to diagnose or exclude pulmonary fibroproliferation as a cause of worsening respiratory failure have included gallium (^{67}Ga) scintigraphy, open-lung biopsy, and laboratory markers of inflammation and fibrosis [141]. The inability to improve gas exchange and lung mechanics by day seven of ARDS reflects progression of fibroproliferation, and in most patients with late ARDS, no test is necessary to confirm the diagnosis. Other frequent causes of radiographic densities in critically ill patients are atelectasis and congestive heart failure, which clear within 24 to 48 hours of adequate treatment.

PARANASAL SINUSES

Plain radiographs, ultrasound, CT scans, and MRI scans are used to diagnose acute sinusitis. Nasal endoscopy can also be helpful in making the diagnosis [142]. Although CT provides the best visualization of the paranasal sinuses, a portable sinus radiograph series may be sufficient in unstable patients. Mucosal thickening, opacification, or air-fluid levels suggest the presence of infection. In one study of 35 CT scans of the sinuses, 33 (94%) were abnormal, and six of these (18%) showed pansinusitis [13]. Because radiographic abnormalities do not always represent infection, microbiologic diagnosis is established with direct aspiration and culture of material from the maxillary sinus. Positive cultures are found in up to 70% of aspirates [13]. Using a nasal disinfection protocol before aspiration and a diagnostic threshold of 10^3 CFU/ml to diagnose infection, one study found positive cultures in 38% of cases [73]. Bacteremia with identical organisms occurs in 17% to 25% of patients with nosocomial sinusitis [13, 73]. Maxillary sinus puncture is not only diagnostic but therapeutic in allowing drainage of infected material. If the patient does not show signs of improvement within 48 hours, more aggressive measures should be taken. In some cases, surgical drainage in the operating room may be required [79]. Because nosocomial sinusitis is a common occurrence, it is advisable to replace nasoenteric tubes orally and to apply decongestants if the diagnostic evaluation is delayed.

INTRAVASCULAR CATHETERS

If catheter-related infection is suspected, evidence of inflammation or purulence at the site of catheter insertion, along the tunnel, connector sites, and ports of infusate should be sought.

URINARY TRACT

When urinary tract infection is suspected, urine should be obtained for direct microscopy, Gram stain and quantitative culture. The urine should not be collected from the drainage bag, because bacteria may multiply in the bag. The catheter should be clamped and urine aspirated from the port. For patients without a bladder catheter, a midstream clean-catch urine specimen should be collected. The collected urine should be transferred to the laboratory rapidly or refrigerated.

ABDOMEN

A patient with clinically septic picture but no obvious source of infection occurs frequently in the ICU. Pneumonia, urosepsis, blood stream infection, and line sepsis can often be ruled out. Attention should then focus on the abdomen, even if the patient has no known preexisting gastrointestinal pathologic condition. Plain abdominal radiograph may detect ileus, megacolon, peritoneal fluid, and free peritoneal air. To identify a focal intraabdominal infection or abscess, ultrasonography and CT are required. CT and ultrasonography are both good screening tests for patients with suspected intraabdominal sepsis. Ultrasonography can be done at the bedside and is most valuable in assessing the liver, perihepatic area, and biliary system [143]. CT can also evaluate these areas and are of greater value in detecting intraabdominal abscesses [144] with a specificity of over 90% [84]. One study reported abdominal CT findings to significantly modify management in 55% of patients and to be misleading in only 9% [145]. However, abscesses may be missed if the bowel is not adequately opacified with contrast or if the abscess is too small to be seen on CT [88]. Because abdominal ultrasound can be done at the bedside, this is perhaps the best initial diagnostic test. Sensitivity of ultrasound is reported to be 67% to 92% with specificity of >90% [146, 147]. If the initial study is negative and the clinical suspicion remains high, sensitivity may be enhanced by serial exams detecting progressive dilatation of the gallbladder and increasing edema of its wall [148, 149]. CT scanning, although not as convenient, may have sensitivity and specificity exceeding 95% and has the additional advantage of detecting pathology present elsewhere in the abdomen [93].

A negative CT scan or ultrasound does not rule out intraabdominal infection. Diagnostic peritoneal lavage is another potentially useful test [150, 151]. Finding pus, bacteria, and elevated leukocyte count in diagnostic peritoneal lavage fluid indicates intraabdominal infection. ^{99}mTc hepatic iminodiacetic acid (HIDA) scan, useful in cases where gallstones are present, have an unacceptably high false-positive rate in acalculous cholecystitis, especially in patients not receiving enteral nutrition [146]. Diagnostic laparoscopy has recently been reported to be safe and definitive in diagnosing acalculous cholecystitis but is not yet widely used [152].

Ascitic fluid should be sampled and cultured. Mesenteric ischemia can be diagnosed by CT, but angiography is the preferred study. Angiography has little value in the diagnosis of ischemic colitis where the optimal investigation is colonoscopy [153].

In critically ill patients with fever and diarrhea, a stool should be tested for *C. difficile*. Because other causes are unlikely in immunocompetent patients, sending stools for bacterial cultures or for ova and parasites is not needed. Although most patients with *C. difficile* colitis present with diarrhea, some patients may present with ileus or toxic megacolon. Endoscopy or CT may reveal colitis. The gold standard for the diagnosis is tissue culture assay for *C. difficile*. EIA provides the answer within 2–3 hours, but sensitivity is 72% on the first and 84% on the second sample compared to 81% and 91%, respectively, for tissue culture toxin assay. Fecal leukocyte examination is sensitive but nonspecific. Cultures for *C. difficile* are technically difficult and require 2–3 days for growth. Although endoscopic visualization may identify the pseudomembranes, it is rarely needed because of its cost and risk of perforation. When all attempts fail to identify the source of sepsis, laparotomy may be needed. However, laparotomy in the absence of localizing clinical and laboratory findings does not improve patient outcome [154].

Conclusion

Because no single test has a high diagnostic yield for most common infections and fever is frequently multifactorial in origin, combinations of tests are often needed in a critically ill patient with fever. The combination of bronchoscopy with protected specimen brush, and/or bronchoalveolar lavage or protected bronchoalveolar lavage, CT scan of the sinuses and maxillary sinus aspirate, cultures of central venous and arterial catheters, urine and blood has a diagnostic yield of 74% in critically ill patients [13]. At times, testing for pneumonia, sinusitis, catheter-related infection and urinary tract infection may have negative results. If no localizing signs are found in such patients, ^{67}Gallium-citrate and ^{111}Indium-labeled leukocyte scintography can be used to identify the sites of inflammation [155, 156]. Radionuclide studies such as ^{67}Ga and ^{111}In-labeled white blood cells are sensitive but not specific and have the further disadvantage of a 24- to 48-hour delay in obtaining results [157]. The greatest strength of these imaging modalities is that the whole body is evaluated, and unexpected sources of fever may be detected in up to 16% of patients [158]. Taken together, CT, ultrasound, and radionuclide studies will diagnose abscesses in greater than 90% of patients [153], and a stepwise approach to their use has been proposed [158]. Although it will not help identify the focus of infection, elevated serum C-reactive protein may correlate with the presence of sepsis [159].

Initially, the combination of tests used in the diagnostic work-up of critically ill patients with fever may be more expensive than empiric, broad-spectrum antibiotic coverage alone. The overall cost of care of patients treated empirically, however, could escalate because of monitoring drug levels, complications of inappropriate antibiotic therapy (bacterial superinfections, fungemia, antibiotic toxicity, etc.), or failure to treat unrecognized serious processes correctly and promptly. Because this assumption has not been evaluated prospectively, it remains an area of controversy [160]. However, until proven otherwise, management of critically ill patients should not be exempted from the rule of knowing what we are treating.

We thank Ms Gail Spake and Dr David Armbruster for reviewing and editing the chapter.

References

1. Dinarello CA, Cannon JG, Wolff SM. New concepts on the pathogenesis of fever. Rev Infect Dis 10:168, 1988.
2. O'Grady NP, Barie PS, Bartlett JG, Bleck T, Garvey G, *et al*. Practice guidelines for evaluating new fever in critically ill adult patients. Task Force of the Society of Critical Care Medicine and the Infectious Diseases Society of America. Clin Infect Dis 26:1042, 1998.
3. Erickson RS, Kirklin SK. Comparison of ear-based, bladder, oral, and axillary methods for core temperature measurement. Crit Care Med 21:1528, 1993.
4. Kluger MJ, Kozak W, Conn CA, Leon LR, Soszynski D. The adaptive value of fever. Infect Dis Clin North Am 10:1, 1996.
5. Cunha BA. Fever in the intensive care unit [editorial]. Intensive Care Med 25:648, 1999.
6. Circiumaru B, Baldock G, Cohen J. A prospective study of fever in the intensive care unit. Intensive Care Med 25:668, 1999.

7. Edgeworth JD, Treacher DF, Eykyn SJ. A 25-year study of nosocomial bacteremia in an adult intensive care unit. Crit Care Med 27:1421, 1999.
8. Sands KE, Bates DW, Lanken PN, Graman PS, Hibberd PL, *et al.* Epidemiology of sepsis syndrome in 8 academic medical centers. Academic Medical Center Consortium Sepsis Project Working Group. JAMA 278:234, 1997.
9. Edmond MB, Wallace SE, McClish DK, Pfaller MA, Jones RN, Wenzel RP. Nosocomial bloodstream infections in United States hospitals: a three-year analysis. Clin Infect Dis 29:239, 1999.
10. Richards MJ, Edwards JR, Culver DH, Gaynes RP. Nosocomial infections in medical intensive care units in the United States. National Nosocomial Infections Surveillance System. Crit Care Med 27:887, 1999.
11. Vincent JL, Bihari DJ, Suter PM, Bruining HA, White J, *et al.* The prevalence of nosocomial infection in intensive care units in Europe. Results of the European Prevalence of Infection in Intensive Care (EPIC) Study. EPIC International Advisory Committee. JAMA 274:639, 1995.
12. Legras A, Malvy D, Quinioux AI, Villers D, Bouachour G, *et al.* Nosocomial infections: prospective survey of incidence in five French intensive care units. Intensive Care Med 24:1040, 1998.
13. Meduri GU, Mauldin GL, Wunderink RG, Leeper KV, Jones CB, *et al.* Causes of fever and pulmonary densities in patients with clinical manifestations of ventilator-associated pneumonia. Chest 106:221, 1994.
14. Craven DE, Steger KA. Epidemiology of nosocomial pneumonia. New perspectives on an old disease. Chest 108(2 Suppl):1S, 1995.
15. Torres A, Aznar R, Gatell JM, Jimenez P, Bonzalez J, *et al.* Incidence, risk, and prognosis factors of nosocomial pneumonia in mechanically ventilated patients. Am Rev Resp Dis 142:523, 1990.
16. George DL, Falk PS, Wunderink RG, Leeper KV Jr, Meduri GU, *et al.* Epidemiology of ventilator-acquired pneumonia based on protected bronchoscopic sampling. Am J Respir Crit Care Med 158:1839, 1998.
17. American Thoracic Society. Hospital-acquired pneumonia in adults: diagnosis, assessment of severity, initial antimicrobial theraphy, and preventive strategies. A consensus statement, American Thoracic Society, November 1995. Am J Respir Crit Care Med 153:1711, 1996.
18. Marik PE, Careau P. The role of anaerobes in patients with ventilator-associated pneumonia and aspiration pneumonia: a prospective study. Chest 115:178, 1999.
19. Baughman RP, Thorpe JE, Staneck J, Rashkin M, Frame PT. Use of the protected specimen brush in patients with endotracheal or tracheostomy tubes. Chest 91:233, 1987.
20. Rodriguez de Castro F, Sole-Violan J, Lafarga Capuz B, Caminero-Luna J, Gonzalez-Rodriguez B, *et al.* Reliability of the bronchoscopic protected catheter brush in the diagnosis of pneumonia in mechanically ventilated patients. Crit Care Med 19:171, 1991.
21. Fagon JY, Chastre J, Hance AJ, Guiguet M, Trouillet JL, *et al.* Detection of nosocomial lung infection in ventilated patients: use of a protected specimen brush and quantitative culture techniques in 147 patients. Am Rev Resp Dis 138:110, 1988.
22. Bryant LR, Mobin-Uddin K, Dillon ML, Griffen WO. Misdiagnosis of pneumonia in patients needing mechanical respiration. Arch Surg 106:286, 1973.
23. Joshi JH, Wang KP, de Jongh CA, Newman KA, Wiernik PH, Schimpff SC. A comparative evaluation of two fiberoptic bronchoscopy catheters: the plugged telescoping catheter versus the single sheathed nonplugged catheter. Am Rev Resp Dis 126:860, 1982.
24. Torres A, Puig Bellacasa JP, Rodriquez-Roisin R, Jimenez De Anta MT, Agusti-Vidal A. Diagnostic value of telescoping plugged catheters in mechanically ventilated patients with bacterial pneumonia using the Metras catheter. Am Rev Resp Dis 138:117, 1988.
25. Meduri GU, Wunderink RG, Leeper KV, Beals DH. Management of bacterial pneumonia in ventilated patients. The role of protected bronchoalveolar lavage. Chest 101:500, 1992.
26. Wunderink RG, Woldenberg LS, Zeiss J, Day CM, Ciemons J, Lacher DA. Radiologic diagnosis of autopsy-proven ventilator-associated pneumonia. Chest 101:458, 1992.
27. Winer-Muram HT, Rubin SA, Ellis JV, Jennings SG, Arheart KL, *et al.* Pneumonia and ARDS in patients receiving mechanical ventilation: diagnostic accuracy of chest radiography. Thoracic Radiology 188:479, 1993.

28. Santos E, Talusan A, Brandstetter RD. Roentgenographic mimics of pneumonia in the critical care unit. Crit Care Clin 14:91, 1998.
29. Niederman MS, Torres A, Summer W. Invasive diagnostic testing is not needed routinely to manage suspected ventilator-associated pneumonia. Am J Respir Crit Care Med 150:565, 1994.
30. Chastre J, Fagon JY. Invasive diagnostic testing should be routinely used to manage ventilated patients with suspected pneumonia. Am J Respir Crit Care Med 150:570, 1994.
31. Fagon JY, Chastre J, Wolff M, Gervais C, Parer-Aubas S, Stephan F, Similowski T, Mercat A, Diew JL, Sollet JP, Tenaillon A. Invasive and noninvasive strategies for management of suspected ventitator-associated pneumonia. A randomized trial. Am Intern Med 132(8):621–630, 2000.
32. Craven DE, Kunches LM, Lichtenberg DA, Kollisch NR, Barry MA, Heeren TC, McCabe WR. Nosocomial infection and fatality in medical and surgical intensive care unit patients. Arch Intern Med 148:1161, 1988.
33. Bryan CS, Reynolds KL. Hospital acquired bacteremic urinary tract infections: epidemiology and outcome. J Urol 132:494, 1984.
34. Platt R, Polk BF, Murdock B, Rosner B. Mortality associated with nosocomial urinary-tract infection. N Engl J Med 307:637, 1982.
35. Warren JW. Nosocomial urinary tract infections. In Mandell GL, Douglas RG, Bennet JE (eds). Principles and Practice of Infectious Diseases. 3 edn, New York: Churchill Livingstone, 1990:2205.
36. Lipsky BA. Urinary tract infections in men. Epidemiology, pathophysiology, diagnosis, and treatment. Ann Intern Med 110:138, 1989.
37. Seiler WO, Stahelin HB. Practical management of catheter-associated UTIs. Geriatrics 43:43, 1988.
38. Shapiro M, Simchen E, Izraeli S, Sacks TG. A multivariate analysis of risk factors for acquiring bacteriuria in patients with indwelling urinary catheters for longer than 24 hours. Infect Cont 5:525, 1984.
39. Haley RW, Hooton TM, Culver DH, Stanley RC, Emori TG, Hardison CD, Quade D, Shachtman RH, Schaberg DR, Shah BV, Schatz GD. Nosocomial infections in US hospitals 1975–1976: estimated frequency by selected characteristics of patients. Am J Med 70:947, 1981.
40. Bromberg K, Gleich S, Ginsberg MB. Clostridia in urinary tract infections. South Med J 75:1298, 1981.
41. Aguado JM, Ponte C, Soriano F. Bacteriuria with a multiply resistant species of Corynebacterium (Corynebacterium group D2): an unnoticed cause of urinary tract infection. J Infect Dis 156:144, 1987.
42. Bergquist D, Bronnestam R, Hedelin H, Stahl A. The relevance of urinary sampling methods in patients with indwelling Foley catheters. Br J Urol 52:92, 1980.
43. Stark RP, Maki DG. Bacteriuria in the catheterized patient: what quantitative level of bacteriuria is relevant. N Engl J Med 311:560, 1984.
44. Michaeli J, Mogle P, Perlberg S, Heiman S, Caine M. Emphysematous pyelonephritis. J Urol 131:203, 1984.
45. Lees JA, Falk RM, Stone WJ, McDougal WS. Pyocystis, pyonephrosis and perinephric abscess in end stage renal disease. J Urol 134:716, 1985.
46. Mermel LA, McCormick RD, Springman SR, Maki DG. The pathogenesis and epidemiology of catheter-related infection with pulmonary artery Swan-Ganz catheters: a prospective study utilizing molecular subtyping. Am J Med 91:197S, 1991.
47. Bjornson HS, Colley R, Bower RH, Duty VP, Schwartz-Fulton JT, Fischer JE. Association between microorganism growth at the catheter insertion site and colonization of the catheter in patients receiving total parenteral nutrition. Surgery 92:720, 1982.
48. Kruse JA, Shah NJ. Detection and prevention of central venous catheter-related infections. Nutr Clin Pract 8:163, 1993.
49. Fry DE, Fry RV, Borzotta AP. Nosocomial blood-borne infection secondary to intravascular devices. Am J Surg 167:268, 1994.
50. Corona ML, Peters SG, Narr BJ, Thompson RL. Infections related to central venous catheters. Mayo Clin Proc 65:979, 1990.
51. Peters G, Loui R, Pulverer G. Adherence and growth of coagulase-negative staphylococci on surfaces on intravenous catheters. J Infect Dis 146:479, 1982.
52. Moro ML, Vigano EF, Cozzi LA. Risk factors for central venous catheter-related infections in surgical and intensive care units. The Central Venous Catheter-Related Infections Study Group. Infect Control Hosp Epidemiol 15:253, 1994.

53. Eyer S, Brummitt C, Crossley K, Siegel R, Cerra F. Catheter-related sepsis: prospective, randomized study of three methods of long-term catheter maintenance. Crit Care Med 18:1073, 1990.
54. Arnow PM, Quimosing EM, Beach M. Consequences of intravascular catheter sepsis. Clin Infect Dis 16:778, 1993.
55. Garrison RN, Wilson MA. Intravenous and central catheter infections. Surg Clin North Am 74:557, 1994.
56. Maki DG, Ringer M, Alvarado CJ. Prospective randomized trial of povidone-iodine, alcohol, and chlorhexidine for prevention of infection associated with central venous and arterial catheters. Lancet 338:339, 1991.
57. Craven DE, Lichtenberg DA, Kunches LM, McDonough AT, Gonzalez MI, *et al.* A randomized study comparing a transparent polyurethane dressing to a dry gauze dressing for peripheral intravenous catheter sites. Infect Control 6:361, 1985.
58. Maki DG, Ringer M. Evaluation of dressing regimens for prevention of infection with peripheral intravenous catheters. Gauze, a transparent polyurethane dressing, and an iodophor-transparent dressing. JAMA 258:2396, 1987.
59. Thomas F, Burke JP, Parker J, Orme JF Jr, Gardner RM, *et al.* The risk of infection related to radial vs femoral sites for arterial catheterization. Crit Care Med 11:807, 1983.
60. Raad I, Umphrey J, Khan A, Truett LJ, Bodey GP. The duration of placement as a predictor of peripheral and pulmonary arterial catheter infections. J Hosp Infect 23:17, 1993.
61. Peters G, Locci R, Pulverer G. Adherence and growth of coagulase-negative staphylococci on surfaces of intravenous catheters. J Infect Dis 146:479, 1982.
62. Pettigrew RA, Lang SD, Haydock DA, Parry BR, Bremner DA, Hill GL. Catheter-related sepsis in patients on intravenous nutrition: a prospective study of quantitative catheter cultures and guide-wire changes for suspected sepsis. Br J Surg 72:52, 1985.
63. Liñares J, Sitges-Serra A, Garau J, Perez JL, Martin R. Pathogenesis of catheter sepsis: a prospective study with quantitative and semiquantitative cultures of catheter hub and segments. J Clin Microbiol 21:357, 1985.
64. Maki DG, Weise CE, Sarafin HW. A semi-quantitative culture method for identifying intravenous catheter-related infection. N Engl J Med 296:1305, 1977.
65. Garner JS, Jarvis WR, Emori TG, Horan TC, Hughes JM. CDC definitions for nosocomial infections. Am J Infect Control 16:128, 1988.
66. Reimer LG. Catheter-related infections and blood cultures. Clin Lab Med 14:51, 1994.
67. Ascher DP, Shoupe BA, Robb M, Maybee DA, Fischer GW. Comparison of standard and quantitative blood cultures in the evaluation of children with suspected central venous line sepsis. Diagn Microbiol Infect Dis 15:499, 1992.
68. Wessler D, Civetta JM. Preventive Care. In Civetta JM, Taylor RW, Kirby RR (eds). Critical Care. 2 edn, Philadelphia: J. B. Lippincott Company, 1992: 1753.
69. White JA. Paranasal Sinus Infections. In Ballenger JJ (ed). Diseases of the Nose, Throat, Ear, Head, and Neck. 14 edn, Philadelphia: Lea & Febiger, 1991: 184.
70. Pittet D, Herwaldt LA, Massanari RM. The Intensive Care Unit. In Bennett JV, Brachman PS (eds). Hospital Infections. 3 edn, Boston: Little, Brown and Company, 1992: 421.
71. Kaplan RJ. Neurological complications of infections of the head and neck. Otolaryngol Clin N Am 9:729, 1976.
72. George DL, Falk PS, Meduri GU, Leeper KV Jr, Wunderink RG, Steere EL, *et al.* Nosocomial sinusitis in patients in the medical intensive care unit: a prospective epidemiological study. Clin Infect Dis 27:463, 1998.
73. Holzapfel L, Chevret S, Madinier G, Ohen F, Demingeon G, *et al.* Influence of long-term oro- or nasotracheal intubation on nosocomial maxillary sinusitis and pneumonia: results of a prospective, randomized, clinical trial. Crit Care Med 21:1132, 1993.
74. Rouby JJ, Laurent P, Gosnach M, Cambau E, Lamas G, *et al.* Risk factors and clinical relevance of nosocomial maxillary sinusitis in the critically ill. Am J Respir Crit Care Med 150:776, 1994.
75. Holzapfel L, Chastang C, Demingeon G, Bohe J, Piralla B, Coupry A. A randomized study assessing the systematic search for maxillary sinusitis in nasotracheally mechanically ventilated patients. Influence of nosocomial maxillary sinusitis on the occurrence of ventilator-associated pneumonia. Am J Respir Crit Care Med 159:695, 1999.
76. Chow AW. Life-threatening Infections of the Head, Neck, and Upper Respiratory Tract. In

Hall JB, Schmidt GA, Wood LDH (eds). Principles of Critical Care. New York: McGraw-Hill, 1992: 1309.
77. Aust R, Drettner B. The patency of the maxillary ostium in relation to body posture. Acta Otolaryngol 80:443, 1975.
78. Michelson A, Schuster B, Kamp HD. Paranasal sinusitis associated with nasotracheal and orotracheal long-term intubation. Arch Otolaryngol Head Neck Surg 118:937, 1992.
79. Seiden AM. Sinusitis in the critical care patient. New Horiz 261:261, 1993.
80. Caplan ES, Hoyt NJ. Nosocomial sinusitis. JAMA 247:639, 1982.
81. Perlman DM, Caplan ES. Nosocomial sinusitis: a new and complex threat. J Crit Illness 2:19, 1987.
82. Ramadan HH, Owens RM, Tiu C, Wax MK. Role of antral puncture in the treatment of sinusitis in the intensive care unit. Otolaryngol Head Neck Surg 119:381, 1998.
83. Kountakis SE, Burke L, Rafie JJ, Bassichis B, Maillard AA, Stiernberg CM. Sinusitis in the intensive care unit patient. Otolaryngol Head Neck Surg 117:362, 1997.
84. Norwood S, Hajjar GB, Younkin SW. Diagnosis and Management of Intraabdominal Sepsis. In Rippe JM, Irwin RS, Alpert JS, Fink MP (eds). Intensive Care Medicine, 2 edn. Boston: Little Brown, 1991: 1315.
85. Seidenfeld JJ, Pohl DF, Bell RC, Harris GD, Johanson WGJ. Incidence, site, and outcome of infections in patients with the adult respiratory distress syndrome. Am Rev Resp Dis 134:12, 1986.
86. Pitcher WD, Musher DM. Critical importance of early diagnosis and treatment of intra-abdominal infection. Arch Surg 117:328, 1982.
87. Fry DE, Garrison RN, Heitsch RC, Calhoun K, Polk HC. Determinants of death in patients with intraabdominal abscess. Surgery 88:517, 1980.
88. Mustard RA, Bohnen JMA, Schouten BD. The Acute Abdomen and Intraabdominal Sepsis. In Hall JB, Schmidt GA, Wood LDH (eds). Principles of Critical Care. New York: McGraw-Hill, 1992: 990.
89. Zingas AP. Computed tomography of the abdomen in the critically ill. Crit Care Clin 10:321, 1994.
90. Bartlett JG. *Clostridium difficile*: history of its role as an enteric pathogen and the current state of knowledge about the organism. Clin Infect Dis 18(Suppl 4):S265, 1994.
91. Runyon BA, Hoefs JC. Culture-negative neutrocytic ascites: a variant of spontaneous bacterial peritonitis. Hepatology 4:1209, 1984.
92. Runyon BA, Umland ET, Merlin T. Inoculation of blood culture bottles with ascitic fluid. Improved detection of spontaneous bacterial peritonitis. Arch Intern Med 147:73, 1987.
93. Bilhartz LE. Acute acalculous cholecystitis, adenomyomatosis, cholesterolosis, and polyps of the gallbladder. In Gastrointestinal Disease. Pathophysiology/Diagnosis/Management. 5 edn. Philadelphia: W. B. Saunders Company, 1993: 1858.
94. Cornwell EE, Rodriguez A, Mirvis SE, Shorr RM. Acute acalculous cholecystitis in critically injured patients. Ann Surg 210:52, 1989.
95. Johnson EE, Hedley-White J. Continuous positive pressure ventilation and portal flow in dogs with edema. J Appl Physiol 33:385, 1972.
96. Johnson EE, Hedley-White J. Continuous positive pressure ventilation and choledochoduodenal flow resistance. J Appl Physiol 39:937, 1975.
97. Savino JA, Scalea TM, Del Guercio LRM. Factors encouraging laparotomy in acalculous cholecystitis. Crit Care Med 13:377, 1985.
98. Johnson LB. The importance of early diagnosis of acute acalculous cholecystitis. Surgery, Gynecology Obstetrics 164:197, 1987.
99. Eggermont AM, Lameris JS, Jeekel J. Ultrasound-guided percutaneous transhepatic cholecystostomy for acute acalculous cholecystitis. Arch Surg 120:1354, 1985.
100. Long TN, Heimbach DM, Carrico CJ. Acalculous cholecystitis in critically ill patients. Am J Surg 136:31, 1978.
101. Reily CA, Dean PJ, Park AL, Levinson MJ. A distinct syndrome of liver disease with multisystem organ failure associated with bile ductular cholestatis. Hepatology 10:739, 1989.
102. Flancbaum L, Alden SM, Trooskin SZ. Use of cholescintigraphy with morphine in critically ill patients with suspected cholecystitis. Surgery 106:668, 1989.
103. Shirai Y, Tsukada K, Kawaguchi H, Ontani T, Muto T, *et al.* Percutaneous transhepatic cholecystostomy for acute acalculous cholecystitis. Br J Surg 80:1440, 1993.
104. McGahan JP, Lindfors KK. Percutaneous cholecystostomy: an alternative to surgical cholecystostomy for acute cholecystitis? Radiology 173:481, 1989.

105. Johlin FC Jr, Neil GA. Drainage of the gallbladder in patients with acute acalculous cholecystitis by transpapillary endoscopic cholecystotomy. Gastrointest Endosc 39:645, 1993.
106. Flancbaum L, Majerus TC, Cox EF. Acute posttraumatic acalculous cholecystitis. Am J Surg 150:252, 1985.
107. Bleck TP, Smith MC, Pierre-Louis SJ, Jares JJ, Murray J, Hansen CA. Neurologic complications of critical medical illnesses. Crit Care Med 21:98, 1993.
108. Schliamser SE, Backman K, Norrby SR. Intracranial abscesses in adults: an analysis of 54 consecutive cases. Scand J Infect Dis 20:1, 1988.
109. Adelson-Mitty J, Fink MP, Lisbon A. The value of lumbar puncture in the evaluation of critically ill, non-immunosuppressed, surgical patients: a retrospective analysis of 70 cases. Intensive Care Med 23:749, 1997.
110. Garibaldi RA, Brodine S, Matsumiya S, Coleman M. Evidence for the non-infectious etiology of early postoperative fever. Infect Control 6:273, 1985.
111. Freisschlag J, Busuttil RW. The value of postoperative fever evaluation. Surgery 94:358, 1983.
112. Galicier C, Richet H. A prospective study of postoperative fever in a general surgery department. Infection Control 6:487, 1985.
113. Meduri GU, Headley S, Kohler G, Stentz F, Tolley E, *et al.* Persistent elevation of inflammatory cytokines predicts a poor outcome in ARDS. Plasma IL-1β and IL-6 levels are consistent and efficient predictors of outcome over time. Chest 107:1062, 1995.
114. Meduri GU, Belenchia JM, Estes RJ, Wunderink RG, ElTorky M, Leeper KV. Fibroproliferative phase of ARDS: Clinical findings and effects of corticosteroids. Chest 100:943, 1991.
115. Andrews CP, Coalson JJ, Smith JD, Johanson WG Jr. Diagnosis of nosocomial bacterial pneumonia in acute, diffuse lung injury. Chest 80:254, 1981.
116. Ashbaugh DG, Maier RV. Idiopathic pulmonary fibrosis in adult respiratory distress syndrome. Arch Surg 120:530, 1985.
117. Meduri GU, Headley AS, Golden E, Carson SJ, Umberger RA, *et al.* Effect of prolonged methylprednisolone therapy in unresolving acute respiratory distress syndrome: a randomized controlled trial. JAMA 280:159, 1998.
118. Mackowiak PA, LeMaistre CF. Drug fever: a critical appraisal of conventional concepts. Ann Intern Med 106:728, 1987.
119. Oizumi K, Onuma K, Watanabe A, Motomiya M. Clinical study of drug fever induced by parenteral administration of antibiotics. Tohoku J Exp Med 159:45, 1989.
120. Mackowiak PA, LeMaistre CF. Drug fever: a critical appraisal of conventional concepts. An analysis of 51 episodes in two Dallas hospitals and 97 episodes reported in the English literature. Ann Intern Med 106:728, 1987.
121. Johnson DH, Cunha BA. Drug fever. Infect Dis Clin North Am 10:85, 1996.
122. Lipsky BA, Hirschmann JV. Drug fever. JAMA 245:851, 1981.
123. Mackowiak PA. Drug fever: mechanisms, maxims and misconceptions. Am J Med Sci 294:275, 1987.
124. Keynes M. Heretical thoughts on the pathogenesis of acute pancreatitis. Gut 29:1413, 1988.
125. Wilson RH, Moorehead RJ. Current management of trauma to the pancreas. Br J Surg 78:1196, 1991.
126. Bardenheier JA, Kaminski DL, Willman VL. Pancreatitis after biliary tract surgery. Am J Surg 116:773, 1968.
127. Peterson LM, Collins JJ Jr, Wilson RE. Acute pancreatitis occurring after operation. Surg Gynecol Obstet 127:23, 1968.
128. White MT, Morgan A, Hopton D. Postoperative pancreatitis. A study of seventy cases. Am J Surg 120:132, 1970.
129. Rosenbaum RC, Frieri M, Metcalfe DD. Patterns of skeletal scintigraphy and their relationship to plasma and urinary histamine levels in systemic mastocytosis. J Nucl Med 25:859, 1984.
130. Adiseshiah M, Wells FC, Cory-Pearce R, Wallwork J, English TA. Acute pancreatitis after cardiac transplantation. World J Surg 7:519, 1983.
131. Alexander JA, Demetrius AJ, Gavaler JS, Makowka L, Starzl TE, *et al.* Pancreatitis following liver transplantation. Transplantation 45:1062, 1988.
132. Frick TW, Fryd DS, Sutherland DE, Goodale RL, Simmons RL, Najarian JS. Hypercalcemia associated with pancreatitis and hyperamylasemia in renal transplant recipients. Data

from the Minnesota randomized trial of cyclosporine versus antilymphoblast azathioprine. Am J Surg 154:487, 1987.
133. Cotton PB. ERCP. Gut 18:316, 1977.
134. Victor DW Jr, Rayburn JL, McCready RA, Hyde GL. Pancreatitis following aneurysmectomy. J Ky Med Assoc 86:285, 1988.
135. Greenberger NJ, Toskes PP, Isselbacher KJ. Acute and chronic pancreatitis. In Fauci AS, Braunwald E, Isselbacher KJ, Wilson JD, Martin JB, Kasper DL, Hauser SL, Lago DL (eds). Harrison's Principles of Internal Medicine. 14th edn, New York: McGraw Hill, 1998: 1741.
136. Leisure MK, Moore DM, Schwartzman JD, Hayden GF, Donowitz LG. Changing the needle when inoculating blood cultures. A no-benefit and high-risk procedure. JAMA 264:2111, 1990.
137. Ilstrup DM, Washington JAD. The importance of volume of blood cultured in the detection of bacteremia and fungemia. Diagn Microbiol Infect Dis 1:107, 1983.
138. Mermel LA, Maki DG. Detection of bacteremia in adults: consequences of culturing an inadequate volume of blood. Ann Intern Med 119:270, 1993.
139. Fagon JY, Chastre J, Hance AJ, Domart Y, Trouillet JL, Gibert C. Evaluation of clinical judgment in the identification and treatment of nosocomial pneumonia in ventilated patients. Chest 103:547, 1993.
140. Miller WT Jr, Tino G, Friedburg JS. Thoracic CT in the intensive care unit: assessment of clinical usefulness. Radiology 209:491, 1998.
141. Meduri GU. Fever in late ARDS. Etiology, pathophysiology, and diagnostic evaluation. Seminars in Respiratory Medicine 15:308, 1994.
142. Roberts DN, Hampal S, East CA, Lloyd GA. The diagnosis of inflammatory sinonasal disease. J Laryngol Otol 109:27, 1995.
143. Marton KI, Doubilet P. How to image the gallbladder in suspected cholecystitis. Ann Intern Med 109:722, 1988.
144. Lundstedt C, Hederstrom E, Brismar J, Holmin T, Strand SE. Prospective investigation of radiologic methods in the diagnosis of intra-abdominal abscesses. Acta Radio 27:49, 1986.
145. Roche J. Effectiveness of computed tomography in the diagnosis of intra-abdominal abscesses. Med J Aust 25:85, 1981.
146. Mirvis SE, Vainright JR, Nelson AW, Johnston GS, Shorr R, *et al.* The diagnosis of acute acalculous cholecystitis: a comparison of sonography, scintigraphy and CT. Am J Roentgenology 147:1171, 1986.
147. Shuman WP, Rogers JV, Rudd TG, Mack LA, Plumley T, Larson EB. Low sensitivity of sonography and cholescintigraphy in acalculous cholecystitis. Am J Roentgenology 142:531, 1984.
148. Orlando R, Gleason E, Dreener AD. Acute acalculous cholecystitis in the critically ill patient. Am J Surg 145:472, 1983.
149. Jeffrey RG Jr, Sommer FG. Follow-up sonography in suspected acalculous cholecystitis: preliminary clinical experience. J Ultrasound Med 12:183, 1993.
150. Potter MA, Paterson-Brown S. Open diagnostic peritoneal lavage. Br J Surg 83:87, 1996.
151. Gow KW, Haley LP, Phang PT. Validity of visual inspection of diagnostic peritoneal lavage fluid. Can J Surg 39:114, 1996.
152. Brandt CP, Priebe PP, Jacobs DG. Value of laparoscopy in trauma ICU patients with suspected acute acalculous cholecystitis. Surg Endosc 8:361, 1994.
153. Teplick SK, Brandon JC, Shah HR, McKenzie R, Itzkoff RL, Harshfield DL. Acute Gastrointestinal Disorders. In Goodman LR, Putman CE (eds). Critical Care Imaging. 3rd edn, Philadelphia: W. B. Saunders Company, 1992: 313.
154. Sinanan M, Maier RV, Carrico CJ. Laparotomy for intra-abdominal sepsis in patients in an intensive care unit. Arch Surg 119:652, 1984.
155. Meduri GU, Belenchia JM, Massie JD, Eltorky M, Tolley EA. The role of gallium-67 scintigraphy in diagnosing sources of fever in ventilated patients. Intensive Care Med 22:395, 1996.
156. Davis LP, Fink-Bennett D. Nuclear medicine in the acutely ill patient–II. Crit Care Clin 10:383, 1994.
157. Connell TR, Stephens DH, Carlson HC, Brown ML. Upper abdominal abscess: a continuing and deadly problem. Am J Roentgenology 134:759, 1980.
158. Gagliardi PD, Hoffer PB, Rosenfield AT. Correlative imaging in abdominal infection: an algorithmic approach using nuclear medicine,

ultrasound, and computed tomography. Semin Nucl Med 18:320, 1988.

159. Povoa P, Almeida E, Moreira P, Fernandes A, Mealha R, *et al*. C-reactive protein as an indicator of sepsis. Intensive Care Med 24:1052, 1998.

160. Chalfin DB, Niederman MS, Fein AM. Protected specimen brush (PSB) or empiric therapy (ET) for the diagnosis and treatment of nosocomial pneumonia (NP)? A decision analysis. Chest 102:96S, 1992.

3. CARDIOPULMONARY RESUSCITATION AND INFECTION

Jean-François Timsit

The prognosis of out-of hospital cardiac arrest is poor [1, 2]. For every eight patients suffering from cardiac arrest, there were three immediate survivors, two at 24 hours, 1.5 leaving hospital alive, and one alive at one year [3]. Continuous information of the public and the health care workers about cardiopulmonary resuscitation (CPR) in the 1970s have led to a dramatic improvement in immediate survival from cardiac arrest.

But, the AIDS epidemic as well as the rapid progression of hepatitis C have changed this situation. Even if CPR with mouth to mouth ventilation (MTMV) is associated with a five to thirty-fold increase in survival, due to fear of transmitted infectious diseases, rescuers became rare. After initial CPR, survivors are at risk of nosocomial pneumonia, especially aspiration pneumonia and bacteremia, which must be recognized and treated promptly.

These two sides of the relationship between CPR and infection will be discussed in this chapter. We will review the risk of acquisition of infection in patients surviving from initial CPR and the risk of transmission of infection between the patient and the caregivers and the way to prevent it.

Infection Acquired During CPR: Estimating the Risk for the Caregiver

RELUCTANCE OF CAREGIVERS IN PERFORMING CARDIOPULMONARY RESUSCITATION AND MOUTH TO MOUTH VENTILATION

The only interventions that have been shown unequivocally to improve long-term survival after cardiac arrest are basic life support and defibrillation [4].

The value of MTMV is currently under discussion because of a widespread fear of transmission of infectious diseases. Healthcare professionals have stated in several studies that they may withhold when confronted with a cardiac arrest in a stranger. Although an infection with Mycobacterium tuberculosis is more likely than one with HIV via MTMV, people's fear is understandable. An expert committee of the American Heart Association stated that MTMV may be omitted in the initial phase of cardiac arrest, and considered recommending chest compressions only if the emergency medical support would arrive rapidly. However, in paralized volunteers, ventilation was not able to provide sufficient gas exchange, especially when the airway was not protected.

For example, a reluctance of lay and medical personnel to perform MTMV in hospital and community settings has been documented, with 45% of respondents declining to perform MTMV on a stranger [5].

Hew *et al.* examined whether the perceived risk and fear of contracting infectious diseases diminishes the willingness of paramedics and emergency medical technicians (EMTs) to perform MMR [6]. Seventy-seven EMTs and 27 paramedics responded to a questionnaire, administered by one of two physicians, containing mock cardiac arrest scenarios that were designed to assess willingness to perform MTMV as a citizen responder. Faced with a situation in which an adult stranger required MTMV, 57% of the participating EMTs and all of the paramedics stated that they would refuse to perform MTMV. None of the paramedics and only 32.5% of the EMTs stated that they would perform MTMV on a man in a gay neighborhood. In addition, 23% of the EMTs and 37% of the paramedics indicated that they would refuse to perform MTMV on a child. Twenty-nine per cent of the prehospital-care providers had been in situations requiring MTMV in the community, and 40% either had walked away or only did external compression. Of those participating paramedics and EMTs who had performed MTMV in emergency situations, only 45% indicated that they would do so again. The respondents indicated that they would not be willing to administer MTMV because of the fear of contracting infectious agents, especially the human immunodeficiency virus (HIV). Despite the proven effectiveness of MMR in saving lives, paramedics and EMTs are highly reluctant to perform MMR as citizen responders. Their perceived risks of contracting infectious agents during MMR are high, despite the low actual risks.

RISKS OF INFECTION FOR THE CAREGIVERS

The possibility of transmission of infection between a victim and a rescuer has caused much concern, especially more recently with heightened anxiety over hepatitis and AIDS.

Even if cases are probably under-reported, the number of infections convincingly related to the resuscitation is estimated to be less than 1/200,000 [7].

There are two main ways of acquiring infectious diseases while performing CPR: MTMV and needlestick transmission.

Mouth to mouth transmission:
Neisseria meningitidis: The risk for salivary transmission of *N. meningitidis* is high especially in the case of systemic infection [8] and may explain why four cases of meningococcal infections have been linked to MTMV performed by healthcare workers. One case of menongococcal meningitis after tracheal intubation of a child suspected to have meningoencephalitis has also been described [9]. Providers who have such an exposure should be offered chemoprophylaxis.
Mycobacterium tuberculosis: Although the risk of acquisition of tuberculosis after performing MTMV to a patient with active tuberculosis should likely be very high, a unique case of tuberculosis to a healthcare worker was described. However, a rescuer who has given MTMV should be followed for conversion and or active tuberculosis. It seems logical to recommend serial tuberculin tests and/or chest radiograph in this case [10].

Enteric pathogens:
Mouth to mouth transmission of enteric pathogens has been described for *Shigella sonnei*, *Salmonella infantis* and possibly for *Helicobacter pylori*.

Risk of transmission of viruses through MTMV:
HIV is rarely isolated from the saliva of HIV infected patients and then in very low concentrations. This finding might explain the low risk of salivary transmission. For example, 1309 dental professionnals who had no behavioral risk factors for HIV infection but have cared for multiple patients known to have AIDS were screened. Only one dentist was seropositive for HIV [11].

On the other hand, hepatitis B virus (HBV) poses substantial risks to caregivers. Although no case of HBV transmision has been ever reported, salivary exchange is considered to be one of the mechanisms of non-parenteral transmission of HBV within families [12] and human bites are responsible for acquisition of HBV [13].

Little is know about the risk of hepatitis C (HCV) transmission during MTMV. The prevalence of HCV positivity in saliva is ranged between 20 to 62% of the HCV infected patients [7]. However, only a single case of saliva transmission after a human bite has been reported.

Needlestick transmission:
Although the risk of acquisition of infection should be considered as very low, the risk of acquisition of infection during emergency cardiopulmonary resuscitation exists especially because the scene of resuscitation is often chaotic resulting in a high risk of needlesticks or other sharps injuries.

In general, the risk resulting for parenteral exposure is greatest with HBV (13.1%), intermediate with HCV (5.8%) and lowest with HIV (0.32%) [14–16]. Particular effort to prevent sharps injuries in this situation is the main and essential way to prevent infection acquisition for the caregivers (see pages 52–53).

Nosocomial Infections After CPR

PATHOPHYSIOLOGY OF INFECTION AFTER CPR

Interruption of blood flow after cardiac or vascular surgery but also after cardiopulmonary rescucitation predispose to the occurrence of systemic inflammatory response syndrome, multiple organ dysfunction and adult respiratory distress syndrome. This could be due to the intensity of the ischemia and reperfusion which is know to activate nuclear factor κB [17] or other signaling pathways and then induce the production of cytokines such as TNF-α, IL-1 or IL-8 [18] as well as oxygen radicals. Ischemia-reperfusion also promotes the adhesion of leukocytes to the endothelium.

TABLE 1. Sequential events leading to immune depression after ischemia-reperfusion injury

Ischemia-reperfusion (bacterial translocation)
Activation of NF kappa B
Release of pro-inflammatory mediators
Release of anti-inflammatory mediators
Decrease in fibronectin and opsonic activity
Depressed neutrophil function (i.e.: Chemotaxism, phagocytosis, intracellular killing)
Shift from T-helper 1 lymphocytes to T-helper 2 lymphocytes
Reduced monocytes and macrophage function
Loss of skin reactivity
Decreased production of B lymphocytes and immunoglobulin

The pro-inflammatory cascade might explain fever occurring after CPR [19].

After the initial phase of injury, negative feedback downregulate early systemic inflammatory response syndrome (SIRS) to limit potential autodestructive inflammation. The early hypo-inflammatory response consists of a release of anti-inflammatory cytokines (IL-4, IL-10) and is followed by a long-lasting hypo-inflammatory state called "compensatory anti-inflammatory response syndrome" (CARS) [20] (Table 1). This could lead to a delayed immunosuppression [21] which could be associated with major infectious complications. This potential mechanism has not yet been demonstrated clinically.

PROBLEMS IN DIAGNOSING NOSOCOMIAL INFECTIONS AFTER CPR

After CPR, fever is a poor marker of infection. It is frequently encountered, as well as sepsis syndrome, after successful CPR and is more frequently considered as a marker of poor neurological outcome [22]. Hyperthermia is responsible for an increase of the volume of the cerebral infarction after occlusion of the cerebral blood flow in animal models [23]. Fever, even moderate in the day following brain ischemia may markedly exacerbate brain injury. It is probably due to ischemia related factors, thermo-dysregulation of central nervous system origin and/or decreased heat loss or altered distribution of body heat due to vasoconstriction [24]. For example, Takino and Okada [19] found 18 patients with a resaturation of a spontaneous circulation and who were not considered brain-dead within the first 48 hours. Forteen had hyperthermia (temperature > 38°C) occurring in the initial 48 hours after resuscitation. Eight patients with later brain death showed significantly appearance of hyperthermia and a high peak temperature (median 39.8°C) and six out the seven patients with prolonged coma have had a peak body temperature greater than 38°C (median: 38.3°C). None of these patients have had evidence of infection. On the contrary, in another study, only six out of 13 patients with bacteremia after cardiac arrest have had hypothermia (<36°C, n = 3) or hyperthermia (>38.5°C, n = 3) [25].

On the other hand, hypothermia is often used by intensivists to prevent brain injuries. The efficacy of hypothermia in preserving neurologic function when instituted before and during certain no flow cardiovascular state has been well documented both clinically and experimentally since the 1950s. Recent experimental evidence in dogs has shown that hypothermia induced after cardiac arrest does indeed mitigate the effects of post-resuscitation syndrome and improves neurologic function and reduces histologic brain damage [24]. Such benefit can be demonstrated with mild (34–36°C) hypothermia [26], thus minimizing complication and requiring less time for induction of hypothermia. Mild hypothermia is considered as an important and secure component for cerebral preservation and resuscitation during, and after, global ischemia and it is often considered as a useful method of cerebral resuscitation after global ischemic states, thereby promoting the prevention of neuromental diseases.

Consequently, after CPR, barbiturates and antipyretic therapies are frequently used and could interfere with body temperature and delay the diagnosis of subsequent infections [27].

THE ROLE OF THE DIGESTIVE TRACT

The importance of intestinal injury is directly related to the duration of ischemia and to the reperfusion injury via O_2 free production [28].

Infection is considered to be partly due to digestive ischemia and bacterial translocation occurring during CPR. After CPR, early onset of nosocomial infections are frequent. In 67 patients who survival from CPR at least 72 hours, 51 developed early onset nosocomial infections (76% pneumonia and 9% bacteremia). Microorganisms responsible for these infections were *Enterobacteriaceae* (32%), *Enterococcus* (9%), *Staphylococcus* spp (12%) and *S pneumoniae* (9%), [29] which correspond mainly to endogenous flora. These patients present digestive symptoms in two thirds of cases (vomiting or hiccough 52%, diarrhea or ileus 16%, digestive hemorrhage 32%). In another study [25] Gaussorgues *et al.* found that 12 out of 13 patients with early onset bacteremia after CPR had fetid diarrhea a few hours after their ICU admission. Moreover, the same microorganisms were found in blood and feces. Moreover, 13 out of 19 patients underwent digestive endoscopy with proven oesophageal, stomacal or colonic ischemia, profound ulceration or necrosis. Non-occlusive mesenteric infarction could also be involved in the genesis of these bacteremia [30].

The digestive lesions together with the microorganisms recovered are strong arguments for the predominant role of digestive tract in the genesis of infection.

LOWER RESPIRATORY TRACT INFECTIONS FOLLOWING CARDIAC ARREST AND SUCCESSFUL CPR

Patients surviving CPR are at high risk of lower respiratory tract infections. They cumulate major risk factors as emergency tracheal intubation, decreased level of consciousness and broncho-aspiration. Animal models indicate that lower oesophageal sphincter pressure may decrease rapidly to 5 cm H_2O during cardiac arrest, which may further increase the risk of gastric inflation and subsequent regurgitation, aspiration and pneumonia during ventilation with an unprotected airway [5]. Gastric regurgitation was recorded to have occurred in 180 out of 797 (22.6%) patients with cardiac arrest [31].

Complications of tracheal intubation performed on emergency have been prospectively evaluated: among 297 tracheal intubations, radiological pictures of pulmonary aspiration have been found in 4% of the cases and might partly explain the high rate of early onset pneumonia after CPR [32].

The incidence of lower respiratory tract infection in CPR survivors was as high as 28.1% using protected specimen brush and bronchoalveolar lavage culture techniques [33] and was higher than that observed in other general ICU ventilated population [34, 35]. Pneumonia occurred mainly in the first week of ICU stay and was due to methicillin sensitive *S. aureus*, *S pneumoniae*, *H influenzae* and *E. coli*. *P. aeruginosa* was isolated relatively late and almost exclusively from infected patients who had received antimicrobial therapy.

In a recent paper [36], Rello *et al.* have shown that cardiopulmonary resuscitation is independently associated with development of very early-onset pneumonia (within the first 48 hours of intubation). CPR (odds ratio: 5.13 (2.14–12.26), continuous sedation (odds ratio: 4.4 (1.8–10.6)) were significant risk factors of pneumonia, while antibiotic use (odds ratio: 0.29 (0.12–0.69)) showed a protective effect.

CATHETER-RELATED INFECTIONS AND BACTEREMIA

After 7.5 minutes-experimental cardiac arrest in dogs, bacteremia was present in all animals [37]. Bacteremia was demonstrated in patients admitted to ICU after successful CPR. Gaussorgues and colleagues [25] found that 13 out of 33 patients had at least two positive peripheral blood cultures in the first 12 hours after admission. Bacteremia were considered as due to mesenteric ischemia as 12 patients had fetid diarrhea during three to five hours following cardiac arrest. The microorganisms isolated were found in both blood and feces in 12 cases. One *S. aureus* catheter-related septicemia occurred after emergency insertion of a central line.

In most cases during CPR, maximal sterile barriers are not used during insertion of central venous catheters. Moreover, the femoral route is frequently chosen. This could explain the high risk of catheter-related infection in this situation [38, 39]. In a study involving prospectively 300 catheters inserted into 204 patients, Goetz *et al.* [39] found that emergent insertion was associated with a six-fold increase in the risk of catheter contamination (clinical infection or colonization with >15 colonies on semiquantitative culture) (odds ratio, 6.2; 95% confidence interval (CI95), 1.1–36.7; P = 0.04).

Even if reasonable, there is no recommendation for the removal of central catheters inserted under emergency conditions, where breaks in aseptic technique are likely to have occurred [40].

OTHER INFECTIONS

Other anecdotal infectious complications have been described such as acute *S. aureus* mediastinitis complicating sternal fracture during chest compressions and a resulting retrosternal hematoma [41–43].

Prevention of Infection

FOR THE PATIENT

During ventilation of unprotected airways, tidal volumes of 0.5 l instead of 0.8–1 L may have an advantage as it decreases the risk of gastric inflation and subsequent aspiration and pneumonia [5]. The use of the laryngeal mask airway alone or after bag valve mask ventilation has been show to reduce the risk of regurgitation [31].

In the study of Rello *et al.* [36], exposure to antibiotic independently prevented development of pneumonia during the first two days of ventilation but has no effect on late onset pneumonia frequently related to multi-resistant strains.

Indeed, other studies have reported the protective effect of antibiotics specifically on episodes caused by primary endogeneous flora [44]. However, protective effect of antibiotics has been shown to attenuate when the time in the ICU increases [45]. Moreover, antibiotic use increases the risk of antimicrobial resistance. Antimicrobial intravenous prophylaxis cannot be recommended. However, in case of fever, after microbiological samples, the threshold for instituting antimicrobial therapy, if there is any suspicion for developing pneumonia or sepsis, should be lowered.

PRECAUTIONS TO REDUCE THE RISK FOR THE CAREGIVERS DURING CPR

Health care workers know "universal precautions" for prevention of cross-transmission of infectious diseases. Guidelines for prevention and management of biohazardous exposures during CPR are summarized in the annex. However, in urgent situations, such as cardiac arrest it is often difficult to take the time to respect these precautions. So, to decrease the risk for caregivers, it is important to facilitate the use of new devices such as needleless systems. One-way valve mouth-to-mask systems or bag-valve-masks [46] are interesting in preventing direct mouth-to-mouth contact between rescuer and patient. It seemed to prevent transmission from the oral flora to the rescuer's side of the device.

Adequate training in CPR is one of the determinants of the efficacy of CPR [47]. This training must address protection from infection during CPR, with a great focus on measures for avoiding sharps injuries.

Conclusion

The benefit of initiating lifesaving resuscitation in a patient in cardiac arrest greatly outweighs the risk for secondary infection in the rescuer or the patient. Nevertheless, use of simple infection-control measures during CPR can reduce a very low level of risk even further.

Instruction in CPR for providers of prehospital care, the medical community, and the general public should emphasize the benefits of providing MTMV, the actual low risks of contracting infectious diseases during administration of MTMV, and the use of widely available and effective barrier masks to minimize any risks due to administration of MTMV. The strategy to compress the thorax first and then maintain the airway and perform ventilation may only have advantages for the first 30 s of CPR.

After successful initial CPR, hyperthermia is frequent and might be due to early onset nosocomial infection which required immediate diagnosis and treatment.

Annex: Guidelines for Prevention and Management of Biohazardous Exposures During Cardiopulmonary Resuscitation (adapted from Mejicano and Maki [7])

1. Health care workers and public protection personnel likely to be called on to give CPR must be aware of the potential catastrophic sequelae of biohazardous exposures, especially needlestick injuries, and of guidelines for prevention. This can be effected through inclusion in all CPR training programs.
   - Recapping or resheathing used needles must be strongly discouraged. Effective and safe needle-disposal units should be made widely and conveniently available throughout the hospital, especially in locations that facilitate their immediate use.
   - Receptacles in metal or other impervious material be available and emptied according to an established routine.
   - Needleless systems now available should be encouraged and made available in various sites, including resuscitation carts and emergency transport vehicles.
   - Health care workers and public protec-

tion professionals must be apprised of the importance of obtaining adequate assistance when administering injections or infusion therapy to patients.
- Personnel must be apprised of the need to use extreme care in cleaning up after CPR and other procedures that involve needles, such as insertion of central lines.

2. Oral barrier devices should be widely and conveniently available throughout hospitals and clinics and in emergency transport vehicles where CPR is likely to be performed.
   - After every CPR procedure, especially if mouth-to-mouth ventilation was done, an effort should be made to determine whether the patient may have had a dangerous, contagious infection, such as pulmonary tuberculosis, meningococcal or streptococcal sepsis, or overwhelming pneumonia. If the patient does not survive, cultures and blood specimens should be obtained. If an autopsy is carried out, evidence of undiagnosed infection should specifically be sought.
3. If a clear-cut biohazardous exposure to a patient's blood occurred through a needlestick, a blood splash into the mouth or eyes, or broken skin, or if blood or open sores were seen in the patient's mouth and mouth-to-mouth ventilation was given, the patient must be tested for evidence of infection with HIV, HBV, and HCV to determine the need for postexposure prophylaxis.
   - With biohazardous exposures, especially needlestick injuries, the exposure should be immediately reported to the employee health service, where the exposed person can be evaluated and managed most consistently and inexpensively and surveillance of all work related injuries can be facilitated.
   - Management of biohazardous injuries must be possible 24 hours a day, seven days a week, by emergency department personnel trained in the institutional biohazardous injury protocol.
   - Particular attention should be given to persons who have sustained repeated injuries to identify accident-prone activities or persons.
4. Institutions should maintain continuous surveillance of all biohazardous injuries. This can form the basis for preventive programs and for assessment of their effectiveness.
5. It is imperative that every hospital have a protocol that provides unambiguous management guidelines that specifically provide the following:
   - Clear definitions of biohazardous exposures
   - Procedures for immediate care of the injury at the time of occurrence, such as squeezing the puncture wound to induce bleeding and using immediate cutaneous disinfection with a virucidal agent, such as an iodophor.
   - Procedures to expeditiously determine the magnitude of risk (for example, screening the resuscitated patient for evidence of active HBV, HCV, and HIV).
   - Guidelines for post-exposure evaluation and treatment, where indicated, especially for exposures to Hepatitis A virus, HBV, HCV, HIV, Mycobacterium tuberculosis, and Neisseria meningitidis.
   - Provisions for long-term follow-up of the exposed rescuer, especially after exposures to HBV, HCV and HIV.
   - Provisions for administrative follow-up of all injuries (to minimize recurrences).
   - Review and revision of the protocol at least annually.
   - Public protection professionals who are likely to provide CPR in the community must also have access to an educational program and post-exposure protocol, which will be most efficiently and consistently effected through a local hospital.

References

1. Kuisma M, Alaspaa A. Out-of-hospital cardiac arrest of non-cardiac origin: Epidemiology and outcome. Eur Heart J 18:1122, 1997.
2. Van Hoeyweghen RJ, Bossaert LL, Mullie A, Martens P, Delooz HH, *et al*. Survival after out-of-hospital cardiac arrest in elderly patients. Ann Emerg Med 21:1179, 1992.
3. Tunstall-Pedoe H, Bailey L, Chamberlain DA, Mardsen AK, Ward ME, Ziderman DA. BMJ 304:1347, 1992.
4. Advanced life support working group of the European resuscitation council. The 1998 European resuscitation council guidelines for adult advanced life support. BMJ 37:81, 1998.
5. Wenzel V, Lindner KH, Prengel AW. Ventilation during cardiopulmonary resuscitation. A literature study and analysis of ventilation strategies. Anaethesist 46:133, 1997.
6. Hew P, Brenner B, Kaufman J. Reluctance of paramedics and emergency medical technicians to perform mouth-to-mouth resuscitation. J Emerg Med 15:279, 1997.
7. Mejicano GC, Maki DG. Infections acquired during cardiopulmonary resuscitation: estimating the risk and defining strategies for prevention. Ann Intern Med 129:813, 1998.
8. Jacobson JA, Fraser DW. A simplified approach to meningococcal disease prophylaxis. JAMA 236:1053, 1976.
9. Gehanno JF, Kohen-Couderc L, Lemeland JF, Leroy J. Nosocomial meningococcemia in a physician. Infect Control Hosp Epidemiol 20: 564, 1999.
10. Bass JB Jr, Farer LS, Hopewell PC, O'Brien R, Jacobs RF, Ruben F. Treatment of tuberculosis and tuberculosis infection in adults and children. American Thoracic Society and the Center for Disease Control and Prevention. Am J Respir Crit Care Med 149:1359, 1994.
11. Klein RS, Phelan JA, Freeman K, Schable C, Friedland JH, Trieger N. Low occupational risk of human immunodeficiency virus infection among dental professionals. N Eng J Med 318: 86, 1988.
12. Powell E, Duke M, Cooksley WG. Hepatitis B virus infection within families: potential importance of saliva as a vehicle of spread. Aust N Z J Med 15:717, 1985.
13. MacQuarrie MB, Forghani B, Wolochow DA. Hepatitis B transmitted by a human bites. JAMA 230:723, 1974.
14. Gerberding JL. Prophylaxis of occupational exposure to HIV. Ann Intern Med 125:497, 1996.
15. Seef LB, Wright HL, Zimmerman HJ, Alter HJ, Dietz AA, *et al*. Type B hepatitis after needlestick exposure: prevention with hepatitis B immune globulin. Final report of the veteran administration cooperative study. Ann Intern Med 88:285, 1978.
16. Kiyosawa K, Sodeyama T, Tanaka E, Nakayano Y, Furuta S, *et al*. Hepatitis C in hospital employees with needlestick injuries. Ann Intern Med 115:367, 1991.
17. Moine P, Shenkar R, Kaneko D, Le Tulzo JY, Abraham E. Systemic blood less affects NF kappa B regulatory mechanisms in the lung. Am J Physiol 273:L185, 1997.
18. Wan S, Leclerc JL, Vincent JL. Inflammatory response to cardiopulmonary bypass: mechanisms involved and possible therapeutic strategies. Chest 112:676, 1997.
19. Takino M, Okada Y. Hyperthermia following cardiopulmonary resuscitation. Intens Care Med 17:419, 1991.
20. Bone RC. Sir Isaac Newton, sepsis, SIRS and CARS. Crit Care Med 24:1125, 1996.
21. Soppi E, Lindroos M, Nikoskelainen J, Kalliomaki JL. Intens Care Med 10:287, 1984.
22. Torres A, Pickert CB, Firestone J, Walker WM, Fiser DH. Long term functional outcome of inpatient pediatric cardiopulmonary resuscitation. Pediatr Emerg Care 13:369, 1997.
23. Kim Y, Busto R, Dietrich WD, Kraydieh S, Ginsberg MD. Delayed postischemic hyperthermia in awake rats worsens the histopathological outcome of transient focal cerebral ischemia. Stroke 27:2274, 1996.
24. Safar P. Resuscitation from clinical death: pathophysiologic limits and therapeutic potentials. Crit Care Med 16:923, 1988.
25. Gaussorgues P, Gueugniaud PY, Vedrinne JM, Salord F, Mercatello A, Robert D. Bacteremia following cardiac arrest and cardiopulmonary resuscitation. Intens Care Med 14:575, 1988.
26. Sterz F, Zeiner A, Kurkciyan I, Janata K, Mullner M, Domanovits H, Safar P. Mild resuscitative hypothermia and outcome after cardiopulmonary resuscitation. J Neurosurg Anesthesiol 8:88, 1996.
27. Gustafson I, Edgren E, Hulting J. Brain oriented intensive care after resuscitation from cardiac arrest. Resuscitation 24:245, 1992.
28. Haglund U, Hulten L, Lundgren O. Mucosal

lesions in the human small intestine in shock. Gut 16:979, 1975.

29. Fourel D, L'Her E, Garo B, Renault A, Boles JM. Infections nosocomiales après arret cardiocirculatoire extra-hospitalier: ***rôle du tube digestif***. Ann Fr Anesth Reanim 18:292S, 1999.
30. Morgan RJ, White PW, Temesy-Armos PN, Davis JT. Treatment of non occlusive mesenteric infarction after cardiopulmonary resuscitation. Crit Care Med 13:53, 1985.
31. Stone BJ, Chantler PJ, Baskett PJ. The incidence of regurgitation during cardiopulmonary resuscitation: a comparison between the bag valve mask and laryngeal mask airway. Resuscitation 38:3, 1998.
32. Schwartz DE, Matthay MA, Cohen NH. Death and other complications of emergency airway management in critically ill adults: a prospective investigation of 297 tracheal intubations. Anesthesiology 82:367, 1995.
33. Rello J, Valles J, Jubert P, Ferrer A, Domingo C, *et al.* Lower respiratory tract infections following cardiac arrest and cardiopulmonary resuscitation. Clin Infect Dis 21:310, 1995.
34. Timsit JF, Chevret S, Valcke J, Misset B, Renaud B, *et al.* Does nosocomial pneumonia increase the risk of death in mechanically ventilated patients? Am Rev Respir Crit Care Med 154:116, 1996.
35. Fagon JY, Chastre J, Domart Y. Nosocomial pneumonia in patients receiving continuous mechanical ventilation: prospective analysis of 52 episodes with use of a protected specimen brush and quantitative culture technique. Ann Rev Respir Dis 139:877, 1989.
36. Rello J, Diaz E, Roque M, Valles J. Risk factors for developping pneumonia within 48 hours of intubation. Am J Respir Crit Care Med 159:1742, 1999.
37. Cerchiari EL, Safar P, Klein E, Diven W. Visceral, hematologic and bacteriologic changes and neurological outcome after cardiac arrest in dogs. The visceral post-resuscitation syndrome. Resuscitation 25:119, 1993.
38. Richet H, Hubert B, Nittnberg G, *et al.* Prospective multicenter study of vascular catheter-related complications and risk factors for positive central catheter cultures in intensive care unit patients. J Clin Microbiol 28:2520, 1990.
39. Goetz AM, Wagener MM, Miller JM, Muder RR. Risk of infection due to central venous catheters: effect of site of placement and catheter type. Infect Control Hosp Epidemiol 11:842, 1998.
40. Pearson, ML. Guidelines for prevention of intravascular-device-related infections. Infect Control Hosp Epidemiol 17:438, 1996.
41. Mensah GA, Gold JP, Schreiber T, Isom OW. Acute purulent mediastinitis and osteomyelitis after closed chest cardiopulmonary resuscitation: a case report and revue of the literature. Ann Thorac Surg 46:353, 1988.
42. Werhens XH, Doevendans PA, Van Dantzig JM, Snoep G, Wellens HJ. Infected sternal fracture hematoma after cardiopulmonary resuscitation initially seen as pericarditis. Am Heart J 132: 685, 1996.
43. Mallinson RH, Tremlett CH, Payne BV, Richards JE. Sternal osteomyelitis after cardiopulmonary resuscitation. J R Soc Med 92:87, 1999.
44. Sirvent JM, Torres A, El-Ebiary M, Castro P, de Battle J, Bonet A. Protective effect of intravenously administered cefuroxime against nosocomial pneumonia in patients with structural coma. Am J Respir Crit Care Med 155: 1729, 1997.
45. Cook DJ, Walter SD, Cook RJ, Griffith LE, Guyat GH, *et al.* Incidence and risk factors for ventilator associated pneumonia in critically ill patients. Ann Intern Med 129:433, 1998.
46. Cydulka RK, Connor PJ, Myers TF, Pavza G, Parker M. Prevention of oral bacterial flora transmission by using mouth to mask ventilation during CPR. J Emerg Med 9:317, 1991.
47. Cobb LA, Fahrenbruch CE, Walch TR, Copass MK, Olsufka M, *et al.* Influence of cardiopulmonary resuscitation prior to defibrillation in patients with out-of-hospital ventricular fibrillation. JAMA 281:1182, 1999.

4. FUNGAL INFECTIONS

Rosemary A. Barnes

Introduction

Fungal infections are a significant problem and represent a major cause of morbidity and mortality in a variety of patients. Improvements in supportive care and widespread use of antimicrobial agents have resulted in an expanding population of at-risk patients. This trend concerns not only severely compromised hosts such as transplant recipients, neutropenic and HIV-positive patients but also non-compromised patients on surgical and medical intensive care units (ICUs), burns and neonatal units with specific risk factors for infection.

Many studies have identified a marked increase in the incidence of fungal infection over the last decade with a major impact on outcomes in critically ill patients. The National Nosocomial Infections Surveillance (NNIS) program has provided nation-wide information from the USA for the past two decades [1]. Data from 1980–1990 show that nosocomial infections increased from 2.0–3.8 infections per 1000 patients discharged during that period and that critical care patients were at highest risk. The studies also demonstrate differences between community-acquired endemic fungi such as *Histoplasma capsulatum* and *Blastomyces dermatidis* which are restricted to specific geographical locations and nosocomial infections with *Candida* and *Aspergillus* spp that prevail in large health-care facilities and largely account for the increasing problem [2]. The NNIS data, collected from self-selecting hospitals as part of a sentinel surveillance system, identified *Candida* as the fourth most common pathogen in the ICU with fungaemia rates increasing five fold over the ten year period. More recently, comprehensive population-based surveillance has begun to define the problem more accurately. In the San Franscisco area the cumulative incidence of invasive mycotic infection was 178.3 per million per year with *Candida* accounting for 72.8 per million per year of this [3]. Whilst human immunodeficiency virus infection was an important contributing factor in this population (being an underlying factor in 47%) other studies have confirmed the extent of the problem. In Canada the incidence of invasive fungal infection varied from 35.4–66.4 per million population with *Candida* responsible for 66% of reports, *Cryptococcus neoformans*, *Aspergillus* species and *Histoplasma capsulatum* accounting for 5–10% of cases and all other fungi responsible for less than 5% (Table 1A) [4].

No comprehensive surveillance of nosocomial fungal infection exists in Europe and the true incidence of fungal infection is unknown. The EPIC study comprised a single day point prevalence study of over 1400 ICUs in Western Europe. Fungal isolates were reported from 17% of patients of whom half were receiving antifungal treatment [5]. Yeasts were reported as the major causative organism in 9% of bloodstream infections, 21% of urinary tract infections, 14% of pneumonia and 11% of other respiratory tract infections (Table 1B) [6]. Although many of these may have represented colonization rather than infection, highlighting problems in diagnosis, there is no doubt that fungi have emerged as significant nosocomial pathogens in critically ill patients.

TABLE 1.A Population-based studies

	Incidence per million population per year						
Reference	Total	Candida	Cryptococcus	Coccioides	Aspergillus	Histoplasma	Other
3	178.3	72.8	65.5	15.3	12.4	7.1	1–1.7
4	35.4–66.4	66%	5–10%	<5%	5–10	5–10	<5%

TABLE 1.B Hospital/ICU-based surveillance of Candida

Reference	Bloodstream infection %	Urinary tract infection %
NNIS [1]	10.2	25
EPIC [5, 6]	9	20

Most systemic fungal infections in the UK and Western Europe involve opportunist fungi such as *Candida*, *Aspergillus*, *Cryptococcus* spp. and *Pneumocystis carinii*. This is in contrast to parts of the USA and the developing world where endemic pathogens such as *Histoplasma*, *Blastomyces* and *Coccidioides* spp. may cause community-acquired infection and contribute to the fungal burden. However, in all geographical areas, infections in critical care patients are predominantly nosocomial and candidosis accounts for nearly 80% of these.

Candida Infections

Yeasts account for 11% of all bloodstream infections in the ICU [1] and 8–15% of nosocomial septicaemias in the USA [7]. Rates from Europe suggest that candidaemia rose from 4.7 cases per 1000 patient days to 7.4 cases between 1987 and 1990 [8]. An incidence of one candidaemia per 500 admissions has been documented in medical and surgical ICUs [9] and *Candida* accounted for 8% of blood culture isolates from a tertiary neonatal ICU [10]. Intensive care treatment is an independent risk factor for fungaemia even when other risk factors are taken into account. Candidaemia has a substantial impact on mortality. Attributable mortality has been estimated at around 38% [11]. This is considerably higher than other nosocomial bloodstream infections. In one large study, candidaemia was the only bloodstream pathogen that independently influenced the outcome of nosocomial infection in ICU patients [12].

Paralleling the rise of nosocomial infection has been a marked "pathogen shift" with a significant decrease in the proportion of *C. albicans* infections (falling from around 90% to 30–50% of all yeast blood culture isolates) over the last five to 10 years coinciding with the emergence of non-*albicans* species such as *C. tropicalis*, *C. parapsilosis*, *C. glabrata* and *C. krusei* [13]. The widespread use of azoles has been implicated [14–16] in this trend but does not fully explain the shift [17] and other factors such as the increased use of intravenous long-lines, total parenteral nutrition and mucositis are probably involved. There is a generally accepted hierarchy of pathogenicity of *Candida* species with *C. albicans* at the top of the league and *C. glabrata* (formerly *Torulopsis glabrata*) bringing up the rear. Nonetheless, even less virulent forms of candidosis can have significant implications for morbidity in critically ill patients and may be more refractory to treatment.

RISK FACTORS FOR CANDIDOSIS

Candida are ubiquitous yeasts that colonize our skin and mucosal surfaces. *C. albicans* is part of the endogenous flora of the oropharynx and gastrointestinal tract of normal healthy individuals and may colonize skin surfaces in small numbers. Other *Candida* spp may colonize hospitalized patients and the hands of healthcare workers allowing horizontal spread and the potential for hospital-acquired infection. Many studies have identified risk factors for invasive disease (Table 2) but since these factors are common to most critical care patients they lack discrimination and are of limited use in identifying high-risk patients. Use of central venous catheters, colonization, broad-spectrum antibiotics and haemodialysis are independent risk factors for disseminated infection [18] but are common to many hospitalized patients. Better understanding of risk factors for individual groups and knowledge of which risk factors are predictors of mortality [19] will enable more rational use of preventative measures. Obviously degree and duration of neutropenia is a significant factor in classically immunocompromised patients [20] whilst operative time, retransplantation, reoperation and cytomegalovirus infection are relevant to liver and solid organ transplant recipients [21]. In neonates, low birth weight is the major factor [22] whilst on medical and surgical ICUs length of stay, severity of illness, peritonitis and pancreatitis [23, 24] may be more useful predictors of invasive Candida infection than other commonly cited risk factors.

TABLE 2. Risk factors for candidosis

Length of stay
Immunosuppression (neutropenia*, corticosteroids)
Central venous catheterization*
Broad-spectrum antimicrobial therapy* (rises with duration of use and no. of agents)
Total parenteral nutrition
Candida colonization*
Haemodialysis*
Previous surgery
Severity of acute illness** (APACHE II score >20)
Very low birth weight
Acute pacreatitis**
Multi-organ failure**

* Independent risk factor.
** Risk factor for mortality.

In all risk groups, *Candida* colonization is an independent risk factor for infection and precedes invasive disease in most cases. However, more than 50% of ICU patients will become colonized during hospitalization and distinguishing infection from colonization may be difficult. Risk of infection increases with the number of sites colonized and is dependent on the colonizing species. One study demonstrated that 15% of patients colonized with *C. albicans* at one site developed fungaemia rising to 17% when two or more sites were colonized. However, patients colonized with *C. tropicalis* at one site had a 58% risk of subsequent fungaemia rising to 100% when two or more sites were colonized with this species [25]. Further studies in surgical ICU patients have confirmed this trend [26] and advocate the use of a candida colonization index to assess the degree of colonization. A ratio of ≥0.5 (representing the number of distinct sites colonized with the same strain over the number of sites tested) has been shown to have a positive predictive value of 66% for determining infection and sensitivity can be further increased if quantitation (based on semi-quantitative fungal load) is simultaneously applied [27]. Increasing fungal load in serial specimens is also predictive of invasive disease [24]. In neonates, a carriage index representing semi-quantitative yeast concentrations in saliva or faeces has been devised: only neonates with $>10^5$ yeast cells/ml saliva or gram of faeces developed fungaemia [28]. Many risk factors involve altered host defences that allow fungal overgrowth, whilst others provide a portal of entry through translocation across mucosal surfaces or direct invasion via intravenous lines or wounds.

Raised gastric pH due to sedation, antacids, H_2 antagonists and exocrine abnormalities may lead to *Candida* overgrowth in the bowel. Widespread use of broad-spectrum antibiotic agents compounds this. Severity of illness, splanchnic ischaemia, impaired gut mobility or ileus will contribute to translocation of yeasts through the bowel mucosa. Total parenteral nutrition is a risk factor over and above the presence of the central line and intravenous lipids promote fungal growth.

IMMUNE RESPONSE TO *CANDIDA*

Candida contain immunodominant mannoproteins on their cell walls capable of binding to CD14 and stimulating a proinflammatory T-helper (Th1) cytokine response such that acute fungaemia may present as profound sepsis. Conversely, exposure to fungal mannoproteins may result in a down-regulatory response associated with anti-inflammatory (Th2) cytokines and persistent fungal infection. This chronic form is more likely to be associated with other causes of monocyte deactivation following immunosuppression, trauma/surgery, immaturity, head-injury or sepsis ("second-hit phenomena"). The application of this Th1/Th2 paradigm to human infection is far from clear [29, 30], but patterns of T cell cytokine production may predict which patients are at risk of infection following immunocompromise or trauma. Critically ill patients frequently display signs of immuneparesis. Mechanisms of this are poorly understood but probably involve dysregulated monocyte function and a switch from Th1 pro-inflammatory pathways to the Th2 anti-inflammatory pathways that may facilitate fungal infection and persistence in these patient groups. The theory that virulent fungi may modulate and thereby evade host immunity through the inability of the host to mount a proinflammatory T cell cytokine response is substantiated by animal models [31, 32] and anecdotal evidence in humans [33]. Thermally injured mice have been shown to generate a burn-associated type two response resulting in a 50-fold increase in susceptibility to *C. albians* infection [34]. Lymphocytes from neonates show a marked reduction in their capacity to inhibit growth of *C. albicans* [35].

Humoral responses are important in determining recovery from fungal infection and a variety of antibodies to *Candida* have been identified by immunodiffusion, counterimmunoelectrophoresis and Western blot analysis [36, 37] but appear to be of little value in identifying at-risk patients in the ICU. Antibody responses to immunodominant highly conserved heat-shock proteins [38] or cell wall protein determinants [39] may be more relevant in protecting the host from infection.

CLINICAL PRESENTATION

Candida infection in critically ill patients presents non-specifically. Fever, moderate leucocytosis and fever that fail to respond to broad spectrum antimicrobial agents may be the only clinical signs and some of these may be absent in immunocompromised individuals or those undergoing haemfiltration. Fever is present in up to 80% of individuals and leucocytosis occurs in only 50% [40]. Acute phase protein responses are generally markedly elevated. A rising C-reactive protein (CRP) level in the absence of any other identified cause should alert the clinician to the possibility of yeast infection [41, 42].

Systemic infection may present according to the portal of entry and candidaemia may result from a number of sources.

Candidaemia is defined as the isolation of any Candida species from at least one blood culture specimen [18]. This is commonly line-associated (candidaemia is not infrequently associated with colonized intravascular devices). The concept of benign candidaemia (i.e. fungaemia that requires line-removal only and forgoes the need for systemic antifungal treatment) is flawed [43]. It is well recognized that even transient candidaemia requires both line removal and a course of antifungal treatment if metastatic complications and excessive mortality are to be avoided. This applies regardless of the species involved as "non-pathogenic" species of *Candida* cannot be identified accurately in critically ill hosts.

Acute dissemination can occur to multiple organs with the formation of microabscesses. Skin and muscle may be involved with the development of a characteristic erythematous papular rash [44]. Dissemination to other non-contiguous organs may be more difficult to identify [45]. Retinal lesions and ophthalmitis are relatively rare occurring in only 9–15% of ICU patients [46, 47], and skin lesions and septic arthritis are similarly infrequently reported [18].

The reticuloendothelial system is the most common site for dissemination but micro-abscesses within the liver and spleen are often only be detected at autopsy. Chronic disseminated candidosis (hepatosplenic candidosis) is seen in classically immunocompromised patients following resolution of neutropenia.

Intra-abdominal candidosis occurs following leakage of commensal gut yeasts into the peritoneal cavity following gastrointestinal perforation or abdominal surgery. Frequently this is a transient phenomenon that is rapidly cleared provided effective surgical repair is achieved [24]. A continued abdominal focus due to recurrent perforation or anastomotic breakdown may lead to invasive disease and disseminate into the bloodstream [48]. Abnormalities in liver enzymes may indicate hepatic involvement and acalculous *Candida* cholecystitis has been reported in critically ill patients [49].

Renal candidosis may be difficult to distinguish from colonization of the urinary tract in catheterised patients. Candiduria is a frequent finding in ICU patients and is consistent with both colonization and infection [45]. The diagnostic thresholds developed for bacterial urinary tract infection (quantitative bacteruria, and pyuria) cannot be applied to fungi [40]. However, funguria in patients with urological pathology or which persists despite changes of urinary catheters is strongly predictive of infection [50, 51].

Other organ involvement is also difficult to identify clinically. The EPIC study reported a 14% incidence of pneumonia due to yeasts [5, 6]. However, the diagnostic criteria used were non-specific and many of these cases probably represented colonization or contamination with oropharyngeal flora. In a five-year review of consecutive cases of ICU patients with *Candida* species isolated from bronchoalveolar lavage, contamination was confirmed or probable in 80% of cases. The majority of patients had counts equal to or exceeding the threshold of 10^3 cfu/ml from protected brush specimens but none had clinical signs consistent with candidal pneumonia [52]. Candidal pneumonia is a rare condition associated with a high mortality rate. The condition may arise following haematogenous dissemination and presents as miliary lesions throughout the lung fields, or may occur as a primary condition following aspiration of oropharyngeal contents. This latter condition presents as a patchy, haemorrhagic bronchopneumonia [53]. Isolation from bronchoscopic specimens has poor predictive value due to the high rates of colonization in mechanically ventilated patients and should not be used to as the sole criteria to initiate treatment. Diagnosis depends on histological demonstration of fungus within the tissues [54].

DIAGNOSIS

The non-specific clinical features of invasive candidal infections mean that demonstration of fungi in clinical specimens must be combined with good clinical acumen. Serology has a relatively small role to play but molecular techniques are under increasing scrutiny.

Historically, blood cultures are reported to be insensitive markers of candidaemia [55] but recent changes in automated culture systems utilizing large volume, lytic methods have greatly improved detection rates and largely obviated the need for specialized systems such as semi-quantitative lysis centrifugation cultures [56].

Detection of antibodies is unreliable in this patient population and seroconversion, if detected, occurs late in the course of disease and is of prognostic significance with a limited role in diagnosis [57]. One recent study of 1751 serum samples from 391 long-term intensive care patients showed that significant antibody production against a number of antigens (including apparently immunodominant 47 and 58 kDa antigens) in various subgroups of patients failed to discriminate between deep and superficial infection and colonization [37].

Detection of fungal components or metabolites in body fluids has been a major area of interest. Antigen detection is well established in the diagnosis of cryptococcosis but has been less successful in other fungal infections. A wide variety of antigens are known to circulate in candidosis but most attention has focused on the detection of circulating cell wall mannan. The immunodominant epitopes have been characterized and the development of monoclonal antibodies has enabled their incorporation into commercially available antigen detection systems. Latex-agglutination kits and more recently an enzyme immunoassay have been marketed with detection limits of 10 and 0.1 ng/ml respectively [58]. Although promising, evaluation in critically ill patients is limited and results from the neutropenic patient population have been disappointing [59, 60]. This apparent lack of sensitivity has been attributed to the fluctuating levels of the low molecular weight antigens and the rapid clearance of mannan from the circulation with the net result that frequent testing of patients (2–3 times a week) is necessary if the test is to have a useful clinical application. Attempts to improve sensitivity of fungal antigen detection through ultrasound–enhancement of latex-based assays [61] have the potential to greatly improve sensitivity. Further developments and characterization of other antigens may identify potential targets for detection [62].

Other fungal metabolites such as mannitol and arabinitol can be detected in fungal infection and elevated serum D-arabinotol : creatinine rations have been reported in the patients with deep-seated candidosis [63] but the routine use of these diagnostic tests is not widespread. Beta (1–3)-D-glucan a characteristic fungal cell wall constituent could be rapidly detected in invasive fungal infection using a modification of the chromogenic limulus lysate test [64]. False positive and negative results occur for all these imunoassays such that a single result cannot be interpreted in isolation. Careful evaluation of all these tests is required in parallel to assess the diagnostic clinical utility in different patient groups [65].

Molecular techniques have opened the way for rapid and sensitive diagnosis of a variety of opportunist pathogens but progress with the detection of fungal DNA by the polymerase chain reaction (PCR) has been hampered by problems with extracting fungal DNA from human samples and with contamination of specimens [66]. A variety of *Candida* genes have been identified as targets for amplification including HSP-90 [67], actin [68] and cytochrome P-450 lanosterol-alpha-demethylase genes [69] but few if any have succeeded in detecting less than 10 cfu/ml particularly in biological specimens. Most exciting is the possibility of screening specimens using a "universal" fungal primer to amplify highly conserved multicopy ribosomal DNA followed by differentiating by hybridization using species-specific probes or amino acid sequencing. Early studies using this technique reported it to the highly sensitive (1 cfu/ml blood) and with high specificity for a wide range of fungal pathogens [70]. Larger studies to compare various methods and confirm the usefulness of this approach in the rapid diagnosis of infection are awaited [71].

TREATMENT

Several phases of treatment have been proposed [72] representing a continuum of therapy of increasing intensity.

Prophylaxis is reserved for severely immunocompromised patients such as liver transplant patients and those with prolonged neutropenia. The ideal antifungal for prophylaxis should be broad-spectrum, fungicidal, well tolerated and cheap with good bioavailability and a low risk of resistance developing. Unfortunately, few if any of the currently available preparations fulfil these criteria. Randomized studies have suggested that azoles are superior to topical agents in the prevention of superficial and systemic infections and fluconazole is most frequently used in this situation. Several studies have shown a decrease in superficial and systemic candidosis in patients with haematological malignancy [73] and usage is frequent in high-risk liver transplant patients [74]. Fluconazole is the only agent that has been proven to be cost effective as prophylaxis [75]. Against this is the study by Schaffner and Schaffner that suggested that fluconazole prophylaxis increased the duration of neutropenia and infection-related health care costs [76]. Despite an uneasy consensus on this approach there is no randomized evidence to support a survival benefit [77]. Increasing concerns that overuse of azole agents will contribute to the pathogen shift and emergence of resistance suggests that systemic prophylaxis in critical care patients should be reserved for those subgroups in whom a clear benefit can be demonstrated. Pre-emptive therapy represents the most logical approach to treatment of fungal infection in the ICU. It involves identifying patients likely to have fungal infection through evaluation of risk factors and surveillance of colonizing flora. Typical patients for consideration of pre-emptive therapy are shown in Table 3.

Empirical therapy is associated with the management of neutropenic fever but may occasionally be used in other ICU patients considered to be at extreme risk of morbidity and mortality but in whom there is no direct evidence of fungal infection. Definitive therapy is reserved for patients with conclusive evidence of invasive disease in the form of fungaemia, histological evidence of invasion or isolation from another sterile site. A large number of new antifungal agents some utilizing novel targets or new preparations of existing drugs [78] have appeared in recent years. Nevertheless, the practical choice in critical care patients lies between amphotericin B preparations and the azole drugs particularly, fluconazole [79].

The triazoles fluconazole and itraconazole, like other azole antifungals, block ergosterol synthesis by inhibiting cytochrome P450 enzymes. Both have a good safety and tolerability profile. Itraconazole has a broader spectrum of activity and is active against *Candida* and *Aspergillus* sp. and other filamentous and dimorphic fungi.

TABLE 3. Criteria for pre-emptive therapy

Persistent pyrexia and leucocytosis and grossly elevated CRP
Persistent funguria or repeated isolation from abdominal drain specimens
Patients colonised with *C. tropicalis*
Patients colonized with other yeast species at two or more non-contiguous sites
or
Patients with a colonization index greater than 0.5 or isolation from intravascular catheter tips

Until recently the lack of an intravenous preparation limited the usefulness of itraconazole in critically ill patients and experience in the ICU is limited. Fluconazole has been has been widely used and randomized controlled trials support its use in the treatment of yeast infections in ICU patients showing equivalent efficacy and a superior safety profile compared to amphotericin B [80]. It can be used safely in neonates [81] where the pharmacokinetics after oral administration paralleled those after intravenous dosing [82]. Much of the published data pre-dates the significant pathogen shift that has occurred and it may be unwise to extrapolate results to the present situation. The spectrum of activity of fluconazole is more limited and whilst active against most *C. albicans* strains in non-HIV positive individuals some non-albicans species (*C. krusei*) are intrinsically resistant and some (*C. glabrata*) rapidly acquire resistance. Yet other species such as *C. tropicalis* show variable susceptibility patterns. Resistance may develop due to a number of mechanisms, notably mutations in the cytochrome P450 enzymes (which confers cross-resistance to other azole drugs) or the presence of an efflux pump mechanism (which may be selective for a fluconazole or a multidrug transporter causing loss of susceptibility to other azoles). Resistant *C. albicans* strains are reported only after prolonged courses of treatment and are rarely a problem in non-HIV infected critically ill patients. Failure of fluconazole therapy is usually due to inadequate dosage or duration of therapy [83]. Dosages of 400 mg/day (6 mg/kg/day in neonates) are recommended in the UK but higher dosages may be needed in hypercatabolic patients particularly those receiving continuous renal replacement therapy which will remove the drug effectively [84]. Dosages of 800 mg/day can be used safely [79, 85] and haemofiltration [83] or continuous peritoneal dialysis [86] are not necessarily an indication for dose reduction. Nevertheless, debate continues on whether fluconazole should be used as a first-line agent in empirical treatment of documented yeast infections before speciation and susceptibility is available [41].

New triazoles are under development. Voriconazole is currently under evaluation in clinical trials. Results are encouraging, and the agent has a broad spectrum of activity. Amphotericin B remains the drug of choice for resistant yeast infections, aspergillosis, cryptococcosis and most other fungal infections due to its broad spectrum of activity. Amphotericin B (AmB) was first introduced in the later 1960s. Amphotericin has fungicidal activity against most molds and yeasts and resistance is rare. A significant drawback to this drug has been toxicity, both immediate and delayed. Up to 90% of patients will experience immediate infusion-related adverse events, which include headache, fever, chills, muscle and joint pains, gastro-intestinal symptoms and hypotension. More serious side effects include nephrotoxicity, with reported rates ranging from 15 to 90%. Nephrotoxicity is manifested by a reduction in glomerular filtration rate, increasing creatinine levels and renal tubular acidosis resulting in severe electrolyte loss and a rising creatinine. Dosages of 1 mg/kg/day are generally used for empirical treatment but 0.7 mg/kg/day is usually adequate for most yeast infections (although *C. lusitaniae* may acquire resistance).

Conventional amphotericin should be given in 500 ml of 5% dextrose over 4 h and it is not necessary to protect the drug from light in infusion bags as it is stable on exposure [87]. There is no need to escalate from lower dosages over several days as this will delay establishment of effective treatment. Test doses (1 mg in 80 ml of 5% dextrose over 30–60 min) can identify hypersensitive patients. Alternatively a small portion of the first dose may be infused slowly over 10 min and then, if no reactions occur after 20 min, the rest of the infusion can be given [88].

Early reactions such as chills and fevers ("shakes and bakes") are mediated by cytokine and prostaglandin release [89]. Such reactions may be self-limiting and disappear if treatment is continued. They may be ameliorated with pethidine [90] or non-steroidal anti-inflammatory agents and antihistamines [89]. Corticosteroids, which are frequently recommended for these side effects are best avoided in patients with infection. Other acute reactions such as severe hypotension, cyanosis or bradycardia can occur and are indications for switching to alternative preparations.

Renal toxicity is the major side effect of conventional amphotericin B treatment. Although usually reversible, provided total cumulative doses do not exceed 4 g, it may take many months for the renal function to return to normal and concomitant therapies such as aminoglycosides exacerbate toxicity. Intravenous supplements of potassium and magnesium are frequently required and amiloride may be used to block the tubular loss of these electrolytes but is seldom completely effective. Dose-limiting toxicity may result in suboptimal therapy and as a result, less toxic preparations of amphotericin B have been developed. The entrapment of amhotericin B within a lipid carrier formulation has been shown to reduce early reactions and nephrotoxicity. A variety of liposomes and lipid complexes have been developed to carry the insoluble amphotericin B within a biodegradable vesicle or lipid bilayer. Liposomes are vesicles consisting of an aqueous environment surrounded by a sphere of phospholipid bilayers. Changing characteristics such as size, electrical charge, permeability and lipid composition can alter the biological and pharmacological properties of the liposomes. Three commercial preparations are available: Amphotericin B lipid complex (Abelcet®), or ABLC, consists of Amphotericin complexed with lipid bilayers in a "ribbon-like" structure. Amphotericin colloidal dispersion (Amphocil®), or ABCD, consists of a lipid complex in a disc-like structure. Finally, liposomal Amphotericin (AmBisome®), or L-AmB, is the only formulation that contains true liposomal structures [91, 92]. These presentations are costly (10–50 times the cost of conventional amphotericin) and consequently, suspensions of amphotericin B in 20% intralipid have been used. This is outside the product license of either product and results do not support this practice [93]. The pharmacokinetics of the different licensed preparations depend on the size, charge, stability and clearance lipid complex/liposome. The increased selectivity of the lipid preparations for fungal ergosterol is thought to account for the decreased toxicity associated with these products but efficacy is not necessarily increased. The improved therapeutic index that has been reported comes from the ability to administer much higher dosages of the drug and possibly from selective targeting of the liposome, through uptake by macrophages and concentration in the reticular endothelial system to sites of infection and the fungal cell wall [94].

All commercially prepared lipid-associated preparations show markedly reduced renal toxicity and dosages of 3–6 mg/kg/day can be given in the face of deteriorating renal function. Following intravenous administration, uptake of the lipid-complexed formulations of amphotericin B appears to be primarily by the reticulo-endothelial system, although plasma lipopro- teins may also have a role to play. Hence, the lipid formulations achieve higher tissue concentrations in the spleen, liver and lungs and relatively lower levels in the kidney, heart and brain. The three lipid formulations appear to have different incidences of side effects. L-AmB appears to have the lowest incidence of early reactions (reported at *c* 5–20%), despite having the fastest infusion rate of all three preparations. ABLC and ABCD appear to have a roughly equivalent incidence of early reactions as conventional amphotericin.

All three lipid formulations have a lower rate of nephrotoxicity than conventional amphotericin B, with reported incidences of 0–30%. Nephrotoxicity may be dose-related in L-AmB, while stabilization of renal function has been reported in emergency-use patients despite continuation of antifungal therapy with ABLC. An increased nephrotoxicity in association with concurrent use of tacrolimus or cyclosporin has been reported for ABCD. The mechanism for reduced renal toxicity is due partly to the lack of concentration of lipid preparations in phagocyte-poor tissues like the kidney and also to preferential binding of negatively-charged liposomal amphotericin to high-density lipoproteins (HDL), receptors, which are lacking in renal tissue [95]. This mechanism is supported by studies showing increased toxicity of amphotericin in patients with raised LDL [96]. Transient elevations of bilirubin and alkaline phosphatase have been reported with both L-AmB and ABLC, and in addition, increases in serum transaminases sufficient to warrant discontinuation of therapy have been reported.

Although all amphotericin products may be associated with a risk of anaphylaxis, allergic-type reactions may be more common with L-AmB infusions (reported rate 2%), including rash, flushing, bronchospasm, rigors and back pain [92].

Because of the significant differences in the various lipid formulations, dose-to-dose equivalence has not been demonstrated and hence, dosage recommendations should be followed for each type of preparation used.

Both liposomal and amphotericin B lipid complex have been used effectively in neonates [97–99]. However, the rationale for using expensive lipid-associated products in critical care patients and those on total renal support (haemodialysis, haemofiltration) is dubtous, especially since little is known about clearance of lipid preparations in these situations. Few randomized trials of the different products have been published and the results of comparative clinical trials [100] are necessary before the full impact and health economics of these agents can be assessed.

Other antifungal drugs may have a role in infections in critical care patients: The pyrimidine analogue flucytosine has a limited spectrum of activity confined mainly to yeast species and resistance can develop rapidly. The drug is myelosuppressive but may be useful in the combination treatment of CNS infections meningitis due to good penetration of the CSF, and infections due to *C. glabrata* or *C. lusitaniaea*. Terbinafine is an allylamine compound widely used for the treatment of superficial dermatophyte infections. However, *in vitro* susceptibility data suggest it may have a broader spectrum of activity and could be of use in the treatment of candidosis and other systemic mycoses [101]. Synergy with azole and amphotericin has been demonstrated but this has yet to be explored in the clinical situation.

New antifungal drugs in development include the echinocandidins, which inhibit beta 1,6 glucan synthesis, and the sordarins, which inhibit fungal protein synthesis. Liposomal nystatin is also under evaluation.

Chemotherapy alone is likely to be unsuccessful if other measures to control a focus of infection are not taken e.g. removal of potentially infected intravascular catheters or surgical repair of abdominal leakage. Other adjunctive therapies have advocated the use of biological response modifiers such as cytokines and growth factors to modulate the immune system in cases of fungal infection. Much attention has focused on growth factors such as G-CSF and GM-CSF, which have the potential to augment the phagocytic response to infection [102]. Of the growth factors, GM-CSF has the broadest range of activities in terms of stimulating phagocytes and fungicidal killing capacity, followed by M-CSF and G-CSF [103, 104]. Clinical data are limited but adjunctive therapy with GM-CSF in neutropenic patients and M-CSF in marrow transplant patients [105] was beneficial, especially in patients with candidosis. It is likely that growth factors and antifungal agents, including lipid preparations, act synergically.

A trial of G-CSF plus fluconazole versus fluconazole alone in the treatment of candidosis in non-neutropenic patients has been performed [106]. Although the results are not fully evaluated, early reports suggest a possible benefit in reducing ICU stay in patients with acute candidaemia. However, the anti-inflammatory effects of G-CSF (decreased TNF, increased IL1ra) [107] may be significant and such treatment could be detrimental in chronic fungal infection. Proinflammatory cytokines are likely to be more rational. Interferon-gamma is established as a useful agent in the prevention of fungal and other infections in patients with chronic granulomatous disease [108] and is effective in mouse models of disseminated candidosis [109, 110]. It is likely to be of benefit in patients with chronic infections such as patients with impaired T-cell mediated immunity [33] where other agents such as IL-12, anti-IL-4 and anti-IL-10 alone or in combination, may also have a role [111].

PREVENTION

Preventative strategies should target both exogenous and endogenous sources of infection.

It is recognized that horizontal transmission of yeasts can occur from patient to patient and via the hands of healthcare workers representing a potent source of infection. Up to 75% of nursing staff carry *Candida* on their hands with *C. parapsilosis* the most frequent species isolated [112]. This species has been implicated in outbreaks particularly on neonatal units. Basic infection control practices including good hand hygiene and attention to aseptic technique can reduce transmission of yeasts [113]. Genomic analysis of strains show that patients may become colonized with multiple strains simultaneously and several different modes of transmission may be involved [114]. DNA typing methods comparing patient strains generally reveal patient-unique strains although instances of cross-infection may be demonstrated occasionally [115]. Reduction of endogenous fungal carriage may also reduce the colonization load and prevent infection via the skin, gut and mucous membranes. Rational use of broad-spectrum antimicrobials will avoid overusage which could lead to fungal overgrowth and increase the risk of infection [116]. Selective decontamination of the digestive tract including non-absorbable antifungal agents such as nystatin and amphotericin have been suggested [117] and are advocated in many liver transplant [118] and neonatal units [119]. Further evidence from large randomized trials is required before it can be determined which subgroups of patients are likely to benefit from this approach.

Other Fungal Infections

ASPERGILLOSIS

Aspergillosis in non-neutropenic ICU patients is uncommon; a rate of 1.3% has been reported from the NNIS study and this includes immunocompromised patients [1]. *Aspergillus* species are ubiquitous environmental fungi and disease follows exposure to airborne fungal spores. Building work and hospital renovation can generate large quantities of dust that contaminate patient care areas and this has been associated with outbreaks of invasive disease [120]. Air sampling is an insensitive way of detecting this: it is often carried out only after clusters of cases appear this is generally many weeks after the contamination has occurred and a source is rarely documented.

Awareness of the problem is crucial and high-risk patients should be nursed away from areas where the potential for dust contamination exists. Outbreaks associated with building construction and renovation can affect ICUs [121] and contamination of air filters [122] and false ceiling spaces [123] have given rise to clusters of cases amongst ventilated patients and liver transplant patients [124]. Liver transplant patients represent a high risk group for invasive aspergillosis [21, 125]. Neutropenia is the major risk factor in the bone marrow transplant situation. However, more than 30% of cases of aspergillosis occur late in the transplant period after neutropenia has resolved, often in association with graft-versus-host disease and corticosteroid usage [126, 127].

Aspergillosis can occur in apparently immunocompetent hosts [128] and has been associated with steroid inhalers [129], topical application of corticosteroids [130] and influenza A disease [131]. Cutaneous disease can occur following contamination of wounds or implantation in the skin through the use of contaminated splints or dressings [132].

Diagnosis of invasive aspergillosis is difficult; many cases remain undiagnosed during life and are only revealed at autopsy. Clinical signs and symptoms are non-specific and refractory fever may be the only manifestation. Despite the frequency of pulmonary involvement, chest radiography changes are frequently unhelpful and the chest x-ray may be normal in a large proportion of patients. Cough and pleuritic chest pain are common symptoms in non-ventilated patients. CT and MRI scanning of the chest has greatly improved the clinical diagnosis and the presence of single or multiple enhancing nodules with cavitation, air crescent formation or the early CT-halo sign are strongly suggestive of filamentous fungal infection of which pulmonary aspergillosis remains by far the most common [133]. Pleural involvement and wedge-shaped infarcts are also characteristic. Since other opportunist infections (notably fusariosis, pseudallerischiosis, and nocardiosis) may occasionally give rise to similar CT appearances, diagnostic bronchoalveolar lavage remains a useful tool for attempted isolation of the organism but cultures may be negative especially in focal disease [134]. Dissemination to any organ can occur but the brain, liver and skin are common sites. In the brain, disseminated lesions may present as areas of infarction. Embolic cerebrovascular accidents are rare in thrombocytopenic patients following transplantation and CNS infarction, particularly multiple lesions, should alert the clinician to the possibility of invasive fungal disease. Skin lesions may appear as ecthyma gangrenosum-like lesions.

Blood cultures are negative (except occasionally in cases of aspergillus endocarditis). Invasive procedures to establish a definitive histological diagnosis carry a high-risk of complications and are rarely performed. Mortality remains very high in transplant patients although there is some evidence that early initiation of high-dose amphotericin (before the appearance of pulmonary infiltrates) improves outcome. Isolation from respiratory specimens including bronchoalveolar lavage (BAL) is specific but relatively insensitive. Isolation of *Aspergillus* spp from specimens including sputa, BALs and endotracheal aspirates has a positive predictive value of 82% in BMT patients [126]. This is less sensitive in other patient groups (e.g. ICU patients where colonization without invasion is not uncommon).

High-resolution CT scans of the chest are now considered the investigation of choice in the diagnosis of IPA. The proximity of lesions to major structures such as the pulmonary artery, the risk of haemorrhage and the feasibility of surgery can also be assessed. Detection of antigens, metabolites or nucleic amplification techniques has not been evaluated in critical care patient groups other than those with haematological malignancy.

CRYPTOCOCCAL INFECTION

Cryptococcal infections are generally restricted to patients with profound cellular immunodeficiency such as HIV disease but a proportion occur in apparently normal hosts. Systemic spread from a primary focus usually involves the central nervous system. Meningitis or meningoencephalitis is the typical presentations but primary pulmonary, cutaneous [135] or prostatic [136] disease can occur. Hydrocephalus secondary to meningitis is associated with increased morbidity and mortality [137]. The disease may follow a chronic relapsing course and the prostate may be a site of persistent infection and a source of recurrent relapse [138]. Diagnosis is made by detection of the cryptococcal antigen in blood and cerebrospinal fluid and treatment with amphotericin B plus flucytosine is usually effective. Patients with continued immunosuppression require long-term secondary prophylaxis with triazoles to prevent relapse.

PNEUMOCYSTIS CARINII

Pneumocystis carinii pneumonia is associated with HIV disease, post-transplant immunosuppression and other cellular immunodeficiencies. Patients on high dose corticosteroids and those with low CD4 counts due to vasculitic disease such as Wegeners granulomatosis are also at risk [139]. Infection usually presents as an interstitial pneumonitis but features can vary considerably. Progressive dyspnoea, and a dry cough are the commonest presenting symptoms but *Pneumocystis carinii* pneumonia (PCP) can also present as a fulminant infection mimicking bacterial sepsis. Fever is usually, but not invariably present. Chest radiographs show interstitial or acinar infiltrates but may be normal in the early stages [140]. Hypoxia is a feature in more than 90% of patients at presentation and may worsen rapidly on exercise and as the patient progresses to respiratory failure. Extrapulmonary pneumocystosis has occasionally been reported.

It is unclear whether PCP is a primary infection arising *de novo* or reactivation of previous asymptomatic infection. Seroprevalence studies tend to support the reactivation theory [141] but post-mortem studies using sensitive PCR techniques have failed to find evidence of *P. carinii* in the lungs of asymptomatic individuals [142]. Clusters of cases of PCP representing apparent point-source outbreaks have also been reported and support the argument for patient-to-patient transmission via the respiratory route [143]. Until it is possible to cultivate the organism reliably and identify environmental reservoirs, it is unlikely that these controversies can be resolved. PCP must be distinguished from other causes of respiratory infection. Induced sputum examination has proved useful in the HIV-positive setting but the differential diagnosis tends to be wider in transplant patients and the fungal load is less such that bronchoalveolar lavage is the preferred diagnostic procedure in this group. Diagnosis depends on demonstration of the organism in the BAL fluid using a variety of staining and immunofluorescence techniques. Molecular diagnosis by PCR is highly sensitive and specific but the test is not rapidly available at every center and so has a limited role in clinical management.

Trimethoprim-sulfamethoxazole (TMP-SMZ, 20 mg/kg trimethoprim) remains the treatment of choice for PCP. It may take several days for a response to become apparent. Patients can be switched to oral therapy after 7–10 days if responding. Pentamidine, clindamycin-primaquine and atovaquone are all suitable agents for patients unable to tolerated TMP-SMZ. The addition of corticosteroids is beneficial in the treatment of severe PCP in AIDS but efficacy has not been evaluated fully outside of this risk group.

EMERGING FUNGAL INFECTIONS

A variety of emerging pathogens have been reported as causes of infections in critical care patients. Non *Candida* yeasts including *Rhodotorula rubra*, *Malassezia furfur*, *Trichosporon beigelii* and *Hansenula anomala* are rare causes of line-associated infection [144]. *Malassezia furfur* is a lipophilic yeast whose presence may go undetected unless culture media is overlaid with olive oil to permit growth from clinical specimens. It is a recognized pathogen in neonatal units and is associated with central venous lines and lipid infusions [145]. Recently it was implicated in an outbreak of folliculitis in an adult ICU [146]. Molds such as *Fusarium* spp and the mucorales can cause syndromes similar to aspergillosis and *Scedosporium apiospermum* (*Pseudallescheria boydii*) infection may follow near-drowning incidents [147].

Conclusion

As we progress in the new millennium, there is little doubt that the problems of fungal infections in critically ill patients will go forward with us. Better surveillance techniques, effective preventative measures and prompt diagnosis and treatment of these infections is our fundamental duty.

References

1. Beck-Sague CM, Jarvis WR, and the National Nosocomial Infections Surveillance System. Secular trends in the epidemiology of nosocomial fungal infections in the United States, 1980–1990. J Infect Dis 167:1247, 1993.
2. Jarvis WR. Epidemiology of nosocomial fungal infections with emphasis on *Candida species*. Clin Infect Dis 20:1526, 1995.
3. Rees JR, Pinner RW, Hajjeh RA, Brandt ME, Reingold AL. The epidemiological features of invasive mycotic infections in the San Franscisco Bay area 1992–1993: Results of a population-based laboratory active surveillance. Clin Infect Dis 27:1138, 1998.
4. Nicolle LE, Rotstein C, Bourgault AM, St-Germain G, Garber G, *et al*. Invasive fungal infections in Canada from 1992 to 1994. Can J Infect Dis 9:347, 1998.
5. Vincent J-L, Bihari DJ, Suter PM, Bruining HA, White J, *et al*. The prevalence of nosocomial infection in intensive care units in Europe: Results of the European Prevalence of Infection in Intensive Care (EPIC) study. J Am Med Assoc 274:639, 1995.
6. Spencer RC. Predominant pathogens found in the European prevalence of infection in intensive care study. Eur J Clin Microbiology Infect Dis 15:281, 1996.
7. Pfaller M, Wenzel R. Impact of the changing epidemiology of fungal infections in the 1990s. Eur J Clin Microbiology Infect Dis 11:287, 1992.
8. Voss A, Le Noble JLML, Lunel FMV, Foudraine NA, Meis JFGM. Candidemia in intensive

care unit patients: Risk factors for mortality. Infection 25:8, 1997.
9. Nolla-Salas J, Sitges-Serra A, Leon-Gil C, Martinez-Gonzalez J, Leon-Regidor MA, *et al.* Candidemia in non-neutropenic critically ill patients: Analysis of prognostic factors and assessment of systemic antifungal therapy. Intensive Care Med 23:23, 1997.
10. Ronnestad A, Abrahamsen TG, Gaustad P, Finne PH. Blood culture isolates during 6 years in a tertiary neonatal intensive care unit. Scan J Infect Dis 30:245, 1998.
11. Wey SB, Mori M, Pfaller MA, Woolson RF, Wenzel RP. Risk factors for hospital acquired candidemia. A matched case-control study. Archives Internal Med 149:2349, 1989.
12. Pittet D, Li N, Woolson RF, Wenzel RP. Microbiological factors influencing the outcome of nosocomial bloodstream infections. A six year, validated, population based model. Clin Infect Dis 24:1068, 1997.
13. Price MF, LaRocca MT, Gentry LO. Fluconazole susceptibilities of *Candida species* and distribution of species recovered from blood cultures over a 5-year period. Antimicrobial Agents Chemo 38:1422, 1994.
14. Wingard JR, Merz WG, Rinaldi MG, Johnson TR, *et al.* Increase in *Candida krusei* infection among patients with bone marrow transplantation and neutropenia treated prophylactically with fluconazole. New England J Med 325:1274, 1991.
15. Wingard JR, Merz WG, Rinaldi MG, Miller CB, Karp JE, Saral R. Association of *Torulopsis glabrata* infections with fluconazole prophylaxis in neutropenic bone marrow transplant patients. Antimicrobial Agents Chemo 37: 1847, 1993.
16. Odds FC. Epidemiological shifts in opportunistic and nosocomial Candida infections: Mycological aspects. Int J Antimicrobial Agents 6:141, 1996.
17. Boschman CR, Bodnar UR, Tornatore MA, Obias AA, Noskin GA, *et al.* Thirteen-year evolution of azole resistance in yeast isolates and prevalence of resistant strains carried by cancer patients at a large medical center. Antimicrobial Agents Chemo 42:734, 1998.
18. Vincent J-L, Anaissie E, Bruining H, Demajo W, El-Ebiary M, *et al.* Epidemiology, diagnosis and treatment of systemic *Candida* infection in surgical patients under intensive care. Intensive Care Med 24:206, 1998.
19. Fraser VJ, Jones M, Dunkel J, Storfer S, Medoff G, Dunagan WC. Candidemia in a tertiary care hospital: Epidemiology, risk factors, and predictors of mortality. Clin Infect Dis 15:414, 1992.
20. Jantunen E, Ruutu P, Niskanen L, Volin L, Parkkali T, *et al.* Incidence and risk factors for invasive fungal infections in allogeneic BMT recipients. Bone Marrow Transplantation 19:801, 1997.
21. Collins LA, Samore MH, Roberts MS, Luzzati R, Jenkins RL, *et al.* Risk factors for invasive fungal infections complicating othotopic liver transplantation. J Infect Dis 170:644, 1994.
22. Huang Y-C, Li C-C, Lin T-Y, Lien R-I, Chou Y-H, *et al.* Association of fungal colonization and invasive disease in very low birth weight infants. Ped Infect Dis J 17:819, 1998.
23. Petri MG, Konig J, Moecke HP, Gramm HJ, Barkow H, *et al.* Epidemiology of invasive mycosis in ICU patients: A prospective multicenter study in 435 non-neutropenic patients. Intensive Care Med 23:317, 1997.
24. Calandra T, Bille J, Schneider R, Mossiman F, Francoli P. Clinical significance of *Candida isolated* from the peritoneum in surgical patients. Lancet ii:1437, 1989.
25. Voss A, Hollis RJ, Pfaller MA, Wenzel RP, Doebbeling BN. Investigation of the sequence of colonization and candidemia in nonneutropenic patients. J Clin Microbiology 32:975, 1994.
26. Garbino J, Pittet D. Candida infections in the ICU. Clin Intensive Care 8:187, 1997.
27. Pittet D, Monod M, Suter PM, Frenk E, Auckenthaler R. Candida colonization and subsequent infections in critically ill surgical patients. Annals Surgery 220:751, 1994.
28. VanSaene HKF, Damjanovic V, Pizer B, Petros AJ. Fungal infections in ICU. J Hospital Infect 41:337, 1999.
29. Romagnani S. The Th1/Th2 paradigm. Immunology Today 18:263, 1997.
30. Allen JE, Maizels RM. Th1–Th2: Reliable paradigm or dangerous dogma? Immunology Today 18:387, 1997.
31. Cenci E, Mencacci A, Spaccapelo R, Tonnetti L, Mosci P, *et al.* T helper type 1 (TH1) and TH2-like responses are present in mice with gastric candidasis and protective immunity is associated with TH1 development. J Infect Dis 171:1279, 1995.
32. Romani L, Cenci E, Mencacci A, Spaccapelo R, Grohmann U, *et al.* Gamma-interferon modifies

CD4+ subset expression in murine candidiasis. Infect Immunity 60(ii): 4950, 1993.
33. Poynton CH, Barnes RA, Rees J. Interferon gamma in the treatment of deep-seated fungal infection in acute leukemia. Clin Infect Dis 26:239, 1998.
34. Utsunomiya T, Kobayashi M, Herndon DN, Pollard RB, Suzuki F. Effects of glycyrrhizin, an active component of licorice roots, on *Candida albicans* infection in thermally injured mice. Clin Experimental Immunology 116:291, 1999.
35. Shareef MJ, Myers TF, Mathews HL, Witek-Janusek L. Reduced capacity of neonatal lymphocytes to inhibit the growth of *Candida albicans*. Biol Neonate 75:31, 1999.
36. Freidank H, Thiel L, Henninger S. Comparison of immunodiffusion and counterimmunoelectrophoresis in demonstrating precipitating antibodies against Candida and *Aspergillus* antigens. Mycoses 37(suppl 1):79, 1994.
37. Weis C, Kappe R, Sonntag H-G. Western blot analysis of the immune response to *Candida albicans* antigens in 391 long-term intensive care patients. Mycoses 40:153, 1997.
38. Matthews RC, Maresca B, Burnie JP, Cardona A, Carratu L, *et al*. Stress proteins in fungal diseases. Medical Mycology 36(suppl):45, 1998.
39. Martinez JP, Gil ML, Lopez-Ribot JL, LaJean Chaffin W. Serologic response to cell wall mannoproteins and proteins of *Candida albicans*. Clin Microbiology Rev 11:121, 1998.
40. Pittet D, Garbino J. Fungal infections in the critically ill. Current Opinion Crit Care 1:369, 1995.
41. Flanagan PG, Barnes RA. Fungal infections in the intensive care unit. J Hosp Infect 38:163, 1998.
42. Ronnestad A, Abrahamsen TG, Gaustad P, Finne PH. C-reactive protein (CRP) response patterns in neonatal septicaemia. APMIS 107: 593, 1999.
43. Henderson VJ. Emerging and reemerging microbial threats. Nosocomial fungal infections. Archives Surg 131:330, 1996.
44. Walsh TJ, Chanock SJ. Laboratory diagnosis of invasive candidiasis: a rationale for complementary use of culture- and non-culture based detection systems. Intl J Infect Dis 1(suppl 1):S11, 1997.
45. Dean DA, Burchard KW. Fungal infections in surgical patients. Am J Surg 171:374, 1996.
46. Donahue SP, Greven CM, Zuravleff JJ, Eller AW, Nguyen MH, *et al*. Intraocular candidasis in patients with candidemia: clinical implications derived from a prospective, multicenter study. Ophthamology 101:1302, 1994.
47. Rex JH, Bennett JE, Sugar AM, Pappas PG, van der Horst CM, *et al*. A randomized trial comparing fluconazole with amphotericin B for the treatment of candidemia in patients without neutropenia. New England J Med 331:1325, 1994.
48. Calandra T. Candida infection in the intensive care unit. Current Opinion Crit Care 3:335, 1997.
49. Hiatt JR, Kobayashi MR, Doty JE, Ramming KP. Acalculous candida cholecystitis: a complication of critical surgical illness. Am J Surg 57:825, 1991.
50. Nassoura Z, Ivatury RR, Simon RJ, Jabbour N, Stahl WM. Candiduria as an early marker of disseminated infection in critically ill surgical patients: the role of fluoconazole therapy. J Trauma 35:290, 1993.
51. Ang BB, Telenti A, King B, Steckelberg JM, Wilson WR. Candidemia from a urinary tract source: microbiological aspects and clinical significance. Clin Infect Dis 17:662, 1993.
52. Rello J, Esandi M-E, Diaz E, Mariscal D, Gallego M, Valles J. The role of *Candida spp* isolated from bronchoscopic samples in nonneutropenic patients. Chest 114:146, 1998.
53. Haron E, Vartivarian S, Anaissie E, Dekmezian R, Bodey GP. Primary Candida pneumonia: Experience at a large cancer center and review of the literature. Med 72:137, 1993.
54. Bauer TT, Torres A. Candida pneumonia. Clin Intensive Care 10:33, 1999.
55. Geha DJ, Roberts DT. Laboratory detection of fungaemia. Clin Lab Med 14:83, 1994.
56. Wilson ML, Davis TE, Mirrett S, Reynolds J, Fuller D, *et al*. Controlled comparison of the BACTEC high-blood-volume fungal medium, BACTEC Plus 26 aerobic blood culture bottle, and 10 milliliter isolator blood culture system for detection of fungemia and bacteremia. J Clin Microbiology 31:865, 1993.
57. Burnie JP. Early diagnosis of fungal infection. Current Opinion Infect Dis 8:258, 1995.
58. Girmenia C, Martino P, De Bernardis F, Cassone A. Assessment of detection of Candida mannoproteinemia as a method to differentiate central venous catheter-related candidemia from invasive disease. J Clin Microbiology 35:903, 1997.
59. Sendid B, Tabouret M, Poirot JL, Mathieu D, Fruit J, Poulain D. New enzyme immunoassays

for sensitive detection of circulating Candida albicans mannan and antimannan antibodies: Useful combined test for diagnosis of systemic candidiasis. J Clin Microbiology 37:1510, 1999.
60. Tokunaga S, Ohkawa M, Takashima M, Seto C, Nakamura S. D-arabinitol versus mannan antigen and candidal protein antigen as a serum marker for Candida pyelonephritis. Eur J Clin Microbiology Infect Dis 14:118, 1995.
61. Grundy MA, Barnes RA, Coakley WT. Highly sensitive detection of fungal antigens by ultrasound-enhanced latex agglutination. J Med Vet Mycology 33:201, 1995.
62. Walsh TJ, Lyman CA, Pizzo PA. Laboratory diagnosis of invasive fungal infections in patients with neoplastic diseases. Baillieres Clin Infect Dis 2:25, 1995.
63. Reiss E, Morrison CJ. Nonculture methods for diagnosis of disseminated candidiasis. Clin Microbiological Rev 6:311, 1993.
64. Obayashi T, Yoshida M, Mori T, Goto H, Yasuoka A, *et al.* Plasma (1-3)-beta-D-glucan measurement in diagnosis of invasive deep mycosis and fungal febrile episodes. Lancet 345:17, 1995.
65. Mitsutake K, Miyazaki T, Tashiro T, Yamamoto Y, Kakeya H, *et al.* Enolase antigen, mannan antigen, Cand-Tec antigen, and beta-glucan in patients with candidemia. J Clin Microbiology 34:1918, 1996.
66. Loeffler J, Hebart H, Bialek R, Hagmeyer L, Schmidt D, *et al.* Contaminations occurring in fungal PCR assays. J Clin Microbiology 37:1200, 1999.
67. Crampin AC, Matthews RC. Application of the polymerase chain reaction to the diagnosis of candidosis by amplification of a HSP 90 gene fragment. J Med Microbiology 39:233, 1993.
68. Kan VL. Polymerase chain reaction for the diagnosis of candidemia. J Infect Dis 168:779, 1993.
69. Burgener-Kairuz P, Zuber J-P, Jaunin P, Buchman TG, Bille J, Rossier M. Rapid detection and identification of *Candida albicans* and *Torulopsis* (*Candida*) *glabrata* in clinical specimens by species-specific nested PCR-amplification of a cytochrome P-450 lanosterol-alpha-demethylase (L1A1) gene fragment. J Clin Microbiology 32:1902, 1994.
70. Einsele H, Hebart H, Roller, Loffler J, Rothenhofer I, *et al.* Detection and identification of fungal pathogens in using molecular probes. J Clin Microbiology 35:1353, 1997.
71. Chryssanthou E, Klingspor L, Tollemar J, Petrini B, Larsson L, *et al.* PCR and other non-culture methods for diagnosis of invasive Candida infections in allogeneic bone marrow and solid organ transplant recipients. Mycoses 42:239, 1999.
72. British Society for Antimicrobial Chemotherapy Working Party. Management of deep *Candida* infection in surgical and intensive care unit patients. Intensive Care Med 20:522, 1994.
73. Uzun O, Anaissie EJ. Antifungal prophylaxis in patients with haematological malignancies: a reappraisal. 86:2063, 1995.
74. Tollemar J. Prophylaxis against fungal infections in transplant recipients: Possible approaches. Biodrugs 11:309, 1999.
75. Stewart A, Powles R, Hewetson M, Antrum J, Richardson C, Mehta J. Costs of antifungal prophylaxis after bone marrow transplantation: A model comparing oral fluconazole, liposomal amphotericin and oral polyenes as prophylaxis against oropharyngeal infections. Pharmaco-Economics 8:350, 1995.
76. Schaffner A, Schaffner M. Effect of prophylactic fluconazole on the frequency of fungal infections, amphotericn B use and health care costs in patients undergoing intensive chemotherapy for hematologic neoplasias. J Infect Dis 172: 1035, 1995.
77. Gotzsche PC, Krogh Johansen H. Meta-analysis of prophylactic or empirical antifungal treatment versus placebo or no treatment in patients with cancer complicated by neutropenia. Brit Med J 314:1238, 1997.
78. Andriole VT. Current and future antifungal: new targets for antifungal agents. J Antimicrobial Chemo 44:151, 1999.
79. Edwards JE Jr, Bodey GP, Bowden RA, Buchner T, De Pauw BE, *et al.* International conference for the development of a consensus on the management and prevention of severe candidal infections. Clin Infect Dis 25:43, 1997.
80. Rex JH, Bennett JE, Sugar AM, Pappas PG, van der Horst CM, *et al.* A randomized trial comparing fluconazole with amphotericin B for the treatment of candidemia in patients without neutropenia. New England J Med 331:1325, 1994.
81. Huttova M, Hartmanova I, Kralinsky K, Filka J, Uher J, *et al.* Candida fungemia in neonates treated with fluconazole: Report of forty cases. Ped Infect Dis J 17:1012, 1998.

82. Nahata MC, Tallian KB, Force RW. Pharmacokinetics of fluconazole in young infants. Eur J Drug Metabolism Pharmacokinetcs 24:155, 1999.
83. Flanagan PG, Barnes RA. Hazards of inadequate fluconazole dosage to treat deep-seated or systemic *Candida albicans* infection. J Infect 35:295, 1997.
84. Pittrow L, Penk A. Dosage adjustment of fluconazole during continuous renal replacement therapy (CAVH, CVVH, CAVHD, CVVHD). Mycoses 42:17, 1999.
85. Martins M, Rex JH. Resistance to antifungal agents in the critical care setting: problems and perspectives. New Horizons 4:338, 1996.
86. Wong S-F, Leung MP, Chan M-Y. Pharmacokinetics of fluconazole in chidren requiring peritoneal dialysis. Clin Therapeutics 19:1039, 1997.
87. Shadomy S, Brummer DL, Ingroff AV. Light sensitivity of prepared solutions of amphotericin B. Am Rev Resp Dis 197:303, 1973.
88. British Society for Antimicrobial Chemotherapy Working Party. Therapy of deep fungal infection in haematological malignancy. J Antimicrobial Chemo 40:779, 1997.
89. Gigliotti F, Shenep JL, Lott L, Thornton D. Induction of prostaglandin synthesis in the mechanism responsible for the chills and fevers produced by infusing amphotericin. J Infect Dis 156:784, 1987.
90. Bunks LC, Aisner J, Fortner CL, Wiernik PH. Meperidine for the treatment of shaking chills and fever. Archives Internal Med 140:483, 1980.
91. van Burik JH, Bowden RA. Standard antifungal treatment, including role of alternative modalities to administer amphotericin B. Balliere's Clin Infect Dis 2:89, 1995.
92. Wong-Beringer A, Jacobs RA, Guglielmo BJ. Lipid formulations of amphotericin B: Clinical efficacy and toxicity. (Review). Clin Infect Dis 27:603, 1998.
93. Moreau P, Milpied N, Fayette N, Ramee J-F, Harousseau J-L. Reduced renal toxicity and improved clinical tolerance of amphotericin B in neutropenic patients. J Antimicrobial Chemo 30:535, 1992.
94. Adler-Moore JP, Proffitt RT. Development, characterization, efficacy and mode of action of AmBisome, a unilamellar liposomal formulation of amphotericin B. J Liposome Research 3:429, 1993.
95. Wasan KM, Motron RE, Rosenblum MG, Lopez-Berestein G. Decreased toxicity of liposomal amphotericin B due to association of amphotericin B with high-density lipoproteins: Role of lipid transfer protein. J Pharmaceutical Sci 83:1006, 1994.
96. Wasan KM, Conklin JS. Enhanced amphotericin B nephrotoxicity in intensive care patients with elevated levels of low-density lipoprotein cholesterol. Clin Infect Dis 24:78, 1997.
97. Scarcella A, Pasquariello MB, Giugliano B, Vendemmia M, De Lucia A. Liposomal amphotericin B for the treatment of neonatal fungal infections. Ped Infect Dis J 17:146, 1998.
98. Weitkamp J-H, Poets CF, Sievers R, Musswessels E, Groneck P, *et al.* Candida infection in very low birth-weight infants: Outcome and nephrotoxicity of treatment with liposomal amphotericin B (AmBisome™). Infect 26:11, 1998.
99. Herbrecht R, Letscher V, Andres E, Cavalier A. Safety and efficiency of amphotericin B colloidal dispersion: an overview. Chemotherapy: 45(suppl 1):67, 1999.
100. Walsh TJ, Hiemenz JW, Seibel NL, Perfect JR, Horwith G, *et al.* Amphotericin B lipid complex for invasive fungal infections: Analysis of safety and efficacy in 556 cases. Clin Infect Dis 26:1383, 1998.
101. Balfour JA, Faulds D. Terbinafine: A review of its pharmacodynamic and pharmacokinetic properties and therapeutic potential in superficial mycoses. Drugs 43:259, 1992.
102. Roilides E, Walsh TJ, Pizzo PA. Clinical use of cytokines during fungal infection. In Van Furth R (ed). Hemopoietic Growth Factors and Mononuclear Phagocytes Basel: Karger.
103. Stevens DA, Walsh TJ, Bistoni F, Cenci E, Clemons KV, Del Sero G, Fe d'Ostiani C, Kullberg BJ, Mencacci A, Roilides E, Romani L. Cytokines and mycoses. Med Mycology Suppl 36:174, 1998.
104. Bodey GP, Anaissie E, Gutterman J, Vadhan-Raj S. Role of granulocyte-macrophage colony-stimulating factor as adjuvant therapy for fungal infection in patients with cancer. Clin Infect Dis 17:705, 1993.
105. Nemunaitis J, Shannon-Dorcy K, Appelbaum FR. Long-term follow-up of patients with invasive fungal disease who received adjunctive therapy with recombinant human macrophage colony-stimulating factor. Blood 82:1422, 1993.
106. Kullberg BJ, Vandewoude K, Aoun M, Jacobs

F, Herbrecht R, Kujath P for the European filgrastim candidiasis study group. A double-blind, randomised, placebo-controlled, phase II study of filgrastim (recombinant granulocyte colony-stimulating factor) in combination with fluconazole for treatment of invasive candidiasis and candidemia in non-neutropenic patients. 38th Interscience Confenernce on Antimicrobial agents and Chemotherapy, San Diego; abstract J-100, 1998.
107. Hartung T, Docke W-D, Gantner F, Krieger G, Sauer A, *et al.* Effect of granulocyte colony-stimulating factor treatment on *ex vivo* blood cytokine response in human volunteers. Blood 85:2482, 1995.
108. Gallin JI, Malech HL, Weening RS, Curnutte JT, Quie PG, *et al.* The International Chronic Granulomatous Disease Cooperative Study Group. A controlled trial of interferon gamma to prevent infection in chronic granulomatous disease. New Engl J Med 324:509, 1991.
109. Kullberg BJ, van't Wout JW, Hoogstraten C. Recombinant interferon gamma enhances resistance to acute disseminated *Candida albicans* infection in mice. J Infect Dis 168:436, 1993.
110. Van der Meer JWM, Vogels MTE, Netea MG, Kullberg BJ. Proinflammatory cytokines and treatment of disease. Annals New York Acad Sci 856:243, 1998.
111. Cenci E, Mencacci A, Del Sero G, Bistoni F, Romani L. Induction of protective Th1 responses to *Candida albicans* by antifungal therapy alone or in combination with an Interleukin-4 antagonist. J Infect Dis 176:217, 1997.
112. Strasbaugh LJ, Sewell DL, Ward TT, Pfaller MA, Heitzman T, Tjoelker R. High frequency of yeast carriage on the hands of hospital personnel. J Clin Microbiology 32:2299, 1994.
113. Pfaller MA. Epidemiology and control of fungal infection. Clin Infect Dis 19(suppl 1):S1, 1994.
114. Khatib R, Thirumoorthi MC, Riederer KM, Sturm L, Oney LA, Baran J Jr. Clustering of Candida infections in the neonatal intensive care unit: Concurrent emergence of multiple strains simulating intermittent outbreaks. Ped Infect Dis J 17:130, 1998.
115. Pfaller MA, Messer SA, Houston A, Rangel-Frausto MS, Wiblin T, *et al.* National epidemiological of mycoses survey: A multicentre study of strain variation and antifungal susceptibility among isolates of *Candida species*. Diagnostic Microbiology Infect Dis 31:289, 1998.
116. Van Saene R, Fairclough S, Petros A. Broad- and narrow-spectrum antibiotics: A different approach. Clin Microbiology Infect 4:56, 1998.
117. Lingnau W, Berger J, Javorsky F, Fille M, Allerberger F, Benzer H. Changing bacterial ecology during a five year period of selective intestinal decontamination. J Hosp Infect 39: 195, 1998.
118. Arnow PM, Carandang GC, Zabner R, Irwin ME. Randomized controlled trial of selective bowel decontamination for prevention of infections following liver transplantation. Clin Infect Dis 22:997, 1996.
119. Damjanovic V, Connolly CM, van Saene HKF, Cooke RWI, Corkill JE, *et al.* Selective decontamination with nystatin for control of a Candida outbreak in a neonatal intensive care unit. J Hosp Infect 24:245, 1993.
120. Manuel RJ, Kibbler CC. The epidemiology and prevention of invasive aspergillosis. J Hosp Infect 39:95, 1998.
121. Harvey IM, Leadbeatter S, Peters TJ, Mullins J, Philpot CM, Salaman JR. An outbreak of disseminated aspergillosis associated with an intensive care unit. Community Med 10:306, 1988.
122. Pittet D, Huguenin T, Dharan S, Sztajzel-Boissard J, Ducel G, *et al.* Unusual cause of lethal pulmonary aspergillosis in patients with chronic obstructive pulmonary disease. Am J Resp Crit Care Med 154:541, 1996.
123. Humpreys H, Johnson EM, Warnock DW, Willatts SM, Winter RJ, Spelller DCE. An outbreak of aspergillosis in a general ICU. J Hosp Infect 18:167, 1991.
124. Fitzpatrick F, Prout S, Gilleece A, Fenelon LE, Murphy OM. Nosocomial aspergillosis during building work – A multidisciplinary approach. J Hosp Infect 42:170, 1999.
125. Lorf T, Braun F, Ruchel R, Muller A, Sattler B, Ringe B. Systemic mycoses during prophylactica use of liposomal amphotericin B (ambisome(TM)) after liver transplantation. Mycoses 42:47, 1999.
126. Von Eiff M, Roos N, Fegeler W, Von Eiff C, Zuhlsdorf M, *et al.* Pulmonary fungal infections in immunocompromised patients: Incidence and risk factors. Mycoses 37:329, 1994.
127. Ribaud P, Chastang C, Latge J-P, Baffroy-Lafitte L, Parquet N, *et al.* Survival and prognostic factors of invasive aspergillosis after allogeneic bone marrow transplantation. Clin Infect Dis 28: 322, 1999.

128. Hovenden JL, Nicklason F, Barnes RA. Invasive aspergillosis in non-immunocompromised patients. Brit Med J 302:583, 1991.
129. Fairfax AJ, David V, Douce G. Laryngeal aspergillosis following high dose inhaled fluticasone therapy for asthma. Thorax 54:860, 1999.
130. Lewis MB, Henderson B. Invasive intracranial aspergillosis secondary to intranasal corticosteroids. J Neurology, Neurosurgery Psychiatry 67:416, 1999.
131. Funabiki Y, Ishii K, Kusaka S, Hakamata Y, Wakatsuki Y, *et al.* Aspergillosis following a influenza infection. Jap J Geriatrics 36:274, 1999.
132. Munn S, Keane F, Child F, Philpott-Howard J, Du Vivier A. Primary cutaneous aspergillosis. Brit J Dermatol 141:378, 1999.
133. Barloon TJ, Galvin RG, Mori M, Stanford W, Gingrich RD. High-resolution ultrafast chest CT in the clinical management of febrile bone marrow transplant patients with normal or nonspecific chest roentgenograms. Chest 99:928, 1991.
134. McWhinney PHM, Kibbler CC, Hamon MD, Smith OP, Gandy L, *et al.* Progress in the diagnosis and management of aspergillosis in bone marrow transplantation: 13 years experience. Clin Infect Dis 17:397, 1993.
135. Bellosta M, Gaviglio MR, Mosconi M, Cavanna C, Viglio A, Rabbiosi G. Primary cutaneous cryptococcosis in an HIV-negative patient. Eur J Dermatol 9:224, 1999.
136. Caballes RL, Caballes RA. Primary cryptococcal prostatitis in an apparently uncompromised host. Prostate 39:119, 1999.
137. Park MK, Hospenthal DR, Bennett JE. Treatment of hydrocephalus secondary to cryptococcal meningitis by use of shunting. Clin Infect Dis 28:629, 1999.
138. Yip SKH, Cheng C, Wong MYC, Tan BH, Sim CS, Lim SH. Cryptococcal prostatic abscess in an immunocompromised patient: A case report and review of the literature. Annals Acad Med Singapore 27:873, 1998.
139. Sneller MC. Wegeners granulomatosis. J Am Med Assoc 273:1288, 1995.
140. Opravil M, Marincek B, Fuchs WA, Weber R, Speich R, Battegay M, *et al.* Shortcomings of chest radiography in detecting *Pneumocystis carinii* pneumonia. J Acquired Immune Deficiency Syndromes 7:39, 1994.
141. Peglow SL, Smulian AG, Linke MJ, Pogue CL, Nurr S, *et al.* Serologic response to *Pneumocystis carinii* antigens in health and disease. J Infect Dis 161:296, 1990.
142. Peters SE, Wakefield AE, Sinclair K, Millard PR, Hopkin JM. A search for *Pneumocystis carinii* in post-mortem lungs by DNA amplification. J Pathology 166:195, 1992.
143. Helweg-Larsen J, Tsolaki AG, Miller RF, Lundgren B, Wakefield AE. Clusters of *Pneumocystis carinii* pneumonia: Analysis of person-to-person transmission by genotyping. Qjm-Monthly J Assoc Physicians 91:813, 1998.
144. Klein NC, Gill MV, Cunha BA. Unusual organisms causing intravenous line infections in compromised hosts: II. Fungal infections. Infect Dis Clin Practice 5:303, 1996.
145. Gueho E, Boekhout T, Ashbee HR, Guillot J, Van Belkum A, Faergemann J. The role of *Malassezia species* in the ecology of human skin and as pathogens. Med Mycology Suppl 36: 220, 1998.
146. Archer-Dubon C, Icaza-Chivez ME, Orozco-Topete R, Reyes E, Baez-Martinez R, *et al.* An epidemic outbreak of Malassezia folliculitis in three adult patients in an intensive care unit: A previously unrecognized nosocomial infection. Int J Dermatol 38:453, 1999.
147. Wilichowski E, Christen H-J, Schiffmann H, Schulz-Schaeffer W, Behrens-Baumann W. Fatal *Pseudallescheria boydii* panencephalitis in a child after near-drowning. Ped Infect Dis J 15:365, 1996.

5. INFECTIONS IN CRITICALLY ILL SOLID ORGAN TRANSPLANT RECIPIENTS

Nina Singh

Introduction

The advent of modern immunosuppressive drugs, improvement in surgical technique, availability of rapid and reliable diagnostic assays, and advances in prophylactic strategies against a number of pathogens have collectively contributed towards a striking decline in infectious morbidity in transplant recipients in recent years. The epidemiologic trends in infectious diseases through the last decade have been most notable for a dramatic decrease in the incidence of several opportunistic infections, e.g. cytomegalovirus and *Pneumocystis carinii*, due largely to the advent of effective prophylaxis. However, recognition of novel microorganisms as potential pathogens and escalating rates of antimicrobial resistance, that largely parallels the more widespread national and global trends in nosocomially acquired infections, has altered the spectrum and therefore our approach towards the management of infections in transplant recipients.

Nosocomial infections, primarily bacterial, have now emerged as leading sources of infections after transplantation. Fifty-three per cent of all infections in heart transplant recipients in one report were nosocomially acquired and of these, 63% were bacterial [1]. In a report in liver transplant recipients, 82% of all febrile episodes over a two year period were nosocomial, of which 62% were bacterial in etiology [2]. Within the same institution, transplant recipients have been shown to have a significantly higher incidence of nosocomial infections than nontransplant patients [3].

Intensive care units (ICU) are an integral part of the management of organ transplant recipients. These critical care areas have also come to represent the most common source of nosocomial infections, with infection rates several fold higher than in other hospitalized patients. Thus, the vulnerability of transplant recipients to opportunistic infections compounded by the superimposed risk of nosocomial infections in critical care setting, poses unique diagnostic and therapeutic challenges in these patients.

Risk Factors for Infections

UNDERLYING DISEASE AND ITS SEQUELAE AS RISK FACTORS FOR POST-TRANSPLANT INFECTIONS. IMPACT OF PRETRANSPLANT ANTIBIOTIC USE

Transplant recipients, even prior to transplantation, are compromised hosts by virtue of preexisting underlying diseases that render them vulnerable to infections. Consequently, these patients are exposed to frequent and often prolonged courses of antibiotics. Antibiotics exposure in pretransplant setting has significant implications for the emergence and subsequent infections due to antimicrobial resistant bacteria in the post-transplant period. Prophylaxis for spontaneous bacterial peritonitis with quinolones in patients with endstage liver disease has been associated with a significantly higher risk of infection due to Gram-positive cocci and quinolone resistant enteric Gram-negative bacteria [4].

The recent and alarming problem of extended-spectrum beta-lactamase (ESBL) production by Gram-negative bacteria also has implications relevant for transplant recipients. ESBLs are mutations of simple beta-lactamases (TEM or SHV-1) which hydrolyze all penicillins and other beta-lactam agents. The genes encoding these beta lactamases are carried on large plasmids, which in over 50% of the cases harbor resistance to trimethoprim and aminoglycosides as well. Up to 33% of these isolates may also be resistant to quinolones. ESBLs are most frequently detected in *K. pneumoniae*, but have been reported in several Gram-negative bacilli. In one report, 28% of all *K. pneumoniae* blood isolates from patients in transplant units produced ESBL [5].

The impact of antibiotics in promoting antimicrobial resistance is perhaps best illustrated by the emergence of VREF as a major pathogen in institutions performing organ transplantation. VREF colonization once acquired, is usually a persistent event. Vancomycin, third generation cephalosporins, and notably metronidazole, have been associated with the acquisition of VREF infection [6]. Furthermore, the number and duration of antibiotics administered preoperatively has been shown to correlate significantly with the risk of VREF infection in liver transplant recipients [6].

Colonization with multiply antibiotic-resistant species of *Pseudomonas aeruginosa* and *Burkholderia cepacia* has been associated with serious morbidity, and even fatal postoperative infections in lung transplant recipients in the early post-transplant period. One-year survival rate of 34% was reported in one study in patients colonized preoperatively with resistant isolates of *Pseudomonas*. Consequently, many centers would not routinely transplant such patients [7].

Length of Hospitalization. Duration of stay in hospital is not only an indirect marker of greater severity of illness, but also renders the transplant candidates susceptible to colonization and infections with nosocomially acquired infections. Nasal carriage with *S. aureus* has been shown to be a predictor of subsequent invasive infections due to *S. aureus* in liver transplant recipients [8]. It is, however, notable that 46% of the patients were nasal carriers of *S. aureus* even prior to transplantation [9]. Prolonged length of hospitalization was significantly associated with MRSA carriage [9]. Length of hospitalization has also been shown to be predictive of a greater risk of ESBL producing *K. pneumoniae* and VREF infections in transplant candidates [5, 6].

Pretransplant Immunosuppression. Given the high mortality associated with fulminant hepatic failure, liver transplantation has been proposed as primary treatment for this entity. Fulminant organ system failure as indication for transplantation and requirement of immunosuppressive therapy prior to transplantation renders these patients uniquely susceptible to opportunistic infections in the early post-transplant period. Patients with fulminant hepatic failure receiving a short trial of corticosteroids were shown to be at high risk for the development of invasive aspergillosis [10].

Systemic fungal infections were reported in 21% of the patients undergoing liver transplantation for acute liver failure and was a major cause of mortality in these patients [11].

Use of pretransplant azathioprine and corticosteroids in lung transplant recipients with idiopathic pulmonary fibrosis was associated with a higher incidence of CMV infection at the time of transplantation [12]. These patients had a significantly higher rate of subsequent CMV disease than those without detectable CMV infection on the day of transplantation [12].

Renal Dysfunction. A variety of host defense defects inherent to uremia, e.g. chemotactic defects, impaired complement activation, opsonization and depressed cell mediated immunity, may increase susceptibility to infection not only in renal, but also nonrenal transplant recipients. Renal dysfunction, particularly requirement of dialysis prior to liver transplantation, identified patients at a significantly higher risk for early infections and death after liver transplantation [13]. Requirement of dialysis has been shown to be a significant risk factor for fungal infections, particularly invasive aspergillosis in liver transplant recipients [14]. Although it is possible that renal failure was merely a marker of overall complicated course, in a recent study requirement of dialysis was the most significant independent predictor for invasive aspergillosis, even when controlled for the severity of illness of patients [15].

Artificial Support Devices. The requirement of invasive circulatory support devices, such as intra-aortic balloon pumps, left ventricular assist devices or artificial hearts are required in many potential heart or heart lung transplant patients. Their prolonged placement is a major risk factor for bacterial colonization and subsequent nosocomial infection after transplantation in these patients (Table 1). Forty-seven per cent of patients requiring total artificial hearts in one report died within 60 days of implantation; 80% of the deaths were due to infections, including mediastinitis [16].

ROLE OF IATROGENIC IMMUNOSUPPRESSION

The specific component of the host defense impaired by the iatrogenic immunosuppressive agent influences the susceptibility to a particular opportunistic pathogen. Corticosteroids primarily affect T lymphocyte activation by inhibiting the release of IL-2 and other related cytokines. Increased susceptibility to fungal infections with high dose maintenance corticosteroid therapy, employed in the early years of transplantation, has been amply documented. Corticosteroids also have nonspecific anti-inflammatory effects and inhibit leukocyte migration. Corticosteroids have varying effects on susceptibility to viral infections. While replication of hepatitis B virus (HBV) and human herpes virus-8 is accelerated by corticosteroids

TABLE 1. Sources of infections in critically ill transplant recipients

I. Donor transmission
   A. Latent infections in the donor transmitted with the transplanted allograft
      - Herpesviruses, e.g., CMV, EBV, HHV-6, hepatitis B and C viruses
      - Protozoa, e.g. *Toxoplasma gondii*
      - Bacteria, e.g., *Mycobacterium tuberculosis*
   B. Donor colonization or acquired infections in the donor
      - Fungi, e.g., *Candida* or *Aspergillus* in donor trachea in lung and heart-lung transplant recipients
      - Donor bacteremia
   C. Contamination during organ procurement and preservation
      - Bacteria, e.g., *Pseudomonas aeruginosa*, *S. aureus*, and fungi, e.g., *Candida*

II. Infections acquired from environmental sources
   - *Legionella* (infected potable water system, humidifiers, and ice machines, etc.)
   - *S. aureus* and vancomycin-resistant enterococci (nosocomial transmission via personnel).
   - *Aspergillus*, e.g., construction activities, contaminated or poorly maintained ventilating ducts, grids, and air filters.
   - Zygomycoses, e.g., infection of surgical wounds via contaminated bandages or dressing.

III. Transmission via blood products
   - Herpesviruses, e.g., CMV
   - Hepatotropic viruses

IV. Reactivation or endogenous infections in the recipients
   A. Reactivation of latent infections
      - Herpesviruses, e.g., CMV, VZV, HHV-6, HSV
      - Hepatitis B and C viruses
      - *M. tuberculosis*
      - *Toxoplasma gondii*
      - *Pneumocystis carinii*
   B. Endogenous colonization in the recipient
      - Candida (gastrointestinal or respiratory tract colonization)
      - *S. aureus* (nasal carriage) and vancomycin-resistant enterococci (gastrointestinal carriage)
      - *Pseudomonas aeruginosa* or *Burkholderia cepacia*, e.g., in cystic fibrosis

[17, 18], these agents *per se* do not activate cytomegalovirus (CMV).

Cyclosporine exerts its major therapeutic effect by inhibition of T cell activation by blocking transcription of IL-2, IL-3, and interferon gamma; a differential inhibition of T helper cells over T suppressor cells is observed [19]. A lower incidence of CMV disease has been reported in transplant recipients receiving cyclosporine as compared with azathioprine containing regimens [20]. It is, however, believed that the inclusion of antithymocyte globulin may have been more important in potentiating CMV rather than the basic immunosuppressive regimen itself. A lower incidence of bacterial infections and *Pneumocystis carinii* pneumonia has been documented in patients receiving cyclosporine [21]. Cyclosporine enhances the ability of macrophages to clear toxoplasma infection, although no effect has been observed clinically [20]. Cyclosporine containing regimens have also been associated with a higher risk of Kaposi's sarcoma after organ transplantation.

Tacrolimus is chemically distinct from cyclosporine and has different cytosolic binding sites. However, like cyclosporine, it inhibits T lymphocyte activation by blocking IL-2 production [22]. On a molar basis, tacrolimus is 30–100 times more potent then cyclosporine [22]. Tacrolimus has been associated with significantly fewer episodes of acute rejection, corticosteroid-resistant or refractory rejection as compared to cyclosporine [23]. Despite its potent immunosuppressive effect, significantly fewer CMV infections were observed with tacrolimus as compared with cyclosporine containing regimens [23]. This is likely due to a lower incidence of rejection and thus requirement of additional immunosuppression with tacrolimus [23].

In recent years, mycophenolate mofetil, an ester prodrug of mycophenolic acid which is derived from the mold *Penicillium brevicompactum*, has been increasingly used as an adjunctive immunosuppressive agent. By allowing a reduction in tacrolimus dosage, the use of mycophenolate mofetil has been associated with a lower incidence of nephrotoxicity and neurotoxicity. Mycophenolic acid, by blocking the production of guanosine nucleotides, serves as a selective inhibitor of T and B cell proliferation and interferes with the glycosylation of adhesion molecules. Mycophenolate mofetil use has been shown to correlate with a higher incidence of CMV infection in some, but not all reports [24]. It has also been proposed that the drug may exacerbate HCV recurrence. On the other hand, a significantly lower incidence of *Pneumocystis carinii* infections has been reported in patients receiving mycophenolate mofetil [24].

T-cell monoclonal antibodies and antithymocyte globulin have been associated with a higher incidence and severity of CMV disease after transplantation. A higher incidence of symptomatic herpes simplex virus infections, aspergillosis, *Pneumocystis carinii* pneumonia, *M. tuberculosis* and post-transplant lymphoproliferative disease has also been reported with the use of OKT3 [20].

IMMUNOMODULATORY VIRUSES

Herpesviruses. Viruses, particularly those belonging to the herpesvirus family, exhibit a variety of immunomodulatory and immunosuppressive characteristics that may facilitate superinfections by other opportunistic pathogens, promote oncogenesis or allograft rejection.

The novel herpesvirus, human herpesvirus-6 (HHV-6) is being increasingly recognized as a significant pathogen in organ transplant recipients. HHV-6 preferentially infects CD4 + T lymphocytes, a characteristic that it shares with HIV and a feature that separates it from all other viruses [25]. Mitogen-driven proliferative responses of both CD4+ and CD8+ lymphocytes are inhibited by HHV-6. HHV-6 is a potent inducer of immunomodulatory cytokines, e.g. IL-1 beta, TNF-alpha, and INF-alpha [25]. HHV-6 is also associated with functional defects of phagocytes. HHV-6 has been documented to be an independent predictor of invasive fungal infections and mortality in organ transplant recipients [15, 26]. It has also been shown to activate other viruses, e.g. EBV and CMV [27, 28].

CMV has been shown to facilitate superinfections with opportunistic pathogens, e.g. *Pneumocystis carinii*, fungi, and Gram-negative bacteria [29, 30]. The precise mechanism of CMV mediated immunosuppression is unclear, although CMV induced production of suppressive cytokines (e.g. transforming growth factor B) which alter lymphocyte and macrophage function, are suspected [31]. Impaired immunity occurring during CMV infection is confined not only to the period in which CMV occurs, but may persist for up to 60 months [32]. CMV may also provoke allograft rejection. CMV upregulates class I and II MHC antigen expression, which may precipitate rejection [33]. Asymptomatic CMV infection was documented to be a significant cause of late-onset acute allograft rejection in renal transplant recipients [34].

Gammaherpesviruses, e.g., EBV and human herpesvirus-8 (HHV-8) are not directly immunosuppressive but are potentially oncogenic. Impairment of EBV-specific cytotoxic T-cell responses in transplant recipients allows uncontrolled proliferation of infected B cells resulting in tumors that range from hyperplasia to polyclonal or monoclonal B cell lymphomas. Oncogenic potential of EBV is further illustrated by the reports of spindle cell tumors in transplant recipients, a novel EBV related malignant condition [35].

The newest herpesvirus to be discovered as a pathogen in transplant recipients is human herpesvirus-8, also known as Kaposi's sarcoma herpesvirus (KSHV). KSHV is now believed to be causally associated with post-transplant Kaposi's sarcoma [36]. KSHV is unique amongst herpesviruses in that it encodes for an unprecedented number of genes that have been incorporated from the host cell genome, a phenomenon known as viral piracy [37]. These include cellular homologs that promote angiogenesis, inhibit apoptosis and counteract host defense mechanisms.

Hepatotropic Viruses. A major cause of death in the early post-transplant period in HBsAg positive transplant recipients is sepsis. Forty-nine per cent (11/23) of the deaths in patients undergoing liver transplantation for HBV were due to sepsis; 91% (10/11) of infection-associated deaths occurred within the first three months [38]. Early deaths due to sepsis have also been observed following retransplantation for HBV infection.

Liver transplant recipients with HCV recurrence post-transplant also have a higher incidence of infections, mainly due to pathogens associated with depressed cell-mediated immunity [39]. Renal transplant recipients with non-A, non-B hepatitis (the majority of whom presumably had hepatitis C) had a significantly higher rate of life threatening infections than those without hepatitis [40]. That hepatitis itself had an immunosuppressive effect was suggested by the fact that allograft survival was better in patients with hepatitis [40].

SURGICAL FACTORS AND TYPE OF TRANSPLANTATION

The site, severity and type of bacterial and fungal infections in the early post-transplant period are strongly influenced by the anatomic barriers breached and technical complications unique to different types of organ transplantation [41].

Technically complex nature of liver transplant surgery renders these patients susceptible to a number of biliary and vascular thrombotic or anastomotic complications. Hepatic artery thrombosis may lead to the development of hepatic infarcts with subsequent gangrene and abscess formation. The clinical presentation is usually acute or fulminant, although hepatic artery occlusion may occasionally be occult and present a clinical picture of unexplained fever and relapsing subacute bacteremia. Hepatic artery thrombosis may also lead to liver abscess formation by compromising the biliary vascular supply. Impaired arterial flow to the hepatic allograft preferentially effects the biliary tree because of the biliary tract's almost total reliance upon hepatic arterial blood supply. Hepatic artery thrombosis may thus lead to biliary tract ischemia and biliary leaks, eventually resulting in intrahepatic abscess formation. Thrombosis of the portal vein, detected prior to transplantation or intraoperatively, was shown to be an independently significant predictor of early bacterial infections after liver transplantation [41].

Biliary composition is altered after liver transplantation, leading to supersaturation with cholesterol and thus, sludge/stone formation which may predispose to infections, e.g. cholangitis. T-tubes, commonly used to protect duct-to-duct biliary anastomosis, are prone to microbial colonization and may form a nidus for the deposition of biliary sludge.

Liver transplant recipients are uniquely susceptible to invasive candidiasis [31]. Most cases originate from endogenous sources; deficient reticuloendothelial function and translocation across the gut mucosa are considered important pathogenetic factors predisposing to invasive candidiasis. Urinary tract and postoperative wound infections are one of the most frequent and serious nosocomial infections in renal transplant recipients. Urinary tract infections occur in more than 50% of the patients during the first three months after transplantation and are the foremost source of bacteremia during this time [42]. Multiple factors including underlying diabetes mellitus, renal failure, malnutrition and prolonged vesical catheterization may contribute towards this risk. A higher risk of infections in cadaveric as compared to living allograft recipients is likely related to renal trauma with nephrectomy, and graft contamination during transportation.

Surgical site infections, abscesses, or urinary tract infections are the most common complication in critically ill pancreatic transplant recipients; these are discussed in greater detail in the section on surgical site infections [43–46].

Heart and lung transplant recipients are uniquely susceptible to nosocomial bacterial pulmonary infections, particularly in the first month after transplantation. Bacterial pneumonia has been reported in 35%–48% of the lung and heart-lung transplant recipients [47, 48]. Impaired mucociliary clearance, loss of cough reflex, postoperative pain with splinting, and donor tracheal colonization are amongst the factors contributing to a high risk of postoperative pneumonia in lung transplant recipients.

Characteristics predisposing to infections in small bowel transplant recipients include the fact that the contents of the transplanted organ are nonsterile and these patients require higher intensity of immunosuppressive therapy to prevent graft rejection [49–53]. Virtually all small bowel transplant recipients experience at least one episode of infection; the number of infectious episodes per patient may range from 1 to 11 (median 5) [50]. Multivisceral transplant recipients and those undergoing colonic segment transplantation with small bowel transplantation are more likely to develop infections [50]. Bacterial translocation in small bowel transplant recipients predisposes these patients to intraabdominal infections (peritonitis and abscesses). Selective decontamination of the gut has been proposed to reduce early postoperative infections in small bowel transplant recipients [50].

It is noteworthy that small bowel transplant recipients remain susceptible to infections, even in the late post-transplant period, i.e., more than six months after transplantation [50].

Major Infectious Complications in Critically Ill Transplant Recipients

BACTEREMIA

Bacteremia remains one of the most serious frequent major infections in critically ill organ transplant recipients. The incidence of bacteremia ranges from 6–10% in renal, 11% in heart, 11% in pancreatic, and 20–25% in liver transplant recipients [54, 55]. The portal and consequently the etiologic pathogen varies with the type of solid organ transplanted. Pneumonia in heart and heart-lung transplant patients, urinary tract infections in renal, abdominal/biliary infections in liver and surgical site/urinary tract in pancreatic transplant recipients respectively, have been the most commonly identifiable sources of bacteremia. A vast majority (56–94%) of the bacteremias after organ transplantation are nosocomially acquired. Heart and liver transplant recipients developing bacteremia, however, are generally more critically ill than renal transplant recipient [55].

Bacteremias in the early post-transplant period in renal transplant recipients are usually due to aerobic Gram-negative bacilli (*E. coli*, *Klebsiella*, and other enterobacteriaceae). Use of trimethoprim-sulfamethoxazole for up to four months post-transplantation, has been associated with a striking decline in the incidence of early bacteremias after renal transplantation [56]. It is notable that up to 50% of all bacteremias in renal transplant recipients may occur more than one year after transplantation. This risk appears to be confined to those requiring a return to dialysis, with Gram-positive bacteria (e.g. *S. aureus*) being the predominant pathogens.

Bacteremias account for 22% to 36% of all major infections after liver transplantation and are by far the most frequent infection in these patients [41, 57, 58]. Twenty-seven to 55% of the bacteremias in liver transplant recipients have been due to an intraabdominal portal. Up to 75% of the bacteremias in liver transplant recipients occur within the first two months post-transplantation. In reports published prior to the 1990s, nearly 50% of the bacteremias were due to aerobic Gram-negative bacilli, including *Pseudomonas aeruginosa* and *Enterobacter* species [59].

The sources and etiologic pathogens causing bacteremias in transplant recipients appear to have undergone a striking evolution in the recent years. Many transplant centers have documented a declining incidence of intra-abdominal infections, largely as a result of improvement in surgical techniques [41]. Intravascular cannulae instead, have now emerged as a leading cause of bacteremia, accounting for 36–45% of these infections in the 1990s. In a recent study, bacteremia accounted for 45% of the febrile episodes occurring in critically ill liver transplant recipients; the leading sources of bacteremias in the ICU were intravascular catheter (29%), pneumonia (18%), and biliary tree (18%) [60]. Paralleling these trends has been an exponential rise in the proportion of infections due to antibiotic resistant staphylococci and enterococci [6, 61].

Pneumonia due to aerobic Gram-negative bacilli was the most commonly identifiable source of bacteremia in heart transplant recipients [55]. Other sources of bacteremia uniquely observed in heart and heart-lung transplant recipients include pseudoaneurysm, mediastinitis, and infections of mechanical assist devices. These infections are predominantly due to Gram-positive bacteria (e.g., *S. aureus*). Direct transmission from graft in a donor with positive blood cultures also poses a risk for bacteremia in heart transplant recipients. Donor bacteremia, however, does not appear to adversely impact the outcome if perioperative prophylaxis is adequate to treat the bacterial pathogen detected [62].

In a study in small bowel transplant recipients, 72% of the patients had at least one episode of bloodstream infection [50]. Intravascular cannulae accounted for 43% of these infections and were the most frequently identifiable portal. Sixty-two per cent of all blood stream infections were due to Gram-positive bacteria [50]. In another report, 45% of all bacterial infections and 72% of all bacteremias after small bowel transplantation, were also due to staphylococci [53].

INFECTIONS OF THE CENTRAL NERVOUS SYSTEM

Although minor neurologic complications may occur in 20–82% of organ transplant recipients, up to 5–8% of such patients have major neurologic sequelae or central nervous system (CNS) lesions [63]. Diverse etiologies, e.g., vascular events, immunosuppressive associated leukoencephalopathy and most significantly infections may account for such lesions. Up to 18 to 22% of central nervous lesions in organ transplant recipients have been due to infections [63].

Brain abscesses, documented in up to 0.63 to 1% of liver transplant recipients, 0.36% of renal and 1.17% of heart and heart-lung transplant recipients, are among the most worrisome and serious of CNS complications [63, 64]. A vast majority of the brain abscesses in organ transplant recipients are fungal in etiology, with invasive aspergillosis accounts for over 90% of fungal brain abscesses in these patients [63, 64]. Organ transplant recipients developing *Aspergillus* brain abscesses are often critically ill with evidence of poorly functioning allograft, requirement of dialysis, and ventilator dependency [64].

Fungal CNS lesions may also be caused by dematiaceous fungi, mucormycosis, *Cryptococcus neoformans*. The timing of onset post-transplantation, however, is distinctive for different fungal pathogens. Whereas, brain-abscesses caused by *Aspergillus*, and Mucor generally occur early (within 30 days) of transplantation, those caused by dematiaceous fungi and Cryptococcus occur later (a median of 21 months after transplantation) [63]. A predilection for frontoparietal lobe involvement has been noted in CNS fungal lesions, even in the absence of sinus disease [63].

A frequent dilemma in the management of CNS lesions suspected to be due to infections, is the need for diagnostic brain biopsies. It has been shown that up to 73% of the patients with fungal brain abscesses after liver transplantation had concomitant extraneural (predominantly pulmonary involvement) due to the same fungus [63]. It was suggested that liver transplant recipients with an enhancing CNS lesion suspected to be due to infection, and with documented pulmonary fungal infection, need not routinely undergo a diagnostic brain biopsy [63]. These lesions were a result of the same fungal pathogen detected in the lung in all cases. A diagnostic brain biopsy, however, is recommended for such lesions in the absence of an extraneural focus because of the diversity of the causal fungal pathogens and the varying susceptibility of fungi to different antifungal agents. Empiric coverage of brain abscesses in liver transplant recipients should include antifungal and not antibacterial or antiviral therapy [63].

Nonfungal brain abscesses are usually due to *Nocardia* and *T. gondii*. They tend to occur later in the post-transplant course in the setting of chronic stable immunosuppression [64]. Heart transplant recipients appear to be more likely to develop brain abscesses due to nocardiosis and toxoplasmosis than other solid organ transplant recipients [64]. *Listeria monocytogenes* may present as isolated bacteremia or meningitis at any time after transplantation. CNS infections due to *Listeria monocytogenes* generally also occur later in the post-transplant course and is unlikely to be observed in the early post-transplant period in critically ill transplant recipients. Brain abscesses due to other bacteria, e.g., *S. aureus*, have been reported, but are usually due to mycotic aneurysms in the setting of endocarditis.

Despite frequent occurrence of systemic CMV disease in organ transplant recipients, CMV meningitis or encephalitis is rare after transplantation [65]. Likewise, the incidence of herpes simplex virus encephalitis does not appear to be higher in transplant recipients as compared with the general population [65]. The most neuroinvasive member of the herpesviruses family, however, is HHV-6. Numerous studies have implicated CNS infection due to HHV-6 as a major cause of CNS disease in the non-transplant setting. In transplant recipients, mental status changes ranging from confusion to coma, seizure and headache have been the predominant presenting features of HHV-6 encephalitis; focal neurologic findings were rare. As with other herpesviruses, viral isolation or detection of HHV-6 DNA by PCR in the cerebrospinal fluid, is widely regarded as the standard for diagnosis of HHV-6 encephalitis [66].

A recent study in liver transplant recipients documented that mental status changes without an identifiable etiology were significantly more likely to occur in patients with HHV-6 viremia, as compared to those without HHV-6 [15]. Confusion and mental status changes in the early postoperative period in transplant recipients are often attributed to immunosuppressive medications. It is well recognized that often lowering the immunosuppression may be enough to reverse the manifestations of herpesviruses in transplant recipients. Thus, it is conceivable that some of the cases with post-transplant mental status changes attributable to immunosuppressive toxicity may, in fact, be due to HHV-6 [67].

PNEUMONIA

The risk of pneumonia in lung transplant recipients is 1.5 to four-fold greater than in other organ transplant recipients. Bacteria account for 48–51% of all pneumonitis after lung transplantation, with nearly one-third of the episodes occurring in the first two weeks post-transplant [68–70]. Gram-negative bacteria, including *Pseudomonas aeruginosa*, accounted for a vast majority of the pneumonias occurring during this time period in one report. Pulmonary infiltrates in critically ill lung transplant recipients, within the first week of transplantation, could also be due to "ischemic reperfusion injury," and less likely due to rejection [68].

In the absence of antifungal prophylaxis, fungal infections were documented in 14% of the lung transplant recipients; 56% of these were due to *Candida* and 33% due to *Aspergillus*. A vast majority of the *Candida* infections are associated with tracheobronchitis and *Aspergillus* with invasive pulmonary infections [71, 72]. The highest risks for invasive aspergillosis in lung transplant recipients are within six months post-transplantation. Patients with *Aspergillus* airway colonization during the first six months were 11 times more likely to develop invasive disease as compared to those not colonized [73].

Pulmonary infiltrates have been documented in 41 to 70% of the critically ill liver transplant recipients with pneumonitis accounting for 36–70% of all pulmonary infiltrates [74]. Pulmonary edema (40%), pneumonia (38%), acute lung injury (8%), and contusion (3%) were the predominant etiology of pulmonary infiltrates in the ICU. Thirty-day mortality in critically ill liver transplant recipients developing pulmonary infiltrates was 35%; pneumonia as etiology, creatinine >1.5 mg/dl, higher APACHE II scores, and length of ICU stay were significant predictors of mortality [74].

Bacterial infections, e.g., *S. aureus*, *Pseudomonas aeruginosa*, and enteric Gram-negative bacteria represent the most frequent etiologic pathogens associated with pneumonia after liver transplantation whereas viral pneumonia due to CMV accounted for 47–50% and HSV for 13–25% of the pneumonias in critically ill liver transplant recipients in the studies in the 1980s, this incidence has declined to less than 5% in recent reports [74]. Invasive aspergillosis remains a significant cause of early pneumonia in liver transplant patients in the ICU. Nearly 50% of the pulmonary infiltrates in critically ill liver transplant recipients occurred within 30 days of transplantation; 75% of the MRSA pneumonias, all cases of invasive aspergillosis, but only 14% of the Gram-negative pneumonias, occurred within this time period [74]. Early onset of *S. aureus* pneumonia likely resulted from high colonization rate in these patients prior to liver transplantation.

The incidence of pneumonia in heart transplant recipients has declined from 50–62% in the precyclosporine era to 24–35% in the studies performed in the 1980s. However, pneumonia remains one of the most frequent infections after heart transplantation with two recent studies reporting an incidence of 14% [75] and 21% [76]. Pneumonia is also amongst the leading causes of death in heart transplant recipients with overall mortality in patients with pneumonia ranging from 23 to 31% [76]. The mortality rate in patients requiring mechanical ventilation, however, may be as high as 50% [76].

In most studies conducted prior to 1990, CMV accounted for 23 to 32% of all the pneumonias after heart transplantation [77, 78]. On the other hand, the etiologic pathogen in nearly 50% of the cases of pneumonia in a large study since 1990 were bacterial [79]. Non-fermenting Gram-negative bacteria were the predominant bacterial pathogens associated with pneumonia. Fungal pneumonia has been documented in 1 to 45% of the heart transplant recipients with virtually all cases being due to *Aspergillus*. In the absence of specific prophylaxis for *P. carinii*, up to 3–5% of the heart transplant recipients may develop *P. carinii* pneumonitis. Nosocomial pneumonias after heart transplantation appeared a median of 20 days post-transplant, CMV a median of 35.5 and *Aspergillus* a median of 36 days post-transplant respectively [76].

Pulmonary complications have been reported in 18–24% of the renal transplant recipients and pneumonia in 8–16% of the patients [80–82]. Bacteria (enteric Gram-negative, *P. aeruginosa* and *S. aureus*) account for virtually all pneumonitis in the early post-transplant period in these patients.

Diagnostic Approach. Early and aggressive pursuit of the etiology of pulmonary infiltrates is warranted in critically ill transplant recipients. Radiographic appearance of the lesions may be distinctive or suggestive of certain entities. Nodular pulmonary infiltrates are suggestive of *Aspergillus*, Cryptococcus and *Nocardia* but may also be observed in *Legionella*, *S. aureus*, *zygomycosis*, and M. tuberculosis [83]. Noninfectious causes of pulmonary nodules included metastatic hepatocellular carcinoma, lymphoma, and pulmonary calcification in liver transplant recipients. Pulmonary infarcts, rounded atelectasis and pulmonary varix in cardiac transplant patients, and acute or chronic rejection in lung transplant recipients may also have a nodular appearance [83]. Cavitary pneumonia in transplant recipients may be due to *Aspergillus*, *Cryptococcus*, *Legionella*, *M. tuberculosis*, *Nocardia*, or *Rhodococcus equi*. Nosocomial bacterial pneumonia most frequently presented as alveolar infiltrates [84]. Interstitial infiltrates with reticular or reticulonodular infiltrates are most likely due to *P. carinii*, CMV or other herpesvirus.

Computerized tomography offers a number of advantages over conventional radiographs, including detection of additional lesions, precise morphology of the lesion, delineation of mediastinal adenopathy, and guiding location for diagnostic intervention. CT scan improved the information obtained by plain radiographs in 33% of the cases of pneumonia in heart transplant recipients [84].

Although isolation or detection of *P. carinii*, *Legionella*, *Nocardia*, *M. tuberculosis* and *Cryptococcus* in the sputum is diagnostic of pulmonary infection due to these pathogens, sputum and respiratory tract secretions yield a diagnosis in fewer than 50% of the transplant recipients with pneumonia. Blood cultures were positive in 40% of the liver transplant patients with pneumonia in the ICU and 29% of the heart transplant recipients with nosocomial pneumonia [84, 85].

Patients in whom noninvasive tests remain nondiagnostic, the choice lies between empiric antibacterial therapy or a diagnostic procedure; we recommend early bronchoscopy with bronchoalveolar lavage. In patients with focal nodular infiltrates, percutaneous needle aspiration is superior to bronchoalveolar lavage with a diagnostic accuracy of 70% to 90%. In patients with diffuse pulmonary infiltrates, bronchoalveolar lavage with or without transbronchial biopsy is the preferred approach. Transbronchial biopsy is particularly valuable for the diagnosis of rejection in lung transplant recipients and for the differentiation of allograft rejection and CMV pneumonitis in these patients. Open lung biopsy should be reserved only for patients with progressive disease refractory to antimicrobial agents in whom bronchoalveolar lavage or percutaneous needle aspiration is nondiagnostic.

All cases of invasive aspergillosis in one study [64], and 87% in another [14], occurred in liver transplanted recipients in the ICU; the median time to onset of aspergillosis was 17 days and 24 days, respectively.

SURGICAL SITE INFECTIONS

Nosocomial postoperative wound infections in transplant recipients may be associated with significant morbidity including prolonged duration of hospitalization and allograft loss (e.g. in renal and pancreatic transplant recipients). Surgical wound infections in renal transplant recipients are usually due to staphylococci or Gram-negative bacilli [42, 86]. Staphylococcal infections tended to be associated with superficial wound infections and occurred earlier, whereas those due to Gram-negative bacilli occurred later, were deep-seated and often led to bacteremia, graft loss, or death. Prolonged urinary catheterization, surgical wall hematoma, reopened wound, and cadaveric donor graft are risk factors for nosocomial urinary or wound infections in renal transplant recipients [87, 88]. Improvements in surgical technique and antimicrobial prophylaxis have proven highly effective in reducing the rate of urinary tract and wound infections in renal transplant recipients. Single perioperative dose of antibiotics led to a reduction in the incidence of wound infections from 25% to 2% [89]. Prophylaxis with trimethoprim-sulfamethoxazole in the early post-transplantation period has also been shown to significantly lower the incidence of urinary tract infections, bacteremias and infections caused by Gram-negative bacilli as well as *S. aureus*, when compared to placebo [56].

Sternal wound infections occur in 2 to 20% of heart and heart-lung transplant recipients. Gram-positive cocci, enterobacteriaceae and *Pseudomonas aeruginosa* are the most common causative organisms. Sternal wound infections may directly extend into the mediastinum and lead to mediastinitis or mycotic aneurysms at the suture sites. Mediastinitis has been reported in 2 to 9% of heart and heart-lung transplant recipients [90]. An unusual cause of mediastinitis in transplant recipients is *Mycoplasma hominis* [91]. Hematologic spread from genitourinary or respiratory source is the suspected source of infection. Most such infections have been treated with a combination of doxycycline, clindamycin and an aminoglycoside [91].

One of the most challenging infections after lung transplantation are those encountered in cystic fibrosis patients colonized with resistant *Pseudomonas* species. Although the infected lung is removed during transplantation, residual colonization of the nasopharynx and sinuses remains a potential nidus for subsequent infections. Pretransplant bilateral maxillary sinus drainage followed by monthly irrigation with tobramycin led to an improved outcome in cystic fibrosis patients in one study [92]. Some centers utilize this approach only if clinically significant sinus infection occurs after transplantation [93]. An innovative approach employing aerosolized colistin and discontinuation of systemic antibiotics led to the emergence of sensitive *Pseudomonas* in patients who previously harbored resistant *Pseudomonas* isolates [7]. Of 20 cystic fibrosis patients with resistant *Pseudomonas* who received aerosolized colistin, all became colonized with sensitive isolates of *Pseudomonas* within a mean of 45 days. In contrast, only 30% (3/10) of the control candidates who received only systemic anti-Pseudomonal activity became colonized with the sensitive isolates. Five of six patients who received colistin and underwent transplantation continued to harbor sensitive organisms after transplantation.

Wound infections are a particularly serious complication after pancreatic transplantation; their incidence ranges from seven to 50% [43, 45, 94]. Deep wound infections are one of the most common causes of graft loss in pancreatic transplant recipients [94]. Unique features of pancreatic transplantation that facilitate deep wound infections include its predisposition to ischemia/infarction (due to inherently low vascular flow of the pancreas) and liberation of digestive juices into the surgical fossa that provoke inflammation and necrosis. *S. epidermidis* and *Candida* species are the most common causative organisms. *Candida* wound infections are a particular problem in pancreatic transplant recipients with bladder drainage procedures; high incidence of candidal urinary colonization (due to diabetes) along with the nonacidic environment in the bladder created by exocrine pancreatic bladder drainage favors candidal infections. Most infections occur within a month of transplantation. Older donor age, retroperitoneal positioning of the pancreas, enteric versus bladder drainage (because the anastomosis cannot be protected by the equivalent of a urinary catheter) are significant risk factors for wound infections in pancreatic transplant recipient [95]. Significant risk factors for surgical site infections have included previous transplant and renal disease. Despite salvage procedures, deep wound infections after pancreatic transplants usually lead to allograft loss; one year allograft survival as low as 16–20% has been reported in patients who develop deep wound infections [94].

Wound infections may occur in 5–15% of liver transplant recipients and account for up to 10% of the bloodstream infections in these patients.

INFECTIVE ENDOCARDITIS

Although relatively rare, endocarditis is a significant infectious complication in critically ill transplant recipients. Up to 74% of the cases of endocarditis after transplantation have been reported to be nosocomially acquired [96]. A prevalence rate of 1.7% amongst liver transplant recipients and 6% in heart transplant recipients has been reported [96]. *S. aureus* is the most common cause of endocarditis after solid organ transplantation, accounting for 30% of all cases. *S. aureus* endocarditis in transplant recipients was commonly associated with previous isolation of the organisms and, in some cases, inadequate treatment of prior infection [96]. Fungi were the etiologic pathogen in 28% of the cases of infective endocarditis in transplant recipients as compared to approximately 2–4% in nontransplant setting. *Aspergillus fumigatus* was the most common cause of endocarditis within 30 days after transplantation and *S. aureus* was the most frequent pathogen after this time. In contrast, only 4% of the cases of endocarditis in transplant recipients were due to viridans streptococci.

Most (80%) organ transplant recipients who developed endocarditis had no history of valvular disease or abnormality [96]. Overall, mortality rate in transplant patients with endocarditis was 57%; the mortality associated with bacterial endocarditis was 40% and that with fungal endocarditis 77% [96].

Major Pathogens in Critically Ill Transplant Recipients

FUNGAL INFECTIONS

Invasive fungal infections have been reported in 0–14% of renal, 5–21% of heart, 15–35% of lung and heart-lung, 18–38% of pancreatic, and 7–42% of liver transplant recipients. Fungal infections most likely to be encountered in critically ill transplant recipients include those due to invasive aspergillosis, candidiasis, and rarely cryptococcosis, zygomycosis, dematiaceous fungi and *Pneumocystis carinii*.

Aspergillosis. Invasive aspergillosis remains a devastating fungal infection in all types of transplant recipients. It has, however, unique clinical characteristics and risk factors in different types of solid organ transplant recipients.

Epidemiology. Lung transplant recipients are more likely than other solid organ recipients to develop infection with *Aspergillus*. Up to 8% of the lung transplant recipients have been shown to develop invasive aspergillosis with an additional 10% demonstrating *Aspergillus* colonization [72, 97–99]. Risk factors for *Aspergillus* infection after lung transplantation include CMV infection and single lung transplantation [72, 100] (Table 3). Colonization with *Aspergillus* is frequently detected in patients with cystic fibrosis. However, isolation of *Aspergillus* species from respiratory secretions of the patients with cystic fibrosis pretransplant has not been shown to predict subsequent development of invasive disease [99, 101]. Most cases of in-vasive aspergillosis in lung transplant recipients occur within the first nine months post-transplantation. A unique form of

TABLE 2. Incidence and risk factors for invasive aspergillosis in organ transplant recipients

Type of Transplant	Incidence of invasive aspergillosis % (range, average)	Unique risk factors
Lung	3–19 (8.4)	Single lung transplant, cytomegalovirus infection
Heart	0–11 (6.2)	No data
Liver	1–8 (1.7)	Poor allograft function, renal failure, OKT3 use
Renal	0–0.9 (0.7)	Graft failure, augmented immunosuppression
Small-bowel	0–3.6 (2.2)	No data
Pancreas	0–2.9 (1.3)	No data

TABLE 3. Incidence, predisposing factors and unique clinical presentation of invasive candidiasis in transplant recipients

Type of transplant	Incidence	Risk-factors	Predominant Clinical presentation
Liver	5–20%	Duration of surgery, reoperation, transfusion	Intra-abdominal infections, peritonitis, candidemia requirements, Roux-en-Y duct anastomosis, renal failure, CMV infection
Lung*	2.5–33%	–	Pneumonia, anastomotic infections, candidemia
Pancreas	5.5–34%	Enteric exocrine drainage, operation time longer than four hours	Deep wound infections, abdominal abscesses, candidemia
Small-bowel*	40–45%	–	Abdominal abscesses, candidemia
Heart*	0.15–8%	–	Pneumonia, vascular anastomotic infections, mediastinitis
Renal	2.3–11.8%	Bladder catheters, diabetes mellitus	Urinary tract infections, candidemia

*Unique risk factors for invasive candidiasis have not been well-defined in these patients.

invasive aspergillosis occurring in lung transplant recipients is ulcerative tracheobronchitis. Local inflammation at the bronchial anastomotic site may form a nidus for *Aspergillus* infection and lead to anastomotic dehisence or bronchoarterial fistula formation.

The incidence of invasive aspergillosis in liver transplant recipients ranges from 1–4% [14, 102–105]. The infection is most often diagnosed between two and four weeks after transplantation. Poorly functioning hepatic allograft and renal insufficiency, particularly the requirement of hemodialysis are considered important risk factors for invasive aspergillosis in liver transplant recipients (Table 2). Although OKT3 use was shown in early studies to be a risk factor for invasive aspergillosis, a recent large study showed that only 8% of liver transplant recipients with invasive aspergillosis had received OKT3 [14]. Approximately 25% of the cases of invasive aspergillosis in liver transplant recipients occur after retransplantation [14]. Rarely, the *Aspergillus* infection is confined to the surgical wound (producing necrotizing fasciitis) or intra-abdominal sites in liver transplant recipients.

Invasive aspergillosis occurs in 1–6% of the heart transplant recipients [106–109]. The median time to development of invasive aspergillosis in these patients is one to two months. Most infections originate in the lungs, and 20–35% disseminate to other organs. Invasive aspergillosis has been reported in 0.7% to 1% of the patients undergoing renal transplantation [106, 110, 111]. Cases of invasive aspergillosis in renal transplant recipients have usually been of pulmonary infection, and occasionally disseminated disease. Augmented immunosuppression and graft failure requiring hemodialysis are risk factors for invasive aspergillosis in renal transplant recipients [111].

Diagnosis. Early diagnosis is critically important in reducing the mortality from invasive aspergillosis. *Aspergillus* can be cultured from sputum in only 8–34% and from bronchoalveolar lavage fluid in 45–62% of patients with invasive pulmonary aspergillosis [112]. Respiratory cultures, therefore, may not detect *Aspergillus* before significant vascular invasion has occurred. High-resolution thoracic computed tomographic (CT) scans may be suggestive of invasive pulmonary aspergillosis soon after the development of symptoms and before culture results are available. Such imaging in neutropenic patients whose fever persisted for more than two days despite empiric antibiotic treatment, showed findings highly suggestive of invasive pulmonary aspergillosis (halo-sign and air-crescent sign) five days earlier than the use of chest roentgenograms [113]. Unfortunately, while the halo-sign is commonly observed in neutropenic and bone marrow transplant recipients, it is not frequently seen in solid organ transplant recipients.

Surveillance serological tests are emerging as a potentially useful tool for the early diagnosis of invasive aspergillosis. Detection of galactomanan of the *Aspergillus* cell wall by Enzyme-linked immunoassay (ELISA) has been shown to have a sensitivity of 50–90% and specificity of 81–93% for the diagnosis of invasive aspergillosis [112, 114, 115]. Furthermore, the galactomannan detection test may be positive as long as 28 days before clinical and radiographic signs of invasive aspergillosis become apparent [114]. However, unlike bone marrow transplant recipients, the efficacy of *Aspergillus* galactomannan for the early diagnosis of invasive aspergillosis, has not been extensively evaluated in solid organ transplant recipients.

Prophylaxis. An effective prophylaxis against invasive aspergillosis is currently not available. Low dose intravenous amphotericin deoxycholate (0.1 mg/kg/day) or intravenous amphotericin B liposome (1 mg/kg/day) have also not been shown to be consistently efficacious. On the contrary, it has been proposed that low-dose amphotericin B may promote the emergence of *Aspergillus* [116]. Aerosolized amphotericin B prophylaxis, administrated during post-transplant hospital stay was shown to reduce the incidence of fungal infections, including aspergillosis in lung, heart-lung and heart transplant recipients in one report [117]. Others have not found it to be effective. Studies in murine model have suggested that aerosolized liposomal amphotericin B may be superior to amphotericin B deoxycholate as prophylaxis for invasive aspergillosis. In a report in lung and heart-lung transplant recipients, nebulized ABLC was administered daily for four days post-transplantation, followed by four weekly treatments. Only one of 20 patients (5%) was documented to have an invasive fungal infection. These data, while encouraging, are preliminary and warrant larger comparative trials. Given the lack of availability of effective prophylaxis, preemptive therapy or empiric therapy in selected high risk patients may be considered as an alternative to prophylaxis.

Although itraconazole is highly active *in vitro* against *Aspergillus*, its efficacy has not yet been demonstrated in clinical trials. Furthermore, the absorption of itraconazole in capsule form can be erratic in transplant recipients. Itraconazole solubilized in cyclodextrin is better absorbed; its efficacy as prophylaxis, however, remains unproven.

Therapy. Amphotericin B deoxycholate in dosages ranging between 1.0 and 1.5 mg/kd/day has been the standard of therapy against invasive aspergillosis. Unfortunately, such a dosing regimen is often limited by the development of nephrotoxicity, particularly in organ transplant recipients receiving tacrolimus. A diminished potential for nephrotoxicity has been amply demonstrated with the liposomal preparations of amphotericin B. However, the expense associated with these agents has led to another relevant question, i.e., whether these drugs should be considered first line therapy against invasive aspergillosis. In animal models of invasive aspergillosis, a survival advantage with lipid preparations of amphotericin B at doses of 5–12.5 mg/kg/day as compared to amphotericin deoxycholate at 0.8–1 mg/kg/day, has been demonstrated [118]. Retrospective study of patients with invasive aspergillosis treated with amphotericin B colloidal dispersion, showed a significantly greater survival in patients treated with amphotericin B colloidal dispersion as compared with historic controls [119]. Another retrospective study in liver transplant recipients showed significantly greater survival in patients treated with high dose liposomal-amphotericin B from 1995 to 1998 as compared to patients treated with amphotericin B deoxycholate between 1992 and 1995 (24/29 *versus* 2/12, p = 0.0003) [120]. Thus, the diminished nephrotoxicity, higher tissue levels achievable with liposomal preparations of amphotericin B and a possible survival advantage, have led many investigators to consider liposomal amphotericin B preparations as first line drugs for invasive aspergillosis in transplant recipients. The role of itraconazole as initial therapy for invasive aspergillosis is unproven. However, it may be used as follow-up therapy for patients who have experienced initial improvement with amphotericin B. A number of new antifungal agents with activity against *Aspergillus in vitro*, are undergoing clinical trials, e.g., voriconazole, and echinocandins.

Although proposed to be potentially beneficial for the prevention, and adjunct to antifungal agents as therapy for fungal infections, the precise role of immunomodulatory agents and hematopoetic growth factors in transplant recipients with invasive aspergillosis, remains undefined. Additionally, in an animal model of invasive aspergillosis, G-CSF not only proved ineffective, but antagonized potent antifungal agents [121].

Candidiasis. With the exception of heart and lung transplant recipients, invasive candidiasis is the most frequently occurring fungal infection in solid organ transplant recipients [31]. The incidence of candida infections is highest in liver and pancreatic transplant recipients. Virtually all candida infections are nosocomially acquired, although the source may vary depending upon the type of organ transplant recipients. Whereas in liver transplant recipients, candidiasis results from endogenous (generally gut) colonization, donor organs are the potential source in heart-lung and lung transplant recipients. Karyotypic analysis has demonstrated candida infection originating in the donor lung as a cause of disseminated disease in a lung transplant recipient [71].

In earlier studies, 15–20% of the liver transplant recipients were documented to have invasive candidiasis [104, 122]. Intraabdominal infections, with or without subsequent dissemination are the usual clinical manifestations (Table 3). Prolonged operation time, retransplantation, greater transfusion requirements, high serum creatinine, and CMV infection are the proposed risk factors for candida infections. More recently, however, many transplant centers have documented a decline in the incidence of invasive candidiasis, even in the absence of specific antifungal prophylaxis [57, 123, 124]. More conservative immunosuppression but, more importantly, improvement in surgical technique likely accounts for this decline.

After pancreatic transplantation, candida infections occur in 15–30% of the patients and manifest predominantly as surgical site or blood stream infections. In heart-lung or lung transplant recipients, the clinical pattern of candida infections may range from tracheobronchitis to systemic invasive disease. Invasive candidiasis in these patients may also result in anastomotic dehiscence, mediastinitis and mycotic aneurysm. The anastomotic site is particularly vulnerable because of poor blood supply and the presence of suture material. Invasive bronchial infection can then result with breakdown of the anastomosis.

Precise patient population to be targeted, optimal regimen, and duration of antifungal prophylaxis for candida remains controversial. Nystatin containing selective bowel decontamination regimens have been proposed to lead to a lower incidence of invasive candidiasis in liver transplant recipients [123, 124]. Its efficacy, however, has never been assessed in a controlled trial. Currently, fluconazole is being used as prophylaxis at many liver and pancreatic transplant centers. A randomized trial from Europe compared fluconazole (100 mg once a day) with nystatin (10^6u every six hours) for 28 days after liver transplantation [125]. Although the incidence of Candida decolonization and superficial fungal infections (thrush and cystitis) decreased, no difference in the incidence of invasive candidiasis was observed in the two groups [125].

Universal employment of azole prophylaxis must be undertaken with caution for the following reasons: a major concern with routine azole antifungal prophylaxis is the emergence of azole-resistant candidiasis, a scenario already documented in liver transplant recipients [126]. Azole-resistant invasive *Candida glabrata* infection occurred in 4% (4 out of 101) of the liver transplant recipients receiving fluconazole prophylaxis and was the direct cause of death in one patient [126]. The routine use of fluconazole is also suspected to have the potential of selecting fungi innately resistant to fluconazole, e.g., *Aspergillus*. Although this association has not been proved, an unusually high incidence of invasive aspergillosis (8%, eight out of 101), in the liver transplant recipients who routinely received fluconazole prophylaxis prospectively, is intriguing [126]. Finally, the need for fluconazole prophylaxis should be assessed on the basis of the institutional trends in the incidence of invasive candidiasis. Given the low incidence of invasive candidiasis at certain transplant centers, the widespread employment of fluconazole prophylaxis for all patients may not be warranted to prevent the infection in 5% of the patients. A preferable approach might be prophylaxis targeted towards high risk patients only.

Pneumocystis carinii. Although *Pneumocystis carinii* has long been classified as a protozoan organism on the basis of morphologic features and lack of growth on fungal media, gene sequencing of *P. carinii* has suggested that the organism is indeed a fungus. Most *P. carinii* infections are believed to arise from reactivation of endogenous infections acquired in childhood. However, clusters of *P. carinii* infection occurring in transplant recipients have been reported. In one report, all of the renal transplant recipients affected had attended the same outpatient facility as patients with advanced HIV infection [127–130]. Compared to the matched controls, PCP cases had more outpatient clinic visits coinciding with visits of HIV infected patients with *P. carinii* infection [129]. Furthermore, *P. carinii* DNA has been demonstrated in more than 50% of air samples from the hospital rooms of *P. carinii* infected patients [131].

Lung transplant recipients are at greatest risk of developing pulmonary infection with *P.*

carinii; in the absence of prophylaxis, PCP may develop in up to 80% of patients [132]. The incidence of infection with *P. carinii* in patients not receiving PCP prophylaxis is 2% in renal transplant recipients, 5% in heart, and 9% in liver transplant recipients. Most infections occur between three and six months post-transplantation. Between 10 and 20% of the cases occur longer than six months post-transplantation, usually in those receiving augmented immunosuppression for rejection [133].

Unlike HIV infected patients, *P. carinii* in transplant recipients is rarely diagnosed by examination of an induced sputum sample. Virtually all cases require bronchoalveolar lavage for diagnosis. Coinfection with CMV or bacteria (especially in lung transplant recipients) is common.

Prophylaxis with oral trimethoprim-sulfamethoxazole has proven highly efficacious and is recommended for all transplant recipients. Adverse effects of trimethoprim-sulfamethoxazole are relatively uncommon in solid-organ transplant recipients. Rash occurs in only 1%. Leukopenia is somewhat more common, occurring in 3–20% of patients.

A more controversial issue in prophylaxis of *P. carinii* infection in transplant recipients is the duration of prophylaxis. Many transplant centers (including ours) offer life-long trimethoprim-sulfamethoxazole. Others employ it for the first six months post-transplantation for heart, renal and liver transplant recipients and for the first twelve months in lung transplant recipients. The rationale being that the risk for *P. carinii* in stable patients declines substantially after six months post-transplantation. However, cases of PCP have been described several months after discontinuing prophylaxis. At one center, 36% of cases of PCP occurred more than one year after transplant and 18% occurred longer than two years after transplantation [134]. In patients receiving augmented immunosuppression for late-occurring rejection, PCP prophylaxis should be resumed or continued. An additional advantage of trimethoprim-sulfamethoxazole prophylaxis is that it is also effective against other microorganisms such as *Nocardia*, *Listeria*, *Toxoplasma gondii* and *Legionella* in transplant recipients. Monthly nebulized pentamidine is an alternative prophylaxis in patients intolerant of trimethoprim/sulfamethoxazole. Breakthrough infections, however, have been reported in such patients.

Cryptococcosis. The incidence of cryptococcus in organ transplant recipients ranges from 0.6%–2.6%. However, there are significant regional variations, with some centers reporting cryptococcosis in up to 5% of the transplant recipients [135]. A vast majority of the cases occur more than six months after transplantation, with some cases being detected four or more years after transplantation. The precise pathogenesis of cryptococcosis, whether it is a newly acquired or reactivation infection in transplant settings, remains unresolved. Given the low incidence of cryptococcosis in transplant recipients, the delayed and often unpredictable time of onset after transplantation, fluconazole prophylaxis is not usually considered necessary in transplant recipients.

Zygomycosis. Infections due to the agents of zygomycosis occurs in 0.3% of liver transplant, 0.4% of renal transplant, and 0.8% of lung transplant recipients [136]. Overt pulmonary involvement only occurs in 25% of reported cases [136]. Other sites of infection include the rhinocerebrum (accounting for little over 50% of reported cases), skin and soft tissues and the gastrointestinal tract [136]. Up to 72% of reported cases have been due to *Rhizopus* species. Other reported species include *Cunninghamella*, *Bertholletiae*, *Mucor* and *Absidia* [136].

All reported pulmonary cases have occurred within the first six months post-transplantation, with many cases occurring at times of augmented immunosuppression in the first three months after solid organ transplantation [136]. The median time between initiation of antirejection treatment and onset of zygomycosis was only 16 days [136]. About half of the cases have also been diabetic. Pulmonary disease is usually in the form of nodules or cavities. Usually one or two large (4–7 cm) cavitary lesions are present. Air fluid levels are usually absent.

Treatment consists of reduction in immunosuppression, surgical resection of the pulmonary lesion, and administration of systemic antifungal therapy. Amphotericin is the antifungal drug of choice. Although there is little published experience of use of lipid preparations in treatment of zygomycosis in transplant recipients, these drugs are widely regarded as first line therapy for zygomycosis in transplant recipients.

Dematiaceous Fungi. Dematiaceous fungi or dark-pigmented fungi are being increasingly recognized as pathogens after transplantation; 65% of the dematiaceous fungal infections in organ transplant recipients have been reported in the 1990s [137]. This rise results largely from improved microbiological techniques for their detection and an increasing population of immunocompromised patients at risk for opportunistic infections.

The clinical presentation of dematiaceous fungal infections is distinct from that of other, more commonly observed fungi in transplant recipients. Most infections caused by the dematiaceous fungi occur late, a median of 22 months after transplantation [137]. However, up to 21% of the patients with dematiaceous fungal infections have systemic invasive infections (predominantly brain abscesses) that may occur within three months of transplantation. Dematiaceous fungi, belonging to the genera *Dactylaria* or *Ochroconis* are noteworthy for their neutrotropic potential and their ability to cause brain abscesses. Recognition of these infections is important because they are more amenable to therapy than, for example, invasive aspergillosis after transplantation. Itraconazole is considered to be the drug of choice for skin and soft tissue infections, whereas amphotericin B plus 5 flucytosine is preferred for systemic infections caused by dematiaceous fungi.

BACTERIAL INFECTIONS

Staphylococcus aureus. Methicillin-resistant Staphylococci, particularly *S. aureus*, have emerged as the leading cause of bacterial infections in liver, heart, kidney, and pancreatic transplant recipients at many centers. Although intravascular cannulae, accounting for 42% of all MRSA bacteremias in one study, are the predominant source, wound infections, nosocomial pneumonia, abdominal abscesses and nosocomial endocarditis have also been documented as sources of MRSA infections. *S. aureus* infections are very early occurring infections in transplant recipients; the median time to onset 24 days in one study, with 53% of the infections occurring within 30 days of transplantation [61]. Nearly one-half of these infections occurred in the ICU setting. Mortality in transplant recipients with *S. aureus* bacteremia was shown to differ significantly with the source of infection. Mortality was 86% in patients with MRSA pneumonia or intra-abdominal infections associated with bacteremia, but 6% in those with catheter-related bacteremia [61]. This difference in mortality was independent of the APACHE II scores of the patients or antimicrobial therapy employed (vancomycin monotherapy versus combination therapy). These data underscore the virulent nature of MRSA in the transplant setting, unless a readily removable source of infection, e.g., intravascular catheters, can be identified.

Colonization of the anterior nares with *S. aureus* has been shown to correlate significantly with infections. Whether eradication of nasal carriage would contribute towards decreasing the incidence of *S. aureus* infections, remains to be determined.

Enterococci. Vancomycin resistant *E. faecium* (VREF) have emerged as nosocomial pathogens of grave concern, particularly following liver transplantation. VREF infections have been documented in 10.5%–16% of liver transplant recipients in some studies. Intra-abdominal infections were the most frequent site of infection due to VREF. Infections were documented a median of 39 and 42 days after transplantation in two studies [138, 139] but considerably earlier (a median of 10 days) in another report [140]. VREF fecal carriage prior to transplantation, previous antibiotic usage (including vancomycin), biliary complications, prolonged hospitalization and ICU stay, surgical re-exploration, surgical complications during transplantation, including hypotension, and primary non-function of the allograft have been identified as significant risk factors for VREF infections [138, 139, 141]. Mortality in the infected patients ranges between 23–50%. ICU stay prior to transplantation, hemodialysis, liver failure, and shock have been shown to be independent predictors of mortality in patients with VREF infections [139, 141]. Not surprisingly, antibiotics have not been effective in reducing mortality; outcome did not differ significantly amongst patients who received the drugs with activity against the isolate *in vitro* as compared to those who received no therapy [138].

The largest reported clinical experience for VREF infection is with quinupristin-dalfopristin, an investigational streptogramin with broad Gram-positive activity. A report of the 396 treated patients with VREF infection from an ongoing open-label, noncomparative emergency use program, showed a 73.65 clinical response rate in 193 bacteriologically evaluable patients [6]. In this study, 31.4% of the treated population were either solid organ or bone marrow transplant recipients [6]. A number of novel antibacterial agents (e.g., linezolid, daptomycin, etc.) are being evaluated in clinical trials for the therapy of VREF infections.

Legionella. Legionellosis has been reported in 2–9% of the solid organ transplant recipients with pneumonia [142]. *Legionella pneumophila* and *L. micdadei* are the most common species implicated, however, *L. bozemanii*, *L. birminghamensis*, *L. dumoffi* and *L. cincinnatiensis* have also caused infections in transplant recipients. Aspiration is considered the most likely mode of transmission and legionella contaminated potable water distribution system as the predominant source of legionellosis [142]. Molecular fingerprinting methods have linked *Legionella pneumophila* infection in transplant recipients to hospital drinking water [143]. Ice machines [144] and ultrasonic humidifiers [145] have also been shown to be the sources of Legionella infection after transplantation.

Pneumonia is the predominant clinical manifestation of legionellosis although pericarditis, necrotizing cellulitis, peritonitis, hepatic allograft infection and hemodialysis fistula infections have also been reported after transplantation [142]. Nodular pulmonary densities and cavitation are characteristic radiographic features but may not be invariably present. *Legionella* are fastidious organisms that do not grow on standard bacteriologic media. Selective media containing dyes and antimicrobial agents are needed for optimal growth. Urinary antigen is both sensitive and specific for the detection of *Legionella* and may also be diagnostically useful for detecting *Legionella* in body fluids (e.g. pleural fluids).

It is recommended that hospitals performing large numbers of transplants should routinely culture the hospital water supply for *Legionella* perhaps once a year [146]. If such cultures are positive, specialized *Legionella* laboratory tests, especially culture on selective media and urinary antigen tests, should be made routinely available in the clinical microbiology laboratory. Therapy of legionellosis in transplant recipients can be problematic since erythromycin can increase cyclospoine or tacrolimus levels, and rifampin can lower these. Ciprofloxacin has been recommended as treatment for *Legionella* in the transplant setting. [125].

VIRAL INFECTIONS

Cytomegalovirus. CMV has been recongized as one of the most significant pathogens in organ transplant recipients. The overall incidence of CMV infection ranges between 40–90% in organ transplant recipients. The highest incidence of CMV infection has been documented in lung or heart-lung transplant recipients (60–98%) and the lowest (40–50%) in renal transplant recipients. Liver and heart transplant recipients have an intermediate risk of CMV infection (50–67%). The frequency of symptomatic disease due to CMV ranges from 8–15% in renal, 20–35% in liver, 27–30% in heart, and 55–60% in lung transplant recipients. The incidence of CMV in small bowel transplant recipients approaches that in lung transplant recipients [49]. Small bowel transplant patients also appear to be uniquely susceptible to recurrent episodes of CMV infection [49].

Most CMV infections occur between one to four months post-transplant, and usually between four and six weeks. A febrile mononucleosis syndrome characterized by fever, arthralgias, myalgias, leukopenia, and atypical lymphocytosis, is the most common symptomatic disease caused by CMV although, localized or disseminated tissue invasive disease may also occur. Predilection to involve the transplanted allograft is a peculiar characteristic of CMV. CMV hepatitis occurs most commonly in liver, CMV pneumonitis in lung and enteritis in small bowel transplant recipients. It is proposed that the transplanted allograft may provide a sequestered site for latently infected cells since MHC mismatches at these sites may prevent the generation of virus specific cytotoxic T cell responses [147]. The clinical impact of CMV is by far greatest in the context of newly acquired or primary infection. Primary CMV acquisition is associated with a higher rate of CMV infection and symptomatic disease, earlier onset of CMV infection post-transplantation, higher incidence of recurrent episodes of CMV, greater risk of dissemination and higher mortality [30, 148, 149]. Symptomatic disease, CMV hepatitis, invasive fungal infections and death in liver transplantation were more likely to occur when primary infection in the recipient was acquired from the donor organ as compared to acquisition from transfusions [150]. The time to onset of CMV after transplantation is also shorter with donor versus transfusion associated CMV infection [150].

CMV serologic status of the recipient and donor is the most significant factor influencing the rate and severity of CMV infection. Eighty to 100% of the seronegative recipients of seropositive donor allograft acquire CMV infection after transplantation. The risk of CMV infection is lowest (<10%) in seronegative recipients of seronegative organ donors. CMV seropositive recipients have an intermediate risk (40–60%) of developing CMV infection. The intensity and type of immunosuppression are also important determinants of the risk of CMV [151]. Antilymphocyte preparations, e.g., OKT3 are extremely potent reactivators of CMV. Primary immunosuppressive agents, e.g., cyclosporine and tacrolimus, on the other hand, are not efficient reactivators but reactivated, they interfere with the host's ability to limit viral replication [151].

Primary infection with HHV-6, which is considered an immodulatory virus, has been proposed to be a risk factor for subsequent CMV invasive disease. Intraoperative hypothermia is a common sequelae of liver transplant surgery. In a study in liver transplant recipients, intraoperative hypothermia was an independently significant risk factor for early CMV infection and active warming using a convective heating device appeared to curtail this risk [152]. HLA matching and retransplantation have also been shown to be risk factors for CMV infection [30, 153].

Diagnosis. The diagnosis of CMV infection has traditionally been made by viral isolation, which can take up to four weeks. The currently available tests not only allow rapid and reliable diagnosis of CMV infection, but may also detect viral shedding at an earlier stage. The shell vial assay for viral cultures uses a monoclonal antibody to detect a 72 kd immediate early CMV antigen and allows detection of CMV within 16 to 24 hours [154]. More recently, CMV antigenemia assay with monoclonal antibodies directed against the 63 kd structural late viral protein, has been developed [155, 156]. The CMV antigenemia assay is more sensitive and allows earlier detection of CMV than shell vial culture. Furthermore, results of the antigenemia assay can be quantitated; the number of antigen-positive cells has been shown to correlate with the likelihood of CMV disease and can also be used to monitor response to antiviral therapy. The major drawback of the antigenemia assay is the need for immediate processing of blood samples. Detection of viral DNA by polymerase chain reaction (PCR) in the leukocyte may be an overly sensitive test for the diagnosis of CMV. Because PCR can detect even minute amounts of viral DNA, it may not differentiate between replicating and latent virus. The precise role of quantitative PCR for the diagnosis of CMV remains to be established. Plasma, as opposed to leukocyte PCR, is specific yet not an excessively sensitive test for the detection of CMV infection [157–159]. Its sensitivity appears comparable to CMV antigenemia.

Management. Although several prophylactic strategies have been used for CMV, an optimal approach has not been defined. High dose acyclovir (800 mg orally q.i.d.), administered to renal transplant patients for 12 weeks decreased the rate of CMV disease [160]. A vast majority of subsequent studies in solid organ transplant recipients, including renal transplant patients, showed no benefit of acyclovir in the prevention of CMV [161]. Ganciclovir, administered intravenously for 2–4 weeks, was efficacious against CMV, predominantly in the seropositive patients [162, 163]. Ganciclovir for 100 days after transplantation was effective both in seropositive patients and in seronegative recipients of seropositive allograft, however the feasibility and cost of administration of ganciclovir for 100 days can be prohibitive [164]. Furthermore, the above strategies require administration of ganciclovir to all patients, most of whom will not experience CMV infection. With prolonged ganciclovir usage, antiviral resistance remains a potential concern and is being increasingly documented in transplant recipients [165–167].

A preferred approach to the prevention of CMV is to target the patients at highest risk for serious disease due to CMV. The success of this approach relies on early identification of CMV infection and employing prophylaxis pre-emptively to prevent asymptomatic infection from progressing to CMV disease. The criteria used to identify high-risk patients may either be a laboratory marker (e.g. viral shedding preceding symptomatic disease) or a clinical event (e.g. institution of OKT3 therapy). Surveillance cultures using a sensitive assay, e.g., CMV antigenemia, offer significant advantage over the previous culture methods, e.g., shell vial assay, for earlier detection of CMV infection [161, 168, 169]. Pre-emptive strategy is particularly appealing, and perhaps ideal for seropositive patients in whom CMV disease generally is less severe [161]. With diligent monitoring, CMV disease can also be prevented in 80 to 100% of the patients with primary CMV infection [170].

Herpes Simplex Virus. Although most HSV infections in transplant recipients present as mucocutaneous lesions due to reactivation of the latent virus, visceral or disseminated HSV infection can be donor transmitted and may have a fulminant presentation with a grave outcome without antiviral therapy. HSV hepatitis is the most frequently documented site of disseminated HSV infection; its incidence (cases per thousand) is reported to be 2.11 in renal, 2.23 in heart, and 4.81 in liver transplant recipients. In a report comprising 12 cases of HSV hepatitis in solid organ transplant recipients, 33% were due to primary HSV infection, believed to be acquired from the donor [171]. The median time to onset of HSV hepatitis was 18 days, although it occurred as early as five days post-transplantation [171]. This characteristic time of onset is in contrast with CMV hepatitis, which usually occurs 30–40 days after transplantation. Clinical manifestations of HSV hepatitis include fever, leukocytosis, thrombocytopenia, and marked elevation of hepatocellular liver enzymes. Mortality from primary visceral HSV infection in seronegative recipients was 75%; hypotension, disseminated intravascular coagulation, metabolic acidosis, low platelet count and high creatinine were significant predictors of mortality [171].

Herpes simplex virus accounted for 41% of all non-cytomegalovirus isolates from the respiratory tract in lung transplant recipients; 80% of the isolates were deemed clinically significant and were associated with pneumonitis [172]. Another clinical presentation of HSV, predominantly reported in intubated lung and cardiac transplant recipients, is HSV tracheobronchitis that manifested as fever, bronchospasm, leukocytosis, and difficulty weaning. Paradoxically, HSV tracheobronchitis had a more severe presentation and worse outcome in immunocompetent as compared to immunosuppressed patients [173]. It was proposed that this maybe due to a more exuberant local immune response in the immunocompetent patients [173].

Low dose acyclovir (200 to 400 mg orally tid) generally employed for 3–4 weeks post-transplant, is highly effective as prophylaxis for HSV in transplant recipients. At one institution, HSV hepatitis was documented in 12/3536 of solid organ transplant recipients prior to the routine employment of acyclovir prophylaxis and in none of the 1144 patients since the utilization of acyclovir prophylaxis [171]. Longer durations (up to three months) are employed for lung transplant recipients in some centers [172].

Varicella Zoster Virus. Up to 70% of pediatric and 5% of adult transplant recipients have been reported to be seronegative for VZV [174, 175]. Exposure to VZV infection may result in primary varicella in these susceptible patients. Median time to onset of varicella was two years after transplantation in one report [174] and 2.4 years in another [176]. Visceral dissemination, frequently documented in transplant recipients is the primary cause of mortality in patients with VZV. Hepatitis, pneumonitis, pancreatitis, gastroenteritis, or meningoencephalitis are the most commonly documented sites of visceral dissemination. Varicella may initially present with acute abdominal pain and in the absence of skin lesions, can defy early recognition [176, 177].

Human Herpesvirus-6. The newest herpesvirus to be identified as a pathogen in transplant recipients is a human herpesvirus-6. Its closest phylogenetic relative is CMV; nucleotide sequencing has revealed 66% DNA homology between CMV and HHV-6.

Most HHV-6 infections, therefore result from endogenous reactivation of the recipient's latent virus; however, donor transmission has also been documented. Although the precise incidence and clinical sequelae of HHV-6 after transplantation remains to be fully elucidated, HHV-6 infection has been reported in 30–40% of liver transplant recipients. Symptomatic disease has been reported in fewer than half of the patients with HHV-6 infection or shedding. The usual timing of onset is between two and three weeks post-transplantation. In transplant recipients, bone marrow suppression, interstitial pneumonitis, and fever of unknown origin, resembling CMV viral syndrome, have been reported due to HHV-6. HHV-6 is a strongly neurotropic virus and its propensity to cause CNS disease has previously been noted in bone marrow transplant patients in the nontransplant setting. Liver transplant recipients and patients with HHV-6 infection were significantly more likely to have mental status changes of unidentifiable etiology, as compared to those without HHV-6 infections.

Viral culture remains the gold standard for diagnosis of HHV-6. A shell vial culture assay (analogous to that for CMV), based on the detection of immediate early antigen of HHV-6 in cell culture, can significantly expedite the time required for detection of HHV-6. Since latent HHV-6 infection occurs commonly in the general population, the role of PCR to diagnose active HHV-6 infections has not been fully ascertained. The antiviral susceptibilities of HHV-6 resemble CMV. HHV-6 is sensitive to both ganciclovir and foscarnet and resistant to acyclovir at achievable serum concentrations. Treatment is indicated if active HHV-6 infection along with clinical disease attributable to HHV-6 is documented as per criteria previously published.

Fever in Transplant Recipients

Fever is common but nevertheless a worrisome clinical event in organ transplant recipients. Sources of fever in transplant recipients are diverse and may, at times, be obscure. Etiologies of fever must be evaluated in temporal context of the time elapsed since transplantation, intensity of immunosuppression and the location of the patient (whether in ICU or non-ICU setting). Most infections in critically ill transplant recipients or those occurring within the first four weeks of transplantation, are related to surgical or technical complications of transplantation and are nosocomially acquired. Bacterial infections are by far the most commonly occurring infection during this period; vascular-catheter related infections, nosocomial pneumonia, and wound or surgical site infections being the frequent source.

The incidence and types of infection also vary with the duration of ICU stay of the patients. For example, 45% of all febrile infections in the ICU in one study occurred within seven days of patients' ICU stay [60]. Pneumonia accounted for 41% of the febrile infections in the ICU during the first seven days of ICU stay, but only for 14% of these after seven days of stay in the ICU [60]. This early risk may be reflective of the universal requirement of intubation after transplant surgery. The risk of catheter-related bacteremia, however, tripled after the first week of ICU stay [60].

Infections in immunocompromised hosts may not be invariably accompanied by a febrile response. Indeed, 27% of transplant recipients with infections in one report were euthermic and 5% were hypothermic [60]. Severity of illness as assessed by APACHE II scores and APS score in hypothermic patients was significantly greater than in those who were febrile or euthermic [178]. Bacteremia was documented in 51% of febrile, 15% of euthermic but 80% of the hypothermic patients [178]. Mortality at 30 days was significantly higher in hypothermic (100%) as compared to febrile (20%) and euthermic patients (23%) ($p = 0.0006$).

Prior to the availability of effective antiviral therapy for CMV, 70% of the prolonged febrile episodes of unknown etiology after the first post-transplant month were due to CMV. The incidence of CMV, as a cause of fever, however, has declined dramatically in recent years.

Fever is also considered an important sign of allograft rejection after transplantation. Fever within the first 16 days post-transplant was more likely to be due to rejection than infection in one study [179, 180]. Peripheral blood eosinophilia may be a clue to rejection in transplant patients. However, rejection episodes in the era of modern immunosuppressive agents have become less florid and hence less likely to be associated with signs of acute inflammation, e.g. fever, leukocytosis, etc. In fact, 85% of the acute rejection episodes in renal transplant recipients receiving cyclosporine were not associated with fever [179].

Therapy with OKT3 monoclonal antibody for the treatment of rejection may be accompanied by flu-like symptoms, including fever in up to 80% of the patients. These symptoms are believed to be due to the release of cytokines, e.g. TNF, interferon-gamma and IL2. The cytokines are elevated within 1–2 hours of OKT3 administration and return to baseline by 24 hours; fever usually resolved in 2–5 days. Three to 15% of the OKT3 recipients may also have aseptic meningitis.

Other causes of fever of obscure etiology after transplantation are drug reactions (e.g. due to interferon-alpha), hematomas, pulmonary emboli, tissue infarction, malignancies (most commonly post-transplant lymphoproliferative disorder), hemolytic-uremic syndrome, or adrenal insufficiency. Major physiologic stress with the concurrent use of drugs such as anticonvulsants (i.e. phenytoin, phenobarbital) and/or rifampin that may lower endogenous corticosteroid levels can provoke acute adrenal insufficiency in critically ill transplant recipients with marginal adrenal reserve, i.e. in those not receiving corticosteroids as part of an immunosuppressive regimen [181]. In up to 7% of febrile transplant recipients, an etiology may remain elusive [2]. It is likely that some of these febrile episodes may be due to the newly recognized viruses, e.g. HHV-6 [2].

References

1. Waser M, Maagiorini M, Luthy A, Laske A, vor Sequesser L, Mohassi P. Infectious complications in 100 consecutive heart transplant recipients. Eur J Clin Microbiol Infect Dis 13:12, 1994.
2. Chang FY, Singh N, Gayowski T, Wagener MM, Marino IR. Fever in liver transplant recipients: changing spectrum of etiologic agents. Clin Infect Dis 26:59, 1998.
3. Sawyer RG, Crabtree TD, Antevil JL, Gleason TG, Pruett TL. Transplantation suppresses leukocytosis but not fever in patients with bacterial or fungal infection. Seventeenth Annual Meeting of the American Society of Transplant Physicians, Chicago, IL 1998; Abstract #602.
4. Novella M, Sola R, Soriano G, Andreu M, Gana J, Oritz J, *et al.* Continuous inpatient prophylaxis of the first episode of spontaneous bacterial peritonitis with norfloxacin. Hepatology 97 A.D.; 25:532.
5. Paterson DL, Ko W, Von Gottberg A, Klugman K, Mohapatra S, *et al.* Epidemiology of bacteremia due to multiply resistant extended-spectrum beta-lactamase (ESBL)-producing *Klebsiella pneumoniae* in transplant unit patients. 39th Interscience Conference on Antimicrobial Agents and Chemotherapy, San Francisco, September 1999; Abstract 1426.
6. Linden P. The emergence of vancomycin-resistant organisms in transplantation. Current Opinion in Organ Transplantation 3:130, 1998.
7. Bauldoff GS, Nunley DR, Manzetti JD, Dauber JH, Keenan RJ. Use of aerosolized colistin sodium in cystic fibrosis patients awaiting lung transplantation. Transplantation 64:748, 1997.
8. Chang FY, Singh N, Gayowski T, Drenning SD, Wagener MM, Mariono IR. Staphylococcus aureus nasal colonization and association with infections in liver transplant recipients. Transplantation 65:1169, 1998.
9. Chang FY, Singh N, Gayowski T, Wagener M, Marino IR. *Staphylococcus aureus* nasal colonization in patients with cirrhosis: prospective assessment of association with infections. Infect Control Hosp Epidemiol 19:328, 1998.
10. Grems JJ, Hiatt JR, Klein AS, Hart J, El-Khoury G, *et al.* Disseminated aspergillosis complicating orthotopic liver transplantation for fulminant hepatic failure refractory to croticosteroid therapy. Transplantation 46:479, 1988.
11. Sampathkumar S, Plevak DJ, Paya MD. Systemic fungal infections following orthotopic liver transplantation for acute liver disease. Transplantation Abstract 352, 1999.
12. Milstone AP, Brumble LM, Loyd JE, Loyd JE, Ely EW, *et al.* Active CMV infection before lung transplantation: risk factors and clinical implications. Transplantation 67:598, 1999.
13. Gayowsksi T, Marino IR, Singh N, Doyle H, Wagener MM, *et al.* Orthotopic liver transplantation in high risk patients: risk factors associated with mortality and infectious morbidity. Transplantation 65:499, 1997.
14. Singh N, Arnow PM, Bonham A, Dominguez E, Paterson DL, *et al.* Invasive aspergillosis in liver transplant recipients in the 1990s. Transplantation 64:716, 1997.
15. Rogers J, Singh N, Carrigan DR, Rohal S, Kusne S, *et al.* Clinical relevance of human herpesvirus-6 infection in liver transplant recipients: role in pathogenesis of fungal infections, neurologic complications, and impact on outcome. 39th Interscience Conference on Antimicrobial Agents and Chemotherapy, San Francisco 1999.
16. Petri WA. Infections in heart transplant recipients. Clin Infect Dis 18:141, 1994.
17. Turkaspa R, Burk RD, Shaul Y, Shafritz DA. Hepatitis B virus contains a glucocorticoid responsive element. Proc Natl Acad Sci 83:1627, 1986.
18. Hudnall SD, Rady PL, Tyring SK, Fish JC. Hydrocortisone activation of human herpesvirus 8 viral DNA replication and gene expression *in vitro*. Transplantation 67:648, 1999.
19. Kim JH, Perfect JR. Infection and cyclosporine. Rev Infect Dis 11:677, 1989.
20. Singh N. Infections in solid organ transplant

recipients. In Wenzel RP (ed). Prevention and Control of Nosocomial Infections. Williams and Wilkins, 1997:1100.

21. Hofflin JH, Potasman I, Baldwin JC, *et al.* Infectious complications in heart transplant recipients receiving cyclosporine and corticosteroids. Ann Intern Med 106:209, 1987.
22. Ochiai TA, Nakajima K, Nagatar M, Suzuki T, Asano T, *et al.* Effect of a new immunosuppressive agent, FK506 on heterotropic cardiac allotransplantation in the rat. Transplant Proceed 19:1284, 1987.
23. The U.S. Multicenter FK506 Liver Study Group. A comparison of tacrolimus (FK506) and cyclosporine for immunosuppression in liver transpalntation. New Engl J Med 332:1110, 1994.
24. Paterson DL, Singh N, Panebianco A, Wannstedt CF, Wagener MM, *et al.* Infectious complications occurring in liver transplant recipients receiving mycophenolate mofetil. Transplantation 66:593, 1998.
25. Singh N, Carrigan DR. Human herpesvirus-6 in transplantation: an emerging pathogen. Ann Intern Med 124:1065, 1996.
26. Dockrell DH, Mendez JC, Jones M, Harmsen WS, Ilstrup DM, *et al.* Human herpesvirus 6 seronegativity before transplantation predicts the occurrence of fungal infection in liver transplant recipients. Transplantation 67:399, 1999.
27. DesJardin JA, Gibbons L, Cho E, Supran SE, Falagas ME, *et al.* Human herpesvirus 6 reactivation is associated with cytomegalovirus infection and syndromes in kidney transplant recipients at risk for primary *cytomegalovirus* infection. J Infect Dis, 1999.
28. Dockrell DH, Prada J, Jones MF, Patel R, Badley AD, *et al.* Seroconversion to human herpesvirus 6 following liver transplantation is a marker of *cytomegalovirus* disease. J Infect Dis 176:1135, 1997.
29. Chatterjee SN, Fiala N, Weiner J. Primary cytomegalovirus and opportunistic infections: Incidence in renal transplant recipients. JAMA 240:2446, 1978.
30. Stratta RJ, Shaeffer MS, Markin RS, Wood RP, Langnas AN, *et al.* *Cytomegalovirus* infection and disease after liver transplantation, an overview. Dig Dis Sci 37:673, 1992.
31. Paya CV. Fungal infections in solid-organ transplantation. Clin Infect Dis 16:677, 1993.
32. Roenhorst HW, Beelen JM, Middeldrop JM, Schrim J, Tegzess AM. Maintenance of CMV latency and host immune responses of long-term renal allograft survivors. Clin Exp Immunol 61:72, 1985.
33. Grattan MT, Moreno-Cabral CE, Starnes VA, Oyer PE, Stinson EB, Shumway NE. *Cytomegalovirus* infection is associated with cardiac allograft rejection and atherosclerosis. JAMA 261:3561, 1989.
34. Reinke P, Fietze E, Ode-Hakim S, Prosch S, Lippert J, *et al.* Late accute renal allograft rejection and symptomless *cytomegalovirus* infection. Lancet 344:1737, 1994.
35. Lee H, Locker J, Nalesnik M, Reyes J, Jaffe R, *et al.* The association of Epstein-Barr virus with smooth muscle tumors occurring after organ transplantation. N Engl J Med 332:19, 1995.
36. Alkan S, Karcher DS, Ortiz A, Khalil S, Akhtar M, Ashraf Ali M. Human herpesvirus-8/Kaposi's sarcoma-associated herpesvirus in organ transplant patients with immunosuppression. Br J Haematology 96:412, 1997.
37. Boshoff C, Weiss RA. Aetiology of Kaposi's sarcoma: current understanding and implications for therapy. Molec Med Today 3:488, 1997.
38. Eason JD, Freeman RB, Rohrer RJ, Lewis WD, Jenkins R, *et al.* Should liver transplantation be performed for patients with hepatitis B? Transplantation 57:1588, 1994.
39. Singh N, Gayowski T, Wagener MM, Marino IR. Increased infections in liver transplant recipients with recurrent hepatitis C virus hepatitis. Transplantation 61:402, 1996.
40. LaQuaglia MP, Tolkoff-Rubin NE, Dienstag JL, Cosimi AB, Herrin JT, *et al.* Impact of hepatitis on renal transplantation. Transplantation 32:504, 1981.
41. Singh N, Gayowski T, Wagener MM, Marino IR. Predictors and outcome of early-versus late-onset major bacterial infections in liver transplant recipients receiving tacrolimus (FK506) as primary immunosuppression. Eur J Clin Microbiol Infect Dis 16:821, 1997.
42. Hoy WE, May AG, Freeman RB. Primary renal transplant wound infections. New York State J Med 81:1469, 1981.
43. Sollinger HW, Ploeg RJ, Eckhoff DE, Stegall MD, Isaacs R, *et al.* Two hundred consecutive simultaneous pancreas-kidney transplants with bladder drainage. Surgery 114:736, 1993.
44. Evrett JE, Wahoff DC, Statz GKJ, Gruessner A, Gruessner RWG, *et al.* Characterization and impact of wound infection after pancreas transplantation. Arch Surg 129:1310, 1994.
45. Hesse UJ, Sutherland DER, Simmons RL,

Najarian JS. Intra-abdominal infections in pancreas transplant recipients. Clin Transplantation 4:287, 1990.

46. Tesi RJ, Henry ML, Elkhammas EA, Sommer BG, Ferguson RM. Decreased wound complications of combined kidney/pancreas transplants using intraabdominal pancreas graft placement. Clin Transplantation 4:287.
47. Dauber JH, Paradis IL, Dummer JS. Infectious complication in pulmonary alograft recipients. Clin Chest Med 11:291, 1990.
48. Kramer P, Ten Kate FWJ, Bijnen AB, Jeckel J, Weinar W. Recombinant leukocyte in interferon A induces steroid resistant acute vascular rejection episodes in renal transplant recipients. Lancet 1:989, 1989.
49. Manez R, Kusne S, Green M, Abu-Elmagd K, Irish W, *et al.* Incidence and risk factors associated with the development of *cytomegalovirus* disease after intestinal transplantation. Transplantation 59:1010, 1995.
50. Kusne S, Furukawa H, Kabu-Elmagd W, Irish W, Rakela J, *et al.* Infectious complications after small bowel transplantation in adults: an update. Transplan Proceed 5:2761, 1996.
51. Woodward JE, Mayer D. The unique challenge of small intestinal transplantation. Brit J Hosp Med 285, 1996.
52. Reyes J, Bueno J, Kocoshis S, Green M, Abu-Elmagd K, *et al.* Current status of intestinal transplantation in children. J Pediatr Surg 33:243, 1998.
53. McAlister V, Grant D, Wall W, Roy A, Ghent C, *et al.* Immunosuppressive requirements for small bowel/liver transplantation. Transplan Proceed 25:1204, 1993.
54. Lumbreras C, Fernandez I, Velosa J, Munn S, Sterioff S, Paya CV. Infectious complications following pancreatic transplantation: incidence, microbiological, clinical characteristics and outcome. Clin Infect Dis 20:514, 1995.
55. Wagener MM, Yu VL. Bacteremia in transplant recipients: a prospective study of demographics, etiologic agents, risk factors, and outcomes. Am J Infect Control 20:239, 1992.
56. Fox BD, Sollinger HW, Belzer FO, Maki DG. A prospective, randomized double-blind study of trimethoprim-sulfamethoxazole for prophylaxis of infection in renal transplantation: clinical efficacy, absorption, effects on microflora and the cost-benefit of prophylaxis. Am J Med 89:255, 1990.
57. Wade JJ, Rolando N, Hallar K, Philpott-Howard J, Casewell MW, Williams R. Bacterial and fungal infections after liver transplantation: an analysis of 284 patients. Hepatology 21:1328, 1995.
58. Lumbreras C, Lizasoain M, Moreno E, Aguado JM, Gomez R, *et al.* Major bacterial infections following liver transplantation. Hepatology-Gastroenterology 39:362, 1992.
59. George DL, Arnow PM, Fox AS, Baker AL, Thistlewaite JR, *et al.* Bacterial infection as a complication of liver transplantation: epidemiology and risk factors. Rev Infect Dis 13:387, 1991.
60. Singh N, Chang FY, Gayowski T, Wagener MM, Marino IR. Fever in liver transplant recipients in the intensive care unit. Clin Transplantation, 2000.
61. Singh N, Paterson DL, Gayowski T, Chang FY, Wagener M, Marino I. Methicillin-resistant *Staphylococcus aureus*: the other emerging gram positive coccus in liver transplant recipients. Clin Infect Dis, 2000.
62. Mossad SB, Avery RK, Goormastic M, Hobbs RE, Stewart RW. Significance of positive cultures from donor left atrium and postpreservation fluid in heart transplantation. Transplantation 64:1209, 1997.
63. Bonham CA, Dominguez EA, Fukui MB, Paterson DL, Pankey GA, Wagener MM. Central nervous system lesions in liver transplant recipients: prospective assessment of indications for biopsy and implications for management. Transplantation 66:1596, 1998.
64. Selby R, Ramirez CB, Singh R, Kleopoulos I, Kusne S, *et al.* Brain abscess in solid organ transplant recipients receiving cyclosporine-based immunosuppression. Arch Surg 132:304, 1997.
65. Singh N, Yu VL, Gayowski T. Central nervous system lesions in adult liver transplant recipients: clinical review with implications for management. Medicine 73:110, 1994.
66. Wang F-Z, Linde A, Hagglund H, Testa M, Locasciulli A, Ljungman P. *Human herpesvirus* 6 DNA in erebrospinal fluid specimens from allogeneic bone marrow transplant patients: does it have clinical significance? Clin Infect Dis 28:562, 1999.
67. Paterson DL, Singh N, Gayowski T, Carrigan DR, Marino IR. Encephalopathy associated with human herpesvirus 6 in a liver transplant recipient. Livr Trans Surg 5:1, 1999.
68. Chaparro C, Kesten S. Infections in lung transplant recipients. Clin Chest Med 18:339, 1997.

69. Paradis IL, Williams P. Infection after lung transplantation. Sem Respir Infect 8:207, 1999.
70. Kramer MR, Marshall SE, Starnes VA, Gamberg P, Amitai Z, Theodore J. Infectious complications in heart-lung transplantation, analysis of 200 episodes. Arch Intern Med 153:2010, 1993.
71. Kanj SS, Welty-Wolf K, Madden J, Tapson V, Baz MA, *et al*. Fungal infections in lung and heart-lung transplant recipients, report of 9 cases and review of the literature. Medicine 75:142, 1996.
72. Westney GE, Kesten S, De Hoyos A, Chapparro C, Winton T, Maurer JR. *Aspergillus* infection in single and double lung transplant recipients. Transplantation 61:915, 1996.
73. Cahill BC, Hibbs JR, Savik K, Juni BA, Dosland BM, *et al*. *Aspergillus* airway colonization and invasive disease after lung transplantation. Chest 112:1160, 1997.
74. Singh N, Falestiny M, Rogers P, Reed MJ, Pulaski J, *et al*. Pulmonary infiltrates in the intensive care unit: predictors and outcome. Chest 114:1129, 1998.
75. Miller R, Naftel DC, Bourg RC, Kirklin JK, Brozena SC, *et al*. Infection after heart transplantation: a multi-institutional study. J Heart Lung Transplant 13:381, 1994.
76. Cisneros JM, Muñoz P, Torres-Cisneros J, Gurgui M, Rodriguez-Hernandez MJ, *et al*. Pneumonia after heart transplantation: a multiinstitutional study. Clin Infect Dis 27:324, 1998.
77. Wreghitt TG, Hakim M, Gray JS, Kucia S. *Cytomegalovirus* infections in heart and heart and lung transplant recipients. J Clin Pathol 41:660, 1988.
78. Dummer JS, Armstrong J, Somers J, *et al*. Transmission of infection with herpes simplex virus by renal transplantation. J Infect Dis 155:202, 1987.
79. Crumpacker CS. Ganciclovir. N Engl J Med 335:721, 1997.
80. Martinez-Marcos F, Cisneros J, Gentil M, Algarra G, Pereira P, *et al*. Prospective study of renal transplant infections in 50 consecutive patients. Eur J Clin Micro Infect Dis 13:1023, 1994.
81. Peterson PK, Andersen RC. Infection in renal transplant recipients. Amer J Med 81:2, 1986.
82. Edelstein CL, Jacobs JC, Moosa MR. Pulmonary complications in 110 consecutive renal transplant recipients. S Afr Med J 85:160, 1995.
83. Paterson DL, Singh N, Gayowski T, Marino IR. Pulmonary nodules in liver transplant recipients. Medicine 77:50, 1998.
84. Cisneros JM, Muñoz P, Torre-Cisneros J, Gurgui M, Rodriguez-Hernandez MJ, *et al*. Pneumonia after heart transplantation: a multiinstitutional study. Clin Infect Dis 27:324, 1998.
85. Singh N, Gayowski T, Wagener MM, Marino IR. Pulmonary infiltrates in liver translant recipients in the intensive care unit. Transplantation 67:1138, 1999.
86. Lobo PI, Rudolf LE, Kreiger JN. Wound infections in renal transplant recipients – a complication of urinary tract infections during allograft malfunction. Surgery 92:491, 1982.
87. Lapchik MS, Filho AC, Restana JO, Filho AP, Wey SB. Risk factors for nosocomial urinary tract and prosoperative wound infections in renal translant patients: a matched pair case control study. J Urology 147:994, 1992.
88. Muakkassa WF, Goldman MH, Mendez-Picon G, Lee HM. Wound infections in renal transplant patients. J Urology 130:17, 1983.
89. Tilney NL, Strom TB, Vineyard GC, Merrill JP. Factors contributing to the declining mortality rate in renal transplantation. New Engl J Med 299:1321, 1978.
90. Wright TL, Combs C, Kim. Metal. Interferon-alpha therapy for hepatitis C virus infection after liver transplantation. Hepatology 20:773, 1994.
91. Tsiquaye KN, Slomka MJ, Maung M. Oral famciclovir against duck hepatitis B virus replication in hepatic and nonhepatic tissues of ducklings infected in ova. J Med Virol 42:306, 1990.
92. Lewiston N, King V, Umetsu D. Cystic fibrosis patients who have undergone heart-lung transplantation benefit from maxillary sinus antrostomy and repeated sinus lavage. Transplant 23:1207, 1991.
93. Finkelstein S, Sayegh R, Uchman S, Christensen S, Swalsky P. HCV undergoes extensive mutational change in N55 region in association with relapse/breakthrough following alpha-interferon therapy. Hepatology 16:132, 1992.
94. Everett JE, Wahoff DC, Statz C, Gillingham KJ, Gruessner A, *et al*. Characterization and impact of wound infection after pancreas transplantation. Arch Surg 129:1310, 1994.

95. Rosen HR, Martin P, Shackelton CR, Farmer DA, Holt C, Busuttil RW. OKT3 use associated with diminished graft and patient survival in patients transplanted for chronic hepatitis. Hepatology 22(Suppl):132A, 1996.
96. Paterson DL, Dominguez E, Chang FY, Snydman DR, Singh N. Infective endocarditis in solid organ transplant recipients. Clin Infect Dis 26:689, 1998.
97. Horvath J, Dummer S, Lloyd J, Walker B, Merrill WH, Frist WH. Infection in the transplanted and native lung after single lung transplantation. Chest 104:681, 1993.
98. Yeldandi V, McCabe MA, Larson Real. *Aspergillus* and lung transplantation. J Heart Lung Transplant 14:883, 1995.
99. Paradowski LJ. Saprophytic fungal infections and lung transplantation – revisited. J Heart Lung Transplant 16:524, 1997.
100. Husni R, Gordon S, Quereshi M. Risk factors for invasive aspergillosis in lung transplant recipients (Abstract 33). In Program and Abstracts of 34th Annual Meeting of the Infectious Diseases Society of American. New Orleans, LA. 34th Ann Meet Infect Dis Soc Amer 1996.
101. Kanj SS, Tapson V, Davis D, Madden J, Browning I. Infections in patients with cystic fibrosis following lung transplantation. Chest 112:924, 1997.
102. Castaldo P, Stratta RJ, Wood RP. Clinical spectrum of fungal infections after orthotopic liver transplantation. Arch Surg 126:149, 1991.
103. Briegel J, Forst H, Spill B, Haas A, Grabein B, *et al.* Risk factors for systemic fungal infections in liver transplant recipients. Eur J Clin Microbiol Infect Dis 14:375, 1995.
104. Collins LA, Samore MH, Roberts MS, Luzzati R, Jenkins RL, *et al.* Risk factors for invasive fungal infections complicating orthotopic liver transplantation. J Infect Dis 170:644, 1994.
105. Kusne S, Torre-Cisneros J, Mañez R. Factors associated with invasive lung aspergillosis and significance of positive cultures after liver transplantation. J Infect Dis 166:1379, 1992.
106. Munoz P, Torre J, Bouza E, *et al.* Invasive Aspergillosis in transplant recipients: a large multicentric study (abstract no. J128). Program and Abstracts of the 36th Interscience Conference on Antimicrobial Agents and Chemotherapy Washington DC: American Society for Microbiology 1996:242.
107. Faggian G, Livi U, Bortolotti U. Itraconazole therapy for acute invasive pulmonary aspergillosis in heart transplantation. Transplant Proc 21:2506, 1989.
108. Rabito FJ, Pankey GA. Infections in orthotopic heart transplant patients at the Ochsner Medical Institutions. Med Clin N Am 76:1125, 1992.
109. Podzimkova M, Gebauerova M, Malek I, Pirk J, Stanek V, *et al.* Infectious complications in patients after heart transplantation. Cor et Vasa 35:263, 1993.
110. Brown RS, Lake JR, Katzman BA, Ascher NL, Sombert KA, *et al.* Incidence and significance of *Aspergillus* cultures following liver and kidney transplantation. Transplantation 61:666, 1996.
111. Cofan F, Iñigo P, Ricart MJ, *et al.* Invasive aspergillosis following kidney and kidney-pancreas transplantation. Nefrologia 16:253, 1996.
112. Paterson DL. Invasive aspergillosis. In Yu VL, Merrigan T (eds). Antimicrobial Therapy and Vaccines. Baltimore: Williams and Wilkins, 1998.
113. Heussel CP, Kauczoe HU, Heussel G, Fischer B, Mildenberger P, Thelen M. Early detection of pneumonia in febrile neutropenic patients: use of thin-section CT. Radiology 169:1347, 1997.
114. Verweij PE, Dompeling EC, Donnelly JP, Schattenberg AV, Meis JF. Serial monitoring of *Aspergillus* antigen in the early diagnosis of invasive aspergillosis. Preliminary investigations with two examples. Infection 25:86, 1997.
115. Swanink CMA, Meis JFGM, Rijs AJMM, Donnelly JP, Verweij PE. Specificity of a sandwich enzyme-linked immunosorbent assay for detecting *Aspergillus* galactomannan. J Clin Microbiol 35:257, 1997.
116. Singh N, Mieles L, Yu VL, Gayowski T. Invasive aspergillosis in liver transplant recipients: association with candidemia, consumption coagulopathy, and failure of prophylaxis with low-dose amphotercin B. Clin Infect Dis 17:906, 1993.
117. Reichenspurner H, Gamberg P, Nitschke M, Valentine H, Hunt S, *et al.* Significant reduction in the number of fungal infections after lung, heart-lung, and heart transplantation using aerosolized amphotericin B prophylaxis. Transplant Proceed 29:627, 1997.
118. Paterson DL, Singh N. Invasive aspergillosis in transplant recipients. Medicine 78:123, 1999.

119. White MH, Wingard JR, Gurwith M, Du Mond C, Mamelok RD, Bowden RA. Amphotericin B colloidal dispersion vs. amphotericin B as therapy for invasive aspergillosis. Clin Infect Dis 24:635, 1997.
120. Linden P, Coley K, Kramer D, Kusne S, Fung J. Invasive aspergillosis in liver transplant recipients: comparison of outcome with amphotericin B LIPID complex and conventional amphotericin B therapy. Transplantation 67:S232, 1999.
121. Graybill J, Loebenberg R, Bocanegra R, Najvar L. Granulocyte colony stimulating factor (G-CSF) and azole antifungal therapy in murine aspergillosis: surprises. 38th International Conference on Antimicrobial Agents and Chemotherapy, San Diego, CA 1998:Abstract J48.
122. Tollemar J, Ericzon BG, Barkhold L, Anderosn J, Ringden O, Groth CG. Risk factors for deep candida infections in liver transplant recipients. Transplant Proceed 22:1826, 1990.
123. Singh N, Gayowski T, Wagener MM, Doyle H, Marino IR. Invasive fungal infections in liver transplant recipients receiving tacrolimus as primary immunosuppressive agent. Clin Infect Dis 24:179, 1997.
124. Patel R, Portelar D, Bradley AD, Harmsen WS, Larson-Keller JJ, *et al.* Candida and non-Candida fungal infections after liver transplantation. Transplantation 62:926, 1996.
125. Lumbreras C, Cuervas-Mons V, Jara P, de/Palacio A, Turrion VS, *et al.* Randomized trial of fluconazole versus nystatin for the prophylaxis of Candida infection after liver transplantation. J Infect Dis 174:583, 1996.
126. Fortun J, Lopez-San Roman A, Velasco JJ, Sanchez-Sousa A, DeVincente E, *et al.* Susceptibility of *Candida glabrata* strains with reduced susceptibility of azoles in four liver transplant patients with invasive candidiasis. Eur J Clin Microbiol Infect Dis 16:314, 1997.
127. Bensousan T, Garo B, Islam S, Bourbigot B, Cledes J, Garre M. Possible transfer of *Pneumocystis carinii* between kidney transplant recipients (letter). Lancet 336:1066, 1990.
128. Branten AJ, Beckers PJ, Tiggeler RG, Hoitsma AJ. *Pneumocystis carinii* pneumonia in renal transplant recipients. Nephrol Dial Transplant 10:1194, 1995.
129. Chave JP, David S, Wauters JP, Van Melle G, Francioli P. Transmission of *Pneumocystis carinii* from AIDS patients to other immunosupressed patients: a cluster of *Pneumocystis carinii* pneumonia in renal transplant recipients. AIDS 5:927, 1991.
130. Hennequin C, Page B, Roux P, Lengendre C, Kreis H. Outbreak of *Pneumocystis carinii* pneumonia in a renal transplant unit. Eur J Clin Microbiol Infect Dis 14:122, 1995.
131. Olsson M, Sukura A, Lindburg L, Lindu E. Detection of *Pneumocystis carinii* DNA by filtration of air. Scand J Infect Dis 28:279, 1996.
132. Gryzan S, Paradis IL, Zeevi A, Duuesnoy RJ, Dummer JS, *et al.* Unexpectedly high incidence of *Pneumocystis carinii* infection after lung-heart transplantation. Implications for lung defense and allograft survival. Am Rev Respir Dis 137:1268, 1988.
133. Arend SM, Westendorp RGJ, Kroon FP, van't Wout JW, Vandenbroucke JP, *et al.* Rejection treatment and *cytomegalovirus* infection as risk factors for *Pneumocystis carinii* pneumonia in renal transplant recipients. Clin Infect Dis 22:920, 1996.
134. Gordon SM, LaRosa SP, Kalmadi S, Arroliga AC, Avery RK, *et al.* Should prophylaxis for *Pneumocystis carinii* pneumonia in solid organ transplant recipients ever be discontinued? Clin Infect Dis 28:240, 1999.
135. Singh N, Gayowski T, Wagener MM, Marino IR. Clinical spectrum of invasive cryptococcosis in liver transplant recipients receiving tacrolimus. Clin Transplantation 11:66, 1997.
136. Singh N, Gayowski T, Yu VL. Invasive gastrointestinal zygomycosis in a liver transplant recipient: case report and review of zygomycosis in solid-organ transplant recipients. Clin Infect Dis 20:617, 1995.
137. Singh N, Chang FY, Gayowski T, Marino IR. Infections due to dematiaceous fungi in organ transplant recipients: case report and review. Clin Infect Dis 24:369, 1997.
138. Newell KA, Millis JM, Arnow PM, Bruce DS, Woodle ES, *et al.* Incidence and outcome of infection by vancomycin-resistant *Enterococcus* following orthotoic liver transplantation. Transplantation 65:439, 1998.
139. Linden PK, Pasculle AW, Manez R, *et al.* Differences in outcome for patients with bacteremia due to vancomycin-resistant *Enterococcus faceium* or vancomycin susceptible *E. faceium*. Clin Infect Dis 22:663, 1996.
140. Kusne S, Molmenti E, Krystofiak S, Rakela J, Fung J. Risk factors associated with vancomycin resistant *Enterococcus faceium* (VREF) bacteremia in liver transplant recipients. 37th

Interscience Conference on Antimicrobial Agents and Chemotherapy, Toronto, Canada 1997:Abstract J–37.
141. Papanicolaou GA, Myers BR, Meyers J, Mendelson MH, Lou W, *et al.* Nosocomial infections with vancomycin-resistant *Enterococcus faecium in* liver translant recipients: risk factors for acquisition and mortality. Clin Infect Dis 23:760, 1996.
142. Chow JW, Yu VL. Legionella a major oportunistic pathogen in transplant recipients. Seminars Respir Infect 13:132, 1998.
143. Marrie TJ, Johnson WM, Tyler SD, Bezanson GS, Burbridge S. Genomic stability of *Legionella pneumophila* isolates recovered from two cardiac transplant patients with nosocomial Legionnaires' disease. J Clin Microbiol 3085, 1994.
144. Bangsborg JM, Uldum S, Jensen JS, Bruun BG. Nosocomial legionellosis in three heart-lung transplant patients: case reports and environmental observations. Eur J Clin Microbiol Infect Dis 14:99, 1995.
145. Phillips SJ, Zeff RH, Gervick D. Legionnaires' disease. Ann Thorac Surg 44:564, 1987.
146. Singh N, Muder RR, Yu VL. Legionella infection in liver transplant reciepients: implications for management. Transplantation 15:677, 1993.
147. Ho M. Infection and organ transplantation. In Gelman S (ed). Anesthesia and Organ Transplantation. Saunders, 1987:49.
148. Singh N, Dummer JS, Kusne S, Breinig MC, Armstrong JA, *et al.* Infections with *cytomegalovirus* and the herpesviruses in 121 liver transplant recipients: transmission by donated organ and the effect of OKT3 antibodies. J Infect Dis 158:124, 1988.
149. Hibberd PL, Basgoz N, Fishman J, Rubin RH. Primary *cytomegalovirus* disease is a risk factor for recurrent CMV disease in transplant recipients (abstract H28). 34th Intersci Conf Antimicrob Ag Chemother 1995; Orlando, FL.
150. Falagas ME, Snydman DR, Ruthazer R, Griffith J, Werner BG, and the Boston Center for Liver Transplantation CMVIG Study Group. Primary *cytomegalovirus* infection in liver transplant recipients: comparison of infections transmitted via donor organs and via transfusions. Clin Infect Dis 23:292, 1996.
151. Fietze E, Prosch S, Reinke P, Stein J, Docke WD, *et al. Cytomegalovirus* infection in transplant recipients. The role of tumor necrosis factor. Transplantation 58:675, 1994.
152. Paterson DL, Singh N, Stapelfeldt W, Wagener MM, Gayowski T, Marino IR. Intraoperative hypothermia is an independent risk factor for *cytomegalovirus* (CMV) infection in liver transplant recipients. Transplantation 67:1151, 1999.
153. Mañez R, White LT, Linden P, *et al.* The influence of HLA matching on *cytomegalovirus* hepatitis and chronic rejection after liver transplantation. Transplantation 55:1067, 1993.
154. Gleaves CA, Smith TF, Shuster EA, Pearson GR. Comparison of standard tube and shell vial cell culture techniques for the detection of *cytomegalovirus* in clinical specimens. J Clin Microbiol 21:217, 1985.
155. The TH, Vander BIJW, VandenBerg AP, *et al. Cytomegalovirus* antigenemia. Rev Infect Dis 12(suppl):737, 1990.
156. Gerna G, Zavattoni M, Percivalle E, Grossi P, Torsellini M, Grazia-Revello M. Rising levels of human *cytomegalovirus* (HCMV) antigenemia during initial antiviral treatment of solid-organ transplant recipients with primary HCMV infection. J Clin Microbiol 36:1113, 1998.
157. Patel R, Smith TF, Espy M, Portela D, Wiesner RH, *et al.* A prospective comparison of molecular diagnostic techniques for the early detection of *cytomegalovirus* in liver transplant recipients. J Infect Dis 171:1010, 1995.
158. Cunningham R, Harris A, Frankton A, Irving W. Detection of *cytomegalovirus* using PCR in serum from renal transplant recipients. J Clin Pathol 48:575, 1995.
159. Schmidt CA, Oettle H, Peng R, Neuhaus P, Blum G, *et al.* Comparison of polymerase chain reaction from plasma and buffy coat with antigen detection and occurrence of immunoglobulin M for the demonstration of *cytomegalovirus* infection after liver transplantation. Transplantation 59:1133, 1995.
160. Balfour HH, Chace BA, Stepleton JT, Simmons RR, Fryd DS. A randomized, placebo controlled trial of oral acyclovir for the prevention of *cytomegalovirus* disease in recipients of renal allografts. N Engl J Med 320:1381, 1989.
161. Singh N, Yu VL, Mieles L, Wagener MM, Miner RC, Gayowski T. High-dose ayclovir compared with short-course preemptive ganciclovir therapy to prevent *cytomegalovirus* disease in liver transplant recipients, a randomized trial. Annals Int Med 120:375, 1994.
162. Martin MM, Mañez R, Linden P, Estores D, Torre-Cisneros J, *et al.* A prospective random-

ized trial comparing sequential ganciclovir-high dose acyclovir to high dose acyclovir for prevention of *cytomegalovirus* disease in adult liver transplant recipients. Transplantation 58:779, 1994.

163. Merigan TC, Renlund DG, Keay S, *et al.* A controlled trial of ganciclovir to prevent *cytomegalovirus* disease after heart transplantation. N Engl J Med 326:1182, 1993.
164. Winston DJ, Wirin D, Shaked A, Busuttil RW. Randomized comparison of ganciclovir and high-dose acyclovir for long-term cytomegalovirus prophylaxis in liver transplant recipients. Lancet 346:69, 1995.
165. Singh N, Yu VL. Oral Ganciclovir usage for *cytomegalovirus* prophylaxis in organ transplant recipients. Is emergence of resistance imminent? Dig Dis Sci 43:1190, 1998.
166. Alain S, Honderlick P, Grenet D, Stern M, Vadam C, *et al.* Failure of ganciclovir treatment associated with selection of a ganciclovir resistant *cytomegalovirus* strain in a lung transplant recipient. Transplantation 63:1533, 1997.
167. Rosen HR, Brenner KG, Flora KD, Rabkin JM, Orloff SL, *et al.* Development of ganciclovir resistance during treatment of primary *cytomegalovirus* infection after liver transplantation. Transplantation 63:476, 1997.
168. Iberer F, Tscheliessnigg K, Halwache G, Rehak P, Wasler A, *et al.* Definitions of *cytomegalovirus* disease after heart transplantation: antigenemia as a marker for antiviral therapy. Transplant Int 9:236, 1996.
169. Verdonck LF, Dekker AW, Rosenberg-Arska M, van den Hoek M. A risk-adapted approach with a short-course of ganciclovir to prevent *cytomegalovirus* pneumonia in CMV-seropositive recipients of allogeneic bone marrow transpalnts. Clin Infect Dis 24:901, 1997.
170. Grossi P, Kusne S, Rinaldo C, St. George K, Magone M, *et al.* Guidance of ganciclovir therapy with pp65 antigenemia in *cytomegalovirus-free* recipients of livers from seropositive donors. Transplantation 61:1659, 1996.
171. Kusne S, Schwartz M, Breinig MK, Dummer JS, Lee RE, *et al.* *Herpes simplex virus* hepatitis after solid organ transplantation in adults. J Infect Dis 163:1001, 1991.
172. Holt ND, Gould FKI, Taylor CE, Harwood JF, Freeman R, *et al.* Incidence and significance of noncytomegalovirus viral respiratory infection after adult lung transplantation. J Heart Lung Transplant 16:416, 1997.
173. Schuller D, Spessert C, Fraser VJ, Goodenberger DM. *Herpes simplex* virus from respiratory tract secretions: epidemiology, clinical characteristics, and outcome in immunocompromised and nonimmunocompromised hosts. Am J Med 94:29, 1993.
174. McGregor RS, Zitelli BJ, Urbach AH, Malatack JJ, Gartner JC. Varicella in pediatric orthotopic liver transplant recipients. Pediatrics 83:256, 1989.
175. Kusne S, Pappo O, Manez R, Pazin G, Carpenter B, *et al.* Varicella zoster virus hepatitis and a suggested management plan for prevention of VZV infection in adult transplant recipients. Transplantation 619, 1995.
176. Feldhoff C, Balfour H, Simmons SR, Nayarian J, Mauer M. Varicella in children with renal transplants. J Pediatr 98:25, 1981.
177. Kashtan CE, Cook M, Chavers BM, Mauer SM, Nevins TE. Outcome of chicken pox in 66 pediatric renal transplant recipients. J Pediatr 131:874, 1997.
178. Singh N, Gayowski T, Wagener MM, Marino IR. Predictors and outcome of hypothermic and euthermic infections in liver transplant recipients. 39th Interscience Conference on Antimicrobial Agents and Chemotherapy, San Francisco 1999.
179. Toogood GJ, Roake JA, Morris PJ. The relationship between fever and acute rejection or infection following renal transplantation in the cyclosporine era. Clin Transplantation 8:373, 1994.
180. Lloyd-Thomas AR, Dhaliwal HS, Lister TA, Hinds CJ. Intensive therapy for life threatening medical complications of hematological malignancy. Intens Care Med 12:317, 1986.
181. Singh N, Gayowski T, Marino IR, Schlichtig R. Acute adrenal insufficiency in critically ill liver transplant recipients. Transplantation 59:1744, 1995.

6. INFECTIONS IN THE NEUROSURGICAL PATIENT

Anne-Marie Korinek and Claude Martin

Introduction

Two groups of infections may develop after neurosurgery. Superficial infections: cutaneous abcesses and osteitis of the skull. Cutaneous abcesses have an excellent prognostic, are easy to treat and have a low morbidity. Osteitis will require the flat to be removed, a plastie to be done, and a prolonged antibiotic therapy, all the preceeding carrying a heavy morbidity. Deep infections: meningitis, ventriculitis, deep abcesses. These infections may induce some degree of mortality and may be followed by neurologic sequelae, especially in children. Shunt infections are also considered as deep infection.

Incidence of Postoperative Infections in Neurosurgery

Among nosocomial infections, central nervous system infections represent 0.4% [1]. In a neurosurgery unit, the rate of infection ranges from <1% to 10% [2–4]. Respiratory tract infections, bloodstream infections and urinary tract infections are very frequent but are covered elsewhere (pages 535–548, 731–748 and Section 6). More detailed consideration on these infections in head fraume patients and in spinal cord injury patieats can be found in a recent review [4b]. In a multicenter study in France, including 10 neurosurgery departments and 2944 patients who underwent a craniotomy, the global rate of infection was 4%, ranging from 1.5 to 10.2%. There were 38% of superficial infections and 62% of deep infections [5].

Bacteriology of Postoperative Infections in Neurosurgery

Staphylococci are most often isolated and they represent 50 to 80% of the isolates. *Coagulase-negative* staphylococci (CNS) contaminate mostly internal and external derivation [6–8]. *Staphylococcus aureus* are responsible for most superficial infections and 50% of deep infections. Gram-negative bacteria (GNB) are found in 25 to 50% of isolates [2, 8]. *Propionibacterium acnes* has recently been recognized as a pathogen bacteria in neurosurgery [9].

In the French multicenter study on craniotomies, *S. aureus* was the lead bacteria (51% of which 1/3 were methicillin-resistant). CNS were isolated in 4%, GNB in 29% (*Enterobacteriaceae* 61%, *Pseudomonas aeruginosa* 11%, *Acinetobacter* 28%). Deep infections were due to Gram-positive cocci (58%) and Gram-negative bacteria (30%).

Wound contamination comes from the patient's skin. *S. epidermidis* and *P. acnes* develop in the deep layer of the epiderm and in the hair follicles which makes it very difficult to eradicate by skin disinfection [9, 10]. Bacteria responsible for deep infections are often found in naso-pharyngeal mucosa or in the ear in the case of cerebrospinal fluid (CSF) fistula. Bacteria may also come from remote sites (urinary or respiratory tract) and the contamination is bloodborne or hand-borne to the surgical wound [1, 2, 11].

Treatment of Postoperative Infections in Neurosurgery

The central nervous system is isolated from the rest of the organism by the hemato-encephalic and the hemato-meningeal barriers. Diffusion of the antibiotics will be markedly reduced except for some of them. In addition there is no local immunity in neither immunocompetent cells nor immunoglobulins. For clinical practice, one must achieve, and maintain, bacterial titers of antibiotics *in situ*: 8 to 10 times the MICs.

MENINGITIS AND VENTRICULITIS

The diagnosis is a very difficult one: fever can be of multiple origins; it is the same for consciousness abnormalities, headache and stiff neck. CSF sample must be obtained. If Gram-stain is negative (which is often the case), cells and protein are difficult to interprete. Low CSF sugar is of some interest to suspect meningitis. The CSF examination can be repeated, if needed, after several hours. If the treatment is prescribed, the following regimens can be prescribed:

- Negative Gram-stain: a combination of cefotaxime plus fosfomycin is recommended. It is active both against GNB (except *P. aeruginosa*) and methicillin-resistant staphylococci [12]. Treatment is prescribed for two weeks.
- Methicillin-susceptible staphylococci. One can use either quinolone, oxacillin rifampin, fosfomycin or chloramphenicol. Treatment is prescribed for two weeks.
- Methicillin-resistant staphylococci. Vancomycin is prescribed by continuous diffusion after a loading dose of 15 mg/kg. Blood concentrations should be kept above 40 mg/l. In younger, healthy patients, 4 to 6, sometimes 8 g per day are needed. No local vancomycin injection is needed. If CSF cultures cannot be negativated, a second antibiotic should be considered (fosfomycine, rifampin, fusidic acid). Treatment is prescribed for three weeks.
- *Propionibacterium acnes*: the combination amoxicilline-rifampin is usually effective. Treatment is prescribed for two weeks.
- *Enterobacteriaceae*: Third generation cephalosporins are prescribed with doses twice as high as in other infections. A combination with fosfomycine or quinolones can be considered. Treatment is prescribed for two weeks.
- *P. aeruginosa*: ceftazidime or ureropeneum is prescribed; a combination with quinolone can be considered, based on the antibiogram. The treatment is prescribed for three weeks.

Abscesses and Empyema

The surgical treatment is aimed at isolating the pathogen responsible for the infection and at evacuating the purulent collection. The medical treatment is based on antibiotics which have a reliable penetration into the CNS (Table 1). Most of the time, an antibiotic combination is given, with no scientific rationale. Treatment is prescribed for three months. Its efficacy is judged by a clinical improvement and a volume reduction of the abscess on the CT-scan. One month after treatment withdrawal, a CT-scan should be performed to confirm the clinical resolution.

Corticosteroids could be used, during the first few days to decrease cerebral edema. The following antibiotics may be used:

- Methicillin-susceptible staphylococci: quinolones, rifampin, fucidic acid, lincosamides, chloramphenicol, cotrimoxazole, oxacillin.
- Methicillin-resistant staphylococci: same antibiotics as above (except quinolones or oxacillin), fosfomycine, vancomycin.
- P. acnes: amoxicilin, combined to rifampin or lincosamides.
- *Enterobacteriaceae*: third generation cephalosporins, sometimes combined with quinolones, fosfomycin, or cotrimoxazole.

TABLE 1. Antibiotic penetration into the brain tissue

No diffusion	Low diffusion (1)	High diffusion (2)
Penicillin M	Penicillin G and A	Quinolones
CIG, GIIG	Carboxy and ureido penicillines	Rifampin
Aminoglycosides	CIIIG	Fosfomycine
Polymyxins	Carbapenems	Cotrimoxazole
Macrolides, Synergistins	Vancomycin (4)	Metronidazole
Cyclines	Teicoplanin (5)	Tetracyclines
	Lincosamides (3)	Chloramphenicol
Fusidic acid (3)		

(1) 30% of serum concentration, increased in case of inflamed meninges.
(2) 40–50% of serum concentrations.
(3) No diffusion in CSF, but penetration into cerebral tissues and abscess pus.
(4) Penetration into the CSF in case of inflamed meninges and provided that a correct dose is given: loading dose 15 mg/kg and 4 to 6 g per day by continuous infusion.
(5) Experience is limited.
CIG, CIIG and CIIIG = First, Second or Third Generation Cephalosporius.

Volet Infection

The treatment is mostly a surgical treatment. The flap, poorly vascularized, must be removed since antibiotics cannot penetrate it. Then, an antibiotic treatment is prescribed for one month. Secondary cranioplasty can be considered three months after antibiotics are stopped, if the local conditions are perfect.

Shunt Infections

In a review of the literature, it was found that a success rate of 96% is expected after removal of the infected shunt, placement of an external shunt, and targeted antibiotic therapy [13]. The success rate fell to 65% when a new internal shunt was placed, together with antibiotics, or to 36% if the infected shunt was not removed, and the infection was treated with antibiotics [13]. A prospective randomized study was conducted in three groups of 10 children each [14]. In group 1, shunt was removed, a new external derivation, or a reservoir, was put place, antibiotics were given, and later, a new internal shunt was placed. In group 1, all patients were cured and hospital stay was 25 ± 17 days. In group 2, the infected material was removed, a new internal valve was placed during the same surgical procedure and antibiotics were given. A total of 90% of patients were cured and hospital stay was 33 ± 8 days. In the third group, the infected material was left in place, antibiotics were given and the success rate was only 30%, with a hospital stay of 47 ± 37 days [14].

- Valve infection with no ventriculitis (cells, glucose and proteins are normal). The shunt is removed, an external derivation is placed and antibiotics are given. Several days later, a new shunt is placed, if possible on the opposite site, and antibiotics are given for two weeks.
- Valve infection and ventriculitis. The shunt must be removed, an external derivation is placed and antibiotics are prescribed for three weeks. After antibiotics are withdrawn, a CSF sample is obtained after two days, and if normal, a new shunt is then placed.

In both situations, bactericidal antibiotics must be chosen, and high CSF levels achieved and maintained.

References

1. Reingold AL, Broome CV. Nosocomial central nervous system infections. In Bennett JV, Brachman PS (eds). Hospital infections 2nd edn. Boston: Little Brown, 1986:521.

2. Stephens JL, Peacock JE. Uncommon infections: eye and CNS.: In Wenzel RP (ed). Prevention and control of nosocomial infections. 2nd edn. Baltimore:Williams and Wilkins, 1993:746.
3. Balch RE. Wound infections complicating neurosurgical procedures. J Neurosurg 26:41, 1967.
4. Tenney JH, Vladov D, Salcman M, Ducker TB. Wide variation in risk of wound infection following clean neurosurgery. Implications for perioperative antibiotic prophylaxis. J Neurosurg 62:243, 1985.

4b. Bodi M, Bogue MC, Rello J. Infections in head traume, neurosurpery and spinal cord injury patients. Semin Respir Infect 15:206, 2000.

5. Korinek AM, the French Study Group of Neurosurgical Infections, the SEHP and the C.CLIN Pairs-Nord. Risk factors for neurosurgical site infections after craniotomy. A prospective multicenter study in 2944 patients. Neurosurgery 41:1073, 1997.
6. Renier D, Lacombe J, Pierre-Khan A, Sainte-Rose C, Hirsch JF. Factors causing acute shunt infection. Computer analysis of 1174 operations. J Neurosurg 61:107, 1984.
7. Saravolatz LD. Infection in implantable prosthetic devices. In Wenzel RP (ed). Prevention and control of nosocomial infections. 2nd edn. Baltimore:Williams and Wilkins, 1993:683.
8. Korinek AM, Bismuth R, Dagreou F. Les infections à staphylocoques à coagulase négative en neurochirurgie. Med Mal Infect 20 (Hors série mars) : 91, 1990.
9. Van EK B, Bakker FP, Van Dulken H, Dijkmans BAC. Infections after craniotomy: a retrospective study. J Infect 12:105, 1986.
10. Van EK B, Dijkman BAC, Van Dulken H, Van Furth R. Antibiotic prophylaxis in craniotomy: a prospective double-blind placebo controlled study. Scand J Infect Dis 201:633, 1988.
11. Mangi RJ, Quintiliani R, Andriole VT. Gram-negative bacillary meningitis. Am J Med 59:829, 1975.
12. Portier H, Armengaud M, Becq-Giaudon B, Bousser J, *et al.* Traitement par l'association céfotaxime-fosfomycine des méningites de l'adults à staphylocoques ou à entérobactéries. Presse Méd 16:2161, 1987.
13. Bisno AL. Infections of central nervous system shunts. In Infections associated with indwelling medical devices. Bisno AL, Waldvogel FA (eds). American Society for microbiology Washington: 1989:93.
14. James HE, Walsh JW, Wilson HD, Connor JD, Beun JR, Tibbs PA. Prospective randomized study of therapy in cerebrospinal fluid shunt infection. Neurosurgery 7:459, 1980.

7. CARDIOVASCULAR MONITORING OF THE SEPTIC PATIENT

J. Andrew Apostle and Juan J. Guardiola

Introduction

The American College of Chest Physicians & Society of Critical Care Medicine Consensus [1] defines sepsis as the systemic inflammatory response syndrome (SIRS) as a result of infection. Septic shock is defined as sepsis-induced hypotension despite adequate fluid resuscitation along with the presence of perfusion abnormalities. These abnormalities may include, but are not limited to, lactic acidosis, oliguria or an acute alteration in mental status. Patients who are receiving inotropic or vasopressor agents may not be hypotensive at the time that perfusion abnormalities are measured. From the years 1950–1991 mortality has soared by 13-fold [2]. Alone sepsis carries a 30–40% lethality [2] but when aggravated by shock, it has a 40–60% mortality [3]. Recently the effectiveness of invasive hemodynamic monitoring in septic shock has undergone intense scrutiny. A lack of well-designed prospective studies assessing this problem has cast a shadow of doubt in regard to the lowering of morbidity or mortality (attributable to the right heart catheterization). A moratorium on their placement was suggested in the literature, which prompted a consensus conference in 1997 to help clarify the role of the pulmonary artery catheter in the critically ill [4]. Minimally invasive and non-invasive cardiovascular monitoring devices are being examined and are increasingly being researched.

Shock States and Differential Diagnosis

Shock is the state in which the circulatory system fails to maintain adequate tissue perfusion. As a consequence of inadequate tissue perfusion, cellular and organ dysfunction ensues, which becomes irreversible unless corrected promptly. Clinical features of shock are arterial hypotension, tachycardia, tachypnea, decreased mentation, oliguria and metabolic acidosis. Blood pressure (BP) is equal to cardiac output (CO) times systemic vascular resistance (SVR). Because hypotension can result from a reduction in either CO or SVR, shock may be categorized as distributive, cardiogenic, extra-cardiac obstructive or hypovolemic. Distributive shock is caused by a maldistribution of blood flow in the microcirculation with a decreased SVR (e.g. sepsis, anaphylaxis, spinal cord injury, barbiturate overdose, etc.). Cardiogenic shock's most common cause is acute myocardial infarction while extra-cardiac obstructive may be caused by cardiac tamponade, massive pulmonary embolus or tension pneumothorax. Hypovolemic shock causes include massive losses of gastrointestinal fluids or frank hemorrhage.

Bedsides clinical assessment provides a good indication of cardiac output and filling pressures of the heart. Based on this clinical assessment an early diagnosis of the type of shock can be made (Table 1).

Invasive hemodynamic monitoring with a pulmonary artery catheter (PAC) allows the classification of a patient with shock into one of four

TABLE 1. Bedside diagnosis of the type of shock [5]

Cardiac output		
Signs	High Cardiac Output	Low Cardiac Output
Pulse pressure	Increased	Decreased (Pulsus Paradoxus in cardiac tamponade)
Skin and digits	Warm and pink	Cool, cyanotic mottling
Capillary refill (nailbed)	Rapid	Slow
Heart sounds	Loud and clear	Soft and muffled
Temperature	Fever or hypothermia	Normal temperature
White blood cell count	Leukocytosis or leukopenia (shift to immature forms)	Normal to mild leukocytosis
Source of infection	e.g. Pneumonia or pyelonephritis	No source of Infection
Possible diagnosis	Septic Shock	Cardiogenic shock Obstructive shock Hypovolemic shock
Filling pressures of the heart [5]		
Filling pressures	Increased filling pressure	Decreased filling pressure
Clinical setting	Chest pain	Bleeding, vomiting or diarrhea
Jugular venous pressure	Jugular venous distension	Jugular veins collapse when supine
Cardiac auscultation	Gallop rhythm	Absent gallop
Pulmonary crepitant rales	Present	Clear lungs
Chest roentgenogram	– Cardiomegaly – Pulmonary venous congestion – Pulmonary edema – Clear in pulmonary embolus and cardiac tamponade	Normal (except when shock is due to pneumonia)
Electrocardiogram	MI – ST segment elevation PE – $S_1Q_3T_3$ Tamponade – decreased voltage	Normal
Cardiac enzymes	Increased in MI	Normal
Possible diagnosis	Cardiogenic shock Obstructive shock	Hypovolemic shock

types: cardiogenic, hypovolemic, distributive or obstructive (Table 2).

Hemodynamics in Septic Shock [6–9]

Septic shock has a characteristic hemodynamic profile consisting of tachycardia, systemic arterial hypotension, low SVR, high CO, low to normal pulmonary capillary wedge pressure (PCWP) and normal or elevated mixed venous oxygen saturation (SvO_2). This "high output-low resistance" state (or hyperdynamic circulation) is seen in more than 90% of patients with septic shock who have been aggressively fluid resuscitated to correct hypovolemia. In a minority of patients, left ventricular dysfunction with a low cardiac output may occur. The responses to sepsis include vascular changes and myocardial dysfunction.

SYSTEMIC VASCULAR RESISTANCE

Severe sepsis is commonly associated with a decrease in SVR which results in hypotension despite a normal or increased cardiac index (CI).

TABLE 2. Hemodynamic profiles in shock

Type of shock	CO	SVR	SvO_2	CVP	PAP	PCWP
Cardiogenic (e.g. MI[1])	↓	↑	↓	↓	↑	↑
Hypovolemic (e.g. hemorrhage)	↓	↑	↓	↓	↓	↓
Distributive (e.g. sepsis[2])	↑	↓	N-↑	N-↓	N-↓	N-↓
Obstructive (massive PE[3])	↓	↑-N	↓	↑	↑	N-↓
Obstructive (cardiac tamponade[3,4])	↓	↑	↓	↑	↑	↑

CO = Cardiac Output, CVP = Central venous pressure (right atrial pressure), PCWP = Pulmonary capillary wedge pressure, SVR = Systemic Vascular Resistance, SvO_2 = Mixed venous oxygen saturation, PAP = Pulmonary artery pressure, N = Normal.

[1] In the presence of a right ventricular infarct PCWP may not increase in cardiogenic shock.

[2] In the late stages of septic shock, CO falls and SVR rises due to myocardial depression.

[3] PCWP is decreased in massive pulmonary embolus, but increased in cardiac tamponade.

[4] Equalization of mean CVP, mean PCWP, right ventricular diastolic pressure and diastolic PAP establishes the diagnosis cardiac tamponade.

Most non-survivors of septic shock demonstrate a persistent vasodilatation and hence refractory hypotension.

GENERALIZED BLOOD FLOW REDISTRIBUTION

Although the CO is increased in sepsis, this flow is not uniformly distributed. There is a reduction in the splanchnic blood flow resulting in mucosal ischemia of the gastrointestinal tract, while blood flow to the other vital organs (e.g. brain and heart) is preserved. Intestinal ischemia has been considered to play a central role in the development of irreversible shock and the multiple organ dysfunction syndrome (MODS).

MICROCIRCULATORY BLOOD FLOW MALDISTRIBUTION

Many vascular beds are dilated but some are constricted while arteriovenous shunts may open and bypass the capillary bed resulting in impaired organ perfusion.

VENOUS CAPACITANCE

Venous tone decreases in the large capacity vessels and pooling occurs resulting in relative hypovolemia.

CAPILLARY PERMEABILITY

A generalized increase in endothelial permeability ("capillary leak") leads to "third-spacing" and intravascular volume depletion thus the effective intravascular volume is reduced in sepsis due to the multiple factors including increase in venous capacitance with venous pooling and decreased intravascular volume secondary to a capillary leak.

MYOCARDIAL DEPRESSION

Depressed myocardial contractile function is a common consequence of severe sepsis. This reversible cardiac dysfunction is manifested by a decrease in left and right ventricular ejection fraction with biventricular dilatation. Since ejection fraction declines, ventricular dilation can be a compensatory mechanism to maintain stroke volume at a constant level by the Frank Starling mechanism. Early septic shock is characterized by an increased cardiac output owing to an increased heart rate and a constant stroke volume. With recovery, CO falls as heart rate decreases and the stroke volume remains constant but there is a reduction in ventricular size and an increase in ejection fraction. Myocardial depression may be the effect of the cytokine – tumor necrosis factor. Myocardial ischemia does not play a significant role since coronary flow is preserved in septic shock [10].

In a minority of patients with septic shock, the left ventricular dysfunction is not compensated and these patients die of myocardial pump failure with a low CI. However, most patients who die of septic shock either succumb in the early stage owing to persistently low SVR with refractory hypotension or die at a later stage as a result of sepsis induced MODS.

Cellular Metabolism in Septic Shock

Distributive abnormalities of systemic blood flow (intestinal ischemia) and maldistribution of blood flow in the microcirculation (arterial-venous shunting) limit effective oxygen extraction during septic shock. In addition to blood flow maldistribution, in some septic patients, a "metabolic block" exists at the cellular level preventing adequate oxygen utilization [11]. As a consequence of the inability of systemic tissues to maximally extract oxygen from the blood, anaerobic metabolism occurs with increased blood lactate concentrations despite near normal mixed venous oxygen saturation and a narrow difference in the arterial-venous oxygen content. The prognostic value of elevated blood lactate concentrations is well established in septic shock [12]. The trend of lactate concentrations is a better prognostic indicator than a single value [13].

Monitoring the Septic Patient

BASIC MONITORING

A. ***Electrocardiogram* (ECG)**: Continuous ECG monitoring is used in almost all patients in the intensive care unit (ICU). ECG monitoring will measure heart rate, detect arrhythmias and myocardial ischemia.

B. ***Non-invasive Blood Pressure Monitoring* (NIBP)**: Automated NIBP is widely available in the ICU, usually as a part of a multicomponent monitor along with continuous ECG and pulse oximetry monitoring. It is frequently used on admission to the ICU before insertion of an arterial cannula. Measurements are unreliable in obesity, in low cardiac output states and in the presence of many arrhythmias.

C. ***Pulse Oximetry***: A pulse oximeter attached to a finger or earlobe allows for transcutaneous estimates of hemoglobin oxygen saturation. Accuracy depends on satisfactory arterial perfusion of the skin. Inaccurate readings are seen with low cardiac output states, vasoconstriction and in hypothermia.

D. ***Urinary Output***: A Foley catheter is inserted and connected to a graduated collecting device (urimeter) so that urinary output can be measured hourly. Urine output is a reliable guide to tissue perfusion. A significant fall in renal perfusion is associated with oliguria, which if allowed to persist, may progress to acute tubular necrosis.

INVASIVE HEMODYNAMIC MONITORING

A. ***Arterial Line***: Intra-arterial monitoring is accurate, allows immediate beat-to-beat analysis and frequent arterial blood gas sampling. In hypotensive septic patients receiving high-dose vasopressor therapy, radial artery pressure underestimates central pressure. Clinical management, based upon radial pressures may lead to excessive vasopressor administration. Awareness of this phenomenon may help minimize the adverse effects of these potent agents by enabling dosage reduction [14].

B. ***Pulmonary Artery Catheter***: Cardiac output is equal to heart rate times stroke volume. Stroke volume depends on preload, afterload and contractility. Preload physiologically is the muscle fiber length at end diastole. Frank Starling's Law of the heart is a fundamental property of heart muscle in which the force of contraction at any given tension depends on the end-diastolic fiber length. Afterload represents the force opposing muscle fiber shortening. This is dictated by the wall tension in the left ventricle (LV) during systole. Tension (T) is directly related to pressure (P) and radius (r) while inversely related to the thickness (h) of the chamber ($T = Pr/2h$). Systemic vascular resistance will affect the afterload by virtue of its direct effect on intraventricular pressure. Contractility or inotropic state is the

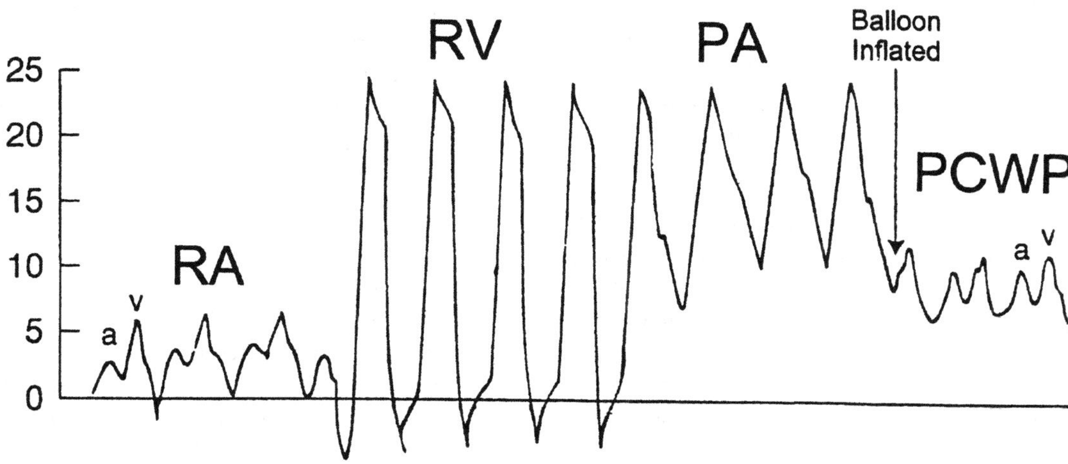

RA = Right Atrium, RV = Right Ventricle, PA = Pulmonary Artery, PCWP = Pulmonary Capillary Wedge Pressure

FIGURE 1. Waveforms and pressures seen during insertion of PAC.

ability of the heart at any given length to generate tension.

The pulmonary artery catheter (PAC) is used to measure pressures (Figure 1) but what pressures are we really measuring? Any indwelling catheter that measures pressures encompasses intravascular pressure, driving pressure and transmural pressure. Intravascular pressure is the pressure inside vessels relative to ambient room pressure at the same level. Driving pressure, in the case of the PA catheter, is the pressure difference between the pulmonary artery and left atrium. Transmural pressure is the pressure differential between the inside and outside of the blood vessel. When we measure the pulmonary capillary wedge pressure (PCWP) we are measuring *estimates* of the left ventricular end diastolic volume (preload). PCWP measures the left atrial pressure, which is an indirect measurement of the left ventricular pressure at end diastole. This in turn is an estimate of the left ventricular end diastolic volume. There is a linear relationship between volume and pressure. This relationship does not always hold true and supposes there is normal left ventricular compliance and juxtacardiac pressure. As we know, this is not always the case with our patients. Left ventricular (LV) compliance is the change in volume per unit of pressure as the LV fills with blood from the left atrium. LV compliance may be compromised (hypertension, LVOF obstructions, dilated cardiomyopathies, restrictive pericarditis, infiltrative processes, fibrosis, nitrates, inotropes, β-blockers, RV overload with septal shift and pulmonary hypertension) leading to a greater elevation in pressure for any given volume. Mitral valve disease may negate this relationship. Transmural pressure (P_{tm}) is the gradient between the intracavitary pressure (PCWP) and the juxtacardiac pressure (P_{jc}) which represents intrathoracic pressure (intrapleural pressure). Juxtacardiac pressures may be elevated by elevated intrathoracic pressures (e.g. mechanical ventilation with PEEP, auto-PEEP, and pneumothorax) or lowered by negative intrathoracic pressure (as in normal or labored breathing). Measurements should be made at end expiration. P_{jc} may be assessed directly by esophageal manometry (a measure of intrapleural pressure).

Proper location of the PAC is important. Measurement should be made in a Zone III condition (where alveolar pressure is less than that of the pulmonary artery or vein). Zone III may be reduced in size with increasing alveolar distension (obstructive lung physiology, auto or excessive PEEP) or diminished pulmonary vascular pressures (severe hypovolemia). AP and lateral films may confirm good position of the catheter. When the patient lies supine Zone III is in the dependent part of the lung therefore the tip of the catheter has to be in this area to have reliable results. The position of the tip should be below the posterior border of the left atrium on a supine lateral chest X-ray. The nasogastric tube is a useful landmark since the esophagus traverses posterior to the left atrium.

The PAC allows for true mixed venous oxygen sampling, whereas central lines do not. The blood returning from the superior vena cava usually has a lower saturation due to increased oxygen extraction. The inferior vena cava usually has a higher saturation owed to shunts such as the renal circulation. Mean venous oxygen saturation (SvO_2) may be the earliest change in the critically ill patient. SvO_2 may decrease with low oxygen delivery (low output states, hypoxia, anemia) or high consumption (e.g. fever, thyrotoxicosis). Elevated SvO_2 may be seen in shunts (left to right), sepsis, hyperbaric oxygen use or excessive inotrope use. SvO_2 may be deceptively normal in septic shock states where there is peripheral shunting and or a "metabolic block" at the cellular level. Sampling errors may occur when the PAC is too distal or in the presence of mitral regurgitation and intracardiac shunt. The first two errors should be recognized promptly when wedging the catheter. There should be no evidence of over wedging with 1.25–1.5 cc of air and the absence of large V waves should be noted. If a shunt is suspected then SvO_2 should be measured from the right atrium, ventricle and pulmonary artery to assess for an abnormal step-up in oxygenation. Lactic acidosis usually marks anaerobic metabolism. Lactic acidosis may indicate inadequate oxygen delivery or dysfunction at the cellular level ("metabolic block").

i. ***Complications***: Cardiac output measurements may also be riddled with inaccuracy. Thermodilution is used but can be inaccurate owing to slow injection of fluid, measurements taken at different times of the respiratory cycle, tricuspid regurgitation, intracardiac shunts or distal location of the PAC.

   Placement of the PAC with its introducer has associated morbidity as noted in Table 3 [15]. This is not an all-inclusive list. The most concerning findings are the last two. If we chose to use the PAC it is incumbent upon the critical care team to resolutely endeavor for correct capture and interpretation of data. For if the data is interpreted incorrectly then inappropriate therapy will likely be prescribed.

ii. ***Controversy & Consensus***: Of late, significant controversy has surrounded the pulmonary artery catheter (PAC). Connors *et al.* suggest that careful consideration should be given as to whether or not one should be placed. Findings that lead to their conclusions were an increased 30-day mortality (4.5% higher), higher cost and protracted intensive care requirement [33]. Proponents of the right heart catheter criticize that this was not a randomized prospective trial. Since it allows for earlier intervention and often leads to a change in therapy that it must logically improve outcome. However, we are reminded of the CAST trial that clearly showed post myocardial infarction anti-arrhythmics are detrimental, counterintuitive to the rational of the time [31]. The risks and its indiscriminate use in the low benefit patient may negate the benefits of the catheter. Compounding this is a high degree of misinterpretation by trained intensive care physicians [31] and nurses [32]. Pulmonary artery occlusion pressure is inaccurate 15% [29, 30] of the time and in the critically ill does not always correlate with left ventricular end diastolic volume [34, 35].

This controversy prompted a consensus statement [4] endorsed by the American

TABLE 3. Complications of pulmonary artery catheterization [11]

Complication	Incidence	Reference
Arterial sticks	10%	15
Pneumothorax	0.5–6%	16
Venous air embolism	0.5%	17
Thoracic duct injury	1% of left–sided attempts	18
Premature ventricular beats	68%	19
Transient ventricular tachycardia	33%	20
Persistent ventricular tachycardia	3%	21
Right bundle branch block	6–12% (resolved in 24 hours)	22
Right bundle branch block with existing left bundle branch block	23%	23
Misplacement of catheter	19% internal jugular	24
Misplacement of catheter	16% subclavian	24
Pulmonary artery rupture	0.034–0.125%	25, 26
Pulmonary artery ruptures that result in death	70%	25, 26
Thrombosis	1–11%	27
Valvular lesions	Up to 31%	27
Infection of catheter or sheath	5.9–29.1%	28
Catheter associated bacteremia	0–4.6%	28
Inaccurate PCWP	15%	29, 30
Inaccurate interpretation doctors	54%	31
Inaccurate interpretation nurses	42%	32

PCWP = Pulmonery Cepilar Wedge Pressure.

Association of Critical Care Nurses, American College of Chest Physicians, American Thoracic Society and Society of Critical Care Medicine. It called for an improved knowledge of interpretation of the data obtained from the pulmonary artery catheter and the complications of the placement. Furthermore, no moratorium should be invoked and the clinician shall carefully weigh the benefits and risks of the catheter before placing it with informed consent. It is agreed that there should be a controlled randomized study to determine indications for placement. Outlined below (Table 4) is a portion of their findings based upon clinical situation.

The Pulmonary Artery Catheter Consensus Conference (PACCC) [4] stated that it is *uncertain* whether pulmonary artery catheter-guided management improves outcomes in patients with sepsis or septic shock. This statement was based upon non-randomized studies with contemporaneous contents. These studies do not answer whether the changes in therapy that are made, based on hemodynamic measurements, alter the outcome of the patient.

The PACCC recommended:

1) The PAC may be useful in patients with septic shock who have not responded to initial aggressive fluid resuscitation and low dose inotropic / vasoconstrictor therapy.
2) Various management strategies for sepsis and septic shock (IV fluids, vasoactive and inotropic drugs, etc.) should be evaluated in prospective, randomized, controlled trials. Investigations should be designed to determine both the effectiveness of the PAC in accurate diagnosis and in monitoring patient response to therapeutic intervention. Management protocols need to be defined for both the PAC-guided and non-PAC-guided groups.

TABLE 4. Summary of consensus statement – based upon clinical situation [4]

Situation	Findings
Improve outcome in MI with cardiogenic shock	Yes
Improve outcome in MI with mechanical complications	Yes
Improve outcome in MI with right ventricular infarction	Yes
Improve outcome in refractory congestive heart failure	Uncertain
Improve outcome in pulmonary hypertension	Uncertain
Improve outcome in shock or hemodynamic instability	Uncertain
Reduce complications and mortality in cardiac surgery – low risk patients	No
Reduce complications and mortality in cardiac surgery – high risk patients	Uncertain
Reduce perioperative complications in peripheral vascular surgery	Yes
Reduce mortality in peripheral vascular surgery	Uncertain
Reduce perioperative complications & mortality in aortic surgery – low risk patients	Uncertain
Reduce perioperative complications & mortality in aortic surgery – high risk patients	Yes
Reduce perioperative complications & mortality in geriatric patients	No
Reduce perioperative complications & mortality in neurosurgical patients	Uncertain
Reduce complications & mortality in patients with pre-eclampsia	No
Alter diagnosis and improve functional outcome in traumatically injured patients	Yes
Alter mortality in traumatically injured patients	Uncertain
Improve outcomes in patients with sepsis or septic shock	Uncertain
Alter diagnosis and treatment in patients with respiratory failure	Yes
Alter outcomes in patients with respiratory failure	Uncertain
Clarify cardiopulmonary physiology in critically ill infants & children	Yes
Improve organ function or survival when PAC used to achieve supranormal oxygen delivery after onset of SIRS from sepsis, trauma or postoperative complication	Uncertain
Improve organ function or survival when PAC used to achieve supranormal oxygen delivery after onset of SIRS from sepsis, trauma or postoperative complication	Uncertain
Are continuous venous oximetry, right ventricular ejection fraction and continuous cardiac output pulmonary artery catheter devices accurate?	Yes

MI = myocardial infarction, PAC = Pulmonary artery catheter, SIRS = Systemic inflammatory response syndrome.

C. ***Non-traditional PACs***: Newer PACs have options that will enhance the understanding of the physiology. Newer devices offer cardiac output measurements from the right as well as the left ventricle. Fiberoptic PACs give continuous cardiac output and SvO_2. Continuous fiberoptic sampling minimizes fluid used and potential introduction of infection with each manipulation.

MINIMALLY & NON-INVASIVE DEVICES

Recent approaches have sought minimally and non-invasive devices. COLD Brand (pulsion) thermodilution, thoracic electrical bioimpedance (Bio-Z/Cardiodynamics), gastric tonometry, transesophageal Doppler stroke volume, transesophageal and transthoracic echocardiogram.

A. *COLD*: Acronym stands for *C*irculation, *O*xygenation, *L*ung water/liver function and *D*iagnosis (Pulsion Medical Systems, Munich, Germany). A dual indicator technique (thermal dye) uses any central vein to inject ice cold indocyanine green dye (ICG-pulsion). A special pulsiocath arterial oximeter with thermal-dye dilution probe in the femoral artery is used for detection. Function and status of systems assessed includes, cardiovascular, lung and liver, as the name implies.

Cardiovascular parameters include, global end diastolic volume, intrathoracic volume, circulating blood volume, cardiac output and cardiac function index (cardiac output/global end diastolic volume). Pulmonary parameters derived include extravascular lung water, pulmonary blood volume and arterial oxygen saturation. Liver status is appraised by rates of disappearance of ICG from plasma and blood. It is cited to aid in management of the critically ill to decrease ventilator days and days in the ICU [36]. It may be used in conjunction with the PAC for more comprehensive volumetric data.

B. *Thoracic electrical bioimpedance (TEB)*: TEB is a form of electrical impedance plethysmography. It utilizes sensors to transmit a small electrical signal through the thorax. Two dual sensors are placed on each side of the patient's neck and chest. The signal travels along the most conductive area, the blood filled aorta. As the volume and velocity of the blood in the aorta changes during systole and diastole a "digital impedance signal quantifier" will measure the changes in impedance to the electrical signal. TEB's measurement of impedance changes over time is similar to the thermodilution measurement of temperature changes over time to calculate cardiac output. Using this method multiple hemodynamic parameters can be measured and calculated, including cardiac output, systemic vascular resistance, contractility indices (velocity index, acceleration index) and thoracic fluid content (CardioDynamics, San Diego, California, USA). The main advantage of this method is being minimally invasive. The main disadvantage is the paucity of studies available and the initial investment in the monitoring unit.

C. *Gastric Tonometry*: The splanchnic bed has countercurrent circulation at the mucosal level rendering it especially vulnerable to ischemia. Global oxygen assessment may underestimate intestinal perfusion. This may lead to endotoxin or bacterial translocation across the gut wall to further compound problems. Intramucosal $CO_2(P_ICO_2)$ may be used to derive intramucosal pH_I using the Henderson-Hasselbach equation. A gastric probe is placed with a balloon and inflated with gas or a buffered solution for 90 min. After this dwell the fluid is removed and analyzed. Low pH_I correlates with a poor outcome. Given its long time between assessments it may prove problematic in titration of inotropes and vasopressors. Fiberoptic gastric pH_I probes remain a possibility. Its role in management is still unclear.

D. *Esophageal Doppler Monitor* [37]: The esophageal Doppler is a flexible ultrasound probe about the size of a nasogastric tube that can obtain a continuous cardiac output by measuring blood flow velocity in the descending thoracic aorta. Stroke volume is calculated as the product of mean velocity and cross-sectional area of the descending aorta. Area of the aorta is estimated using a nomogram based on the patient's age, height and weight. In adults, the measures of cardiac output made simultaneously with the esophageal Doppler monitor and standard thermodilution show good correlation. An attribute of this technique is easy probe insertion since it can be placed within minutes without major complications and requires minimal technical skill. The probe may be left in place for over two weeks. Disadvantages are difficulty in maintaining an optimal probe position and the fact that it cannot provide direct measurements of pulmonary artery and wedge pressures.

E. *Echocardiogram*: Using echocardiography, the same principles may be applied to determine cardiac output. Measurement of the left ventricular out flow tract (LVOT) diameter (d) and time velocity integral (TVI) as determined by Doppler signal a cardiac output (CO) may be calculated. CO in liters/minute = TVI $\times$ (d^2 $\times$ 0.785) $\times$ heart rate [38–41]. There is agreement over a wide range of values, when referenced to the PAC [42]. Sinus rhythm is required for factual results. In the unstable patient it may still be used safely but will not allow for ongoing monitoring to aid in titration of therapy [43]. Transesophageal echocardiogram (TEE), in certain instances, may be more revealing than the transthoracic approach [44]. TEE [45] is assuming an increasingly important role in the non-invasive evaluation of the hemodynamically unstable patient [43]. With experienced personnel, TEE

TABLE 5. Goals of hemodynamic management

Hemodynamic goals	Oxygen delivery goals	Organ perfusion goals
MAP ≥ 60 mm Hg	SpO_2 > 92% & SvO_2 > 70%	CNS – Normal sensorium
PCWP = 14–18 mm Hg	– Hgb = 7–9 g/dl – Hgb = 10–12 g/dl with myocardial infarction or ischemia	Skin – Pink, warm & dry
Cardiac Index > 3 l/m²/min	Serum Lactate < 2 mM/l	Renal – Urine output > 1 ml/Kg/Hr

can be performed safely in critically ill patients with a high success rate. TEE facilitates prompt definitive diagnosis of major cardiac disorders that can be surgically correctable (endocarditis, cardiac tamponade, aortic dissection, mechanical complications of myocardial infarction). TEE can also help to determine the non-surgical cardiac contribution to hemodynamic instability. The patient with hypovolemic hypotension shows a small left ventricular cavity and hyperdynamic function. Intracavitary gradients due to mid-ventricular obstruction or systolic anterior motion of the mitral valve are often identified by Doppler echocardiography in such situations. Administration of fluids and withdrawal of inotropic agents result in paradoxical increases in blood pressure and lessening of pulmonary congestion as the intracavitary gradient decreases [45].

Clinical and Hemodynamic Goals in Patients with Septic Shock

Based upon recent studies [46–48] it seems most reasonable to attempt to achieve a normal oxygen delivery and perfusion pressure that is associated with evidence of adequate organ oxygenation and perfusion. Oxygen delivery is determined by the product cardiac output and oxygen content while perfusion pressure is best reflected by mean arterial pressure. Interventions designed to achieve supranormal oxygen delivery in septic shock (with fluids and inotropes) have not demonstrated a benefit and such therapy may actually be associated with a reduced survival rate. Ideal goals are listed below (Table 5).

Recommendations for Hemodynamic Support of Septic Patients

Practice parameters for hemodynamics [49] have been outlined by the Task Force of the American College of Critical Care Medicine, Society of Critical Care Monitoring.

1. Patients with septic shock should be treated in an ICU, with continuous electrocardiographic monitoring of arterial oxygenation [49].
2. Arterial cannulation should be performed in patients with shock to provide a more accurate measurement of intra-arterial pressure and to allow beat-to-beat analysis so that decisions regarding therapy can be based on immediate and reproducible blood pressure information [49].
3. Resuscitation should be titrated to clinical endpoints of arterial pressure, heart rate, urine output, skin perfusion and mental status and indices of tissue perfusion such as blood lactate and mixed venous oxygen saturation [49].
4. Assessment of cardiac filling pressures may require central venous or pulmonary artery catheterization. Pulmonary artery catheterization also allows for assessment of pulmonary arterial pressures, cardiac output measurement and measurement of mixed venous oxygen saturation [49].

Appendix

Pulmonary Artery Catheter Measurements – Normal

Parameter	Symbols	"Normal" Range
Right Atrial Pressure (Central Venous Pressure)	RAP or CVP	1–7 mm Hg
Right Ventricular Systolic Pressure	RVSP	15–25 mm Hg
Right Ventricular Diastolic Pressure	RVDP	0–8 mm Hg
Pulmonary Artery Systolic Pressure	PASP	15–25 mm Hg
Pulmonary Artery Diastolic Pressure	PADP	8–15 mm Hg
Pulmonary Artery Mean Pressure	PA mean	10–20 mm Hg
Pulmonary Capillary Wedge Pressure	PCWP	6–12 mm Hg
Cardiac Output	CO	3.5–5.5 L/min
Cardiac Index	CI	2.8–3.2 L/min/m^2
Pulmonary Vascular Resistance	PVR	150–250 dyne sec cm^{-5}
Systemic Vascular Resistance	SVR	800–1200 dyne sec cm^{-5}
Right Ventricular Stroke Work Index	RVSWI	7–12 gram meters/m^2
Left Ventricular Stroke Work Index	LVSWI	43–61 gram meters/m^2
Arterial Oxygen Content	CaO_2	20 vol. %
Mixed Venous Oxygen Saturation	SvO_2	75%
Mixed Venous Oxygen Content	CvO_2	15 vol. %
Oxygen Delivery	Do_2	800–1200 ml/min
Oxygen Consumption	Vo_2	225–275 ml/min
Oxygen Extraction	O_2 Extraction	25%

Formulas

Pulse Pressure = SBP − DBP

$$\text{Mean Arterial Pressure} = \frac{SBP + 2(DBP)}{3}$$

CO = SV × HR

CI = CO/BSA

SV Index = SV/BSA

$$PVR = \frac{(PAP - PCWP)80}{CO}$$

$$SVR = \frac{(MAP - CVP)80}{CO}$$

RVSWI = SVI(PA − PAOP)(0.0136)

LVSWI = SVI(MAP − CVP)(0.0136)

$CaO_2 = 1.36(Hgb)(SaO_2) + 0.003(PaO_2)$

$CvO_2 = 1.36(Hgb)(SvO_2) + 0.003(PvO_2)$

$Cc'_{O2} = 1.36(Hgb)(FIO_2) + 0.003(P_{BH2O} - Pa_{CO2})(FIO_2)$

A-V O_2 Content Difference = $CaO_2 - CvO_2$

$Do_2 = CO \times CaO_2$

$Vo_2 = CO\ (CaO_2 - CvO_2)$

Fick CO = $(Vo_2/8.5)(CaO_2 - CvO_2)$

O_2 Extraction = $(CaO_2 - CvO_2)/CaO_2$

$$Q_s/Q_t = \frac{Cc'_{O2} - Ca_{O2}}{Cc'_{O2} - Cv_{O2}} \times 100$$

References

1. American College of Chest Physicians & Society of Critical Care Medicine Consensus Conference. Definitions for sepsis and multiple organ failure and guidelines for the use of innovative therapies in sepsis. Crit Care Med 20:864, 1992.
2. Marik PE, Varon J. The Hemodynamic Derangements in Sepsis. Chest 114:854, 1998.
3. Conners AF. Right Heart Catheterization: Is it Effective? New Horizons 5:195, 1997.

4. Pulmonary Artery Catheter Consensus Conference Participants'. Pulmonary Artery Catheter Consensus Conference: Consensus Statement. Crit Care Med 25:910, 1997.
5. Wood LDH. The pathophysiology of the circulation in critical illness. Hall JB, Schmidt GA, Wood LDH (eds). Principles of Critical Care. New York: McGraw Hill, 2nd Edn, 1998:268.
6. Parillo JE. Pathogenic mechanisms of septic shock. N Engl J Med 328:1471, 1993.
7. Parker MM. Pathophysiology of cardiovascular dysfunction in septic shock. New Horizons 6:130, 1988.
8. Marik PE, Varon J. The Hemodynamic derangements in sepsis: Implications for treatment strategies. Chest 114:854, 1998.
9. Astiz ME, Rackow EC. Septic Shock. Lancet 351:1501, 1998.
10. Cunnion RE, Schaer GL, Parker MM, *et al.* The Coronary Circulation in Human Septic Shock. Circulation 73:637, 1986.
11. Rackow EC, Astiz ME, Weil MH. Cellular Oxygen Metabolism during Sepsis and Shock. JAMA 259:1989, 1988.
12. Weil MH, Afifi AA. Experimental and clinical studies in lactate and pyruvate as indicators of the severity of acute circulatory failure (shock). Circulation 41:989, 1970.
13. Vincent JL, Dufaye P, Berk J. Serial lactate determinations during circulatory shock. Crit Care Med 11:449, 1983.
14. Dorman T, Breslow MJ, Lipsett PA *et al.* Radial artery pressure monitoring underestimates central arterial pressure during vasopressor therapy in critically ill surgical patients. Crit Care Med 26:1646, 1998.
15. Coulter TD, Wiedemann HD. Complications of Hemodynamic Monitoring. Clin Chest Med No 2; June:249, 1999.
16. Herbst CA Jr. Indications, Management and complications of percutaneous subclavian catheters. Arch Surg 113:1421, 1978.
17. Felicano DV, Mattox KL, Graham JM, *et al.* Major complications of percutaneous subclavian vein catheters. An J Surg 138:869, 1979.
18. Haapaniemi L, Slatis P. Supraclavicular catheterization of the superior vena cava. Acta Anaesthesiol Scand 18:12, 1974.
19. Shah KB, Rao TL, Laughlin S, *et al.* A review of pulmonary artery catheterization on 6,245 patients. Anesthesiology 61:271, 1984.
20. Sprung CL, Elser B, Schein RM, *et al.* Ventricular arrhythmias during Swan-Ganz catheterization of the critically ill. Chest 79:413, 1981.
21. Sprung CL, Pozen RG, Rozanski JJ, *et al.* Advanced ventricular arrhythmia during bedside pulmonary artery catheterization. Am J Med 72:203, 1982.
22. Luck JC, Engel TR. Transient right bundle branch block with "Swan-Ganz" catheterization. Am Heart J 92:263, 1976.
23. Aktar M, Danato AN, Gilbert-Leeds CJ, *et al.* Induction of iatrogenic electrocardiographic patterns during electrophysiologic studies. Circulation 56:60, 1977.
24. Kaiser CW, Koornick AR, Smith N, *et al.* Choice of route for central venous cannulation: Subclavian or internal jugular vein? A prospective randomized study. J Surg Oncol 17:345, 1981.
25. Boyd KD, Thomas SJ, Gold J, *et al.* A prospective study of complications of pulmonary artery catheterizations in 500 consecutive patients. Chest 84:245, 1983.
26. Kearney TJ, Shabot MM. Pulmonary artery rupture associated with the Swan-Ganz catheter. Chest 108:1349, 1995.
27. Connors AF Jr, Castele JR, Farhat NZ, *et al.* Complications of right heart catheterization. A prospective autopsy study. Chest 88:567, 1985.
28. Mermel LA, Maki DG. Infectious complications of Swan-Ganz pulmonary artery catheters. Pathogenesis, epidemiology, prevention and management. Am J Respir Crit Care Med 149:1020, 1994.
29. Morris AH, Chapman RH, Gardner RM. Frequency of technical problems encountered in the measurement of pulmonary artery wedge pressure. Crit Care Med 12:164, 1984.
30. Morris AH, Chapman RH, Gardner RM. Frequency of wedge pressure errors in the ICU. Crit Care Med 13:705, 1985.
31. The Cardiac Arrhythmia Suppression Trial (CAST) Investigators. Preliminary report: Effect of ecainide and flecainide on mortality in a randomized trial of arrhythmia suppression after myocardial infarction. N Engl J Med 321:406, 1989.
32. Iberti TJ, Daily EK, Leibowitz AB, Schecter CB, Fischer EP, Silverstein JH. Assessment of critical care nurses' knowledge of the pulmonary artery catheter. Crit Care Med 22:1674, 1994.
33. Connors AF Jr, Speroff T, Dawson NV, *et al.* The effectiveness of right heart catheterization in the initial care of critically ill patients. JAMA 276: 889, 1996.

34. Ellis RE, Mangano DT, VanDyke DC. Relation of wedge pressure to end-diastolic volume in patients undergoing myocardial revascularization. J Thoracic Cardiovasc Surg 78:605, 1979.
35. Calvin JE, Driedger AA, Sibbald WJ. Does the pulmonary capillary wedge pressure predict left ventricular preload in the critically ill patient? Crit Care Med 9:437, 1981.
36. Mitchell JP, Schuller D, Calandrio FS, Schuster DP. Improved outcome based on fluid management in critically ill patients requiring pulmonary artery catheterization. Am Rev Resp Dis 145:990, 1992.
37. Gan TJ, Arrowsmith JE. The esophageal Doppler monitor. A safe means of monitoring circulation. BMJ 315:893, 1997.
38. Nishimura RA, *et al.* Non-invasive measurement of cardiac output by continuous wave Doppler echocardiography: Initial experience and review of the literature. May Clin Proc 59:484, 1984.
39. Hattle and Angelsen. Doppler Ultrasound in cardiology, 2nd edn. Lea and Febiger, Philadelphia, 1985.
40. Baker DW. Applications of pulsed Doppler. Rad Clin North Am 18:79, 1980.
41. Nishimura RA, *et al.* Doppler echocardiography: Theory, instrumentation, technique and application. Mayo Clinic Proc 60:321, 1985.
42. Am J Cardiol 76:392, 1995.
43. Sohn D-W, Shin G-J, Oh JK, Tajik AJ, Click RL, Miller FA, Seward JB. Role of Transesophageal Echocardiography in Hemodynamically Unstable Patients. May Clin Proc 70:925, 1995.
44. Heidenreich J. Am Coll Cardiol 26:152, 1995.
45. Pearson AC. Noninvasive evaluation of the hemodynamically unstable patient: the advantage of seeing clearly. Mayo Clin Proc 70:1012, 1995.
46. Hayes. NEJM 330:1717, 1994.
47. Gattinoni. NEJM 333:1025, 1995.
48. Negland, Cook. Crit Care Med 24:517, 1996.
49. Task Force of the American College of Critical Care Medicine, Society of Critical Care Monitoring Crit Care Med 27:639, 1999.

8. ROLE OF INVASIVE DEVICES IN THE PATHOGENESIS OF NOSOCOMIAL PNEUMONIA

Torsten T. Bauer, Ricard Ferrer and Antonio Torres

Introduction

Nosocomial pneumonia is still a common problem, especially in intubated and mechanically ventilated patients. The endotracheal tube contributes substantially to the pathogenesis of pneumonia in these patients, because it facilitates microaspiration and impairs host defenses. Common nosocomial pathogens like *Pseudomonas aeruginosa* are known to produce exopolysaccharide and generate the complex biofilm structure, which allows adhesion to abiotic surfaces and protection from antibiotic action. Multiple studies have identified bacterial biofilm on the inner lumen of endotracheal tubes, which represent a permanent source of infectious material. Endotracheal tubes, removed from patients with ventilator-associated pneumonia are covered more frequently with biofilm than those of uninfected controls but it remains unclear whether this represents a source of infection or secondary contamination. Bacterial biofilm, however, may play an important role in recurrent pulmonary infections of the intubated and mechanically ventilated patient.

Other invasive devices like bronchoscopes and tracheal suction catheters can also introduce microorganisms into patient's lower respiratory tract and, in some cases, can induce pneumonia.

Nosocomial pneumonia remains a common complication in patients who require mechanical ventilation. Endotracheal intubation has been identified on various occasions as a risk factor for nosocomial pneumonia [1]. This negative effect may be due to four different device/host interactions as it has been summarised by Levine and Niederman [1]:

1. The endotracheal tube can have direct effects on the airway that result in a reduction in local host defences. Thus, mucosal injury can reduce mucociliary function, while upper airway defenses are bypassed and the effectiveness of cough is reduced.
2. Indirectly, intubation can result in an enhanced capacity of tracheobronchial cells to bind Gram-negative bacteria, an effect that favors airway colonization and pneumonia.
3. The injury to the airway can create binding sites for bacteria in the basement membrane of the bronchial tree and the stimulation of the secretion of mucus, which then stagnates and can create potential sites for bacterial adherence.
4. Finally, the endotracheal tube can also enhance bacterial entry to the lung by serving as a reservoir for bacteria to remain sequestered.

Recent studies suggested that microorganisms can adhere to the surface of endotracheal tubes. Some species produce an exopolysaccharide that acts as a slime-like adhesive and the surface lining has been referred to as bacterial biofilm [2].

Other invasive devices like bronchoscopes and tracheal suction catheters can also introduce microorganisms into patient's lower respiratory tract. Although transmission of infections by bronchoscopy depends on many factors, the cleaning and disinfection process is the single element that the clinician can most influence. In spite of the disinfection measures several cases of nosocomial transmission of infections and pneumonia have been detected [3].

This chapter will review the basic research related to bacterial biofilms formation on abiotic surfaces, the possible role of bacterial biofilm on the inner lumen of endotracheal tubes and the possible role of other invasive devices for the pathogenesis of ventilator-associated pneumonia.

Bacterial Biofilm Definition and Formation

Bacterial biofilms are defined as matrix-enclosed bacterial populations' adherent to each other and/or to surfaces or interfaces. This definition includes microbial aggregates and also adherent populations within the pore spaces in porous media [2].

The biofilm can be regarded as a complex matrix with channels that allow nutrients to circulate analogous to tissues of higher organisms [4]. The sessile forms of the bacteria coated in biofilm can give rise to *planktonic* bacteria that may eventually leave the biofilm and disperse into the environment. Among the bacterial species that may generate biofilms are some that are currently regarded to have only low pathogenic potential in the context of nosocomial pneumonia such as *S. epidermidis*. However, *P. aeruginosa* and *S. pneumoniae* are common nosocomial pulmonary pathogens and their potential to aggregate in biofilms has been well described [5]. Four fundamental steps have been identified during the process of biofilm formation and are best described for *P. aeruginosa* [5]. Flagella play an important role for the initial attachment to abiotic surfaces of *P. aeruginosa* during the first step of biofilm formation. Type IV pilli and twitching motility further leads to the formation of microcolonies of these bacteria. Recent research showed that strains of *P. aeruginosa* unable to form these initial microcolonies were also unable to form a mature biofilm on a polyvinylchloride (PVC) plastic surface [6]. Once microcolonies are formed, the attached bacteria have to mature into a differentiated biofilm [5]. Bacteria secrete small molecule pheromones at this stage to determine whether there are enough bacteria to initiate the expression of a particular phenotype ("*quorum sensing*") [7]. If this step is successful, the microcolonies differentiate into a structured, thick, biocide-resistant biofilm.

Bacterial Biofilm and Antibiotic Drug Resistance

Biofilm-covered bacteria in the inner lumen of endotracheal tubes have a decrease susceptibility to antibiotic drugs for three reasons. First, the biofilm reaches into an air-filled lumen that provides almost no host defence mechanisms. Ultrastructural analysis of biofilm in endotracheal tube has shown to harbor also polymorphonuclear leukocytes as well, however until now it is unclear whether this reflects directed migration or simply a contaminating mechanism during coughing or endotracheal suctioning [8]. Second, the biofilm protects the sessile forms of the bacteria physically from antibiotic action. Antibiotics may be either unable to penetrate the biofilm [9, 10] or the decreased diffusing capacity also increases the likelihood of deactivation prior to target contact [11]. The third reason for antibiotic resistance is the slow-growing or starved state of the sessile bacteria and some researchers hypothesize that the bacteria may even adopt a distinct phenotype as a biologically response to growth on a surface [12, 13].

Bacterial Biofilm in Endotracheal Tubes

To date only a few studies have addressed bacterial biofilm formation in endotracheal tubes of mechanically ventilated patients. Most studies tried to prove three important points about biofilm in this medical device: presence and quantity, the ultrastructure, and the viability of the observed microorganisms. In 1986 Sottile *et al.* studied 25 ventilation tubes (PVC, endotracheal or tracheostomy) that had been removed from patients of one multidisciplinary ICU after an average of 9.2 days (range 1 to 46 days) of respirator support [14]. By means of scanning electron microscopy (SEM) they could identify amorphous material on the inner surface that was confluent in 21/25 tubes (84%) and intermittent in 4/25 endotracheal tubes (16%). Rod shaped or coccoid bacteria were seen on the surface of 17/25 devices (68%). Qualitative bacterial cultures were obtained from 23 endotracheal tubes and showed bacterial growth on 19/23 occasions (83%). A total of 92% of the patients had received antibiotic drugs and the following microorganisms were cultured: *S. aureus*, *P. aeruginosa*, *Proteus mirabilis* and *S. epidermidis*. Diaz-Blanco *et al.* observed coccoid structures through SEM on all 29 endotracheal tubes from neonates after mechanical ventilation for 0.5 to 14 days (100%) [15]. *S. epidermidis* could be cultured from 12/29 tubes (41%) and group B hemolytic *S. epidermidis*, *P. aeruginosa* and *K. pneumoniae* from 1/29 tubes (3%), respectively. All patients had received antibiotics (100%).

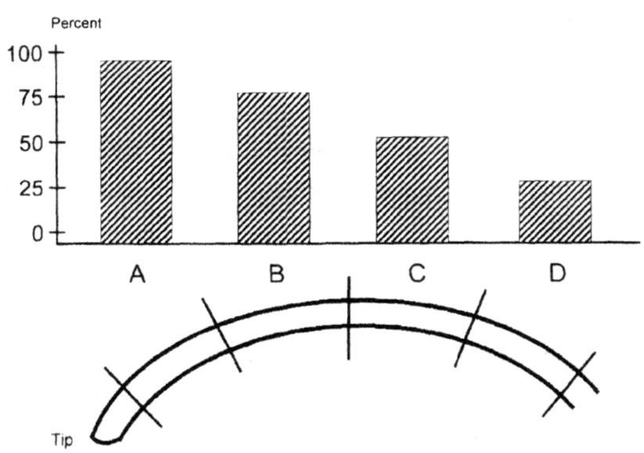

FIGURE 1. Frequency of biofilm formation in relation to sections of the endotracheal tube (n = 50). A total of four sections were analyzed (sections A–D) and bars represent the percentage of tube sections with radiographically identified biofilm. The sections close to the tip of the endotracheal tube (Section A) were more often covered with biofilm than the proximal parts [17].

An attempt was made to quantify the amount of material deposited on endotracheal tubes by Inglis *et al.* [16]. Cotton swabs of all tubes were subjected to quantitative bacterial cultures and the scraped-off material was also weighted. The researchers found more than 50 mg of biofilm dry weight in 30/40 tubes (75%), but the absolute weight seemed to not be associated with the duration of use. In 33/45 tubes (75%), bacteria were cultured (*P. aeruginosa*, *K. pneumoniae*, *Proteus mirabilis*, *E. coli* and *Enterobacter cloacea*) and the bacterial counts were as high as 10^6 colony forming units (cfu) per centimeter of tube length.

In 1993, Inglis radiographically detected biofilm in 45 of 50 endotracheal tubes (90%) removed from patients of a general ICU [17]. The integrity of the tube was maintained in this study and the amount of deposited material could be analyzed according to tube shape. Biofilm thickness was measured with a dialgauge caliper and the distribution assigned to a Magill curve template (Figure 1). They could clearly demonstrate that the presence of biofilm was more likely at the tip of the endotracheal tube (segment A, 45/50 tubes, 90%) and decreased towards the proximal end of the tube (segment D, 14/50 tubes, 28%). No correlation was found with the duration of use for this distribution pattern. The biofilm *in vivo* is probably a combination of microbial biofilm generation and ventilatory secretion deposition during expiration, coughing or endotracheal suctioning. This hypothesis is further supported by the fact that endoluminal biofilm from endotracheal tubes of mechanically ventilated patients is composed not only of bacteria and exopolysaccharides but also contains neutrophils in varying stages of disintegration with an amorphous matrix most likely corresponding to respiratory mucus [8].

Sequence of Colonization of Endotracheal Tubes

It has been shown that oropharyngeal colonization proceeds pulmonary infection and is an independent risk factor of nosocomial pneumonia [18–20]. Microaspiration is probably the most important pathogenic mechanism [1, 21] but oropharyngeal colonization may also facilitate biofilm development in the endotracheal tube [16]. Feldman *et al.* investigated biofilm formation in 21 ICU patients undergoing 24 extubations (mean length of intubation 0.5 to 12 days [22]). Through scanning electronic minoscope (SEM), they identified biofilm on the inner surface of all endotracheal tubes (24/24, 100%) and viable – mostly Gram-negative – bacteria were identified from secretions of all but three tubes (21/24, 88%). In a second part of this study they tried to identify the sequence of colonization by sampling of the oropharynx, the nasogastric tube, the interior of the airway tube and endotracheal secretions in ten uninfected patients on at least five consecutive days [22]. It was interesting that the appearance of microorganisms in lower respiratory tract secretions almost invariably preceded their appearance in the interior of the endotracheal tube. This finding strongly suggests that the sequence of colonization is oropharynx – tracheobronchial tree – endotracheal tube and that the biofilm formation only plays a minor role, at least for the etiology of the first pulmonary infection. This belief is also supported by the more prominent biofilm formation near the tip of the endotracheal tube in this [22] and previous studies (Figure 1) [8].

Bacterial Endotracheal Tube Biofilm and Nosocomial Pneumonia

It has been proposed that bacteria from the biofilm lining of the endotracheal tube might be scattered into the lungs during ventilation gas flow, since dissemination of bacteria from the tube could be demonstrated *in vitro* [16]. Dynamic studies simulating the scattering of tracheal tube biofilm have shown that bacteria can be disseminated many centimeters from the orifice of the endotracheal tube, far into the lung [17].

Sottile *et al.* were among the first to suggest that there may be a relationship between nosocomial pneumonia and bacterial adherence to the interior of the endotracheal tube [14]. A study in neonates undergoing prolonged mechanical ventilation failed to demonstrate a clinical relationship between endotracheal tube colonization and nosocomial pneumonia [15]. However, this study may have lacked sufficient power, because the children were screened for nosocomial infections after extubation. In a recently published case control study, endotracheal tubes from patients with ventilator associated pneumonia were more often covered with biofilm (20/20, 100%) than those of uninfected control patients (6/20, 30%) [23]. Of those patients with ventilator-associated pneumonia, 14/20 (70%) had pathogens that were indistinguishable by genotyping in both endotracheal tubes and tracheal secretions. In contrast, no matching pairs of pathogens were isolated from control patients.

However, this study leaves the question unanswered whether the bacteria at the inner lumen of the endotracheal tube have contributed to the development of ventilator-associated pneumonia or whether they have spread from the tracheobronchial tree to the tube during coughing or endotracheal suctioning.

The contribution of endotracheal tube biofilm for the pathogenesis of ventilator-associated pneumonia is controversial [24, 25], especially if the magnitude of the problem is related to that of other risk factors of ventilator-associated pneumonia [26–29]. Nevertheless, it may be of crucial importance to the pathogenesis of recurrent ventilator-associated pneumonia [5, 22]. Rello *et al.* investigated recurrent episodes of pneumonia caused by *P. aeruginosa* in 37 mechanically ventilated patients [30]. They were able to analyze 16 isolates of five patients and all but one was considered relapses because of the concordance in chromosomal fingerprinting. As pointed out above, *P. aeruginosa* is known to produce bacterial biofilm with reduced antibiotic susceptibility and even withstands topical antibiotic therapy in a clinical setting [31].

Bronchoscope

Bronchoscopy can occasionally transmit infectious lung disease. The bronchoscope traverse the nasopharynx or oropharynx and carry with it the indigenous microbial flora to distal regions and may thus inoculate the tracheobronchial tree and possibly the pulmonary parenchyma. Another potential complication is the bronchoscopic spread of infection from an infected patient to an uninfected patient.

Although transmission of infections by bronchoscopy depends on many factors, the cleaning and disinfecting process is the single key measure to avoid transmission of infections. Some organisms like *Mycobacteria* are inherently more resistant to disinfectants. In addition, the effectiveness of the germicide depends on its type, concentration, and duration of exposure. If residual patient material, such as blood or sputum, remains in the bronchoscope after cleaning, the effectiveness of any subsequent disinfecting procedure will dramatically diminish. Moreover, the complexity of the instrument, with crevices, joints or pores, create problems for both cleaning and disinfecting.

Several studies have tried to estimated this risk of developing lung infection after bronchoscopy. In a large retrospective study of 24,521 patients who underwent bronchoscopy, Credel *et al.* found only two cases of pneumonia [32]. In a prospective study, Pereira *et al.* reported after bronchoscopy the development of fever in 16% of the patients, parenchymal infiltrates in 6%, and one patient developed rapidly progressive pneumonia and died. No organisms were isolated from cultures of blood drawn at the time of the procedure or during complications. Among the patients who developed pneumonia, the isolates from sputum generally consisted of aerobic and anaerobic microorganisms normally found in the mouth [33]. In a third study, using two types of disinfecting solutions to clean the bronchoscope, Suratt *et al.* surveyed 249 bronchoscopic procedures and no patient developed pneumonia in either period [34].

Although these few studies imply that bronchoscopy may be free of the risk of transmitting microorganisms, reports of bronchoscopic transmission of infections clearly have occurred. In 1978, Hussain reported transmission of a *Pseudomonas* species in seven patients who had undergone bronchoscopy. Infection was related to the biopsy-suction attachment and resulted in one patient developing a right lower lobe pneumonia [35]. Sammartino *et al.* reported in 1982 the infection of 11 patients after a bronchoscopic procedure because the presence of *Pseudomonas aeruginosa* in the inner channel of the bronchoscope, despite appropriate cleaning [36]. The contamination was eliminated after sterilizing the bronchoscope with ethylene oxide. Boisjoly *et al.* reported a case in which bronchoscopy for the evaluation of hemoptysis was followed two weeks later by uveitis and four weeks later by endophthalmitis [37]. Both sputum and vitreous cultures yielded *Pseudomonas aeruginosa*. Despite aggressive medical treatment, enucleation was eventually performed.

Bronchoscopic transmission of bacteria other than *Pseudomonas* spp. has also occurred. In one report, investigators isolated a *Proteus* species from an index patient, eight subsequent patients, and the biopsy channel of the bronchoscope; each isolate had the same susceptibility profile, but no patient developed pneumonia [38]. In an outbreak that had serious consequences, Webb and Vall-Spinoza reported three patients who developed infection with *S. marcescens* after undergoing bronchoscopy; two patients died of necrotizing pneumonia caused by this organism, an index patient infected by *S. marcescens* was identified [39].

A case of fatal streptococcal pneumonia and septicemia followed flexible bronchoscopic examination and endobronchial biopsy in a patient with severe chronic congestive heart failure was reported by Beyt *et al.* [40]; a causal relationship was unclear.

Anecdotal reports of development of pneumonia and lung abscess after transbronchial biopsy of a peripheral mass lesion are noteworthy [41, 42]. Whats and Green reported that transbronchial fine-needle aspiration of a subcarinal lymph node was followed by bacteriemia secondary to *Streptococcus viridans* infection [43].

The increasing incidence of tuberculous and nontuberculous mycobacterial infection has increased the likelihood that bronchoscopy may spread these organisms. In addition, Mycobacteria are inherently more resistant to disinfectants. In 1980 Leers [44] and Nelson *et al.* in 1983 [45] reported one case each of cross-contamination with *Mycobacterium tuberculosis* but not developed evidence of tuberculosis. In a subsequent report, Wheeler *et al.* described three cases of bronchoscopic transmission of *M. tuberculosis* that resulted in clinically significant infection [46]. Recently, Agerton *et al.* reported that fatal multidrug resistant tuberculosis was transmitted by bronchoscopy [47]. In the four above mentioned reports were detected problems in the disinfecting procedure. Mycobacteria other than M. *tuberculosis* like M. *chelonae* have been implicated in bronchoscopic transmission of infections [48, 49]. In both cases, they detected problems with the disinfecting procedure.

Spread of pre-existing pulmonary infections is more common than the propagation of an infection from patient to patient by the bronchoscope. Fortunately, in most cases, patients have not shown clinical evidence of infection. Although transmission of infections to an uninfected patient by bronchoscopy depends on many factors like the inmunological status of the patient or the duration of the procedure, the cleaning and disinfecting process is the single key measure to control. Routine procedures to prevent contamination include compliance with recommended cleaning and disinfecting regimens and regular maintenance of bronchoscopes [50].

According to our experience, because the high incidence of airway colonization in intubated patients, bronchoscope is a clear potential transmitter of nosocomial infections. Bronchoscopes in ICU need to follow a very strict policy of cleaning, aeration and disinfection. A specific ICU nursing team taking care of these practices and monthly microbiological surveillance of the inner channel and outer parts of the bronchoscope is strongly recommended.

Tracheal Suction Catheters

Endotracheal suctioning is an essential and common supportive treatment for patients requiring mechanical ventilation. Currently, there are two types of suction-catheter systems, the open single-use catheter system and the closed multi-use catheter system (Figure 2).

Open suctioning uses a single use catheter that can be rapidly inserted and withdrawn from the endotracheal tube. Suction catheters may introduce microorganisms into the lower respiratory tract increasing the risk of colonization of the lower airways, and thus the risk of ventilator-associated pneumonia. Moreover, in patients with respiratory instability, complications associated with this technique include arterial oxygen desaturation, cardiac arrhythmias, inability to maintain PEEP, and sudden death [51]. Sterile gloved technique is mandatory when using the open system because the risk of environmental cross-contamination. Closed multiuse systems have less risk of cross-contamination. However, the multiuse catheter can be contaminated after the initial pass through the endotracheal tube and repeated

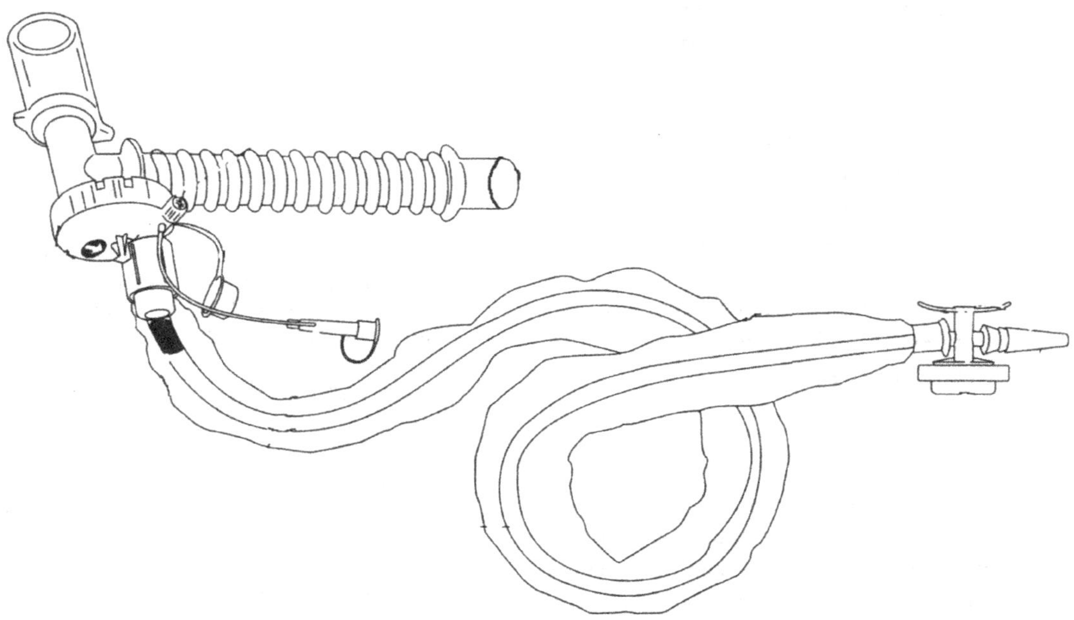

FIGURE 2. Closed multiuse catheter system for tracheal suction.

insertions may increase the chance of lower airway colonization from the suction-catheter tip and endotracheal tube.

Closed suction catheter devices are now used in many hospitals, decreasing the risk of environmental cross-contamination, saving time and eliminating the need to disconnect the patient from the ventilator [52–55]. However, results of comparing the two systems suggest that the risk of catheter contamination or pneumonia is not different comparing the standard procedure with the multiuse system [56, 57]. At present, no rigorously obtained scientific evidence exists to recommend one practice or another. This is also the recommendation reported in the most recent guidelines for the prevention of nosocomial pneumonia published by the Centers for Disease Control and prevention [58].

The optimal procedure of the closed multiuse catheter system is still not clear. On one hand, it is recommended to change the in-line suction catheter every 24 hours. This recommendation is based on the ability of bacteria to aggregate on the surface of suction catheters and endotracheal tubes to form a biofilm that protects the bacteria from the action of microbial agents or host defences [8, 14]. Dislodgement of these bacterial aggregates into the lung has been proposed as a possible mechanism for the development of ventilator-associated pneumonia [16]. Other investigators have suggested that increased manipulation of the ventilator circuit can predispose to the development of ventilator-associated pneumonia [28, 59]. Recently, Kollef *et al.* reported the same incidence of ventilator-associated pneumonia in two groups of patients with or without daily changes of in-line suction catheters [60] suggesting that the practice of avoiding the change every 24 hours of in-line suction catheters during mechanical ventilation is safe.

In our opinion, the closed multiuse catheter system is useful in unstable patients requiring mechanical ventilation with high oxygen concentrations or high levels of PEEP and in immunosuppresed patients for the extremely high risk of infections that these patients have. The in-line suction catheter must be changed when a mechanical failure of the device is detected (e.g., malfunction of the valve resulting in the leakage of air into the protected covering sheath of the catheter) or when visible soil is clotting the inner catheter (such as resulting from aspiration of blood or aspirated emesis). Except the situations mentioned above we use the open system with the single use catheter for the routine suctioning procedure.

Conclusions

Bacterial biofilm has been demonstrated on the inner surface in a high percentage of endotracheal tubes removed from mechanically ventilated patients. The biofilm formation seems to be independent from the duration of mechanical ventilation. However, whether this is due to the rapid formation or whether there are other factors involved has not been investigated systematically. Endoluminal biofilm seems to form either more rapidly or more frequently at the distal end of the endotracheal tube. However, *in vivo* pure biofilm does not develop and factors like mucus deposition also have to be taken into account. Recent research indicates that bacterial biofilm may form more frequently in endotracheal tubes of patients with ventilator-associated pneumonia. Nevertheless, this may represent contamination and the magnitude of the contribution to the pathogenesis of ventilator-associated pneumonia of endoluminal bacterial biofilm may be minimal when other risk factors are taken into account. In contrast, bacterial biofilm of endotracheal tubes may play an important role as a persistent source of infectious material for recurrent episodes of ventilator-associated pneumonia.

Other invasive devices like bronchoscope and tracheal suction catheters can also play a role in the pathogenesis of nosocomial pneumonia. Using the adequate mode of cleaning and disinfecting the bronchoscope is mandatory to prevent infections.

References

1. Levine SA, Niederman MS. The impact of tracheal intubation on host defenses and risks for nosocomial pneumonia. Clin Chest Med 12:523, 1991.
2. Costerton JW, Lewandowski Z, Caldwell DE, Korber DR, Lappin-Scott HM. Microbial biofilms. Annnu Rev Microbiol 49:711, 1995.
3. Prakash UB. Does the bronchoscope propagate infection? Chest 104:552, 1993.
4. Costerton JW, Cheng KJ, Geesey GG, Ladd TI, Nickel JC, *et al.* Bacterial biofilms in nature and disease. Annu Rev Microbiol 41:435, 1987.
5. Costerton JW, Stewart PS, Greenberg EP. Bacterial biofilms: a common cause of persistent infections. Science 21:1318, 1999.
6. O'Toole GA, Kolter R. Flagellar and twitching motility are necessary for *Pseudomonas aeruginosa* biofilm development. Mol Microbiol 30:295, 1998.
7. Parsek MR, Greenberg EP. Quorum sensing signals in development of *Pseudomonas aeruginosa* biofilms. Methods Enzymol 310:43, 1999.
8. Inglis TJ, Lim TM, Ng ML, Tang EK, Hui KP. Structural features of tracheal tube biofilm formed during prolonged mechanical ventilation. Chest 108:1049, 1995.
9. Vorachit M, Lam K, Jayanetra P, Costerton JW. Resistance of *Pseudomonas pseudomallei* growing as a biofilm on silastic discs to ceftazidime and co-trimoxazole. Antimicrob Agents Chemother 37:2000, 1993.
10. Shigeta M, Tanaka G, Komatsuzawa H, Sugai M, Suginaka H, Usui T. Permeation of antimicrobial agents through *Pseudomonas aeruginosa* biofilms: a simple method. Chemotherapy 43:340, 1997.
11. Dibdin GH, Assinder SJ, Nichols WW, Lambert PA. Mathematical model of beta-lactam penetration into a biofilm of *Pseudomonas aeruginosa* while undergoing simultaneous inactivation by released beta-lactamases. J Antimicrob Chemother 38:757, 1996.
12. Costerton JW. Introduction to biofilm. Int J Antimicrob Agents 11:217, 1999.
13. Fletcher M. The physiological activity of bacteria attached to solid surfaces. Adv Microb Physiol 32:53, 1991.

14. Sottile FD, Marrie TJ, Prough DS, Hobgood CD, Gower DJ, *et al.* Nosocomial pulmonary infection: possible etiologic significance of bacterial adhesion to endotracheal tubes. Crit Care Med 14:265, 1986.
15. Diaz-Blanco J, Clawson RC, Roberson SM, Sanders CB, Pramanik AK, Herbst JJ. Electron microscopic evaluation of bacterial adherence to polyvinyl chloride endotracheal tubes used in neonates. Crit Care Med 17:1335, 1989.
16. Inglis TJ, Millar MR, Jones JG, Robinson DA. Tracheal tube biofilm as a source of bacterial colonization of the lung. J Clin Microbiol 27:2014, 1989.
17. Inglis TJ. Evidence for dynamic phenomena in residual tracheal tube biofilm. Br J Anaesth 70:22, 1993.
18. Coalson JJ, Gerstmann DR, Winter VT, Delemos RA. Bacterial colonization and infection studies in the premature baboon with bronchopulmonary dysplasia. Am Rev Respir Dis 144:1140, 1991.
19. Rubenstein JS, Kabat K, Shulman ST, Yogev R. Bacterial and fungal colonization of endotracheal tubes in children: a prospective study. Crit Care Med 20:1544, 1992.
20. Garrouste-Orgeas M, Chevret S, Arlet G, Marie O, Rouveau M, *et al.* Oropharyngeal or gastric colonization and nosocomial pneumonia in adult intensive care unit patients. A prospective study based on genomic DNA analysis. Am J Respir Crit Care Med 156:1647, 1997.
21. Estes RJ, Meduri GU. The pathogenesis of ventilator-associated pneumonia: I. Mechanisms of bacterial transcolonization and airway inoculation. Intensive Care Med 21:365, 1995.
22. Feldman C, Kassel M, Cantrell J, Kaka S, Morar R, *et al.* The presence and sequence of endotracheal tube colonization in patients undergoing mechanical ventilation. Eur Respir J 13:546, 1999.
23. Adair CG, Gorman SP, Feron BM, Byers LM, Jones DS, *et al.* Implications of endotracheal tube biofilm for ventilator-associated pneumonia. Intensive Care Med 25:1072, 1999.
24. Koerner RJ. Contribution of endotracheal tubes to the pathogenesis of ventilator-associated pneumonia. J Hosp Infect 35:83, 1997.
25. van Saene HKF, Damjanovic V, Williets T, Mostafa SM, Fox MA, Petros AJ. Pathogenesis of ventilator-associated pneumonia: is the contribution of biofilm clinically significant? [letter]. J Hosp Infect 38:231, 1998.
26. Torres A, Aznar R, Gatell JM, Jiménez P, González J, Ferrer M, *et al.* Incidence, risk, and prognosis factors of nosocomial pneumonia in mechanically ventilated patients. Am Rev Respir Dis 142:523, 1990.
27. Bonten MJ, Bergmans DC, Ambergen AW, de Leeuw PW, van der Geest S, *et al.* Risk factors for pneumonia, and colonization of respiratory tract and stomach in mechanically ventilated ICU patients. Am J Respir Crit Care Med 154:1339, 1996.
28. Craven DE, Kunches LM, Kilinsky V, Lichtenberg DA, Make BJ, McCabe WR. Risk factors for pneumonia and fatality in patients receiving mechanical ventilation. Am Rev Respir Dis 133:792, 1986.
29. Fernández-Crehuet R, Diáz-Molina C, De Irala J, Martínez-Concha D, Salcedo-Leal I, *et al.* Nosocomial infection in an intensive-care unit: Identification of risk factors. Infect Control Hosp Epidemiol 18:825, 1997.
30. Rello J, Mariscal D, Marco F, Jubert P, Sanchez F, *et al.* Recurrent *Pseudomonas aeruginosa* pneumonia in ventilated patients: relapse or reinfection? Am J Respir Crit Care Med 157:912, 1998.
31. Gorman S, Adair C, O'Neill F, Goldsmith C, Webb H. Influence of selective decontamination of the digestive tract on microbial biofilm formation on endotracheal tubes from artificially ventilated patients. Eur J Clin Microbiol Infect Dis 12:9, 1993.
32. Credle WF Jr, Smiddy JF, Elliot RC. Complications of fiberoptic bronchoscopy. Am Rev Respir Dis 109:67, 1974.
33. Pereira W, Kovnat DM, Khan MA, Iacovino JR, Spivack ML, Snider GL. Fever and pneumonia after flexible bronchoscopy. Am Rev Respir Dis 112:59, 1975.
34. Suratt PM, Gruber B, Wellons HA, Wenzel RP. Absence of clinical pneumonia following bronchoscopy with contaminated and clean bronchofiberscopes. Chest 71:52, 1977.
35. Hussain SA. Fiberoptic bronchoscope-related outbreak of infection with *Pseudomonas*. Chest 74:483, 1978.
36. Sammartino MT, Israel RH, Magnussen CR. *Pseudomonas aeruginosa* contamination of fiberoptic bronchoscopes. J Hosp Infect 3:65, 1982.
37. Boisjoly HM, Jotterand VH, Bazin R, Bergeron MG. Metastatic *Pseudomonas* endophtalmitis following bronchoscopy. Can J Ophthalmol 22:378, 1987.
38. Weinstein HJ, Bone RC, Ruth WE. Contamination of a fiberoptic bronchoscope with a

Proteus species. Am Rev Respir Dis 116:541, 1977.
39. Webb SF, Vall-Spinosa A. Outbreak of *Serratia marcescens* associated with the flexible fiberoptic bronchoscope. Chest 68:703, 1975.
40. Beyt BE Jr, King DK, Glew RH. Fatal pneumonitis and septicemia after fiberbronchoscopy. Chest 72:105, 1977.
41. Hsu JT, Barrett CR Jr. Lung absess complicating transbronchial biopsy of a mass lesion. Chest 80:230, 1981.
42. Muers M, Lane D. Acute pneumonia and pneumothorax as a complication of transbronchial biopsy. Endoscopy 12:183, 1980.
43. Watts WJ, Green RA. Bacteriemia following transbronchial fine needle aspiration. Chest 85:295, 1984.
44. Leers WD. Disinfecting endoscopes: how to not transmit *Mycobacterium tuberculosis* by bronchoscopy. Can Med Assoc J 123:275, 1980.
45. Nelson KE, Larson PA, Schraufnagel DE, Jackson J. Transmission of tuberculosis by flexible fiberbronchoscopes. Am Rev Respir Dis 127:97, 1983.
46. Wheeler PW, Lancaster D, Kaiser AB. Bronchopulmonary cross-colonization and infection related to mycobacterial contamination of suctuon valves of bronchoscopes. J Infect Dis 159:954, 1989.
47. Agerton T, Valway S, Gore B, Pozsik C, Plikaytis B, *et al.* Transmission of a highly drug-resistant strain (strain W1) of *Mycobacterium tuberculosis*. Community outbreak and nosocomial transmission via a contaminated bronchoscope. JAMA 278:1073, 1999.
48. Pappas SA, Schaaff DM, DiCostanzo MB, King FW, Sharp JT. Contamination of flexible fiberoptic bronchoscopes. Am Rev Respir Dis 127:391, 1983.
49. Uttley AHC, Honeywell KM, Fitch LE, Yates MD, Collins CH, Simpson RA. Cross contamination of bronchial washings. Brit Med J 301:1274, 1990.
50. Mehta AC, Minai OA. Infection control in the bronchoscopy suite. Clinics Chest Med 20:19, 1999.
51. Brown SE, Stansbury DW, Merril EJ, Linden GS, Light RW. Prevention of suctioning-related arterial oxygen desaturation. Comparison of off-ventilator and on-ventilator suctioning. Chest 83:621, 1983.
52. Mayhall CG. The Trach Care closed tracheal suction system: a new medical device to permit tracheal suctioning without interruption of ventilatory assistance. Infect Control Hosp Epidemiol 9:125, 1988.
53. Baker T, Taylor M, Wilson M, Rish J, Brazeal S. Evaluation of a closed system endotracheal suction catheter. Am J Infect Control 17:97, 1989.
54. Johnson KL, Kearney PA, Johnson SB, Niblett JB, Mcmillian NL, Mc Clain RE. Closed versus open endotracheal suctioning: costs and physiologic consequences. Crit Care Med 22:658, 1994.
55. Cobley M, Atkins M, Jones FL. Environmental contamination during tracheal suction. A comparison of disposable conventional catheters with a multiple-use closed system device. Anaesthesia 46:957, 1991.
56. Deppe SA, Kelly JW, Thoi LL, Chudy JH, Longfield RN, *et al.* Incidence of colonization, nosocomial pneumonia, and mortality in critically ill patients using a Trach Care closed-suction system versus an open-suction system: prospective, randomized study. Crit Care Med 18:1393, 1990.
57. Ritz R, Scott LR, Coyle MB, Pierson DJ. Contamination of a multiple-use suction catheter in a closed-circuit system compared to contamination of a disposable, single-use suction catheter. Respir Care 31:1087, 1986.
58. Tablan OC, Andreson LJ, Arden NH, Breiman RF, Butler JC, McNeil MM. Guideline for prevention of nosocomial pneumonia. The Hospital Infection Control Practices Advisory Committee, Centers for Disease Control and Prevention. Infect Control Hosp Epidemiol 15:588, 1994.
59. Kollef MH, Shapiro SD, Fraser VJ, Silver P, Murphy M, *et al.* Mechanical ventilation with or without 7-day circuit changes: a randomized controlled trial. Ann Intern Med 123:168, 1995.
60. Kollef MH, Prentice D, Shapiro SD, Fraser VJ, Silver P, *et al.* Mechanical ventilation with or without daily changes of in-line suction catheters. Am J Respir Crit Care Med 156:466, 1997.

9. AIDS IN THE INTENSIVE CARE UNIT

David M. Forrest, Carlos Zala, Marianne Harris, Peter Phillips,
James A. Russell and Julio S.G. Montaner

Introduction

Since Acquired Immunodeficiency Syndrome (AIDS) was first recognized, it has been a leading cause of death among young people in the industrialized world and has had devastating effects in developing nations [1]. With the introduction of modern antiretroviral therapy, there has been a marked decline in the incidence of AIDS among treated Human Immunodeficiency Virus (HIV)-infected individuals. Since 1995, stabilization in the incidence of AIDS-related opportunistic infections in industrialized countries has been followed by a reduction in the rate of new AIDS case and AIDS-related mortality. These changes are thought to be due to the introduction of highly active antiretroviral combination regimens [2–5]. Although the admission rates of HIV-infected persons to the intensive care unit (ICU) are likely to have fallen in conjunction with a decline in the AIDS case-rate, there are no data to substantiate this. Moreover, changes in the rate of HIV infection and demographics of those infected also can be expected to alter the frequency of ICU admission of HIV positive persons [6].

The pandemic of HIV infection is expanding rapidly especially in developing nations [5]. Estimates by the Joint United Nations Program on HIV/AIDS (UNAIDS) and the World Health Organization (WHO), a cosponsor of the Joint Program, indicate that by the beginning of 1998 over 30 million people were infected with HIV, the virus that causes AIDS, and that 11.7 million people around the world had already lost their lives to the disease. Unless a cure is found or life-prolonging therapy can be made more widely available, the majority of those now living with HIV will die within a decade.

These deaths will not be the last; there is worse to come. The virus continues to spread, causing nearly 16,000 new infections a day. During 1997 alone, that meant 5.8 million new HIV infections, despite the fact that more is known now than ever before about how to prevent the spread of the epidemic.

Despite improvements in HIV treatment and access to medical resources in industrialized countries, however, the growth of the epidemic is no less alarming. For example, the rate of new HIV infections almost doubled in Canada between 1992 and 1996 with an increase in infection rates among women, aboriginal peoples and injection drug users. There has been increasing heterosexual transmission of HIV among minorities in the United States, while the incidence of infection has fallen among homosexual men and injection drug users [6]. In Europe, injection drug use accounts for 40% of cases of HIV infection and there have been explosive outbreaks in this population in Eastern Europe [7]. HIV infection is now considered virtually endemic in the United States [8].

Hence, the rate of HIV infection is rising particularly among groups with less access to medical care. Use of opportunistic infection prophylaxis and antiretroviral therapy by individuals in these groups is less likely: their presentation with advanced HIV disease and its complications therefore should be anticipated

[6]. Hence, just as AIDS will not disappear even with the advent of effective antiretroviral regimens, so too is it likely that AIDS-related complications will continue to be encountered in the ICU.

Human Immunodeficiency Virus Infection

VIROLOGY AND COURSE OF INFECTION

AIDS is caused by chronic infection with the lentivirus HIV, which is a member of the family of retroviruses. The virus infects cells principally by binding to the CD4 molecule, a cell surface glycoprotein which acts as receptor for the major histocompatibility (MHC) II molecule, although binding to a chemokine coreceptor is also necessary for viral entry into the cell [9, 10]. Hence, HIV primarily infects cells bearing a CD4 receptor: helper T-lymphocytes and monocytes/macrophages. However, HIV can also infect cells which do not bear the CD4 receptor, including gastrointestinal and cervical mucosal cells, megakaryocytes, renal epithelial cells, cardiac myocytes and neurons, although the clinical significance of this property is unclear [11].

After the virus enters the cell, reverse transcription of the viral ribonucleic acid (RNA) genome occurs by means of a reverse transcriptase contained within the virus, producing pro-viral double-stranded deoxyribonucleic acid (DNA). The DNA particles gain access to the nucleus and are generally integrated into the host genome, where they enter a state of latency. With activation of the cell (such as during an immune response to intercurrent infection), transcription of proviral DNA is initiated and viral RNA and proteins are synthesized. New virions are assembled and bud from the cell, thus spreading infection to other susceptible cells [12] (see Figure 1).

Chronic infection with HIV results in gradual destruction of CD4+ (helper) T-lymphocytes with progressive immune deterioration, culminating in the clinical syndrome of opportunistic infections and malignancies characterizing AIDS. The mechanism of immune destruction is complex and involves both direct HIV-mediated cytopathic effects (such as destruction of individual cells and formation of syncytia) and indirect, nonvirologic mechanisms (reviewed in detail in [10]). The latter include the action of HIV as a superantigen (thus stimulating the T-cell receptor directly); induction of an autoimmune response due to the similarity of HIV to the MHC molecule; stimulation of apoptosis (programmed cell death); and virus-specific cytotoxic immune responses [9, 10].

The clinical course of HIV infection has been delineated clearly [9, 10, 13] (see Figure 2). Approximately 1–6 weeks after primary infection with HIV, 50–70% of patients suffer an acute mononucleosis-like syndrome, often with a rash, but usually the syndrome is not recognized (or only identified retrospectively). During this benign, self-limited seroconversion illness, there is a high level of viremia followed by a cellular and humoral immune response against HIV, which is established within one week to three months of infection. With the establishment of immunity, the level of viremia usually declines. However, the immune response is inadequate to eradicate or contain the infection, and viral replication persists. Even if viremia is undetectable, HIV replication continues unabated in lymphoid tissue.

After initial infection, most patients enter a period of clinical latency for several years (generally 8–12 years, variable with age at seroconversion [14]). Most patients remain asymptomatic or suffer only minor symptoms (such as persistent generalized lymphadenopathy) during this time, but viral replication and destruction of the immune system progress relentlessly with eventual collapse off CD4+ T-lymphocyte number and function. Profound immunosuppression ensues with the development of persistent constitutional symptoms, opportunistic infections and neoplasms typical of the end-stage of HIV infection (AIDS; Figure 2).

The rapidity of immune destruction and hence prognosis in HIV infection is clearly

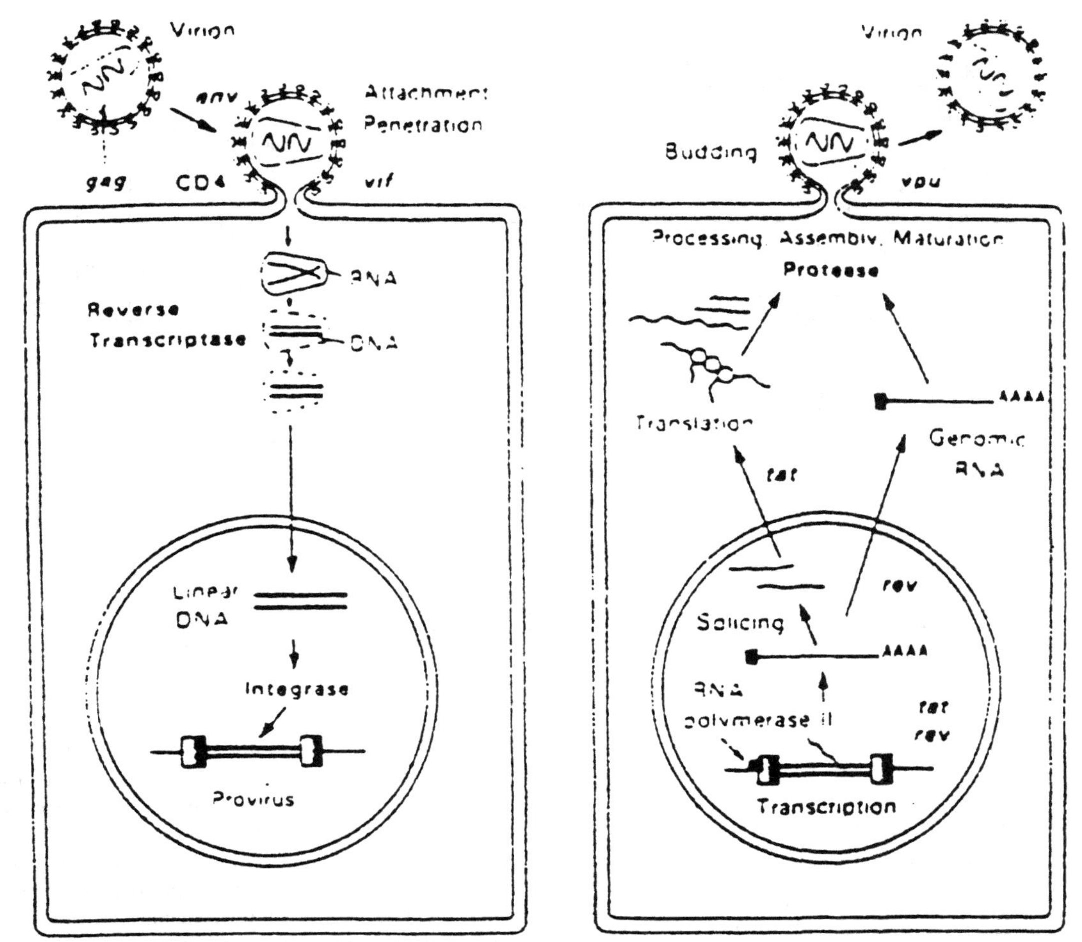

FIGURE 1. The life cycle of the human immunodeficiency virus. (Reproduced with permission from Blattner *et al.* (93).)

linked to the level of viremia as assessed by the plasma viral load [15] (Figure 3). Most untreated patients (approximately 80%) progress to AIDS in 8–12 years. In some (<10%), immune destruction does not progress for an extended period; such patients are characterized by stable, normal CD4+ counts and low plasma viral load, likely the consequence of a more enhanced immune response to HIV infection. Others (1–15%) progress much more rapidly (within 2–3 years) and are typified by a high plasma viral load and lower levels of anti-HIV antibodies. Hence, the natural history of HIV infection is heterogeneous [10]. Ultimately, though, HIV infection carries a 100% mortality rate.

ANTIRETROVIRAL THERAPY

The course of the disease has been altered substantially by the advent of highly active combination antiretroviral therapy (usually with three or more agents) which has been able to reduce plasma viral loads in infected individuals to undetectable levels [16]. Such potent antiviral effects have been associated with increases in CD4+ T-lymphocyte counts, immune reconstitution and reduction in the incidence of AIDS-

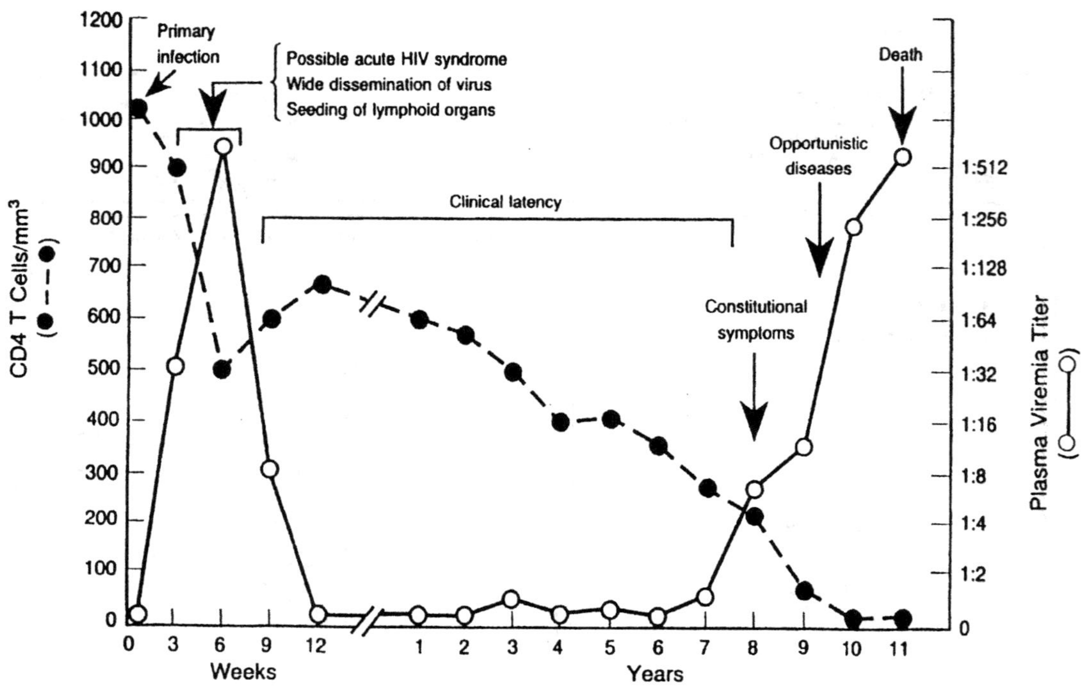

FIGURE 2. The natural history of HIV infection. During the early period of infection, there is widespread dissemination of virus and a sharp decline in the number of CD4+ cells in peripheral blood. An immune response to HIV ensues, with a decrease in detectable viremia followed by prolonged clinical latency. The CD4+ count continues to decrease during subsequent years, until it reaches a critical level, below which there is significant immunocompromise and a substantial risk of opportunistic infections and malignancies characteristic of AIDS. (Reproduced with permission from Pantaleo *et al.* (9).)

defining illnesses among HIV-positive persons and decreased mortality due to AIDS [2–5, 16, 17]. However, initial hope that this might herald a cure for HIV infection has not been realized [16].

The many antiretroviral drugs now available have significant adverse effects and many drug interactions, compounded by their use in combination. Critical care practitioners require an understanding of the potential effects of these agents (*vide infra*). In view of these toxicities, it is generally unwise to initiate combination antiretroviral therapy in critically ill patients. Further, many of the antiretroviral agents are difficult to administer in the critical care setting: some must be taken with food or without, they may be difficult to administer via a nasogastric tube and there are many potential interactions with other medications required in the setting of the acute illness. Thus, although the development of an AIDS-defining illness in a patient naïve to antiretroviral therapy is a clear indication for its institution, usually this should be delayed until the critical illness has resolved.

HIV replication, plasma viral load and destruction of the immune system rebound immediately following discontinuation of antiretroviral therapy [16, 17]. It is reasonable, then, to continue preexisting therapy, provided there are no adverse effects of the agents used which may result in further compromise of the patient's condition and it is possible to administer them. On the other hand, if the reason for admission to ICU is an AIDS-defining illness despite patient

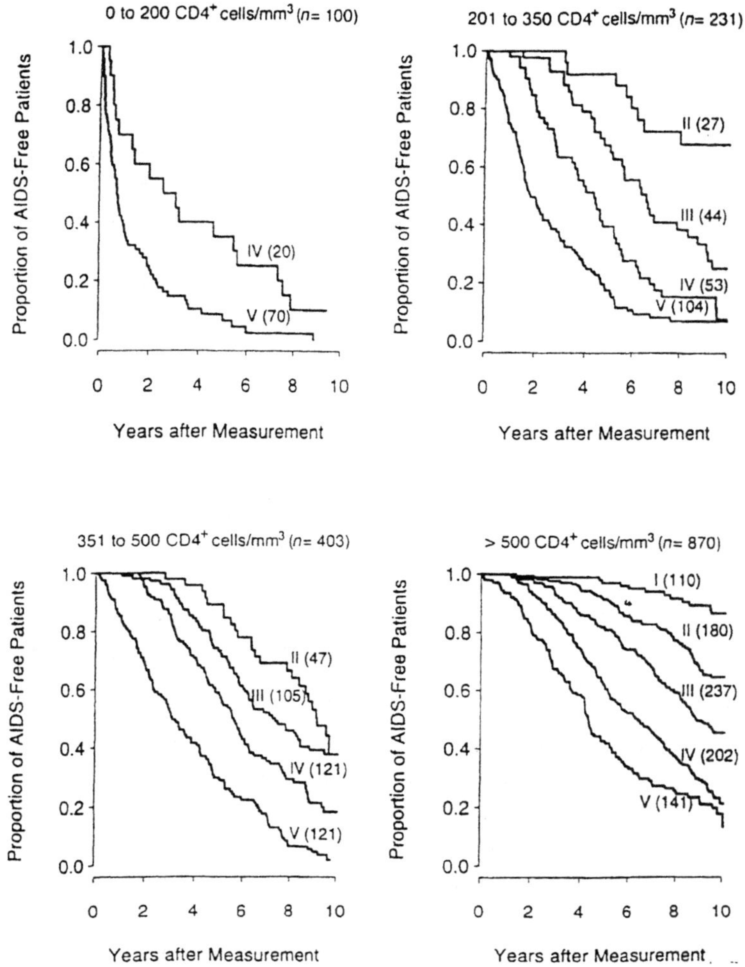

FIGURE 3. Plasma viral load and prognosis in HIV-1 infection. Kaplan-Meier curves showing AIDS-free survival by HIV-1 RNA viral load category among groups with different baseline CD4+ lymphocyte counts. The five categories of HIV-1 RNA were the following: I = 500 copies/mL; II = 501-3000 copies/mL; III = 3001-10000 copies/mL; IV = 10001-30000 copies/mL; V = > 30000 copies/mL. (Reproduced with permission from Mellors *et al.* (15).)

adherence for at least several weeks to the regimen prescribed, it is likely the regimen is ineffective and its continuation will not be beneficial. In any case, whenever antiretroviral therapy is discontinued, *it is imperative that all agents be stopped*. Even temporary interruption of one of the antiretroviral agents in a multi-drug regimen risks induction of viral resistance and can seriously compromise future antiretroviral management [16]. Consultation with a physician who specializes in HIV care and is familiar with antiretroviral agents is recommended.

SURROGATE MARKERS IN HIV INFECTION

A number of laboratory tests correlate with HIV disease prognosis and are called *surrogate markers* of disease progression. Of these, the most important for modern management of the HIV-positive patient are the plasma viral load and the CD4+ T-lymphocyte count [16]. The prognostic value of the former has been demonstrated [15] (Figure 3): since it provides evidence of the level of viral replication, its use primarily is related to monitoring virologic response to antiretroviral therapy [16].

HIV plasma viral load is a measure of circulating viral RNA by polymerase chain reaction (PCR). A low level of circulating HIV RNA implies a lower level of viral reproduction in lymphoid tissue and correspondingly less aggressive immune destruction. Thus, a low HIV plasma viral load portends slower progression of HIV disease and a better prognosis. The median survival of untreated individuals with a plasma viral load less than 5000 copies per ml is 10 years. On the other hand, a high viral load indicates unchecked HIV replication and aggressive destruction of the immune system. HIV-positive individuals with high viral loads have a poorer prognosis; untreated patients with a plasma viral load in excess of 34,000 copies per ml have a median survival of three years [15]. These observations have been confirmed in clinical trials of antiretroviral therapy, which have also shown that plasma viral load is predictive of survival independent of the CD4+ T-lymphocyte count [16].

The primary goal of highly active antiretroviral therapy is to reduce viral replication (as reflected by the plasma viral load) to the lowest level possible, thereby delaying immune system deterioration. By so doing, a second goal of therapy can also be achieved, namely the limitation of emerging viral resistance to antiretroviral agents, since suppression of viral replication limits the opportunity for resistant mutations to occur.

Hence, in the ideal situation, plasma viral load is reduced to levels reported as "undetectable". This does not mean, however, that viral replication, disease activity and thus immune destruction are completely suppressed: viral RNA is simply no longer measurable in the plasma. Detection of circulating viral RNA is dependent on the sensitivity of the assay used and the lowest identifiable level of viral RNA in plasma [18, 19]. More importantly, viral replication may continue in "sequestered sites" within the lymphoid system, even in the complete absence of plasma viral RNA. Indeed, immunologic benefits of antiretroviral agents may reflect more the result of inhibition of viral activity and thus reduced suppression of various mechanisms of nonvirologic immune destruction than their reduction of HIV burden *per se* [17]. Although useful as a tool for monitoring response to antiviral treatment of HIV infection, the plasma viral load therefore has a number of limitations and has no prognostic or diagnostic utility in the ICU setting.

While the HIV plasma viral load is indicative of the level of viral activity and rapidity of destruction of the immune system, the more traditional surrogate marker, the CD4+ T-lymphocyte count, provides evidence of the degree of immunosuppression resulting from HIV infection. Hence, a low number of CD4+ cells corresponds to susceptibility of the HIV-infected individual to opportunistic infections and neoplasms that occur once HIV-induced immune destruction has progressed to its final stage (AIDS) [20]. The CD4+ T-lymphocyte count has been demonstrated to be a useful prognostic marker and therapeutic endpoint in multiple studies [16]. It also serves as an important criterion for staging of HIV infection, for recommendations regarding initiation and goals of therapy, and for institution of prophylaxis against opportunistic infections in HIV disease [1, 16].

The CD4+ count can be measured in traditional units (number of CD4+ cells per microliter) or in metric units (number of CD4+ cells $\times 10^9$ per liter). Thus, for instance, a CD4+ count of 500/μl in traditional units is equal to 0.5×10^9/l in metric units. By convention, however, traditional units have become the standard used. The normal CD4+ count is 400–1400 cells/μl. HIV-positive individuals are at risk of AIDS-related complications at a CD4+ count less than 250 cells/μl and CD4+ count less than 200 cells/μl is now considered consistent with a diagnosis of AIDS in the revised CDC classification (1993) [13]. It is important to consider not just the absolute number of CD4+ cells, but also their number in relation to the total circulating pool of T-lymphocytes. This is usually reported as a fraction or percentage of the total lymphocyte count. Generally, a CD4+ fraction less than 15% suggests significant immunosuppression and may reflect susceptibility to AIDS-defining opportunistic infections, even at an absolute CD4+ count which otherwise would not be considered indicative of such immune dysfunction.

Despite the widespread acceptance of the CD4+ count as a guide to decision making in HIV care and a reflector of immune dysfunction, there are several problems with its use in the acute setting. First, there is considerable diurnal variability in CD4+ lymphocyte counts, even in non-HIV-infected persons: CD4+ counts show circadian variation with counts being lowest in the morning and highest in the evening. This effect is less pronounced in HIV-infected individuals than in healthy ones. While consistent measurement of CD4+ count at a fixed point in the day can limit this variability in the ambulatory setting [16], loss of normal circadian rhythm in the critically ill make the effect of such fluctuations throughout the day impossible to determine in the individual patient.

The CD4+ count can also vary from day to day, so that short-term fluctuations in CD4+ count of up to 30% may occur which are not attributable to a change in disease status [20]. Therefore, it is recommended that at least two measurements be made of CD4+ count on different days in order to better assess the actual state of immune function [16]. Given the daily perturbations in the critically ill population in organ system function, including fluctuations in immune system function, it is not clear that repeated measurements of CD4+ count in a critically ill patient will enhance its predictability of the degree of immunosuppression.

Finally, the CD4+ count can vary with immune stimulation, such as with intercurrent illness. For example, in a non-HIV-infected individual, severe viral infection can cause marked depression of CD4+ count, even to levels indicative of profound immunosuppression in an HIV-infected patient. Yet such depression of CD4+ cell number does not correlate with enhanced susceptibility to the opportunistic infections characteristic of AIDS. Similarly, fluctuations of CD4+ count in an acutely ill HIV-positive individual may also occur regardless of cause and may not be reflective of actual level of immune dysfunction [20].

For these reasons, a CD4+ count (even if repeated) should not be regarded as a reliable indicator of immunosuppression in the critically ill patient. In other words, predicting the likelihood of HIV-related illness in a critically ill patient (regardless of HIV status) on the basis of a low CD4+ T-lymphocyte count (absolute and/or relative) is not dependable. In contrast, a high or normal CD4+ count (i.e., >250 cells/μl) and CD4+ fraction greater than 15% suggest that HIV-related illness is unlikely. Regardless, the most reliable reflector of immune function is a CD4+ count a short time prior to the onset of the presenting illness and such information should be sought. Furthermore, diagnostic and therapeutic decisions should not be driven by the CD4+ count alone. Hence, we feel there is only a limited rôle for CD4+ counts in the critical care setting.

It should be noted that the description of HIV plasma viral load as a marker of viral activity and the CD4+ T-lymphocyte count as a marker of degree of immunosuppression is clearly an oversimplification. The virology and immunopathology of HIV infection is increasingly recognized as complex and is still incompletely understood [10, 17]. There are qualitative defects in lymphocyte function and other aspects of immune function in HIV disease not reflected by the absolute or relative CD4+ T-lymphocyte count. Furthermore, the level of plasma HIV RNA does not precisely reflect the immunopathologic effects of HIV infection. The immunologic responses to antiretroviral therapy in HIV infection demonstrate the complex interactions between viral activity and immune changes in HIV disease [17]. For example, disease activity and immune dysfunction can persist even in the presence of apparent suppression of viral replication; increases in CD4+ counts may not correspond to repair of immune dysfunction and initial increases in CD4+ levels may be associated with exacerbation or development of opportunistic infections. Immunologic and clinical benefits have been observed using antiretroviral regimens which are no longer able to suppress plasma viral load. Thus, the plasma viral load and CD4+ count should preferably be considered as surrogate markers and are imperfect indicators of disease activity and progression.

Spectrum of HIV-Related Disease in the ICU

There are relatively few conditions which lead to ICU admission among HIV seropositive persons. Causes of ICU admission unrelated to HIV infection are similar to those among non-HIV-infected individuals of similar age and demographics. Furthermore, since HIV infection is asymptomatic early in its course when there is relatively normal immune function, patients with unsuspected HIV infection may develop non-HIV-related illness which may require admission to ICU. Given the changing demographics of HIV infection, admission of HIV-positive patients with non-HIV-related critical illness typical of HIV-negative persons with similar risk factors for HIV infection (such as endocarditis, pneumonia and soft tissue infections in injection drug users) is likely to become more common. In addition, as antiretroviral therapies improve and longevity and preservation of immune function increase, it should be anticipated that more HIV-positive patients will be admitted to ICU with illnesses associated with disease found in non-HIV-infected persons. Patients with critical illness not connected to underlying HIV infection have a prognosis similar to individuals without HIV infection who have the same illness and such patients usually respond similarly to management for their condition [20].

It is not clear that the spectrum of HIV-related critical illness has changed from that found in previous years [20]. Recent studies, for example, suggest that *Pneumocystis carinii* pneumonia (PCP) is less prevalent, constituting only 16–27% of admissions [6, 21]. However, these studies were based on data collected prior to 1993 and the modern era of antiretroviral therapy and/or included patients either with low acuity illness (e.g., uncomplicated pneumothorax) or non-AIDS complications (e.g., ischemic heart disease, drug overdose or trauma). Nevertheless, the study by Casalino *et al.* from an Infectious Diseases ICU in a French hospital is instructive [21]. Not surprisingly, 33.5% of admissions to the ICU in the period studied (1990–1992) were HIV-related. Of the 354 patients evaluated, 49% were admitted with respiratory failure (45% of whom were admitted because of PCP; other causes of respiratory failure included bacterial pneumonia (47%), tuberculosis, Kaposi's sarcoma and toxoplasmic pneumonia); 27% of patients had neurologic complications (predominantly toxoplasmic encephalitis (62%), but also meningitis (17%) and other cerebral lesions); 10% had severe sepsis (primarily related to bacteremia or bacterial pneumonia); 5% were admitted with cardiac dysfunction due to opportunistic infection and complications, such as pericarditis, or HIV-related dilated cardiomyopathy, and 9% were admitted for "miscellaneous" reasons, most not directly related to HIV disease, such as drug overdoses and toxic drug reactions. Although this implies a broad spectrum of HIV-related disease in the ICU, the specialization of the ICU in this study as a referral center for critically ill patients with infectious diseases may not be representative of more general systems or even medical ICUs.

In contrast, most studies have shown that PCP is the predominant cause of HIV-related acute respiratory failure (ARF), accounting for 63–93% of admission to the ICU among HIV seropositive patients [6], although this is based again on observations prior to the modern era of HIV treatment. Recent data suggest that the spectrum of AIDS defining illnesses in HIV seropositive patients treated with highly active antiretroviral therapy has not changed and that PCP remains the most common AIDS defining illness in this group (Figure 4) [22]. Finally, combination antiretroviral therapy is associated with reconstitution of immune function [17], with increasingly common recommendations that PCP prophylaxis can be stopped in individuals who have improved CD4+ counts [23]. If indeed immune reconstitution is not sufficient to provide protection against AIDS complications and/or such immune recovery is not sustained, even those patients on highly active antiretroviral therapy may be at risk for development of opportunistic infections. Hence, PCP is likely to remain a common AIDS-related complication precipitating admission to the ICU.

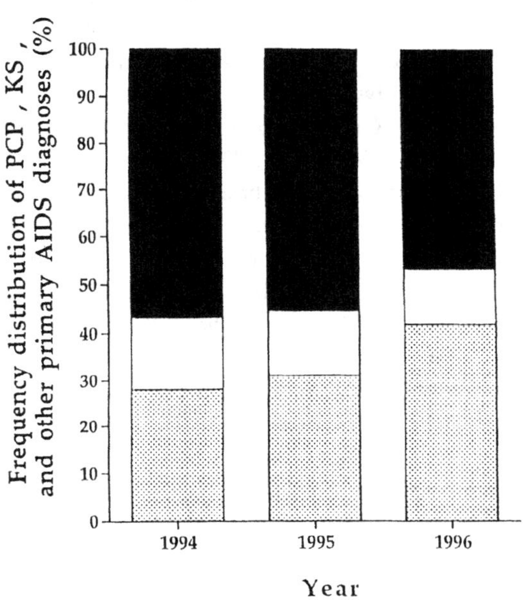

FIGURE 4. Proportion of AIDS index diseases attributed to *Pneumocystis carinii* pneumonia (PCP; gray bar), Kaposi's sarcoma (KS; white bar) and other AIDS-defining illnesses (black bar) among participants in a drug treatment program ever prescribed antiretroviral therapy between January 1, 1994 and December 31, 1996. There was no significant difference in the proportion of patients who developed AIDS due to PCP ($p = 0.048$ for 1994 versus 1996), Kaposi's sarcoma ($p = 0.442$ for 1994 versus 1996) or Other AIDS-defining illness ($p = 0.190$ for 1994 versus 1996). (Reproduced with permission from Forrest *et al.* (22).)

While HIV infection is a multisystem disease and the manifestations of HIV-related immune dysfunction involve multiple organ systems, complications of HIV infection relevant to the intensivist will be discussed according to organ system.

Respiratory Disease

APPROACH

While PCP remains the most frequent cause of acute respiratory failure in HIV seropositive individuals, there is a broad differential diagnosis which should be considered. The differential diagnosis includes bacterial pneumonia (e.g., community acquired pneumonia, atypical pneumonia and mycobacterial infection), fungi, viruses, parasites (such as *Toxoplasma*), and non-infectious etiologies, such as lymphocytic interstitial pneumonitis and neoplastic diseases (Table 1). Following hospital admission, the diagnosis of nosocomial pneumonia should be considered. Occasionally multiple etiologies can coexist (e.g., pneumococcal infection complicating PCP).

There are no specific clinical clues which can differentiate these various causes of respiratory failure. There is sufficient overlap of clinical, radiological and laboratory findings that it is difficult to make a precise diagnosis without definitive evidence of a specific etiology. However, there are several findings which may be helpful. For example, a CD4+ count, preferably obtained

TABLE 1. Differential diagnosis of pulmonary complications of HIV disease

- Infections
  - Bacteria
    - *Streptococcus pneumoniae*
    - *Hemophilus influenzae*
    - *Staphylococcus aureus*
    - *Moraxella catarrhalis*
    - *Mycobacterium tuberculosis*
    - *Mycobacterium avium* complex
    - Other nontuberculous mycobacteria
    - *Rhodococcus equi*
    - *Nocardia asteroides*
  - Fungi
    - *Pneumocystis carinii*
    - *Cryptococcus neoformans*
    - *Histoplasma capsulatum*
    - *Aspergillus fumigatus*
    - *Blastomyces dermatitidis*
  - Protozoa
    - *Strongyloides stercoralis*
    - *Toxoplasma gondii*
  - Viruses
    - Cytomegalovirus
    - Herpes simplex
    - Varicella-zoster
    - Adenovirus
    - Other respiratory viruses
- Noninfectious
  - Malignancies
    - Kaposi's sarcoma
    - Non-Hodgkin's lymphoma
    - Primary lung carcinoma
  - Other pulmonary syndromes
    - Lymphocytic interstitial pneumonitis
    - Nonspecific interstitial pneumonitis
    - Bronchiolitis obliterans and organizing pneumonia
    - Primary pulmonary hypertension

Adapted with permission from [63].

shortly before the presenting illness (*vide supra*), can be of value [24]. If the recent CD4+ T-lymphocyte count is >250 cell/μl, an AIDS-defining illness such as PCP is unlikely. A low CD4+ count is not helpful in ruling out any etiology.

Similarly, the level of lactate dehydrogenase (LDH) can assist in differential diagnosis [24, 25]. The serum LDH level is characteristically elevated in an HIV-positive patient with PCP; the degree of increase tends to correlate with the severity of disease and radiographic change, and changes in the LDH level tend to parallel the course of PCP. Hence, a normal LDH level makes PCP an unlikely diagnosis. However, an elevated LDH level is not diagnostic, because serum LDH can be raised by other causes of respiratory illness and non-respiratory disease, such as pulmonary embolism, lymphoma, liver disease or dysfunction (a common finding in the critically ill population), megaloblastic anemia, hemolysis (as may occur, for example, in HIV-positive patients receiving dapsone) or with various HIV therapies (e.g., antiretroviral medications) [24, 25]. Extreme elevations in LDH are less likely to be due to PCP and more likely to indicate another diagnosis such as disseminated histoplasmosis, disseminated toxoplasmosis, lymphoma, or major hemolysis.

A chest X-ray can provide useful diagnostic clues to etiology [24]. Often at the time of ICU admission, the chest X-ray shows non-specific diffuse pulmonary infiltrate consistent with adult respiratory distress syndrome (ARDS). However, when reviewed retrospectively, the evolution of chest X-ray findings through the course of presenting illness prior to development of respiratory failure can aid in differential diagnosis (see Table 2). The extent of chest radiographic involvement more clearly distinguishes PCP from other causes of pulmonary infiltrate than does the LDH level [25]. Patients who have community acquired bacterial pneumonia will usually have typical signs of asymmetrical, lobar or nonlobar consolidation. Patients who have atypical pneumonia usually have fairly extensive, more symmetric lung involvement that may be out of proportion to clinical signs and symptoms.

It should be emphasized that no finding is sufficiently specific to establish a diagnosis. Hence, definitive determination of the etiology of respiratory failure in the HIV seropositive patient is dependent on the recovery of the causative pathogen and/or histopathologic confirmation [24]. This is especially important when the serostatus of the patient is unknown,

TABLE 2. Major radiologic differential diagnosis of pulmonary involvement in the HIV-positive patient

Chest radiograph appearance	Differential diagnosis
Normal chest X-ray	PCP, CMV, MAC
Diffuse or localized interstitial pattern	PCP, TB, CMV
Diffuse alveolar pattern	PCP, cardiogenic pulmonary edema
Miliary pattern	TB, histoplasmosis
Consolidation	Bacteria, TB, PCP, KS
Nodular opacification	PCP, bacteria, KS, cryptococcosis
Upper lung field predominance	PCP, TB
Cavitary lesions	TB, aspergillosis, PCP, bacteria
Pleural effusion	KS, bacteria, mycobacteria
Pneumothorax	PCP

Abbreviations: PCP = *Pneumocystis carinii* pneumonia; CMV = cytomegalovirus; MAC = *Mycobacterium avium* complex; TB = *Mycobacterium tuberculososis*; KS = Kaposi's sarcoma.
Reproduced with permission from [20].

but also when an HIV-positive patient is not known to have AIDS, because of the serious prognostic and therapeutic implications of a diagnosis of AIDS. Thus, diagnostic investigation should include microbiologic evaluation of tracheobronchial secretions for common bacterial pathogens and mycobacteria and of bronchoscopically obtained specimens (bronchoaveolar lavage and bronchoscopic brush specimens) for bacteria (including *Legionella* and mycobacteria), fungi, *Pneumocystis*, viruses and cytology [24, 26]. Examination for *Pneumocystis* should be requested specifically, as many laboratories do not screen bronchoscopic specimens for this organism routinely. Induction of sputum can increase the sensitivity of noninvasive evaluation for *Pneumocystis* to as high as 94% [27], but its success is highly dependent on the experience of the personnel and laboratory.

Where feasible and with appropriate precautions, bronchoscopy is the preferred diagnostic approach [24, 26] and should certainly be performed if PCP is possible and routine and/or induced sputum examination is negative [27]. Ideally, bronchoscopy should be undertaken prior to institution of empiric therapy. However, as with many other critical infectious illnesses, delay in institution of treatment in favor of a diagnostic procedure is usually not warranted. Nevertheless, even several days of empiric therapy has substantial influence on diagnostic yield of bronchoalveolar lavage (BAL) in HIV-positive persons [28]. Bronchoscopy thus should be performed as soon as possible after institution of treatment, unless a definitive diagnosis is established by other means [26]. Specimens are obtained most easily from the middle lobe, but sampling from the upper lobe has higher yield in patients receiving anti-*Pneumocystis* prophylaxis with aerosolized pentamidine [29].

The sensitivity of BAL for *P. carinii* and other treatable pathogens in the HIV-infected patient is 85–95% [24, 26]; sensitivity can be enhanced by concentrating the specimens [24]. If a definitive etiology is not established by this means, open-lung biopsy may be considered, taking into account the inherent risks and benefits of doing so in the individual case. In our experience, open lung biopsy is rarely necessary. Although transbronchial biopsy can increase the sensitivity of bronchoscopic examination, the complications of the procedure generally render it too risky in the critically ill patient with respiratory failure, particularly if the patient is supported by positive pressure ventilation [20, 26]. Finally, detection of alveolitis (presence of inflammatory cells) and number of CD4+ cells on BAL is predictive of long-term survival in the HIV-seropositive patient, regardless of underlying pulmonary disease [30].

PNEUMOCYSTIS CARINII PNEUMONIA

Based on molecular genetic data, *Pneumocystis carinii* is classified as a fungus [31]. Since *Pneumocystis* cannot be grown in the laboratory, its microbiology is not well understood and *in vitro* antimicrobial sensitivity is thus not possible [32]. The organism is ubiquitous and most healthy children have been infected by *Pneumocystis* at an early age. The organism is distributed worldwide and infects multiple mammalian species, although there are geographic variations in its prevalence and there seems to be no transmission of infection between species; it is not clear whether there is an environmental reservoir [32]. Nevertheless, such differences in prevalence of the microbes are not sufficient to account for differences in the frequency of infection in immunocompromised hosts: this seems more related to the prevalence of more virulent infections (such as tuberculosis), differences in public health and medical system infrastructure, and lack of access to sophisticated medical care [33].

Animal studies suggest that *Pneumocystis* is transmissible by the airborne route, but clearly the organism poses a risk of clinically significant infection only among immunocompromised hosts with impairment of cellular immunity [33]. Indeed, it is likely that most people are exposed frequently throughout their lives; it is thought that *Pneumocystis* may become part of the host's residential microbial flora or infection may be transient but repetitive. It has been theorized that clinical PCP disease in an immunocompromised host results from reactivation of latent infection, but primary or recurrent infection has been documented as an etiology of PCP in HIV-infected persons and may be much more important than earlier recognized [31, 32, 34, 35]. Although there have been no recommendations to date to isolate patients with PCP, given the risk of transmission and the potential role of primary or recurrent infection in producing clinically significant disease, it may be prudent to consider isolation of patients with PCP from other individuals with compromised cellular immunity [31, 34, 35]. In the setting of HIV infection, PCP occurs as a complication of late-stage HIV disease once the CD4+ count has declined below 200 cells/μl.

The site of primary infection with *Pneumocystis* is the lung, where the organism attaches to alveolar type I cells and maintains an extracellular existence within the alveoli. With immunocompromise, *Pneumocystis* organisms proliferate and fill alveolar spaces forming a foamy alveolar exudate. Damage to type I alveolar cells occurs with increased alveolocapillary permeability and hyaline membrane formation with interstitial fibrosis and edema. Changes in the surfactant system occur with a fall in surfactant phospholipids and a rise in surfactant protein; these alterations likely contribute significantly to the alterations in respiratory function in PCP [32, 33].

The host inflammatory response is manifested by proliferation of type II alveolar cells and a scanty mononuclear infiltrate. Comparative histologic data suggest there may be a higher burden of microbes but less tissue damage in HIV-related pneumocystosis than in PCP occurring in non-HIV-infected hosts [33]. Nevertheless, in the setting of HIV infection, the host response seems more complex and potentially harmful and parenchymal injury actually may worsen with therapy [36]. Inflammation, interstitial edema and fibrosis, type II pneumocyte proliferation and cellular infiltration of the alveolar wall are more abundant than in other HIV-related pulmonary diseases [37].

Typically, PCP has an insidious onset in the HIV-infected host with a two- to three-week prodrome consisting of fever, dyspnea and cough (usually described as nonproductive), in contrast to a more fulminant presentation in other immunocompromised individuals [32]. Chills, weight loss, sputum production, chest pain and hemoptysis have also been described and 6–7% of patients report no symptoms. Adventitious breath sounds are heard in only 30–46%. Clinical presentation does not seem to be altered by type of prophylaxis (if any) used prior to development of PCP [32]. With the use of aerosol pentamidine in the late 1980s and early 1990s, extrapulmonary infection with *Pneumocystis* became increasingly recognized. Virtually any organ can be affected, most frequently lymphatic tissue (including spleen), bone marrow, liver, pancreas and gastrointestinal tract, adrenal, thyroid, parathyroid and pituitary glands, genitourinary system, heart, and the eyes and ears [32].

Routine laboratory testing of PCP is nonspecific; the value of the LDH level is discussed above. The hallmark of PCP in a predisposed individual is hypoxemia at rest or with exercise out of proportion to the changes found on clinical examination and on chest radiograph. Arterial hypoxemia may not be apparent at rest, but only with exercise, and continuous pulse oximetry has been shown to be useful in this regard [32]. Arterial blood gas measurements may also show respiratory alkalosis; a decline in pH with an inadequate respiratory compensation (manifest by a rising $PaCO_2$ on serial blood gas measurements) suggests respiratory fatigue and incipient respiratory failure.

There are a variety of chest radiograph findings with PCP [32] (Table 2). Indeed, it is prudent to consider PCP with virtually *any* abnormal radiographic findings in the correct clinical setting, but a normal chest X-ray does not rule out PCP. In early stages in non-critically ill patients, normal chest radiographs are found in up to one third of cases. In approximately 80% of established cases, a "classic" appearance is found of ground-glass perihilar interstitial infiltrates progressing over time to involve all lung fields diffusely, often with an alveolar pattern – consistent with findings typical of ARDS. Pleural disease, vascular engorgement, and asymmetric lobar consolidation are unusual. The use of aerosolized pentamidine as prophylaxis has been associated with an increased incidence of upper lobe infiltrates. Cystic changes can also be seen and are usually apical and subpleural. They are more common in patients previously treated prophylactically with aerosolized pentamidine and are most readily detected on computerized tomographic (CT) scanning of the chest. Pulmonary cystic changes also predispose to the development of pneumothoraces, seen in up to 9% of patients. Pneumothorax has been associated with a poor prognosis and tension pneumothorax with cardiopulmonary arrest has been reported. Rarely, transudative or exudative pleural effusions may be found; these resolve spontaneously with treatment of underlying PCP [32, 38].

Nuclear medicine gallium-67 lung scans may also be a useful adjunctive diagnostic modality with a sensitivity of 94–100% but specificity of only 47–74% [32]. However, they are expensive, time-consuming, may not be readily available, and may require movement and transfer of the patient with attendant risks. Because of the lack of diagnostic specificity, this test has limited utility in the critically ill population.

Acute respiratory failure occurs in 5–30% of cases of AIDS-related PCP [39]. Physiologically, acute respiratory failure complicating PCP is similar to that of ARDS with tachypnea, ventilation-perfusion imbalance, hypoxemia, hyperventilation with low pCO_2, and decreased pulmonary compliance. In association, there is a hemodynamic profile typical of a systemic inflammatory response with high cardiac output and distributive shock [32]. End-organ failure and even death may result from direct involvement by *Pneumocystis* of multiple extrapulmonary organs [32, 40].

Particularly in the critically ill patient, empirical therapy for PCP is warranted pending definitive diagnostic testing. Antimicrobial management options are outlined in Table 3. Primary antimicrobial agents include trimethoprim-sulfamethoxazole (TMP-SMX) and pentamidine isethionate. Both are equally effective [32, 41], but each has distinct advantages, disadvantages and toxicities. Changes in therapy necessitated by drug toxicity are not associated with adverse outcomes, whereas the need for a change in treatment because of clinical failure of one therapeutic agent is associated with lower survival rate [41].

TMP-SMX provides broad-spectrum coverage against a variety of Gram-positive and Gram-negative organisms in addition to PCP. Initially, TMP-SMX should be given intravenously in the critically ill patient, but it is well-absorbed orally, allowing step-down to enteral therapy. However, TMP-SMX is poorly tolerated in HIV-infected patients: adverse reactions are reported in 44–100%, with severe toxicity requiring discontinuation in up to 57% [32]. The most common adverse effects are fever, rash (which may progress to Stevens–Johnson syndrome),

TABLE 3. Antimicrobial therapy of common infections in AIDS patients

Infection	Drug of choice	Dose/Route	Usual duration	Alternative therapy
Protozoa				
Toxoplasmosis (*Toxoplasma gondii*)	Pyrimethamine[1]	200 mg loading dose, then 75–100 mg PO once daily	4–6 wks[2]	Pyrimethamine *plus* (clindamycin 600–900 mg IV q6h until marked clinical improvement, then 450 m PO q6h), *or* (clarithromycin) 1000 mg PO bid), *or* (azithromycin 1200 mg PO once daily)
	Plus Sulfadiazine	1–1.5 gm PO q6h	4–6 wks	
	Maintenance therapy: Pyrimethamine[1]	25–50 mg PO once daily	Indefinite	Pyrimethamine[1] *plus* clindamycin 300–450 mg PO qid (at least 1200 mg daily)
	plus Sulfadiazine	500–1000 mg PO qid	Indefinite	
Cryptosporidiosis (*Cryptosporidium parvum*)	No proven effective therapy			Reports of resolution with antiretroviral therapy induced immune reconstitution. Azithromycin 600 mg PO daily *plus* paromomycin 1 gm PO bid for 4 weeks, then paromomycin alone 1 gm bid for 8 weeks.
Microsporidiosis (*Encephalitozoon intestinalis*, *Enterocytozoon bieneusi*)	Albendazole	400 mg PO bid	3 wks	Efficacy of albendazole demonstrated for *E. intestinalis* Reports of resolution with antiretroviral therapy induced immune reconstitution.
Giardiasis (*Giaria lamblia*)	Metronidazole	250 mg PO tid	5 d	(Albendazole 400 mg PO daily for 5 days) *or* (furazolidone 100 mg qid for 7–10 days), *or* (Tinidazole 2 grams once [not marketed in North America])
Amebiasis (symptomatic) (*Entamoeba histolytica*)	Metronidazole[3]	750 mg PO/IV tid	10 d	(Tinidazole 1 gm bid for 3 days [800 mg tid for 5 days for liver abscess] [not marketed in North America]), *or* (dehydroemetine[4] 1–1.5 mg/kg/d IM [maximum 90 mg/d] for up to 5 d)

TABLE 3 (Continued)

Infection	Drug of choice	Dose/Route	Usual duration	Alternative therapy
	followed by Iodoquinol	650 mg PO tid	20 d	An alternate luminal agent (e.g., diloxanide furoate 500 mg tid × 10 d, or paromomycin 500 mg qid × 7 d)
Isosporiasis (*Isospora belli*)	Trimethroprim, (TMP); sulfamethoxazole (SMX)	TMP 160 mg, SMX 800 mg (1 DS tablet) PO/IV qid	10 d[5]	Pyrimethamine 50–75 mg PO daily plus folinic acid 5–10 mg PO daily × 4 weeks
	Maintenance therapy Trimethoprim; sulfamethoxazole	1 DS tablet 3 ×/wk	Indefinite	Pyrimethamine 25 mg PO daily *plus* folinic acid 5 mg PO daily
Pneumocystosis (*P. carinii*)	*Intravenous therapy* Trimethoprim-sulfamethoxazole (TMP-SMX)	Based on TMP component 15–20 mg/kg/d IV, divided q6h	21 d	(Clindamycin 600 mg IV q6h *plus* primaquine 15–30 mg [base] PO daily) *or* (Pentamidine 4 mg kg/day IV)
	Oral therapy Trimethoprim	200 mg PO qid (or 5 mg/kg tid)	21 d	(Trimethoprim-sulfamethoxazole 2 DS tablets tid or qid), *or* (clindamycin 450 mg PO tid plus primaquine 15 mg [base] PO daily) *or* (atovaquone 750 mg PO tid)
	plus			
	dapsone	100 mg PO daily	21 d	
Fungi				
Candidiasis				
Oropharyngeal	Fluconazole	100 mg PO daily	7–14 d[6]	Itraconazole 100–200 mg/d[7], or Ketoconazole 200 mg/d or Clotrimazole 10 mg troche [dissolve in mouth 5 times/day]
Esophageal	Fluconazole	400 mg loading dose then 200 mg, PO daily	3 wks[6]	Ketoconazole 200–400 mg daily PO, *or* Itraconazole 200 mg daily PO[7], *or* Amphotericin B 0.3–0.6 mg/kg IV daily for 7–14 d
Fluconazole-refractory mucosal candidiasis (oral, esophageal	Itraconazole oral solution[7]	100 mg, PO bid (swish and swallow)	2 wks[6]	Higher dose fluconazole (200–400 mg/day), or Amphotericin B oral suspension 100 mg qid (swallow and swallow), or Amphotericin B 0.3–0.6 mg/kg/day IV for 1–2 weeks

TABLE 3 (Continued)

Infection	Drug of choice	Dose/Route	Usual duration	Alternative therapy
Candidemia	Amphotericin B	0.5–1.0 mg/kg, Daily, IV	Until total dose 0.5–1.0 g (2–3 wks)	Lipid formulation of amphotericin B (e.g. liposomal amphotericin B 3–5 mg/kg/day)
	Or Fluconazole (*C. glabrata* less susceptible, *C. kruseii* resistant)	400–800 mg daily IV (PO after 7 days)	14 days after last positive blood culture	
Focal invasive or disseminated	Amphotericin B	0.5–1.0 mg/kg, Daily, IV	Until total dose ≥ 1–2 g and clinical resolution	Fluconazole 400–800 mg PO/IV *or* lipid formulation of Amphotericin B (e.g. liposomal amphotericin B, 3–5 mg/kg/day)[8]
	Plus/minus 5-Flucytosine[9]	25 mg/kg q6h, PO/IV		
Cryptococcal meningitis (*Cryptococcus neoformans*)	Amphotericin B	0.7 mg kg, Daily, IV	2–3 wks, and clinical response[10]	Lipid formulation of amphotericin B
	Plus/minus 5-Flucytosine	25 mg/kg q6h, PO/IV		
	Then Fluconazole	400 mg, Daily, PO/IV	8 wks	Itraconazole 200 mg bid PO
	Maintenance therapy: Fluconazole	200 mg Daily, PO	Indefinite	Itraconazole 200 mg bid[11]. *or* Amphotericin B 1 mg kg IV, once *or* twice weekly indefinitely
Histoplasmosis (*Histoplasma capsulatum*)	Amphotericin B[12]	0.5–1.0 mg/kg, Daily, IV	Until total dose 1–2 g	Itraconazole 200 mg bid PO (after loading dose of 300 mg bid for 3 days) for 12 weeks for mild to moderate disease
	Maintenance therapy: Itraconazole[7,13]	200 mg, Daily, PO	Indefinite	Fluconazole 400 mg/day (less effective) *or* Amphotericin B 1 mg/kg 1–2 times/week

TABLE 3 (Continued)

Infection	Drug of choice	Dose/Route	Usual duration	Alternative therapy
Coccidioidomycosis: (*Coccidioides immitis*)				
Extrameningeal	Fluconazole	400–800 mg PO/IV, daily	Indefinite	Itraconazole 200 mg bid *or* ketoconazole 400 mg bid[7] *or* amphotericin B 0.5–1.0 mg/kg/day IV until a total dose of 1.0–2.0 mg/kg
Meningitis	Fluconazole	400–800 mg, PO/IV daily	9–12 months	Amphotericin B 0.5–1.0 mg/kg/day IV until total dose 1–2 g IV*plus* intrathecal[14] amphotericin 0.1–0.3 mg 3 times per week long term, or itraconazole 200 mg bid[7], *or* ketoconazole 800–1200 mg/day[7]
	Maintenance therapy: Fluconazole	400 mg, PO daily	Indefinite	Itraconazole 200 mg bid, *or* ketoconazole 400 mg bid[7], *or* (if only extrameningeal disease, then Amphotericin B 1 mg/kg weekly)
Viruses				
Herpes simplex				
Mucocutaneous	Acyclovir	400 mg PO 3–5 times daily	10 d[15]	Famciclovir 500 mg PO bid (*or* 250 mg tid) for 5–10 days *or* valacyclovir 1 gm PO bid
Severe or refractory[16] mucocutaneous	Acyclovir	2.5–5 mg/kg, IV q8h (infused over 1 hr)	7–10 d[15]	Acyclovir 800 mg PO 5 times daily, *or* valacyclovir 1 gm PO bid, or famciclovir 500 mg PO bid or tid, *or* foscarnet 40–60 mg/kg IV q8h (infusion over 1 hr by infusion pump), or trifluridine (topically) in a 5% ophthalmic solution
Visceral or disseminated	Acyclovir	10 mg/kg, IV q8h (infusion over 1 hr)	10 d	Foscarnet 60 mg/kg IV q8h (infusion over 1 hr by infusion pump)
Herpes zoster				
Dermatomal	Famciclovir	500–750 mg, PO q8h	7 d	Acyclovir 800 mg PO 5 times daily or 10–12 mg/kg IV (infusion over 1 hr) q8h, *or* foscarnet 40 mg/kg IV q8h (infusion over 1 hr by infusion pump)
	Or			
	Valacyclovir	1000 mg PO tid	7 d	

TABLE 3 (Continued)

Infection	Drug of choice	Dose/Route	Usual duration	Alternative therapy
Disseminated (cutaneous or visceral) or ophthalmic	Acyclovir	10–12 mg/kg, IV q8h (infusion over 1 hr)	7–14 d	Foscarnet 40–60 mg/kg IV q8h (infusion over 1 hr by infusion pump)
CMV (cytomegalovirus)	Ganciclovir[17]	5 mg kg, IV q12h	14–21 d	Foscarnet 90–100 mg/kg IV q12h (infusion over 2 hr by pump); or cidofovir 5 mg/kg (protocol for probenecid + IV saline pre/post dose) weekly ×2 doses, then q2weeks; on intraocular ganciclovir implant + oral ganciclovir 1.5 gm tid
	Maintenance therapy[18]			
	Ganciclovir	5 mg/kg, IV daily	Indefinite	Ganciclovir 6 mg/kg IV daily (5 days/week); or foscarnet 90–120 mg IV (infusion over 2 hr by pump) once daily 5–7 days/week; or other options for CMV retinitis (ganciclovir 1–1.5 gm PO tid +/− intraocular ganciclovir implant; or cidofovir [as above])
Bacteria				
Streptococcus pneumoniae:				
Uncomplicated pneumonia	Penicillin G[19]	2 million units IV q4–6h	7–10 d	Cephalosporin (e.g. cefuroxime 0.75–1.5 g IV q8h, or ceftriaxone 1–2 gm IV q24h); *or* levofloxacin 500 mg PO/IV daily; or a macrolide (e.g. azithromycin 500 mg IV/PO daily, or erythromycin 500 mg IV q6h); *or* vancomycin
Pneumonia (decreased pneumococcus susceptibility)				
Intermediate resistance (penicillin MIC 0.12–1.2 ug/ml)	Ceftriaxone	2 gm IV daily	7–10 d	Cefotaxime; high dose penicillin G (>10 million units/days); or levofloxacin 500 mg IV/PO daily; or imipenem
High level resistance (penicillin MIC ≥2 ug/ml)	Vancomycin Or	15 mg/kg IV q12h	7–10 d	Imipenem 500 mg IV q6h; *or* cefotaxime or ceftriaxone (if cefotaxime and ceftriaxone MIC ≤2 ug/ml). For empiric

TABLE 3 (Continued)

Infection	Drug of choice	Dose/Route	Usual duration	Alternative therapy
	Levofloxacin	500 mg IV/PO daily	7–10 d	treatment of community-acquired meningitis: 3rd generation cephalosporin (cefotaxime 2 gm IV q4h or ceftriaxone 2 gm q12h) plus high dose vancomycin 15 mg/kg IV q6h
Staphylococcus aureus Pneumonia, bacteremia (uncomplicated)				
• methicillin susceptible (MSSA)	Nafcillin *or* oxacillin *or* cloxacillin[20]	2 g IV q4h	14 d	Vancomycin 15 mg kg IV q12h, or cefazolin 2 g IV q8h
• methicillin resistant (MRSA)	Vancomycin	15 mg/kg IV q12h	14 d	Teichoplanin (not available in North America) or Linezolid
Hemophilus influenzae pneumonia	Ceftriaxone	1–2 g IV q24h	10–14 d	Ampicillin 1–2 g IV q6h (if susceptible) *or* cefotaxime 1–2 g IV q6–8h *or* cefuroxime 0.75–1.5 g IV q8h or trimethoprim-sulfamethoxazole, or ciprofloxacin
Salmonella Bacteremia	Ciprofloxacin	750 mg, PO q12h	2–4 wks	Ampicillin 2 g IV q4–6h for 1–4 weeks (if susceptible), then amoxicillin 500 mg tid to complete a 2–4 week course or therapy[21], or cefotaxime *or* ceftriaxone, *or* trimethoprim-sulfamethoxazole
Listeria Meningitis	Ampicillin *plus*	200 mg/kg/d IV, divided q4h	3–6 wks	Trimethoprim-sulfamethoxazole 20 mg/kg/day (based on the trimethoprim component) divided q6h; or meropenem 1 g IV q8h
	Gentamicin[22]	2 mg/kg, IV q8h	2–6 wks	The risk/benefit considerations may favour stopping the gentamicin after 2–3 weeks there has been a good clinical response
Syphilis[23] Early (primary and secondary)	Benzathine penicillin G[24]	2.4 million units, once, IM		Doxycycline 100 mg PO bid for 4 weeks[25]

TABLE 3 (Continued)

Infection	Drug of choice	Dose/Route	Usual duration	Alternative therapy
Latent (>1 yr duration)				
• spinal fluid studies negative	Benzathine penicillin G[26]	2.4 million units, weekly, IM	3 wks (3 doses)	If no spinal fluid examination then consider one of follow regimens: Aqueous crystalline penicillin G 12–24 million units/day divided q4h IV for 10–14 days; *or* procaine penicillin G 2–4 million units IM *plus* probenecid 500 mg qid PO; or ceftriaxone 1 g IV/IM daily for 10–14 days[26,27]
Neurosyphilis	Aqueous crystalline penicillin G	18–24 million units IV q4h	10–14 d	Ceftrizxone 1 g IM or IV daily for 14 d *or* procaine penicillin G 2.4 million units IM daily *plus* probenecid 500 mg PO qid for 10 d[27,28]
Mycobacteria	Isoniazid[29]	300 mg, PO daily	9 mo[30]	An empiric regimen for suspected multidrug resistant TB (MDR–TB, ie resistant to INH and rifampin) may include: a parenteral drug (amikacin), plus a fluoroquinolone (ciprofloxacin or levofloxacin), plus ethambutol, plus pyrazinamide, plus INH, plus rifabutin, plus cycloserine (or ethionamide, or amino salicylic acid)
Mycobacterium tuberculosis	*plus* Pyridoxine (vitamin B6)	50 mg, PO daily	9 mo	
	plus Rifampin[31]	600 mg, PO/IV daily	9 mo	
	plus Pyrazinamide	20–30 mg/kg, PO daily	2 mo	
	plus/minus Ethambutol[32]	25 mg/kg, PO daily	2 mo	
M. avium complex (MAC)	Clarithromycin	500 mg, PO bid	Indefinite	Azithromycin 500 mg daily *plus* ethambutol 15 mg/kg/d is less effective[33]
	plus Ethambutol	15 mg/kg, PO daily	Indefinite	
	plus/minus Rifabutin	300 mg, 12 h, PO	Indefinite	

[1]Pyrimethamine should be used in conjunction with folinic acid (10–50 mg d for primary therapy, 10–20 mg d for maintenance therapy) in order to minimize hematologic toxicity (anemia, leukopenia, thrombocytopenia). AZT should be used with caution or withheld during the acute phase of treatment of toxoplasmosis.

[2]Primary therapy for toxoplasmosis should be continued until complete resolution or marked improvement has occurred clinically and radiologically (usually 4–6 weeks).

[3]Indicated for intestinal disease and or liver abscess. Asymptomatic cyst passers may be treated with a luminal agent, e.g., iodoquinol 650 mg tid for 20 d (alternative: diloxanide furoate 500 mg tid for 10 d or paromomycin 25–30 mg kg d divided in 3 daily doses for 7 d). Chloroquine phosphate 600 mg base (1 g)/d for 2 d, then 300 mg base (500 mg) d for 2–3 weeks may be used in the management of amebic liver abscess.

TABLE 3 (Notes to Table 3)

[4]Because of the potential for cardiotoxicity, patients receiving dehydroemetine should remain sedentary and have electrocardiographic monitoring.
[5]Continue treatment for 3 more weeks with trimethoprim (160 mg)-sulfamethoxazole (800 mg) 1 DS tablet PO, bid.
[6]Mucosal candidiasis in HIV patients has a high relapse rate. Intermittent or continuous maintenance therapy (systemic or topical) may be required.
[7]Take ketoconazole tablets or itraconazole capsules with food or cola. However, itraconazole solution is best absorbed fasting.
[8]Lipid formulations of amphotericin B are less nephrotoxic than conventional amphotericin B, but more expensive.
[9]Consider addition of 5-flucytosine in patients with overwhelming infection or local involvement with meningitis or endophthalmitis.
[10]Patients should receive amphotericin B with or without 5-flucytosine (100 mg/kg/day in 4 divided doses) until significantly improved and stable (usually by 2–3 weeks), at which time treatment can be changed to fluconazole 400 mg d PO/IV to complete a 10-week course of treatment. Itraconazole 200 mg bid PO is an alternative to fluconazole in this situation provided that drug interactions and poor absorption are not a concern.
[11]High relapse rate (24%) associated with lower dose of itraconazole 200 mg daily.
[12]Amphotericin B is indicated for disease which is moderate to severe or involves the central nervous system. Itraconazole effective for mild disease.
[13]Relapse rate is lowest with itraconazole, 5%; amphotericin B 19%, fluconazole 33%, and ketoconazole 50%.
[14]IT amphotericin B (cisternal, cervical, ventricular, or lumbar) should be started at a low dose (0.01–0.025 mg) and increased gradually as tolerated to a dose of 0.1–0.3 mg 3 times weekly. The best intrathecal route of administration is cisternal. IT amphotericin B should be given 3 times per week for 3 months then 1–2 times per week for several months. Further dosage tapering is based upon clinical course and spinal fluid parameters.
[15]Treatment should be continued until all lesions have crusted. Long-term suppressive therapy (acyclovir 200–400 mg 3–4 times daily) may be required to control frequent relapses.
[16]Foscarnet IV, high dose continuous IV acyclovir, topical trifluridine, or topical cidofovir may be used to treat acyclovir-resistant (thymidine-kinase-deficient) *Herpes simplex* infection.
[17]AZT should be discontinued during ganciclovir treatment in most cases because of additive hematologic toxicity (granulocytopenia). If long-term ganciclovir is indicated, then consider substituting alternate antiretroviral therapy or granulocyte colony stimulating factor to manage dose-limiting neutropenia (<500 cells/mm^3).
[18]Maintenance therapy is required for CMV retinitis but is controversial for gastrointestinal involvement.
[19]Patients receiving sulfa as PCP prophylaxis may develop pneumonia with sulfa-resistant bacterial pathogens.
[20]Vancomycin is the drug of choice for empiric therapy in areas where methicillin-resistant *S. aureus* is encountered, but is less effective than penicillinase-resistant synthetic penicillins against methicillin-susceptible *S. aureus* infections.
[21]If recurrence of bacteremia, then consider indefinite ciprofloxacin 500 mg bid or trimethoprim-sulfamethoxazole.
[22]Some authors also recommend intrathecal gentamicin.
[23]Some authorities advise CSF examination and or treatment with a regimen appropriate for neurosyphilis for all patients coinfected with syphilis and HIV, regardless of the clinical stage of syphilis. HIV-infected patients should have frequent follow-up and serologic testing at 1, 2, 3, 6, 9 and 12 months. Any patient without a 4-fold decline in nontreponemal serology by 3 months for primary or secondary syphilis, or 6 months in early latent syphilis, or a 4-fold rise in titer at any time should have a CSF examination and be treated with the neurosyphilis regimen unless reinfection can be established as the cause of the increased titer.
[24]Failed therapy and development of neurosyphilis has been reported with benzathine penicillin. CSF abnormalities are common in early syphilis in HIV patients and are of uncertain prognostic significance. Some authorities recommend CSF examination and modification of treatment accordingly.
[25]Treponema-cidal antibiotics (e.g. penicillin rather than doxycycline) are preferred for syphilis in HIV-infected patients. Document penicillin allergy (history +/− skin testing) and consider desensitization.
[46a]HIV-infected patients who have late syphilis should undergo cerebrospinal fluid examination. Those patients who have a normal spinal fluid examination (including negative CSF VDRL) do not require high-dose IV penicillin therapy and should receive benzathine penicillin G 2.4 m.u. IM weekly for 3 doses.
[26]Asymptomatic neurosyphilis is present in 1/2 of such patients. Therapy with either benzathine penicillin GIM or ceftriaxone IV/IM is associated with serologic or clinical failures in >20% of HIV-infected patients with latent syphilis or asymptomatic neurosyphilis.
[27]Since the durations of these regimens are shorter than that recommended for latent syphilis, some authorities recommend benzathine penicillin 2.4 million unit IM (once) after completion of any of the 10–14 day regimens (MMWR 1993; 42[RR–14]:36).
[28]Significant failure rate in HIV-related neurosyphilis, even with high dose IV penicillin.
[29]Isoniazid: higher dose of 10 mg/kg recommended for tuberculous meningitis until clinical response observed.
[30]Antituberculous therapy should be continued for 9 months or at least 6 months after conversion to culture negative state.
[31]Rifampin dose of 10 mg/kg if bodyweight below 50 kg.
[32]Ethambutol not required unless regional INH resistance is 4% or higher, or if drug resistance or disseminated disease is known or suspected.
[33]Neither amikacin nor clofazimine have been shown to improve outcomes in randomized clinical trials. Clofazimine has recently been associated with shorter survival in combination therapy.

leukopenia and other cytopenias, hepatic and renal dysfunction, hyponatremia and hyperkalemia, and gastrointestinal upset [20, 32]. However, many adverse effects can be managed successfully with supportive care, antihistamines, antipyretics and even corticosteriods, and desensitization to the drug can be carried out safely [20, 32]. TMP-SMX must be administered several times daily and intravenous doses require a large volume of fluid for dilution. PCP resistant to TMP-SMX is increasingly frequent, is likely to become more common and more clinically significant as the HIV pandemic grows and as TMP-SMX and the similar dihydropteroate synthase inhibitor, dapsone, are used more often for prophylaxis [35, 42]. A recent analysis identified resistance to sulfa drugs as a microbiologic factor associated with a poor outcome in patients with PCP. Mutations in the dihydropteroate synthase (DHPS) gene of *P. carinii* were found in 31 (20.4%) of 152 episodes of PCP. *P. carinii* DHPS mutations were independently associated with significantly lower short-term survival after diagnosis of PCP. Interestingly, the rate of DHPS mutations was closely related with the rate of previous or current use of sulfa drugs as chemoprophylaxis [43].

Pentamidine isethionate, in contrast, is only available parenterally (preferably used intravenously) and is administered once daily; the aerosolized form is appropriate for prophylaxis but not for the treatment of AIDS-related PCP, because of its association with extrapulmonary PCP [20, 32]. Of the various potential respiratory pathogens in AIDS patients, pentamidine has activity only against *Pneumocystis carinii*. Adverse effects are common, may be life-threatening and result in need to change therapy in up to 80% of patients [32]. Immediate reactions (many related to rate of infusion) include tachycardia, hypotension, flushing, syncope and hallucinations. Other reactions include fever, rash, gastrointestinal upset, cytopenias, hyponatremia and renal dysfunction. Hypoglycemia due to stimulation of insulin release may occur and prolonged pancreatic β-cell stimulation may progress to chronic glucose intolerance and even insulin-dependent diabetes. Prolongation of the QTc interval on electrocardiogram has been reported with evolution to polymorphic ventricular tachycardia (torsades de pointes). Magnesium depletion related to chronic malnutrition in the setting of advanced HIV disease may increase the likelihood of cardiotoxicity. Pancreatitis may occur and the risk of this complication may be worsened by the coadministration of pentamidine with antiretroviral agents (such as didanosine) which also are associated with pancreatitis [20]. Didanosine is contraindicated in patients receiving pentamidine.

Alternative anti-*Pneumocystis* agents include dapsone (particularly combined with trimethoprim), clindamycin-primaquine, atovaquone and trimetrexate [20, 32]. Clindamycin-primaquine and dapsone-trimethoprim have similar efficacy to TMP-SMX in patients with mild-to-moderate disease; dapsone-trimethoprim has been found to be better tolerated than TMP-SMX [32]. The spectrum of adverse effects of both drug combinations is similar to those of TMP-SMX, but dapsone and primaquine can produce methemoglobinemia (especially in patients with glucose-6-phosphate dehydrogenase deficiency), which may require discontinuation of the drug. While clindamycin can be administered both intravenously and enterally, the other agents are only available orally. Neither atovaquone nor trimetrexate has been shown to be effective enough to recommend use in the critically ill patient with PCP and both drugs are associated with significant adverse effects [20, 32].

Hence, TMP-SMX and pentamidine represent first-line agents for treatment of PCP. Presently, if tolerated, TMP-SMX remains the preferred first choice in the critically ill patient, because of its broader antibacterial spectrum (an advantage if the diagnosis is not clear or if more than one etiology is suspected). Prior use of sulfa medication as prophylaxis does not abrogate the choice of TMP-SMX as the preferred agent. However, if clinically significant sulfa resistance becomes more prevalent, this recommendation will require reevaluation. If previous sensitivity to TMP-SMX is known or TMP-SMX is not tolerated, then pentamidine isethionate is favored. In that instance, if there is concern of an alternate etiology, such as bacterial infection, additional antibiotic treatment is warranted. If pentamidine is used, appropriate precautions and monitoring for adverse effects are necessary, although the drug can be used safely outside of an intensive care setting.

Corticosteroids were shown initially to be beneficial as an adjunct to anti-*Pneumocystis* drugs in therapy of PCP-related acute respiratory failure [44]. Adjunctive therapy with corticosteroids is recommended in moderate-to-severe PCP (initial PaO_2 on room air of <70 mmHg) [36], but benefit may be seen even in milder PCP [45]. Corticosteroids attenuate the inflammatory response to infection with *Pneumocystis*, which is exacerbated by microbial killing when anti-*Pneumocystis* agents are instituted [46]. The suggested dose is prednisone 40 mg orally twice daily for seven days, followed by 40 mg daily for seven days, and then 20 mg daily for seven days [36]. Initially, the equivalent dose of hydrocortisone is preferred in the critically ill patient. Adjunctive corticosteroid therapy should be started at the time antimicrobial agents are initiated and continued throughout the course of treatment to prevent early deterioration.

Response to PCP therapy may not be seen for five to seven days [32]. Corticosteroids ameliorate initial deterioration in the early treatment phase and there may be significant improvement in the first three days [43]. Thus, patients treated maximally with combined anti-*Pneumocystis* drugs and corticosteroids who fail to improve within three to five days should be evaluated thoroughly to rule out potential intercurrent infections, other complications (such as fluid overload or pneumothorax) or alternative diagnoses. Lack of improvement after seven days suggests resistance and warrants a trial of an alternative anti-*Pneumocystis* agent [20].

As a consequence of the severe compromise of lung compliance in patients who develop respiratory failure due to PCP, in the early years of the HIV epidemic, standard ventilatory strategies often resulted in application of very high mean airway pressures. In addition, infection with *P. carinii* also causes formation of bullae and lung cysts. These factors likely account for the high incidence of pneumothoraces reported previously [6]. Although mechanical ventilation using newer lung protection strategies may limit ventilator-induced lung injury and improve outcome [47], their use remains controversial [48, 49] and changes in outcome related to modality of mechanical ventilation for respiratory failure due to PCP have not been studied.

A recent trial of low (5 ml/kg) versus high tidal volume (12 ml/kg) in ARDS found significantly decreased mortality in the low (approximately 30%) versus the high tidal volume (approximately 40%) [50]. Therefore, we suggest ventilation using lung protective low tidal volume because of the similarities of PCP and ARDS. Continuous positive airway pressure delivered by face mask has been shown to be efficacious for relief of hypoxia and reduces work of breathing among patients with respiratory failure related to PCP, but it is not clear that such treatment affects patient outcome. Patients who fail such support and require intubation have a high mortality rate [51].

Acute respiratory failure (ARF) related to PCP has a very poor prognosis, which thus raises questions regarding the appropriateness of offering critical care support to such patients. However, the outcome of PCP-related ARF has varied through the AIDS epidemic, largely due to changes in patient selection for ICU support and because of increased use of corticosteroids as adjuvant therapy [6]. Thus, investigators have attempted to identify subgroups destined to have a high mortality in order to advise patients about treatment options. Consequently, many tools have been developed to identify predictors of outcome of PCP-related ARF in AIDS [6]. Based on this work, it seems the degree of physiologic dysfunction in multiple organ systems on presentation to ICU is an important determinant of outcome in acute respiratory failure due to AIDS-related PCP [52]. This supports previous findings of the predictability of physiological scores in other critically ill populations [6].

In addition, it has been demonstrated that mortality amongst patients who develop ARF after at least five days of maximal therapy with anti-PCP drugs and corticosteroids is higher than that of patients with fewer than five days of prior maximal therapy [39, 53]. The importance of duration of maximal therapy as a predictor of in-hospital mortality may be related to the pathophysiology of pneumocystosis. Since initiation of anti-PCP therapy may exacerbate the inflammatory response by antimicrobial killing of *Pneumocystis* organisms [36] resulting in deterioration of oxygenation during the first three to five days of treatment [44], such a deterioration in gas exchange may precipitate respiratory failure. Even adjunctive corticosteroids within the first five days of therapy may not be sufficient to prevent early development of respiratory failure. Nevertheless, since acute respiratory failure in the early stages of therapy is due to an acute inflammatory process, it may be reversible. In contrast, development of respiratory failure despite five or more days of maximal therapy may represent the consequence of progression of pulmonary parenchymal inflammation to early fibrosis with poor prognosis.

The long term prognosis of PCP survivors also affects decision making about critical care support for patients with PCP and acute respiratory failure, since anticipated longevity may also influence the value patients place on critical care support. However, while some studies have documented a worse long-term prognosis for patients requiring admission to ICU than for patients who do not develop respiratory failure, others have not found this and excellent potential long-term survival has been emphasized [6]. This is especially relevant in the modern era of antiretroviral therapy. A recent study found that in-hospital survival was lower for patients with PCP who develop acute respiratory failure, but their long-term survival was no different from that of patients with PCP who do not develop respiratory failure [39] (Figure 5).

TUBERCULOSIS AND OTHER MYCOBACTERIAL INFECTIONS

Although tuberculosis itself remains a devastating infectious illness in the developing world, the disease is a major problem in the HIV-infected population globally. It is estimated that about 40% of HIV-seropositive persons worldwide and more than 8% of HIV-infected individuals in North America are co-infected with *Mycobacterium tuberculosis* [54, 55]. In the United States, there are thought to be 6000–9000 new tuberculosis infections annually in HIV-positive persons [54, 55] and at least 21% of persons with tuberculosis are also infected with HIV [56]. In the developed world, tuberculosis is especially common in indigent persons and among those who use illicit drugs, one-third of whom also are infected with HIV [55].

HIV-positive individuals are at high risk of developing tuberculosis through primary or exogenous recurrent infection or reactivation of latent disease. This susceptibility is related to T-lymphocyte cytokine responses, which are altered in the setting of HIV infection [55]. Alteration of cell-mediated immunity by HIV infection therefore reduces host ability to contain latent infection and to resist reinfection and contributes to the rapid progression of clinical disease [56]. Further, co-infection with *Mycobacterium tuberculosis* and HIV seems to have detrimental effects on the natural course of HIV infection. For example, *M. tuberculosis* seems to upregulate HIV replication in alveolar macrophages and lymphocytes, possibly by induction of cytokines with resultant cellular stimulation. Clinical studies have also shown that the mortality rate of HIV-infected individuals with tuberculosis is doubled and seems due to more rapid progression of HIV disease rather than tuberculosis [55]. Hence, all patients with tuberculosis should be tested for HIV infection [55].

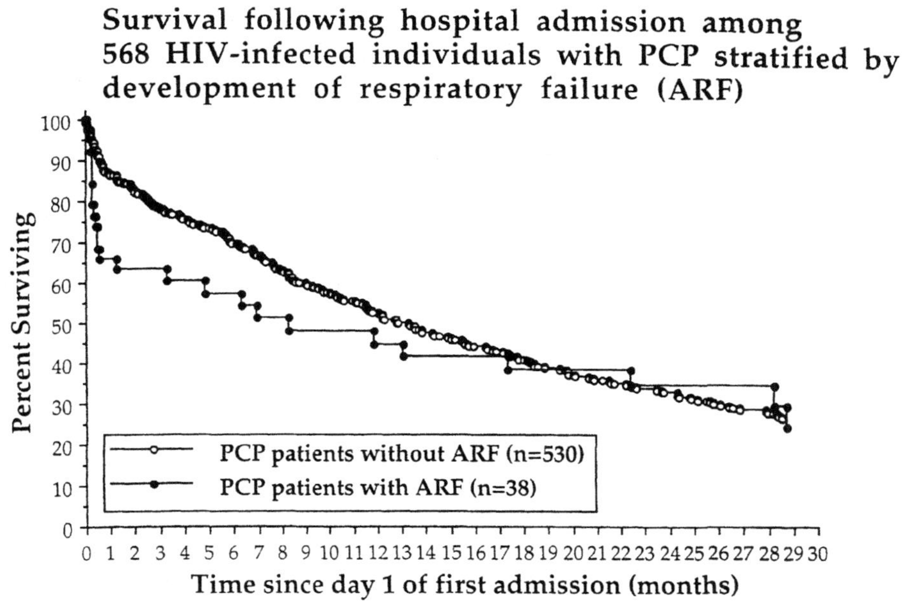

FIGURE 5. Long term survival from date of first hospital admission of patients with AIDS-related PCP and acute respiratory failure (ARF) compared with AIDS patients with PCP who did not develop respiratory failure at St. Paul's Hospital between 1991 and 1996. There is no difference in the survival curves between the two patient groups ($p = 0.798$). PCP patients with ARF ($n = 38$) - closed circles. PCP patients without ARF ($n = 530$) - open circles. (Reproduced with permission from Forrest *et al.* (39).)

Clinical manifestations of tuberculosis in the setting of HIV infection are protean, depending on the level of immunosuppression [55]. Constitutional symptoms characteristic of tuberculosis are nonspecific and similar symptoms are common with HIV infection itself [20]. The presentation of tuberculosis is more typical early in the course of HIV infection, while mycobacteremia and extrapulmonary disease are more common at later stages of immunosuppression [55, 56]. Reactivation tuberculosis in the HIV-infected person may have radiographic features of primary tuberculosis, including intrathoracic lymphadenopathy, mid- and lower-zone infiltrates, pleural effusions and miliary pattern [20]. Upper-zone infiltrates and cavitation found with tuberculosis in the non-HIV-infected individual are more frequent in persons with CD4+ count more than 200 cells/μl [55]. Approximately 5% of patients have a normal chest radiograph with positive sputum smears [20, 55].

Although prospective tuberculin skin testing has been shown to be useful in HIV-infected individuals, it has no clinical utility as a diagnostic test when active tuberculosis is considered, for several reasons [20]. First, the tuberculin skin test is often minimally or not reactive in advanced HIV disease because of suppression of cell-mediated immunity. While skin test reactivity may be preserved early in the course of HIV infection, the prevalence of anergy increases as the CD4+ count declines [56]. Second, active tuberculosis can result in specific anergy to mycobacterial antigens, even in HIV-negative patients, so that the tuberculin skin test may be nonreactive.

Diagnosis of tuberculosis should be based on the identification of the organism on smear and culture of clinically infected tissue or lower respiratory tract secretions [20]. Recently, a number of rapid diagnostic tests have been developed. Using polymerase chain reaction (PCR), ribosomal RNA or DNA of *M. tuberculosis* can be identified in clinical specimens (e.g., sputum) within 24 hours [55]. The tests are used in smear-positive cases in patients who have received fewer than seven days of anti-tuberculous therapy, where sensitivity and specificity of the tests are greater than 95%. However, the availability of these tests does not obviate the need for acid-fast staining of lower respiratory secretions, which is necessary to gauge contagiousness. PCR tests are not indicated for HIV-infected patients with positive acid-fast smears in whom clinical suspicion of tuberculosis is high, since a negative test does not rule out tuberculosis. Similarly, if clinical suspicion of tuberculosis is high and acid-fast smears are negative, anti-tuberculous therapy is indicated regardless of the results of the rapid diagnostic tests. If smears are negative and suspicion of tuberculosis is low, clinical decision making will not be altered by the result of a rapid diagnostic test, since a positive result is likely to be a false positive in this context [55]. Finally, analysis of *M. tuberculosis* by restriction-fragment-length polymorphisms can allow identification of specific strains of *M. tuberculosis*, which can be useful in epidemiologic analysis and identification of multidrug resistant strains [55].

Recommended therapy for tuberculosis in the HIV-infected host is outlined in Table 3. Therapy should be continued for a minimum of six months. Several studies have documented improved effectiveness with more prolonged antituberculous therapy (9–12 months) in the setting of HIV infection [54, 55]. There have been reports of malabsorption of anti-tuberculous medications in HIV-infected patients, but pharmacokinetic studies have produced conflicting results and measurement of plasma drug levels is unwarranted [55].

Explosive outbreaks of multidrug resistant tuberculosis were associated with mortality rates as high as 89% in HIV-infected persons [55, 56]. However, use of two or more effective anti-tuberculous drugs has increased survival among HIV-positive patients. Most deaths among patients treated effectively are due to complications of HIV infection rather than due to tuberculosis [54–56]. Isolated resistance to isoniazid is the most common form of reduced susceptibility, but alternative therapy is associated with a good outcome. Rifampin resistance is uncommon, but when present, it is usually found in the setting of HIV infection; therapy with alternative regimens may need to be prolonged [54]. Multidrug resistance should be suspected in patients with persistent fever or lack of clinical response after 14 days of anti-tuberculous therapy [20].

The treatment of tuberculosis in HIV-positive persons has been affected by the advent of highly active antiretroviral therapy, for a number of reasons. First, there is substantial risk of drug interactions between anti-tuberculous medications and antiretroviral drugs, notably reduction in drug levels of protease inhibitors and non-nucleoside reverse transcriptase inhibitors by rifampin and (to a lesser extent) by rifabutin. Rifabutin seems to be of similar efficacy to rifampin and should be substituted for it if protease inhibitors are to be continued; the dose of the protease inhibitors may need to be increased to prevent emergence of drug-resistant HIV [54, 55]. Consultation with a specialist and/or pharmacist familiar with the treatment of HIV is advised. The second important HIV/tuberculosis interaction is that initiation of antiretroviral therapy shortly after starting treatment of tuberculosis has been associated with worsening of tuberculous disease in up to 36% of patients. Other causes of deterioration should be considered. Such paradoxical reactions are generally self-limited and resolve within 10 to 40 days, but may require a short course of corticosteroids [55].

Standard treatment of drug-susceptible tuberculosis in an HIV-positive patient results in sterilization of sputum and rates of failure similar to non-HIV-infected persons. However, more prolonged therapy may be necessary to prevent relapse [55, 56]. Predictors of poor survival include low CD4+ count, absence of directly observed therapy, multidrug resistant *M. tuberculosis*, and history of injection drug use [54].

Nontuberculous mycobacterial infections have become more common in the setting of HIV infection largely as a consequence of improvements in the care of HIV-infected patients, particularly the advent of prophylaxis for other opportunistic infections and the use of antiretroviral drugs [56]. Over 95% of these infections are due to *Mycobacterium avium* complex (MAC) and usually represent disseminated disease. Significant MAC-related disease generally only occurs in the context of severe immunosuppression (CD4+ count fewer than 50 cells/µl). The recovery of MAC from the respiratory tract is usually not clinically relevant in the HIV-infected patient, unless associated with an endobronchial lesion or localized pulmonary disease in a susceptible host. On the other hand, the isolation of MAC from the respiratory tract in the absence of a localized process is usually associated with eventual disseminated disease and therefore is a marker of advanced HIV-induced immunosuppression [56]. The treatment of MAC infection is outlined in Table 3. Given the occurrence of MAC infection at a late stage of HIV disease and its disseminated nature, it is a rare cause or complication of ICU admission in the HIV-positive individual.

Other mycobacteria account for fewer than 5% of nontuberculous mycobacterial infections. *M. kansasii* can cause infection in patients with CD4+ count less than 200 cells/µl and usually produces pulmonary disease, although one quarter of patients have extrapulmonary involvement. Chest radiographs may show focal upper lobe infiltrates, diffuse interstitial disease or cavitation [56]. In general, isolation of *M. kansasii* from the respiratory tract of an HIV-positive patient warrants treatment. *Mycobacterium genavense* is a rare fastidious species that has been associated with disseminated disease in the HIV-infected patient, while *M. xenopi*, *M. haemophilum* and other miscellaneous nontuberculous mycobacteria can cause pulmonary and/or disseminated disease. Therapy for these infections is reviewed elsewhere [56], but generally they do not respond to standard anti-tuberculous medications and consultation with an Infectious Diseases specialist is recommended.

BACTERIAL PNEUMONIA

Bacterial infections, especially lower respiratory tract infections, occur more frequently than opportunistic infections in HIV-infected individuals and bacterial pneumonia is more common than PCP in the setting of HIV infection [57]. Indeed, more than one third of HIV-positive persons develop a serious bacterial infection during the course of their illness. The case definition of AIDS has been revised such that the occurrence of two or more episodes of bacterial pneumonia within a one-year period is diagnostic of AIDS. Nevertheless, bacterial infection in the HIV-positive patient often presents long before disease due to opportunistic pathogens [57].

Susceptibility to bacterial infection is related to the general immune dysfunction typical even in early HIV disease, although bacterial pneumonia becomes increasingly common as CD4+ count declines [57]. While the exact mechanism is unclear, HIV has deleterious effects on B-lymphocyte performance and hence antibody-mediated immune function. As a consequence, HIV-positive patients are predisposed to infection with encapsulated bacteria, such as *Streptococcus pneumoniae* and *Haemophilus influenzae*. Similar defects in monocyte-macrophage and neutrophil function with abnormal chemotaxis, phagocytosis and intracellular killing predispose to infection with organisms such as *Staphylococcus aureus*. In addition, neutropenia secondary to HIV-related medications (e.g. zidovudine, TMP-SMX, ganciclovir) can also increase the risk of bacterial infection. Finally, local pulmonary defense mechanisms, including alveolar macrophage, complement and surfactant function, are impaired in the setting of HIV infection [57].

The etiologies of bacterial pneumonia in the setting of HIV infection are similar to the causes of community acquired pneumonia in the non-HIV-infected population [57]. In particular, infection with *S. pneumoniae* and *H. influenzae* are common. Bacteremia is more common than in HIV-negative individuals. Previously thought to be a frequent pathogen causing pneumonia in the HIV-seropositive patient, infection with *Legionella* species is rare. On the other hand, while infection with Group B *Streptococcus* (*S. agalactiae*) is unusual in HIV-negative persons, it is more common in those with HIV disease. The incidence of *Staphylococus aureus* as a community acquired pathogen is increasing in HIV-infected injection drug users. The defective cell-mediated immunity characteristic of HIV infection predisposes HIV-positive persons to infection with *Nocardia*, which may cause abscess formation and pulmonary disease indistinguishable from tuberculosis. *Rhodococcus equi* is a Gram-positive bacillus which causes infection in immunocompromised hosts exposed to animals, especially horses. Such infection has been recognized more frequently in HIV-infected persons with a clinical presentation similar to nocardiosis or tuberculosis.

Hospitalized patients may develop nosocomial pneumonia [57]. This occurs most commonly in patients with advanced HIV disease, since these patients are most likely to require care in hospital. Additional predisposing factors include the presence of a central venous catheter and neutropenia. Gram-negative pathogens are the most frequent etiologies. Of note, *Pseudomonas aeruginosa* has been recognized as a more frequent pathogen in community acquired pneumonia in HIV-infected individuals.

The clinical features of bacterial pneumonia in HIV-seropositive persons are similar to those in non-HIV-infected patients [57]. Notably, bacterial pneumonia has a more fulminant presentation than the indolent course characteristic of PCP. While two-thirds of patients with bacterial pneumonia have lobar consolidation, up to 40% can have diffuse disease. Other features typical of bacterial pneumonia which are less frequent with other causes of respiratory disease in the HIV-positive patient include elevation of the white blood cell count with left shift, normal or only mildly elevated LDH levels, and CD4+ count greater than 200 cells/μl.

While recovery of the pathogen from lower respiratory tract secretions is essential, mere isolation of a pathogen does not necessarily signify infection, since colonization of the respiratory tract is common in chronically ill individuals [57]. Hence, a Gram's stain of expectorated sputum showing fewer than 10 epithelial cells and more than 25 white blood cells per high power field with organisms morphologically resembling those cultured subsequently is required to support a particular microbiologic diagnosis. Since bacteremic pneumonia can occur in the absence of positive samples of lower respiratory tract secretions, blood cultures should always be obtained. As noted previously, specimens obtained bronchoscopically are recommended, especially in critically ill patients, both to increase the yield for bacterial pathogens and to rule out co-infection of the lower respiratory tract (for example, with *Pneumocystis*) [20].

Treatment of bacterial pneumonia in the setting of HIV infection is outlined in Table 3. In general, therapy is the same as that for similar infection in immunocompetent hosts. Where PCP is suspected, trimethaprim-sulfamethoxazole provides coverage against many of the bacterial pathogens causing lower respiratory tract infection in the HIV-positive patient. However, since the combination is only bacteriostatic, if bacterial pneumonia is suspected strongly, especially in a critically ill patient, we recommend therapy including agents with bactericidal action, such as cefuroxime or ceftriaxone. Of note, pneumonia due to pneumococcus with intermediate sensitivity to penicillin (minimum inhibitory concentration of 1–4 μg/ml) can be treated adequately with penicillin G. If there is a high prevalence of penicillin-resistant pneumococci (minimum inhibitory concentration of

≥4 μg/ml), initial therapy with ceftriaxone or vancomycin is suggested with modification based on the results of microbiologic testing. Similarly, if *S. aureus* is suspected as the causative pathogen (based on the results of Gram's stain and/or culture) and there is a high prevalence of methicillin resistance, initial empiric therapy with vancomycin is recommended for the critically ill patient.

In general, the mortality due to bacterial pneumonia in the setting of HIV infection is similar to that in HIV-negative persons [58]. Although recurrences are more common, the outcome of pneumococcal pneumonia in HIV-infected individuals may be better than in HIV-seronegative persons [57]. On the other hand, the mortality rate of HIV-positive patients with Gram-negative nosocomial infection is higher [20]. Because of the high incidence of pneumococcal infection in HIV-positive persons, it is recommended they receive pneumococcal vaccine, although vaccine efficacy is less predictable than in HIV-seronegative individuals [57]. When possible, pneumococcal vaccine should be given when the CD4 cell count is greater than 200 cells/μl.

FUNGAL PNEUMONIA

Fungal infections are the most common opportunistic infections in HIV disease [59], but comprise fewer than two pulmonary infectious episodes per 100 person-years [60]. Fungal pneumonia tends to be a complication of late-stage HIV disease [20]. Resistance of fungi to nonimmune killing by polymorphonuclear leukocytes discriminates pathogenic from opportunistic fungi [61]. The former include *Cryptococcus neoformans* and agents of endemic mycoses which cannot be killed effectively by nonimmune phagocytes, so that an intact cellular immune system is necessary for effective host resistance to infection. Such infections occur in normal hosts, often with recovery. In contrast, spores of opportunistic fungi (such as *Aspergillus*) are killed by nonimmune phagocytes, so that infection characteristically occurs in patients with reduced neutrophil number or function; cell-mediated immunity is of little importance to host resistance to these fungi. Finally, *Candida* has features of both types of fungi: mucocutaneous candidiasis is more common with T-cell deficiency, while invasive candidal disease requires neutrophil dysfunction [62].

These divisions are somewhat artificial in the setting of HIV disease, as HIV-infected patients are actually more prone to developing infection by the "pathogenic" group of fungi, which are perhaps better described as T-cell opportunists in this setting. However, since neutrophil function is abnormal in HIV disease (especially late in disease and with concomitant depression of neutrophil number due to HIV-related medication, etc.), such patients are predisposed also to infection with fungi traditionally felt to be opportunists in the setting of phagocyte dysfunction. It is also noteworthy that the burden of fungal infection in patients with AIDS is generally higher than in those without HIV disease and is often systemic, making treatment more difficult [62].

Cryptococcosis is the most common fungal infection complicating AIDS [62]. *Cryptococcus neoformans* is an encapsulated fungus that is found worldwide, particularly in bird droppings, decaying fruit and soil. The organism enters the body by inhalation of spores with initial infection in the lung, although this is usually asymptomatic. However, pulmonary infection can occur with primary infection and the clinical and radiographic features resemble pneumocystosis. Onset is subacute with fever, cough and dyspnea in patients with pulmonary disease; on chest radiograph, diffuse interstitial infiltrates are typical, but radiographic manifestations can be protean. *Cryptococcus* has a remarkable trophism for the central nervous system, so patients with pulmonary disease should be presumed to have concomitant meningitis and systemic infection. Blood cultures for fungi, a serum cryptococcal antigen assay and a lumbar puncture should be performed. The serum cryptococcal antigen has high sensitivity and specificity: the test is positive in more than 98% of cases of cryptococcal meningitis. The organisms may be found on direct smear and culture of BAL specimens from the lower respiratory tract. While cryptococcal antigen can be found in lavage fluid, serum cryptococcal antigen is almost always positive and a negative cryptococcal antigen in lavage fluid does not rule out the disease. Currently recommended therapy is outlined in Table 3.

In highly endemic areas, infection with *Histoplasma capsulatum* exceeds cryptococcosis as an opportunistic fungal infection in patients with AIDS [62]. The organism is endemic to the major river valleys in North, Central and South America and the Caribbean [63], particularly in soil enriched by bird or bat droppings [62]. The organism is acquired by inhalation. Progression of primary infection is the most common mechanism of pulmonary disease in immunocompromised hosts, but pulmonary disease can also occur as a result of reactivation of previous infection [62]. The onset of illness is often subacute with nonspecific symptoms. The chest radiograph may be normal or may show a diffuse or miliary pattern, but localized infiltrates can also be seen [63]. Disseminated disease with diffuse involvement of the reticuloendothelial system and hepatosplenomegaly is common. Serum histoplasma polysaccharide antigen testing is highly sensitive, but cross-reaction can occur with paracoccidioidomycosis, blastomycosis and *Penicillium* infection. The organism can also be recovered by BAL on direct smear and culture. Treatment is amphotericin B for life-threatening or CNS histoplasmosis. Maintenance therapy with itraconazole is required for life. Itraconazole is the treatment of choice for mild to moderately severe disseminated histoplasmosis.

Coccidioidomycosis is endemic to arid and semi-arid climates in the southwestern United States, Central and South America. For most AIDS patients, disease is the result of new infection, acquired by the pulmonary route. The illness is principally respiratory but can be disseminated. Diagnosis can be established by recovery of the organism on BAL. Patients with advanced HIV disease have severe and often fatal illness. Initial treatment is with fluconazole or amphotericin B followed by lifetime maintenance therapy [62]. *Blastomyces dermatitidis* is co-endemic with *Histoplasma* over much of North America, but cases have also been reported in Africa, Central and South America, India and the Middle East. Infection in HIV seropositive individuals is rare and associated with aggressive pulmonary infection and rapid dissemination. The organism can be identified on BAL specimens. The infection has been incurable in AIDS patients [62]. *Paracoccidioidoes brasiliensis* is endemic to Central and South America. Paracoccidioidomycosis is also a rare complication of AIDS and produces aggressive pulmonary infection and widespread dissemination. The organism can be recovered on BAL. Prognosis in HIV positive patients is better, however, and the disease should be treated with amphotericin B and lifetime maintenance therapy with itraconazole [60].

Pulmonary aspergillosis was reported as a more common fungal infection in HIV patients than cryptococcal disease in one series [60] and is said to occur in 0.1–0.5% of patients [62]. The fungus is found worldwide in decaying organic matter. Infection is by the respiratory route and pulmonary disease is usual with primary infection. Intact phagocyte function is necessary for immunity and more than half of AIDS patients with aspergillosis have neutropenia, while most others have advanced HIV disease with CD4+ counts less than 50 cells/μl and severe phagocyte immune dysfunction. While presenting features are usually nonspecific, patients with cavitary and endobronchial lesions may have hemoptysis, which is rare in other pulmonary opportunistic infections [62]. Two distinct forms of pulmonary disease are seen: invasive parenchymal infection with localized or diffuse consolidation or cavitation, especially in the upper lobes, and bronchial disease with endobronchial lesions and even bronchial obstruction [62, 63]. Dissemination is common [63]. Diagnosis is best established by bronchoscopy and biopsy of endobronchial lesions, if identified [62]. The mere recovery of the organism on BAL, however, does not distinguish colonization from invasive disease, although positive cultures of sputum or BAL specimens in the absence of an alternate etiology raise the likelihood of invasive disease. A definitive diagnosis can only be established by histopathologic evidence of tissue invasion on appropriate biopsy specimens; obtaining such biopsies may not be feasible in a critically ill patient. Treatment is outlined in Table 3. The prognosis for recovery in AIDS patients is poor [62], although occasional case reports suggest that survival time may be improved with highly active antiretroviral therapy.

Candidal infection of mucocutaneous sites is common and virtually all HIV-infected patients have mucosal candidiasis at some point during the course of their illness [62]. Infection with *Candida* can involve the trachea and upper bronchi but parenchymal disease is extremely uncommon. Mucocutaneous candidiasis can be treated with fluconazole [62]. Fluconazole-resistant mucosal candidiasis is associated with prolonged exposure to azoles and CD4+ lymphopenia. Management options include itraconazole oral solution and amphotericin B (oral solution or intravenous). Other fungal infections are rare in HIV-positive patients.

VIRAL INFECTIONS

The clinical effect of viral pulmonary infections in HIV disease is poorly defined. HIV itself can cause pulmonary disease and a lymphocytic alveolitis, but such disease is generally mild. It may contribute, however, to the development of lymphoid interstitial pneumonitis or nonspecific pneumonitis [64]. Primary influenza pneumonitis occurs with no greater frequency or severity in the setting of HIV infection than in non-HIV-infected individuals [64]. Treatment with amantadine, rimantadine or zanamivir must be started within 48 hours of symptom onset and is usually not effective. Ribavirin may be used for critically ill patients but is unproven. Infection of the lower respiratory tract with respiratory syncytial virus and rubeola (measles) virus is more common in HIV-infected children than in those without HIV disease. These viruses rarely produce severe pneumonitis in adults. Aerosolized ribavirin can be effective [64]. Adenovirus is an infrequent cause of pulmonary disease in HIV-positive patients, but can cause a fulminant and fatal disease for which there is no available treatment [64].

Infection of the lower respiratory tract with herpes simplex virus (both types 1 and 2) has been observed in 0.2–4% of autopsy series. Varicella-zoster virus (VZV) infection can occur occasionally in adults, but is more common in children. Diagnosis is difficult in the case of herpes simplex virus, since mere recovery of the organism from lower respiratory tract secretions does not signify infection. Instead, identification of histopathologic change (Cowdry type A intranuclear inclusions) in tissue specimens is necessary. Development of diffuse alveolointerstitial infiltrates in a patient with vesicular rash typical of primary VZV infection warrants treatment even in the absence of demonstrable histopathology of pulmonary specimens. Varicella-zoster pneumonitis has not been reported with cutaneous reactivation of infection (shingles) in AIDS patients. Both herpes simplex and VZV infections can be treated effectively with acyclovir. Ganciclovir also has activity against herpes simplex virus [64].

Cytomegalovirus (CMV) is the most frequently isolated virus from the respiratory tract in HIV-infected patients and active infection is found in up to 90% of cases of advanced HIV disease in autopsy series [64]. Its pathogenic importance, however, remains controversial [20]. CMV is seldom implicated clinically as a cause of pneumonitis, even though foci of CMV and inclusion bodies can often be found at autopsy [65]. The course of CMV pneumonitis in the setting of HIV infection certainly is not as fulminant as in the bone marrow transplant population, and it is likely that in most patients with AIDS, infection with CMV produces subclinical disease [64].

Even with the advent of corticosteroid use as adjunctive therapy for PCP, there has not been a rise in the incidence of clinical CMV pneumonitis [20]. The presence of CMV in patients with PCP does not seem to affect short- or long-term survival or length of hospital stay [65].

Seropositivity for CMV in the general population increases with age and homosexual men have a particularly high seroprevalence [64, 65]. Disease is due to reactivation of latent infection, can involve multiple organs and typically occurs at a late stage of HIV disease, when the CD4+ count is less than 50 cells/μl [20]. CMV pneumonitis in the context of AIDS should be diagnosed only if hypoxemia and diffuse pulmonary infiltrates coexist with the presence of CMV cytopathic effect (intranuclear and intracytoplasmic inclusions) in lung tissue without evidence of alternate etiologies [20, 65]. Treatment is suggested only if there is histologic evidence of infection and lack of response to treatment for other pathogens [65]. This is an important consideration in the critically ill, since therapy against CMV is associated with significant side effects (such as neutropenia with ganciclovir and renal dysfunction with foscarnet). Treatment is outlined in Table 3.

MISCELLANEOUS CAUSES OF CRITICAL PULMONARY DISEASE

A variety of other disorders can lead to respiratory failure in the HIV-positive patient. Reactivation of latent infection with *Toxoplasma gondii* is an infrequent cause of pneumonitis [64], though reported in 2% of patients with respiratory failure admitted to ICU in one study [21]. Pulmonary disease may occur as an isolated process or may coexist with disseminated or central nervous system disease. Diffuse bilateral infiltrates are typical, but a coarse nodular pattern may also be seen. The organism can be recovered on BAL [64]. Treatment is outlined in Table 3. Bronchopulmonary cryptosporidiosis has also been reported, although its significance as an isolated cause of pulmonary infection is unclear [64]. Pulmonary strongyloidiasis has occurred in patients with disseminated disease characteristic of autoinfection and is associated with a high mortality rate [64].

Kaposi's sarcoma (KS) is the most common malignancy in HIV-infected persons [63] and has been linked to infection with herpes virus type 8. Mucocutaneous disease is most common, but pulmonary involvement occurs in up to 25% of patients. Pulmonary disease in the absence of mucocutaneous lesions is rare [20]. Pulmonary KS is often indistinguishable from other HIV-related pulmonary disease. Hemoptysis and lymphadenopathy are frequent, pleural effusions are common, and endotracheal or endobronchial lesions can cause airway obstruction. Bronchoscopic visualization of the typical red-violaceous lesions is usually sufficient for diagnosis; BAL can rule out superimposed infection [20, 63]. Parenchymal disease can be difficult to diagnose, since transbronchial and even open lung biopsy are often unhelpful [63]. Chemotherapy with liposomal anthracyclines and paclitaxel can be effective [66], but respiratory failure related to KS has a poor prognosis [20].

Other malignant causes of pulmonary infiltration and disease include non-Hodgkin's lymphoma and solid tumors, including primary lung cancer. Lymphocytic interstitial pneumonitis, nonspecific interstitial pneumonitis, bronchiolitis obliterans and organizing pneumonia, and pulmonary hypertension may also cause respratory failure in HIV-seropositive patients [63]. Pleural effusions are usually parapneumonic or empyemas (including tuberculous) or are related to Kaposi's sarcoma; 20% may be transudates associated with hypoalbuminemia. Pneumothorax is most commonly encountered with PCP [38].

Neurologic Disease

Neurologic disease is the second most common cause for admission to the ICU among HIV-seropositive persons. Most of the cases in one series had space occupying lesions and fewer than 20% had meningitis [21]. Neurologic disease may also be a concomitant problem in patients requiring ICU care for other reasons [20]. Involvement of the nervous system can be considered in terms of site of neuroanatomic localization of clinical dysfunction: meningitis, focal or diffuse central nervous system (CNS) disease and peripheral nervous system disease (myelopathy and peripheral neuropathy), and ocular disease. The assessment of neurologic complications in HIV-positive patient is based on three tenets: neuroanatomic localization of dysfunction, temporal profile of its evolution, and consideration of the stage of HIV infection [67]. Both meningitis and parenchymal CNS disease can present with headache and/or CNS dysfunction; an approach to the management of such patients is outlined in Figure 6.

MENINGITIS AND MENINGOENCEPHALITIS

The clinical presentation of meningitis in the HIV-positive patient may be different from that typical of an immunocompetent host. Fever, headache, photophobia and nuchal rigidity may be of variable duration and severity. Particularly in the case of subacute or chronic forms of meningitis, symptoms and findings may be subtle [20, 68]. Hence, an HIV-positive patient who presents with fever, malaise and/or nonspecific findings, even with mild abnormalities on neurologic inquiry and examination, should be investigated for CNS complications, including meningitis. This is especially important in the critically ill patient if no other cause is readily identifiable for abnormal mental status and/or the presenting condition. Given the increased likelihood of a space occupying lesion in the HIV-positive patient with neurologic abnormalities, radiologic imaging of the CNS with computed tomography (CT) or magnetic resonance (MR) is ideally recommended in all circumstances prior to performing a lumbar puncture. However, if these are not readily available, lumbar puncture may be performed safely without prior CNS imaging in patients in whom papilledema and focal neurologic deficits are absent. In any event, institution of empiric treatment should not be delayed [20].

Aseptic meningitis related to direct meningeal infection by HIV may be a presenting or complicating syndrome during seroconversion, but is more common later in the course of HIV disease as the CD4+ count falls below 250 cells/μl [20, 67]. There is associated mild cerebrospinal fluid (CSF) pleocytosis and mildly increased protein concentration. The CSF pleocytosis may respond to highly active antiretroviral therapy, but clinical benefit is uncertain [67]. Other etiologies of aseptic meningitis common to the HIV-seronegative patient are also possible and neurosyphilis should always be considered.

Acute meningitis may be due to typical agents of bacterial infection (e.g., pneumococcus, meningococcus and *H. influenza*); *Staphylococcus aureus* and *Salmonella* are also important etiologies in the setting of HIV disease. Meningitis due to *Listeria monocytogenes* may present subacutely and is more common with T-cell immune deficiency and hence in patients with HIV disease. Chronic meningitis may be due to *M. tuberculosis*, *Histoplasma*, *Coccidioides* and *Treponema pallidum* [69]. Noninfectious causes of a meningeal syndrome include lymphoma and meningeal carcinomatosis.

The most important treatable form of chronic meningitis in AIDS patients is due to *Cryptococcus neoformans*. CNS disease, a result of dissemination from the primary site of infection in the lungs, occurs as a late complication of HIV disease when the CD4+ cell count has declined below 200 cells/μl. Abnormalities of CSF may be mild or even absent; the CSF white cell count is generally less than 20 cells/μl and predominantly lymphocytic [20, 67, 68]. The serum cryptococcal antigen is highly sensitive and specific; a negative serum cryptococcal antigen virtually excludes cryptococcal meningitis [62]. Serial measurement of antigen titer in serum has not been useful in the management of infected patients and response to therapy should be based on clinical features in addition to spinal fluid culture and antigen titer. The most important predictor of early mortality is abnormal mental status at time of presentation. CSF titer greater

Presenting Symptoms: New or Worsening Headaches or CNS Dysfunction in Immunocompromised HIV-Infected Patients[1]

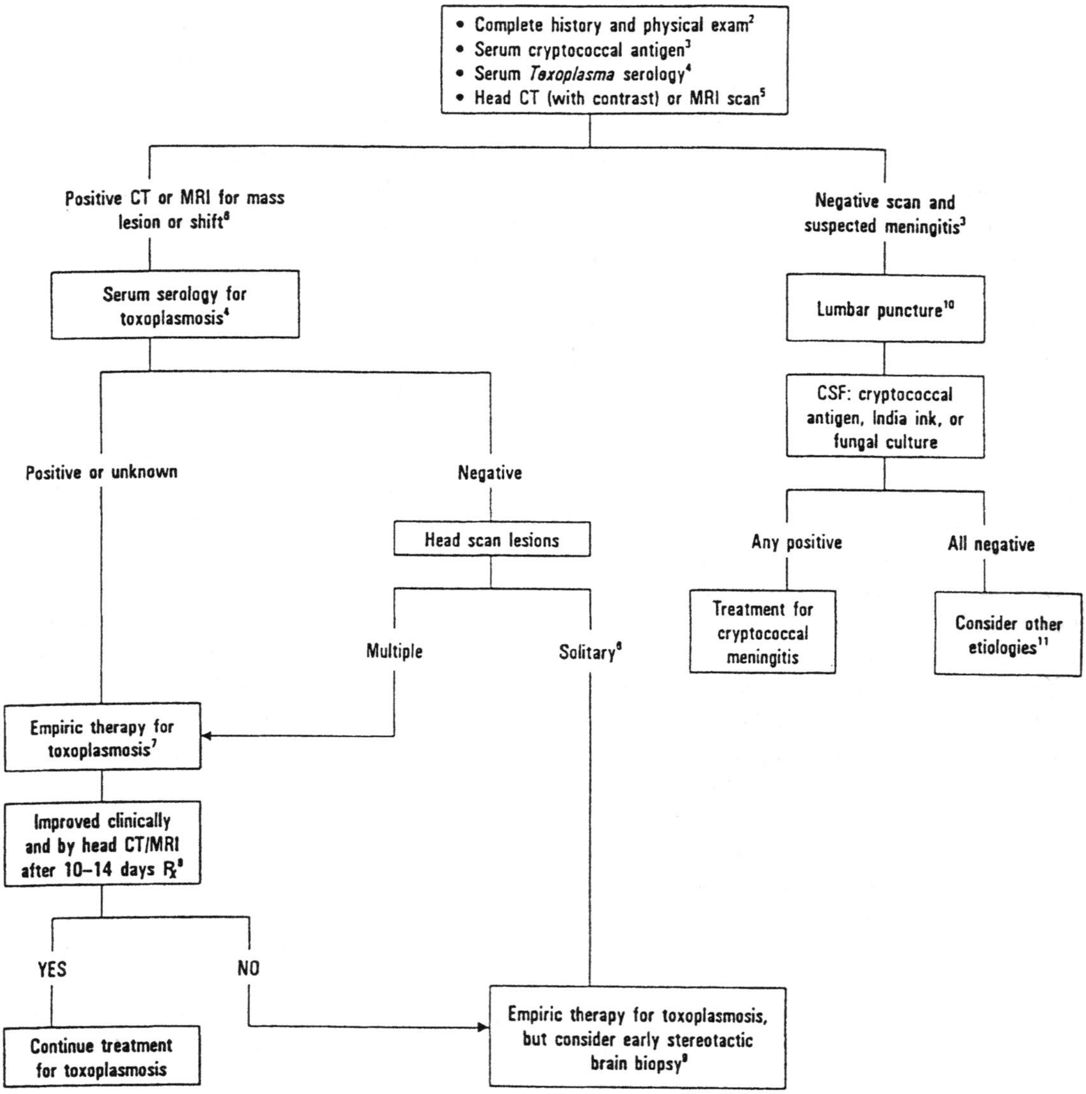

than 1 : 1024 is also associated with poor prognosis [68].

Increased intracranial pressure (ICP) is a potentially life-threatening complication in patients with HIV-related cryptococcal meningitis. In fact, early death or visual loss after the onset of chemotherapy may be related to high CSF pressure, regardless of antifungal therapy. The pathophysiologic mechanisms of increased ICP in cryptococcal meningitis are not fully understood. It has been hypothesized that absorption of CSF via the arachnoid villi is impaired due to an increased viscosity of the CSF or a microscopic plug of polysaccharide directly blocking CSF flow [70]. Symptoms consistent with elevated ICP include headache, mental obtundation, papilledema and cranial nerve palsies. An elevated opening pressure is usually defined as >200 mm CSF. In the recently reported ACTG trial [71], almost all early deaths (13 of 14) were associated with elevated intracranial pressure. Of note, patients presenting with elevated ICP do not show radiologic evidence of hydrocephalus.

Optimal therapy for this complication has not been established. In the absence of obstructive hydrocephalus, serial lumbar punctures provide a mechanism to prevent complications of a high ICP. A practical approach used in the context of the MSG/ACTG study included daily lumbar punctures, use of acetazolamide, and ventriculoperitoneal shunts for asymptomatic patients with ICP greater than 320 mm CSF and for symptomatic patients with ICP higher than 180 mm CSF. The use of lumbar drainage and selective placement of lumbar peritoneal shunts have also been attempted with satisfactory outcomes [72].

Acute meningoencephalitis is characterized by a mix of clinical meningism and CNS dysfunction (either global or focal). Potential etiologies include viruses (e.g., CMV and VZV), bacteria (such as *M. tuberculosis* and *L. monocytogenes*) and parasites (including *Toxoplasma*, *Acanthamoeba*, *Strongyloides* and *Trypanosoma*). Subacute or chronic presentation is more consistent with parenchymal and meningeal fungal infection (e.g., due to *C. neoformans*, *Aspergillus* or *Candida*). Progressive multifocal leukoencephalopathy (PML) due to CNS infection with the JC papova virus may also produce a meningoencephalitic syndrome (*vide infra*) [69].

Therapy for the various forms of meningitis is described in Table 3. Salvage therapy for crypto-

FIGURE 6. An algorithm for the management of the HIV-infected patient with headache or CNS dysfunction. History and physical examination should include neuropsychological testing where feasible. The serum cryptococcal antigen is a rapid, accurate and noninvasive method for identifying cases of cryptococcal CNS infection and a positive test should prompt initiation of therapy pending definitive diagnostic investigation. In acute toxoplasmic encephalitis, IgG is positive in 84-97% of cases, and in association with typical neuroradiological findings, may have a positive predictive value as high as 80%. Seronegative patients should be considered for early biopsy, but treated empirically in the interim for toxoplasmosis. Computed tomographic (CT; preferably with contrast) or magnetic resonance (MR) imaging should be done urgently, particularly in patients with papilledema, focal neurologic findings or seizures. If patients have an acute presentation with symptoms and signs compatible with acute bacterial meningitis, lumbar puncture (LP) should be performed without delay, provided there are no contraindications (such as papilledema or focal findings), since delay in LP and institution of appropriate therapy may affect outcome adversely. Patients presenting with headache and/or lethargy without features of acute illness should have neuroimaging performed as an initial step. However, if there is an unacceptable delay, LP should be considered, provided there are no contraindications. Multiple lesions on neuroimaging suggest toxoplasmosis, while solitary lesions indicate lymphoma, toxoplasmosis or progressive multifocal leukoencephalopthy. Empiric therapy for toxoplasmosis should be started if there are compatible clinical and neuroradiographic features. Steroids should be reserved for lesions associated with life-threatening edema. Stereotactic biopsy should be considered if there is clinical deterioration after 7 days or no response to therapy after 10 days of anti-toxoplasmic therapy. (Reproduced with permission from Tobin *et al.* (73).)

coccal disease which fails to respond to standard treatment includes liposomal amphotericin or high dose fluconazole (800–1200 mg per day) plus 5-flucytosine [20]. However, if a clear etiology is not identified readily or diagnostic testing (especially lumbar puncture) is delayed, empiric therapy should be instituted. This is especially important with regard to bacterial causes of meningitis, which are most life-threatening. Hence, empiric therapy should include high dose ceftriaxone or cefotaxime (e.g., ceftriaxone 2 g IV Q12H) and high dose ampicillin (e.g., 2 g IV Q4H). High dose vancomycin (e.g., 1 g IV Q6H) should be considered in a critically ill patient with meningitis where there is a high prevalence (>2%) of *Streptococcus pneumoniae* that has only intermediate sensitivity or resistance to penicillin. An alternative in penicillin allergic patients is combination chloramphenicol and trimethoprim-sulfamethoxazole; early penicillin skin testing is suggested. Vancomycin should also be considered in predisposed patients if there is a high prevalence of methicillin resistant *S. aureus*. In a critically ill patient with suspected meningitis and advanced HIV disease in whom lumbar puncture and serum cryptococcal assay cannot be performed in a timely fashion, empiric treatment for cryptococcosis is warranted. Therapy should be tailored based on results of microbiologic testing.

Dexamethasone 0.4 mg/kg IV Q12H for two days is suggested for bacterial meningitis, with the first dose administered with or just before the first dose of antibiotic. Development of hydrocephalus as a complication of basal meningitis (e.g., cryptococcosis, tuberculosis or listeriosis) may occur, necessitating ventricular drainage.

CNS DISEASE

Diffuse CNS dysfunction can present with depression of both consciousness and cognition (i.e., encephalopathy) or with preserved alertness in the face of cognitive impairment (i.e., dementia) [67]. In the setting of HIV infection, the latter refers to a condition termed AIDS dementia complex, which is thought likely related to primary infection of the CNS with HIV. In this condition, the CSF profile is nonspecific with normal or mild elevations of protein and mild mononuclear pleocytosis. HIV RNA viral load in the CSF is not a useful diagnostic test. The syndrome is reviewed in detail elsewhere [67].

Encephalopathy in the HIV-infected patient is usually toxic/metabolic or related to adverse medication effects. A primary encephalopathic process may be difficult to distinguish from one due to metabolic and other abnormalities typical of a critically ill patient with multiple organ dysfunction [69]. Many of the alternate causes of encephalopathy are those that cause focal CNS disease (such as toxoplasmosis or lymphoma) or meningoencephalitis. However, viral infections due to herpes simplex and CMV generally do not produce focal disease. Although herpes encephalitis is rare in the setting of HIV infection, it may be less fulminant and more diffuse [67]. CMV encephalitis can produce a syndrome indistinguishable from AIDS dementia complex, but may have a more acute encephalitic presentation. There may be diagnostic changes on neuroimaging (periventricular signal change or enhancement or HR) and the CSF profile is nonspecific, although polymerase chain reaction (PCR) of CSF for CMV may be helpful in distinguishing this process from other etiologies. Diagnosis is important, since specific therapy is available (see Table 3).

Investigation of an HIV-positive patient with a focal CNS lesion should begin with contrast CT or MR imaging of the CNS [20]. The most important etiologic considerations include the causes of meningoencephalitis, toxoplasmosis, primary B-cell lymphoma (and more rarely other neoplasms), and progressive multifocal leukoencephalopathy (PML) [67]. Other focal processes include nocardiosis, tuberculoma, neurosyphilis, fungal infection and herpes or VZV infection [20, 69]. Specific therapy is described in Table 3. A syndrome resembling multiple sclerosis also has been reported [67]. Meningoencephalitis presents with meningism as well as global or focal CNS abnormality, but depending on the location of the lesion, all of the other conditions can present in a similar fashion. There may be differences, however, in the temporal evolution of the illness, effects on mentation, and in concomitant systemic manifestations; neuroimaging usually is most discriminating [67].

Infection with *Toxoplasma gondii* is common and 3–30% of the general population are infected [73]. Reactivation of infection with *T. gondii* leading to focal or global CNS disease is the most common infectious encephalitic process in the HIV-infected patient [67], accounting for 62% of neurologic illness on admission to ICU in one series [21] and occurring in 38% of HIV-infected persons with positive serology [73]. The disease usually occurs at a late phase of HIV disease, usually at a CD4+ count of less than 100 cells/μl [59]. Usually toxoplasmic lesions occur in the cerebral cortex or diencephalic nuclei, less often in the cerebellum, and rarely in the brainstem or spinal cord [67]; multiple lesions are more common than with lymphoma [73]. Focal deficits referable to the abscess location develop over several days. Ring-enhancing lesions with mild surrounding edema may be seen on neuroimaging [67]. Presence of serum antibody (IgG or IgM) to *Toxoplasma* raises suspicion of toxoplasmosis, particularly if a rise in titer is documented (though this is often absent in HIV disease) [69]. Diagnosis can be confirmed on biopsy, but this is rarely necessary, since a presumptive diagnosis can be established by response to therapy; only in the absence of such response does biopsy need to be undertaken to determine an alternate etiology [67]. On the other hand, negative serology should prompt early consideration of brain biopsy [20, 67]. CSF evaluation is usually risky (because of CNS mass effect of toxoplasmic abscesses) and is usually unhelpful, since standard CSF serologic testing and culture are unreliable. A PCR test now available is specific but lacks sensitivity [67]. Treatment is outlined in Table 3. The use of corticosteroids is not recommended unless edema is sufficient to be life-threatening [20, 67]. Since lymphoma may respond transiently to corticosteroids, coadministration with anti-toxoplasmic treatment may confound assessment of therapeutic response [20]. A response to therapy should be detected clinically within several days and radiologically within approximately one week [67].

The principal diagnostic alternative to toxoplasmosis in the HIV-positive patient is lymphoma. CNS lymphoma in this setting is usually primary and of B-cell origin, and virtually all lesions contain genetic material of Epstein-Barr virus [67]. The disease occurs in patients with late-stage disease at a CD4+ count less than 50 cells/μl [59, 67]. Generally, the disease progresses more slowly than does toxoplasmosis, over weeks rather than days. The lesions are usually multicentric and tend to affect the deep brain, especially in the periventricular white matter and along the subependymal surface of the lateral ventricles. Lesions appear more diffusely enhancing than toxoplasmic abscesses and there may be associated edema. If safe, CSF evaluation for cytology and PCR for Epstein-Barr virus may be helpful. PCR appears to be sensitive and specific, but if PCR is negative or not available, brain biopsy is necessary to establish a definitive diagnosis. A SPECT thallium scan may help differentiate CNS lymphoma (increased uptake) from toxoplasmosis or other brain abscess. Biopsy is usually reserved for patients who have failed anti-toxoplasmic therapy. Treatment involves radiotherapy and chemotherapy, but the prognosis is poor [67].

Opportunistic infection with the human papovavirus JC produces the clinical syndrome of PML. Infection of oligodendrocytes leads to widespread demyelination with resultant focal neurologic signs. It usually affects patients with CD4+ count less than 200 cells/μl. Onset is typically slow, over weeks to months. MR is the preferred neuroimaging modality and multiple or single lesions in the white matter are characteristic with high signal on T_2 weighting and low signal on T_1 weighting; lesions do not enhance on CT. Unlike other causes of focal lesions, there is loss of tissue rather than mass effect. Diagnosis is usually established on clinical and radiological grounds, but PCR of CSF for JC virus sequences is specific (though not highly sensitive). Biopsy can establish the diagnosis definitively. No specific therapy exists except treatment of underlying HIV infection with combination antiretroviral medications. Prognosis is generally poor [67].

MYELOPATHY, PERIPHERAL NEUROPATHY AND MYOPATHY

Myelopathy can occur in HIV disease. This may be a vacuolar process likely due to HIV itself and resembling that found in patients infected with human T-lymphotropic virus-1 (HTLV-1) infection. It is usually diffuse and slowly progressive; there is no specific treatment [20]. Less commonly, myelopathy may be rapidly progressive and segmental with clinical transverse myelitis. Etiologic agents include CMV, VZV, *Toxoplasma* and lymphoma [20].

Subacute progressive polyradiculopathy due to CMV may cause a mix of motor and sensory abnormalities that progress over days to weeks. It is associated with abnormal CSF with polymorphonuclear pleocytosis, hypoglycorrhachia and elevated protein. CMV may be cultured or detected by PCR. Treatment is reviewed in Table 3. VZV may also produce a painful polyradiculopathy [20].

Peripheral neuropathy may occur at any stage of HIV infection. An acute or subacute demyelinating polyneuropathy resembling Guillain-Barré syndrome may occur in the HIV-infected individual, typically before there has been a marked decline in CD4+ count. This likely is an autoimmune phenomenon. Treatment with corticosteroids, immunoglobulin or plasma exchange may be beneficial [20, 67]. The disorder may be chronic [67]. A painful polyneuropathy associated with clinical features resembling Sjögren's syndrome and lymphocytic infiltration of multiple organs may also occur at the pre-AIDS stage of HIV disease; there may be response to antiretroviral drugs and corticosteroids. Similarly, a painful polyneuropathy due to vasculitis has been described and can be treated with corticosteroids [67]. The late phase of HIV infection may be associated with an axonal distal sensory polyneuropathy, possible related to HIV infection itself, although a similar syndrome may occur with some antiretroviral medications (especially didanosine, zalcitabine and stavudine). Painful dysesthesias occur in a stocking-and-glove distribution. Treatment is symptomatic [20, 67, 68].

Mononeuritis multiplex may be an autoimmune phenomenon when it occurs early in the course of HIV infection. A second type due to CMV infection occurs when the CD4+ count is severely depressed. It may affect muscles of the shoulder girdle and respiration and may be fatal if not treated early. Diagnosis may be difficult, as the CSF may be negative by culture and PCR for CMV. Anti-CMV treatment can be effective and may need to be started empirically [67].

Myopathic processes reported in the setting of HIV disease include an idiopathic inflammatory process resembling polymyositis. Corticosteroids may be of value. Infectious myopathies may also occur focally or diffusely due to toxoplasmosis or as a localized process due to *S. aureus*. Treatment is supportive and directed against the etiologic organism. Zidovudine can also induce a myositis which may be asymptomatic or present with proximal muscle weakness. Discontinuation of the offending antiretroviral agent usually results in reversal of the condition within two weeks [20, 67]. Rhabdomyolysis may also occur as a result of illicit drug use or pentamidine [74].

OCULAR DISEASE

Fundoscopy should be performed in all HIV patients when they present with acute illness. Fluffy "cotton wool" spots in the retina are common, self-limited, non-sight-threatening, and likely due to HIV itself. CMV retinitis is the most common cause of sight-threatening retinal disease. Areas of whitish exudate surrounded by hemorrhage and edema are characteristic. Treatment can forestall retinal deterioration and loss of vision [68]. A more aggressive form of retinal necrosis affecting the outer layers of the retina (progressive outer retinal necrosis (PORN)) is also reported and is due to herpes simplex or VZ virus. Combination therapy is often needed. Consultation with an ophthalmologist is recommended.

Cardiac Disease

Cardiac involvement in HIV disease is often under-recognized [75], yet primary heart failure accounted for 5% of ICU admissions in one series [21]. Two-thirds of patients with AIDS are found to have cardiac abnormalities at autopsy and cardiovascular disease is reported in 7% of HIV-infected persons, although up to 90% of HIV-infected patients have been reported to have echocardiographic abnormalities. Cardiovascular involvement occurs in over 90% of children who have vertically-acquired HIV infection. However, clinically significant cardiac disease is generally overshadowed by involvement of other organs. Clinical cardiac disease does not affect long-term outcome, and related symptoms may be misinterpreted as being due to noncardiac causes [75, 76]. Nevertheless, primary cardiac disease may of greater importance in the critically ill HIV-positive patient. Cardiac disease may occur at any stage of HIV disease and may include endocardial (valvular), myocardial and/or pericardial involvement.

Infective endocarditis usually occurs in injection drug users and is almost exclusively bacterial and most often right-sided [75, 76]. Three quarters of cases are due to *Staphylococcus aureus*. Fungal infections with *Cryptococcus* and *Candida* are infrequent and seen almost exclusively in injection drug users [76]. Appropriate treatment is dependent on the causative organism. Where there is a high prevalence of methicillin resistant *S. aureus* in the injection drug using population, in a predisposed patient who is critically ill, initial empiric therapy with vancomycin is warranted. Endocarditis in HIV-positive persons who are not injection drug users is usually marantic (noninfectious) and this is the most frequent type of valvular involvement in patients with HIV disease. Since vegetations are sterile, valve leaflets are not destroyed and patients usually present with embolic complications [76]. Infective endocarditis due to *Salmonella* has been described in patients who do not use drugs [75]. Mitral valve prolapse can often be demonstrated on echocardiography in late-stage HIV disease, possibly the result of cachexia and loss of ventricular volume, but is not usually of clinical significance [76].

Myocarditis is found in up to 50% of HIV-infected patients at autopsy [75]. *Toxoplasma gondii* is the most common infectious cause of myocarditis in AIDS patients [76]. Other infectious etiologies include *Cryptococcus*, *Histoplasma*, *Aspergillus*, *Mycobacterium tuberculosis* and other bacteria, coxsackie B virus, Epstein-Barr virus and CMV [75, 76]. Interestingly, *Pneumocystis* seems to spare the heart [75]. HIV itself has been purported to be a cause of myocarditis, but definitive evidence is lacking [76]. Noninfectious infiltration of the myocardium has also been reported with KS and lymphoma [75]. Far more common is a nonspecific lymphocytic myocarditis, which has been found in up to 40% of cases in autopsy series, and in 80% of these cases, no etiologic agent was identifiable [75]. Despite its frequency, the relationship of myocarditis to clinical findings or functional abnormality is unclear and death related to myocarditis is rare [76]. Treatment is predicated on identification of etiology. If etiology cannot be identified, therapy is supportive.

Clinical or subclinical dilated cardiomyopathy is one of the most common cardiac complications of HIV disease [75]. Wall motion abnormalities and ventricular dysfunction are not uncommon in HIV-infected persons, but clinical ventricular failure is found in fewer than 5% of patients [76]. However, long-term survival of patients with clinical myocardial dysfunction is poor [75]. The cause of cardiomyopathy is controversial. It may be due to HIV or opportunistic infection of the myocardium, a postviral phenomenon, the result of autoimmune mechanisms or cytokine effects, a consequence of nutritional abnormalities (such as thiamine, selenium or protein-calorie deficiency) or due to adverse drug effects (such as cocaine and potentially even nucleoside reverse transcriptase inhibitors, which are known to induce myopathy). It is most likely multifactorial. Direct HIV infection itself is felt an unlikely cause [76]. Treatment in the absence of a recognizable etiology includes standard therapy for cardiac failure, including correction of rhythm disturbances, afterload and preload reduction, digoxin and inotropes. Since primary cardiac failure due to HIV-related cardiomyopathy without identification of an underlying treatable cause that leads to need for critical care support has a poor prognosis; alteration of outcome is unlikely to be affected by ventilatory or hemodynamic support.

Pericardial involvement is the most common form of cardiac disease in the setting of HIV infection, found in 20–38% of patients [75, 76]. Most effusions are small and hemodynamically insignificant. Many are asymptomatic, but patients can present with symptoms of pericarditis or even cardiac tamponade. Most effusions are idiopathic, but may be due to infection or malignancy (including lymphoma and Kaposi's sarcoma). HIV infection of the pericardium itself may play a role [75]. Although large, hemodynamically significant pericardial effusions require drainage, small asymptomatic effusions need not be aspirated unless there is clinical evidence of systemic infection. In that case, open drainage is recommended so that pericardial biopsy can also be obtained [76]. Therapy otherwise is determined by underlying cause.

Right ventricular abnormalities and pulmonary hypertension have been reported in as many as 17% of patients. In some cases, this may represent primary pulmonary hypertension due to pulmonary vascular disease. In others, it has been linked to recurrent pulmonary infection and fibrosis [76]. Disturbances of cardiac rhythm can also occur related to medications, especially those that prolong the QTc interval on electrocardiogram (such as fluconazole, pentamidine and macrolides), which can lead to development of torsades de pointes. Malnourished patients who have hypomagnesemia are at particular risk and medications which promote renal magnesium wasting (such as pentamidine, foscarnet and cidofovir) may worsen this predisposition.

Gastrointestinal Disease

As many as 70% of HIV-positive patients develop abnormalities of the gastrointestinal (GI) tract and liver [77]. Many of these processes are chronic and may present clinical manifestations which are unrelated to the presenting critical illness (e.g., diarrhea). Indeed, Casalino *et al.* found no episodes of ICU admission related to GI disease [21]. While opportunistic and other infectious or neoplastic etiologies must be considered, diarrhea and other GI symptoms are often due to treatment effects. Hence, GI disorders are common among HIV-infected patients in the ICU setting, although they may not be the primary cause for admission.

Abdominal discomfort and GI symptoms are frequent causes of emergency room visits among HIV-infected persons [77]. Abdominal pain may be associated with common presentations, such as acute gastroenteritis, appendicitis, hepatobiliary disease, pancreatitis, perforation and obstruction. But symptoms and signs are often atypical and unusual causes must be considered, as well as multiple etiologies and non-gastrointestinal disease [78]. For example, differential diagnosis of right lower quadrant pain and tenderness must include infectious colitis (including pseudomembranous colitis) and GI perforation due to neutropenic typhilitis, CMV colitis or lymphoma. Abdominal plain radiographs, ultrasound and CT scanning are useful diagnostic modalities and endoscopic evaluation (including endoscopic retrograde cholangiopancreatography) is often essential [77, 78]. However, few HIV-positive patients require laparotomy, usually only for complications such as perforation [77].

The most common oral manifestation of HIV disease is thrush, a candidal infection of the orobuccal and lingual mucosa which may also involve the corners of the mouth to cause cheilitis. White plaques which may be scraped away and hyphae on microscopic examination are characteristic. Topical antifungal agents or oral ketoconazole or fluconazole are usually effective therapy [68]. Oral hairy leukoplakia are pathognomonic of HIV disease and are usually observed with advanced HIV infection. Lesions are asymptomatic fine white striations on the undersurface and lateral aspects of the tongue and the condition is likely due to infection with Epstein-Barr virus. The presence of hairy leukoplakia portends a poor prognosis and predicts rapid progression of disease. There is no specific therapy, although podophyllin and desciclovir have been used with some success [68, 79].

An increased incidence of severe necrotizing gingivitis and periodontitis has also been reported [79] and may contribute to pulmonary infection through aspiration. Treatment with daily chlorhexidine mouthwashes is helpful and should be provided to all HIV-positive patients in ICU. Antimicrobial therapy may also be necessary [68, 79]. Aphthous ulceration may also occur, likely due to HIV infection itself and/or autoimmune disease. Differential diagnosis includes CMV, tuberculous and cryptococcal infections, as well as lymphoma and squamous cell carcinoma. Lesions may become secondarily infected with bacteria, especially Gram-negative organisms. Treatment of idiopathic aphthous ulceration includes fluocinonide ointment, systemic corticosteroids and thalidomide [79].

Esophageal disease is also common and up to one-third of HIV-positive patients suffer from esophageal complications. Although not usually life-threatening, esophageal disease is important in the critically ill patient, because symptoms related to esophageal conditions often contribute to antecedent poor oral intake, dehydration and malnutrition. Clinical features of esophageal disease may include odynophagia, dysphagia, singultus (hiccuping), retrosternal chest pain and bleeding [78]. In 40–80% of cases, esophagitis is due to *Candida albicans* infection, usually in conjunction with oropharyngeal candidiasis. Empiric therapy with an azole (e.g., fluconazole) is cost-effective, with further investigation or repeat biopsy if there is no response [68, 78]. If ketoconazole is used, an acid pH in the stomach is necessary for absorption; therefore, medications which raise gastric pH (such as H2 hiatomire blockers and proton pump inhibitors) should be avoided [68]. Fluconazole does not share this property, has fewer adverse effects than ketoconazole and is preferred [78]. Other imidazoles may also be used. Amphotericin B should be considered for patients with infection by a fungus resistant to imidazoles [68].

CMV esophagitis can be identified by biopsy (with relevant histopathologic changes) in 10–40% of cases. CMV may coexist with Candida in up to 20% of patients and may account for lack of response to anti-fungal therapy [78]. It may present as a diffuse esophagitis or as single or multiple ulcers [77]. Other etiologies of esophageal disease include viral infections (herpes simplex, Epstein-Barr, herpes type 6 and papova viruses, as well as HIV itself), rarely bacterial or mycobacterial disease (including nocardiosis, actinomycosis, bacillary angiomatosis (bartonellosis), and infection with *M. tuberculosis* and *M. avium* complex), pneumocystosis, protozoal disease (e.g., cryptosporidiosis) or neoplastic disease (including KS and lymphoma), as well as peptic and idiopathic aphthous esophagitis [77, 78]. Given the broad array of etiologies, endoscopic diagnosis (with tissue biopsy for culture and histopathology) in the critically ill patient is essential, particularly if empiric antifungal therapy has failed. Contrast radiography is seldom useful unless perforation is suspected, in which case CT or MR imaging of the chest (to exclude mediastinal collection) is also suggested. Treatment is determined by established etiology (see Table 3). Corticosteroids may be useful for aphthous esophagitis or in cases where no etiology is identified and there is no response to empiric therapy for common pathogens [68, 78].

In general, the stomach is prone to the same processes which affect the esophagus and there is some overlap with small intestinal disease [77, 78]. However, since *Candida* is sensitive to acid pH, candidiasis is rarely a problem [78]. On the other hand, parietal cell dysfunction in HIV disease can lead to hypochlorhydria and overgrowth of microorganisms [78].

Interestingly, infection with *Helicobacter pylori* and peptic ulcer disease is unusual in HIV-positive persons [78]. CMV can produce extensive gastritis with abdominal pain, nausea, vomiting and even upper GI hemorrhage [68]. KS and lymphoma can result in obstruction [68]. Treatment is determined by underlying etiology (see Table 3). Of note, anti-acid medication may not be effective if there is hypochlorhydria already and sucralfate may be a better choice. Because of the high incidence of diarrhea in this population, magnesium-containing antacids are best avoided [78].

Small and large bowel disease due to malignancy or infection frequently cause GI distress in HIV-infected individuals [68]. Diarrhea occurs in at least half of patients in developed nations and up to 90% of patients in the developing world. Homosexual males and patients with CD4+ counts less than 250 cells/µl are at greatest risk [78]. History (including travel, medications and diet) is important. Infrequent or large volume stools or nocturnal diarrhea suggest a small bowel origin, while bloody or small volume, frequent stools with urgency and/or tenesmus suggest a large bowel process. Initial diagnostic investigation should include multiple stool samples for culture and sensitivity, ova and parasites, and specific tests (e.g., acid fast staining, enzyme-linked immunosorbent assay or PCR), but more intensive investigation including endoscopic evaluation has been shown to be effective [78]. Even if an enteropathogen is identified, its role in producing symptoms is not established and endoscopy is indicated [78]. Patients with symptoms suggestive of small bowel diarrhea should have upper GI endoscopy performed first, including biopsy of distal duodenum and/or proximal jejunum. If symptoms suggest a large bowel source, then lower GI endoscopy is necessary and colonoscopy is preferred, since sigmoidoscopy alone will miss a substantial proportion of lesions [78]. Given the inability to obtain history in a critically ill patient, both upper and lower GI endoscopy may be needed.

A variety of etiologic agents may be responsible. Bacterial enteropathogens, such as *Salmonella*, *Shigella* and *Campylobacter* can produce gastroenteritis with fever. Abnormalities of immune function may result in a prolonged carrier state despite antibiotic therapy [78], which has significant infection control implications in the ICU. Antibiotics are used frequently in HIV-positive patients; therefore, pseudomembranous colitis due to *Clostridium difficile* is not infrequent in this population [77, 78]. Enterotoxin production contributes to inflammation, mucosal sloughing and ulceration which may progress to toxic megacolon and perforation [77]. Since antidiarrheal agents which reduce intestinal motility can precipitate toxic megacolon, patients should not be prescribed such medication until the diagnosis has been ruled out by stool evaluation for culture and toxin assay and/or lower GI endoscopy. In late-stage HIV disease, infection of the GI tract with MAC can occur and is the likely source of disseminated infection. A diarrheal illness can also occur which can be complicated by obstruction, fistula formation, hemorrhage and perforation [78]. Treatment is the same as in immunocompetent persons and is reviewed elsewhere. Treatment of MAC infection is described in Table 3.

CMV can cause disease anywhere in the GI tract, most commonly the colon [77, 78]. Disease is due to vascular infection and inflammation with focal thrombosis, ischemia and eventual ulceration which can involve the full thickness of the bowel wall [77]. Such infection is unusual except in the advanced stages of HIV disease when the CD4+ count has declined below 100 cells/µl [78]. The diagnosis is established by careful histologic examination of multiple tissue biopsy specimens [78]. CMV infection can be life-threatening if it progresses to appendicitis with perforation and sepsis or intestinal hemorrhage, obstruction or perforation [77]. Other viral etiologies include herpes simplex virus, adenovirus, astrovirus, picobirvirus, calcivirus, coronavirus and rotavirus [68, 78]. HIV infects intestinal mononuclear cells and enterocytes, but the diagnosis of HIV-related enteropathy should be entertained only when other etiologies have been excluded, and even then, it is still considered controversial. Treatment of HIV enteropathy is symptomatic [78]. Treatment of CMV intestinal disease is described in Table 3.

Cryptosporidial infection of the small bowel occurs in 20% of HIV-positive patients in the developed world and in a much larger proportion of patients in developing nations [77]. It can occur at any stage of illness. There is better chance of spontaneous resolution in a patient with a CD4+ count greater than 180 cells/μl, but persistent exacerbations and remissions are the rule [77, 78]. At a CD4+ count less than 50 cells/μl, diarrhea may be fulminant [78]. Diagnosis is made by acid-fast stain or enzyme-linked immunsorbent assay of the stool or biopsy [78]. Microsporidiosis of the small bowel is also common, usually at an advanced stage of HIV disease. Diagnosis is generally made by biopsy [77, 78]. There is no effective treatment for either of these conditions [78]. Other protozoal pathogens of the GI tract include *Entamoeba histolytica*, *Giardia lamblia*, *Isospora belli*, and *Cyclospora cayetanensis* [78]. Appropriate therapy for these infections is reviewed elsewhere.

Other conditions involving the bowel in HIV infected persons include KS and lymphoma. These may produce chronic diarrhea and/or intestinal obstruction, but KS is the most common lesion causing upper GI hemorrhage in HIV-positive patients [77]. Hemorrhage from the GI tract is directly attributable to HIV infection in 40–60% of cases. Although the 39% mortality rate is almost five times that of non-HIV-infected patients, many lesions are treatable and an aggressive approach is warranted, including endoscopy, angiography, nuclear medicine studies and local or angiography-guided treatment, in addition to surgery [77]. Other potential causes of upper GI hemorrhage include infection (especially CMV and *Candida*), lymphoma and etiologies common in immunocompetent hosts (including esophageal varices). Lower GI hemorrhage may be due to agents of infectious colitis, KS, lymphoma and hemorrhoids [77].

Hepatobiliary disease is common and virtually all HIV-positive patients have abnormalities of liver enzymes, especially with advanced disease [78]. In addition to the usual causes of viral hepatitis, liver disease may be due to opportunistic infections. MAC infection is a particularly frequent cause, but other mycobacteria can also produce parenchymal liver disease and bacillary peliosis hepatis (due to *Bartonella henselae* or *B. quintana*) with multiple vascular lesions has also been recognized. Granulomatous hepatitis due to fungal infection occurs in advanced disease. CMV, herpes virus and adenovirus can cause hepatitis as well. Finally, *Pneumocystis*, *Toxoplasma* and rarely other protozoal agents can invade the liver. Noninfectious etiologies of hepatic disease include Hodgkin's and non-Hodgkin's lymphoma and KS, although the latter is seldom clinically significant. HIV-related medications are frequent causes of perturbations of hepatic enzymes and liver function. Up to 90% of HIV-positive patients are treated with potentially hepatotoxic agents, and often require dose reduction or discontinuation [78]. Liver biopsy may be necessary to establish the cause of parenchymal disease. Treatment is dependent on identification of the etiologic agent.

Acalculous cholecystitis has been reported and *Cryptosporidium*, microsporidia, MAC and CMV have been implicated as responsible pathogens [68, 78]. Cholangitis (AIDS cholangiopathy) occurs in more than 50% of cases with acalculous cholecystitis and immunosuppression predisposes to superimposed bacterial cholangitis [78]. Sclerosing cholangitis has also been described [77]. Biliary obstruction may also be due to compression of the bile duct by lymphoma or KS [77]. Radiologic imaging with ultrasound or CT scanning is useful and endoscopic retrograde cholangiopancreatography is effective in the diagnosis and management of AIDS cholangiopathy, including sphincterotomy or stent placement. Cholecystitis warrants drainage or cholecystectomy [78].

Pancreatitis occurs in up to 22% of HIV-infected individuals, but most remain asymptomatic [78]. Pancreatic inflammation may be caused by medications (especially pentamidine, didanosine, zalcitabine and TMP-SMX), opportunistic infections (particularly CMV, *Cryptococcus* and *Toxoplasma*, and to a lesser extent, *Cryptosporidium*, HSV, *M. tuberculosis* and MAC), neoplasms (lymphoma and KS) and even HIV itself. The more common associations, such as ethanol use and hypertriglyceridemia (possibly secondary to protease inhibitors) should not be overlooked, especially in predisposed patients [78]. It is important to recognize that hyperamylasemia may not signify pancreatitis: macroamylasemia, due to circulating immune complexes which bind amylase, is common in HIV-infected persons [78]. Treatment of pancreatitis in the HIV-infected patient is the same as in the non-HIV-infected individual. It is imperative that offending medications be recognized and discontinued and HIV-related causes should be identified.

Renal Disease

In the setting of the critically ill patient with HIV infection, there are many potential etiologies for renal dysfunction. Acute renal failure in the HIV-infected patient is more likely to be encountered by the intensivist than chronic renal failure. Acute renal failure is due to volume depletion in one-third of cases, while 40–50% of instances are caused by drugs used to treat HIV infection or its complications, radiocontrast dye, sepsis, tubulointerstitial nephropathies, rapidly progressive glomerulonephritis and obstructive nephropathy [74].

Prerenal azotemia may lead to the development of acute tubular necrosis especially if combined with hemodynamic compromise or nephrotoxic agents. Hence, correction of volume depletion and hemodynamic support are essential, as well as identification and dosage adjustment or discontinuation of nephrotoxic drugs. Tubular necrosis may also be related to myoglobinuria due to rhabdomyolysis, which may be the result of drugs or HIV itself. Acute tubulointerstitial nephritis is usually due to medication (such as TMP-SMX, rifampin or foscarnet) and has a prognosis similar to that in non-HIV-infected persons. Thrombotic thrombocytopenic purpura (TTP) and hemolytic uremic syndrome (HUS) occur with increased frequency in HIV-positive patients and are discussed below. Rapidly progressive proliferative glomerulonephritis is an autoimmune phenomenon rarely seen in HIV-positive patients. Obstructive nephropathy may be the consequence of tubular precipitation of medications, such as acyclovir or indinavir, or ureteric obstruction from tumor or retroperitoneal fibrosis [74]. The outcome of acute renal failure in the HIV-infected population is similar to that of age-matched controls; 85% of patients can be managed without renal replacement therapy and approximately half of patients who require dialysis recover renal function [74].

All types of glomerular lesion have been reported in HIV disease. Chronic glomerulopathies generally occur in asymptomatic persons and the pathologic expression and outcome of renal disease is influenced by genetic, immunologic and other host factors [74]. The most common glomerulopathy is a rapidly progressive form of glomerulosclerosis [74]. This process occurs almost exclusively in blacks, and while it has been reported in otherwise asymptomatic individuals, recent evidence suggests it occurs in advanced disease and may be an AIDS defining illness [80]. The pathogenesis of the disease is unknown, but is not thought to be immunologic [74]. There is no effective treatment and all patients progress to end-stage renal failure. Prognosis of patients with renal replacement therapy is related to stage of HIV disease.

TABLE 4. Causes of cytopenias in HIV-positive patients

Anemia
Anemia of chronic disease
Parvovirus B19 infection
Adverse drug reaction
Thrombotic thrombocytopenic purpura
Hypersplenism
Marrow infiltration (infection or tumor)
Megaloblastic anemia
Autoimmune hemolysis
Iron deficiency or blood loss
Preexisting or coexisting condition
Thrombocytopenia
HIV-associated immune destruction
HIV-associated decreased production
Adverse drug reaction
Thrombotic thrombocytopenic purpura
Hypersplenism
Marrow infiltration (infection or tumor)
Leukopenia
HIV-associated lymphopenia
Neutropenia due to HIV-associated decreased production
Adverse drug reaction
Anti-neutrophil antibodies
Hypersplenism
Marrow infiltration (infection or tumor)

Reproduced with permission from [81].

The prognosis has been improved with antiretroviral therapy and the effect of highly active antiviral combinations is unknown [68, 74].

Immune complex glomerulonephritis occurs more often in white males. This condition may present with more nephritic features than glomerulosclerosis and progression to end-stage renal disease is rapid [74]. The pathogenesis may be related to immune complexes (HIV-related or due to coinfection (e.g., with hepatitis B or syphilis), a lupus-like syndrome or IgA). Again, no specific therapy exists and the outcome of hemodialytic support is related principally to stage of HIV infection [74]. Finally, nephrocalcinosis and opportunistic infection of the kidneys can contribute to chronic renal failure [68, 74].

Hematologic Disease

Hematologic abnormalities (especially cytopenias) are among the most common manifestations of HIV disease [81]. Identification of the cause of a cytopenia is important because specific therapy may be indicated. The various causes of cytopenias are listed in Table 4.

The pathogenesis of cytopenias in HIV disease is generally impaired production due to abnormalities in cytokine regulation and disturbances in the bone marrow microenvironment, as well as peripheral destruction [81]. HIV itself seems responsible for impaired hematopoiesis. Although direct infection of progenitor cells does not occur, HIV infection of marrow accessory cells may be important, perhaps by altering cytokine production [81]; these mechanisms are reviewed in detail elsewhere [82]. Given that cytopenias in HIV disease are usually not due to progenitor cell destruction and there are multiple mechanisms involved, the cellularity of the bone marrow does not correlate with the degree of cytopenia or the stage of HIV infection [81, 82]. Normal or increased cellularity is typical and dysplastic changes are common [82]. Bone marrow aspiration and biopsy can be useful in making a specific diagnosis (such as identifying bone marrow infiltrative disorders, distinguishing thrombocytopenia caused by inadequate production from that due to increased destruction, and assessing iron stores to assist in differentiation of anemia due to iron deficiency from anemia of chronic disease) [81].

The most frequent form of anemia in HIV-infected individuals is typical of anemia of chronic disease [81]. Erythrocyte production and reticulocyte count are depressed. The smear shows normochromia and normocytosis frequently with anisocytosis, and low serum iron, iron binding capacity and transferrin saturation. There are increased marrow iron stores and decreased sideroblasts. Presence of such anemia correlates with survival from the time of diagnosis of AIDS [81]. Therapy is supportive.

Other causes of normochromic, normocytic anemia include adverse drug effects, primarily through myelosuppression (e.g., zidovudine, sulfa medications and ganciclovir). Primaquin and dapsone can induce hemolysis in patients with glucose-6-phosphate dehydrogenase deficiency [81]. A positive direct antiglobulin (Coomb's) test has been reported, but autoimmune hemolytic anemia is rare [81, 82]. However, thrombotic thrombocytopenic purpura with thrombocytopenia, hemolytic anemia with schistocytes on peripheral smear, fever, renal dysfunction and neurological abnormalities has been reported with increased frequency in patients with HIV disease. Response to plasma exchange or plasma transfusion and antiplatelet agents is similar to that in non-HIV-infected persons [81]. Chronic pure red cell aplasia can develop in HIV-positive patients coinfected with parvovirus B19, but symptoms of fifth disease noted in immunocompetent patients are absent. The anemia responds to intravenous immunoglobulin [81]. Although serum B_{12} (cobalamin) levels are often low in the setting of HIV infection and reduced B_{12} absorption is common, patients do not generally respond to B_{12} administration [81]. Paraproteinemias, common in HIV disease, do not seem to contribute to cytopenias in HIV infection [82]. GI hemorrhage from various causes and splenic sequestration may contribute to anemia [68, 81]. Finally, bone marrow infiltration by opportunistic infection or malignancy is an important cause of anemia in the HIV-seropositive patient [68].

Treatment of anemia should be directed at the underlying cause, where one can be identified which is amenable to therapy. Otherwise, the only therapies available are blood transfusion and erythropoietin. Administration of erythropoietin may reverse suppression of erythropoiesis due to inflammatory cytokines [82]. Administration of erythropoietin has been shown to increase hematocrit and decrease transfusion requirements with improvements in quality of life in HIV-infected patients [81]. Erythropoietin therapy does not have immediate effects and is ineffective in the presence of intercurrent opportunistic infection [82]. Hence, it is not likely to be of value in the critical care setting.

Lymphopenia is characteristic of HIV infection, but is nonspecific [68]. Neutropenia is often caused or exacerbated by myelosuppressive medications used in the treatment of HIV infection, [and HIV-related complications] such as zidovudine, sulfa medications, ganciclovir and pentamidine [81]. However, the major reason for leukopenia in HIV infection is impaired production. An autoimmune neutropenia, due to circulating antineutrophilic antibodies, has also been reported and responds to high dose gammaglobulin injections [68]. Bone marrow infiltration is another important cause, usually recognized in association with other cytopenias. Where there is impaired hematopoiesis, colony stimulating factors may be effective [68]. Granulocyte-monocyte colony stimulating factor (GM-CSF) stimulates HIV replication in monocytes; granulocyte colony stimulating factor (G-CSF) does not seem to have this effect. Use of GM-CSF in combination with zidovudine may enhance antiviral effects by increasing the concentration of active drug in monocytes [82], but because of better tolerability, G-CSF is preferred [81]. Although neutropenia in HIV-infected patients seems to be better tolerated than in the setting of chemotherapy (especially with mucositis), neutropenic HIV-positive patients are prone to infection with microorganisms for which host defense is dependent on neutrophil function (*vide supra*) and appropriate isolation precautions and treatment are warranted [81].

The most important cause of thrombocytopenia in HIV is autoimmune destruction, similar to idiopathic thrombocytopenic purpura in non-HIV-infected patients, and typically occurring in the early stages of HIV disease. Antibodies are directed against the gpIIb/IIIa glycoprotein on platelets, which is similar to the gp160/120 antigen of HIV, and there is also increased binding of immune complexes to the platelet surface. Both of these processes result in immune-mediated platelet destruction. However, nonimmune mechanisms of platelet depletion (such as consumption and sequestration) and inadequate platelet production are also important [81, 82]. Various therapeutic options are available and it is not clear which is best [82]. High dose gammaglobulin infusions raise platelet counts promptly but only transiently and repeated infusions are necessary to sustain effect [81]. Corticosteroids elevate platelet counts in 40–80% of patients, but long-term remission occurs in only 10–20% with such treatment [82]. Other therapies include vincristine and anabolic steroids, but these have an overall response rate of only 10%. High dose vitamin C and interferons have also been tried with limited success [82]. Treatment with zidovudine results in elevation of platelet counts in 40–60% and complete normalization of counts in 20%. The mechanism is unclear, although both increased thrombopoiesis and reduced peripheral destruction have been postulated [81]. As yet, other antiretroviral medications have not been shown to have this effect [82]. Finally, in patients failing other therapies, splenectomy has an initial response rate of 60–100% and long-term effect in 40–60% of patients without apparent detrimental effects [81, 82]. Splenic irradiation is an effective alternative [77].

Other mechanisms of thrombocytopenia are important in the later stages of HIV disease. These include hypersplenism and sequestration, bone marrow infiltrative disorders (especially lymphoma and opportunistic infections), thrombotic thrombocytopenic purpura, and myelosuppressive drug effects [81]. A progressive reduction in productive capacity of the bone marrow also occurs as the stage of HIV disease advances [82]. Treatment is determined by underlying etiology.

The "lupus anticoagulant" has also been reported in HIV-positive patients. This is the result of production of antibodies to acidic phospholipids, which prolongs the phospholipid-dependent clotting assay (such as the activated partial thromboplastin time). It is the consequence of the immune dysfunction characteristic of HIV disease [81, 82]. As many as 70% of HIV-seropositive patients may have such antibodies. The presence of these antibodies causes a prolongation of the partial thromboplastin time which cannot be corrected by mixing with normal plasma and may give positive results on nonspecific anti-*Treponema* serotests (e.g., VDRL) [81, 82]. Antibody titers tend to increase in the face of opportunistic infection [82]. The presence of antiphospholipid antibodies may be associated with major thromboembolic events [81, 82]. The prothrombotic state characteristic of HIV infection may also be the result of protein S deficiency, persistent opportunistic viral infections and other abnormalities of coagulation [82].

Endocrine Disease

Endocrine abnormalities are not a typical feature of HIV disease, but certain endocrinopathies encountered in HIV infection are of particular importance in the ICU [68]. The adrenal glands are most often affected, especially by infiltration with CMV, MAC, *Cryptococcus* and KS, but clinical adrenal insufficiency is uncommon. This may not be the case in the critically ill state, where relative adrenal insufficiency may have greater clinical significance, especially in patients with AIDS (who have a blunted cortisol response to adrenocorticotropic hormone). Ketoconazole interferes with cytochrome P-450 and may precipitate adrenal insufficiency, and rifampin may decrease cortisol bioavailability. A sick euthyroid state has been reported but actual clinical hypothyroidism is rare. Abnormalities of glucose can be produced with administration of pentamidine. This drug causes lysis of insulin-containing pancreatic β-cells, initially raising insulin levels and causing hypoglycemia; sustained glucose intolerance and diabetes mellitus may ensue. Medications can produce a variety of effects on electrolyte and mineral metabolism.

Dermatologic Disease

Dermatologic disease is common in the HIV-infected patient. Multiple manifestations of infection, malignancy, autoimmunity and drug sensitivity can be found; these are reviewed in detail elsewhere [83]. The major significance of cutaneous lesions in the HIV-positive patient in the ICU setting is that they may provide clues to the cause of a systemic or more deep-seated disease process, may require specific therapy or may provide evidence of HIV disease in a patient not known to be infected.

Herpes virus infections also produce skin manifestations which are not uncommon in the critical care setting and are important to recognize [68, 83]. These include orolabial or genital herpes simplex infection, which is characterized by the presence of painful grouped vesicles on an erythematous base which rupture and become crusted. They are common and may become chronic and extensive as immunosuppression worsens. Disseminated lesions may be difficult to distinguish from VZV infection (primary [chickenpox] or secondary [shingles]) and can be differentiated by culture of vesicle fluid. Herpes virus infections are treated with thymidine kinase inhibitors (see Table 3). Acyclovir-resistant cases require treatment with foscarnet [83]. Disseminated VZV infection warrants isolation because of the possibility of airborne spread.

Common skin infections can occur with atypical presentations, such as botryomycosis (plaque or papule formation with pustules) related to staphylococcal folliculitis, sometimes with sepsis, or intertriginous impetigo [83]. Bacillary angiomatosis, due to infection with *Bartonella* species, manifests with cutaneous vascular papules (which may resemble pyogenic granulomas and may ulcerate) or subcutaneous nodules. Bone and viscera may be involved (e.g., with peliosis hepatis) and blood cultures may be positive. Bartonellosis can be differentiated from similar lesions by histopathology. Treatment with macrolides, doxycycline, TMP-SMX or quinolones is effective [83]. Other cutaneous infections include cutaneous manifestations of fungal or mycobacterial infection, syphilis or cutaneous viral exanthems, including the maculopapular rash of HIV seroconversion [83].

Noninfectious skin disorders are common. The most important disorders to recognize in the critical care setting are cutaneous drug eruptions, which are the most common manifestation of drug hypersensitivity. A variety of lesions may be seen from morbilliform eruption to Stevens-Johnson syndrome or toxic epidermal necrolysis. Antibiotics, especially sulfa medications, are the most frequent etiologies and antiretroviral agents, such as the non-nucleoside reverse transcriptase inhibitors, are also important causes [83].

Finally, neoplasms (e.g., lymphoma) can also produce cutaneous manifestations [83]. KS is an endothelial neoplasm of capillaries or lymphatics which may involve any part of the body [66] and remains a common AIDS defining illness [22]. The neoplastic process has been linked to infection with herpes virus 8, although other factors also seem to be important [64]. In the setting of HIV disease, the lesions are more common in homosexual men and are rare in other risk groups [68]. The main importance of KS in the critical care setting is that its identification should lead to a suspicion of HIV disease in a patient not known to be HIV-seropositive and that mucocutaneous KS raises the possibility that a pulmonary infiltrate or GI bleed may be due to KS as well [20].

Adverse Medication Effects

Patients with HIV disease are treated with a sometimes bewildering array of prophylactic and therapeutic agents. Many of these are associated with substantial adverse effects, some of which may be relevant to the intensivist. For example, use of TMP-SMX and other sulfa and related drugs is common in HIV-positive patients. These medications have been linked to a systemic inflammatory response syndrome with shock which can be fatal. Associated drug eruption is a useful clue.

Increased use of antiretroviral agents has introduced new risks and potential critical illness. The development of potentially fatal lactic acidosis has been associated with the reverse transcriptase inhibitor zidovudine [84] and other nucleoside analogues [85–87]. The mechanism is thought to be nucleoside-induced mitochondrial dysfunction and alterations in mitochondrial respiration, which result in myopathy, a high lactate/pyruvate ratio, lactate accumulation, and altered fatty acid metabolism with hepatic macrovesicular steatosis [6, 84]. Hepatic failure worsens the lactic acidosis, but sepsis does not seem to play a significant role. Discontinuation of nucleoside therapy may reverse the acidosis, but may not result in recovery. The risk factors for the development of this complication have not been definitively identified. Abacavir, a nucleoside analogue, has been associated with a hypersensitivity reaction which may be fatal if the patient is rechallenged.

Protease inhibitors have been associated with a number of metabolic disturbances, particularly hyperlipidemia (including hypertriglyceridemia and low high-density lipoprotein levels) [88], insulin resistance, glucose intolerance, and new-onset or worsening of pre-existing diabetes mellitus [89]. The long-term implications of these metabolic effects are not yet known, but there have been case reports of avascular necrosis of the hip and premature coronary artery disease in patients receiving therapy with protease inhibitors. These metabolic disturbances in HIV patients on antiretroviral therapy have been associated with a syndrome of peripheral lipodystrophy and central adiposity, the etiology of which remains unclear. The associated changes in fat distribution may be of more than cosmetic significance. In a recent case in our institution, a 41-year old man with HIV and COPD experienced marked improvement in his CD4+ cell count (from 40 to 680) and suppression of his plasma viral load to undetectable (<50 copies/ml) on a regimen of two nucleosides and two protease inhibitors. However, the occurrence of abdominal obesity with thoracic adiposity further compromised his pulmonary function, resulting in his death from respiratory failure (N. Press, personal communication). Antiretroviral agents have many other side effects and toxicities; these are reviewed in Table 5.

Ethical Considerations in the Treatment of the HIV-Positive Patient in the ICU

As in other chronic illnesses, HIV-infected individuals seem not to find their disease debilitating. In one survey, 49% indicated their quality of life after HIV infection was better than before it, and patients strongly preferred longevity in their present state to reduced life expectancy in excellent health [90]. Yet, since AIDS ultimately is a fatal illness, the appropriateness of critical care for such individuals has been questioned [6].

This has been particularly so for PCP, because of the poor prognosis associated with PCP-related acute respiratory failure (ARF). Numerous studies have attempted to address the question of which patients might benefit from critical care support in this setting – or more importantly, what characteristics predict the failure of such treatment [6]. In the case of PCP-related ARF, predictors of in-hospital survival seem to be the degree of global physiological dysfunction and duration of maximal combined anti-*Pneumocystis* and corticosteroid therapy prior to development of ARF. No prognostic feature predictive of in-hospital mortality seems predictive of duration of long-term survival, and long-term survival is no different from that of patients who do not develop ARF [39]. In addition, the study by Casalino *et al.* showed no difference in functional status from baseline prior to the critical illness in HIV positive individuals who survive ICU treatment [21]. It is important also to recognize changes in the outcome of ICU

TABLE 5. Main toxicities of antiretroviral agents

Class/Agent	Toxicities
Nucleoside analogues	All agents in this class: Liver dysfunction, lactic acidosis, hepatic steatosis,
Zidovudine	Macrocytic anemia, neutropenia, nausea, vomiting, headache, rash, myopathy (with elevated CPK), nail pigmentation
Didanosine	Hyperamylasemia, pancreatitis, peripheral neuropathy, diarrhea, nausea, vomiting, hyperuricemia, gout, sicca syndrome
Zalcitabine	Peripheral neuropathy, mouth ulcers, rash, pancreatitis
Stavudine	Peripheral neuropathy, paricreatitis
Lamivudine	Anemia, neutropenia (both rare)
Abacavir	Hypersensitivity reaction[1]
Nonnucleosides	All agents in this class: Rash, Stevens-Johnson syndrome or erythema multiforme (rare), elevated transaminases, hepatitis
Nevirapine	Methadone withdrawal, somnolence
Delavirdine	Nausea, vomiting
Efavirenz	CNS disturbance[2], methadone withdrawal
Protease Inhibitors	All agents in this class: Peripheral lipodystrophy syndrome[3], bleeding episodes in hemophiliacs, liver dysfunction
Saquinavir	Gastrointestinal intolerance, headache
Ritonavir	Gastrointestinal intolerance, taste disturbance, circumoral and/or peripheral paresthesias, headache, hypertriglyceridemia, hepatitis, elevated CPK and uric acid
Indinavir	Gastrointestinal intolerance, benign hyperbilirubinemia, dry skin and lips, nephrolithiasis, crystal nephropathy
Nelfinavir	Diarrhea, abdominal pain, rash
Amprenavir	Diarrhea, rash, paresthesias

[1] Abacavir hypersensitivity is rare (3%) and potentially fatal. Symptoms may include fever, rash, malaise, nausea, vomiting, diarrhea, headache, fatigue, chills, myalgia, and respiratory symptoms (dyspnea, pharyngitis, cough). In cases of suspected hypersensitivity reaction, abacavir should be discontinued. Rechallenge should not be attempted, as it has been associated with life-threatening reactions and death.
[2] Efavirenz is associated with a usually transient disturbance of sleep and/or mood in 52% of patients during the first 4 weeks on therapy. Symptoms include dizziness, light-headedness, impaired concentration, somnolence, insomnia, abnormal dreams, confusion, agitation, depression, depersonalization, or hallucinations.
[3] A syndrome of peripheral lipodystrophy has been associated with protease inhibitor containing regimens, with prevalence rates ranging from 25 to 84%. Features include peripheral subcutaneous fat loss and central fat accumulation, hypercholesterolemia, hypertriglyceridemia, insulin resistance, and (rarely) hyperglycemia.

treatment for PCP (and other HIV-related illness) over time, which reflect changes in treatment strategy, general patient care, patient selection and demographics or comorbidities [39].

Recent investigations have attempted to address the outcome of non-PCP critical illnesses in HIV-infected individuals. For instance, in one study, as with PCP and other critical illnesses, in-hospital mortality for non-PCP critical illness was related to severity of organ dysfunction on presentation and the duration of AIDS diagnosis prior to ICU admission. Markers of severity of immunosuppression were not predictive of short-term survival. On the other hand, long-term survival was dependent only on the severity of underlying AIDS [91]. Similarly, Casalino *et al.* found short-term, in-hospital mortality (39%) was comparable to that of non-HIV infected patients admitted to ICU [21]. Further, across all categories, functional status among survivors was similar to that prior to their critical illness. The investigators also showed that in-hospital mortality is related to severity of physiologic organ dysfunction on admission to ICU and the nature of presenting illness (lowest for respiratory (34%) and miscellaneous (such as drug reactions and overdoses and renal failure; 24%) groups; highest for neurologic (41%), cardiac (69%) and sepsis (58%) groups). Duration and severity of AIDS prior to ICU was also predictive of short-term outcome, but CD4+ count was not. In addition, HIV-related variables (other than CD4+ count) were associated with long-term survival [21]. However, the severity of AIDS as a determinant of outcome is difficult to judge in the present era and previous antiretroviral use is likely of greater significance [6].

Despite refinements in the development of prognostic tools, they are not sufficiently predictive to direct decision making in the individual patient. Furthermore, respect for patient autonomy dictates that patient values be paramount in the decision making process. Preliminary results of a decision analysis suggest that these values are important in the decision making of patients, particularly with regard to advanced directives. While the values patients place on outcomes are important in determining treatment choices where there is an intermediate chance of survival, in this model of rational decision making, those values become exponentially less influential on the favored decision where the chance of survival is very poor [92]. This implies that other values, such as consideration of efficient use of costly resources, may become more important [6]. Defining the risks and benefits of ICU care where outcome is less certain is thus especially important in assisting patients to judge the value of such support and help in their decisions about its institution [6, 21].

Thus, it is important to recognize that outcome from critical illness in the setting of HIV disease dose not render provision of such support futile. Indeed, given documentation of good long-term outcomes in many situations and the improved prognosis for those suffering from HIV disease, critical care support for HIV-positive patients may not just prolong life but also may preserve good quality of life. As with any chronic illness, the worth patients place on their life quality should not be underestimated. It is paramount that patients' wishes and values should be sought and respected in decisions about their medical care.

Conclusions

In spite of reductions in mortality due to HIV disease as a consequence of powerful antiretroviral regimens, changing demographics and increasing infection rates suggest HIV-positive patients will continue to require ICU support, so that the relevance of HIV disease in critical care medicine will not diminish. While the spectrum of critical HIV disease likely will change, respiratory failure related to PCP undoubtedly will remain an important reason for ICU admission. However, HIV-related illness in the critical care setting has protean manifestations affecting virtually every organ system. Furthermore, new drug-related diseases are likely to become an increasing problem. Thus, the intensivist must maintain a familiarity with the clinical features of HIV disease as they may appear in the critically ill HIV-positive patient. Such knowledge is also important in recognizing manifestations of HIV-related illness in the patient who is not known to be infected, so that appropriate therapy can be provided.

The degree of physiologic dysfunction in multiple organ systems in particular is an important predictor of in-hospital mortality of ARF due to PCP, and for other HIV-related illnesses requiring ICU admission. The duration of maximal combined anti-*Pneumocystis* and corticosteroid therapy in PCP prior to ICU admission is also an important determinant of short-term outcome. The long-term survival of patients with ARF due to PCP is comparable to that of patients with PCP who do not develop ARF and variables predictive of in-hospital mortality do not predict long-term survival. In general, long-term survival of AIDS patients who require ICU admission is largely determined by the stage and progression of their underlying HIV disease, but this is difficult to ascertain in the modern era of highly active antiretroviral therapy. Importantly, the functional status of patients who survive ICU appears similar to their baseline prior to developing critical illness. Hence, as more is learned of the evolving spectrum and outcomes of critical illness in HIV disease, such knowledge should inform a discussion between patients and their caregivers about the circumstances, role and desirability of critical care support.

References

1. Horowitz H, Telzak E, Sepkowitz K, Wormser G. Human immunodeficiency virus infection, Part I. Disease-a-Month 44:545, 1998.
2. Hogg R, Heath K, Yip B, *et al.* Improved survival among HIV-infected individuals following initiation of antiretroviral therapy. J Am Med Assoc 279:450, 1998.
3. Palella F, Delaney K, Moorman A, *et al.* Declining morbidity and mortality among patients with advanced human immunodeficiency virus infection. New Engand J Med 338:853, 1998.
4. Fleming P, Ward J, Karon J, Hanson D, De Cock K. Declines in AIDS incidence and deaths in the USA: A signal change in the epidemic. AIDS 12(Suppl A):S55, 1998.
5. Klein R, Gourevitch M. Overview of HIV and AIDS: biology and epidemiology of the virus. Gastrointestinal Clinics of N Am 8:751, 1998.
6. Forrest D, Russell J, Montaner J. AIDS in the intensive care unit: Focus on *Pneumocystis carinii* pneumonia. Current Opinion in Critical Care 5:368, 1999.
7. Hamers F, Downs A, Infuso A, Brunet J-B. Diversity of the HIV/AIDS epidemic in Europe. AIDS 12(Suppl A):S63, 1998.
8. Graham N. Epidemiology of acquired immunodeficiency syndrome: Advancing to an endemic era. Am J Med 102(Suppl 4A):2, 1997.
9. Pantaleo G, Graziosi C, Fauci A. The immunopathogenesis of human immunodeficiency virus infection. New England J Med 328:327, 1993.
10. Ahsan N, Langhoff E. Immunopathogenesis of human immunodeficiency virus. Seminars in Nephrology 18:422, 1998.
11. Watkins B, Klotman M, Gallo R. Human immunodeficiency virus. In Mandell G, Bennett J, Dolin R (eds). Principles and Practice of Infectious Diseases. New York: Churchill Livingstone, 1996: 1590.
12. Hardy W. The human immunodeficiency virus. Med Clin N Am 80:1239, 1996.
13. Chaisson R, Volberding P. Clinical manifestations of HIV infection. In Mandell G, Bennett J, Dolin R (eds). Principles and Practive of Infectious Diseases. New York: Churchill Livingstone, 1996: 1217.
14. Muñoz A, Sabin C, Phillips A. The incubation period of AIDS. AIDS 11(Suppl A):S69, 1997.
15. Mellors J, Muñoz A, Giorgio J, *et al.* plasma Viral load and CD4+ lymphocytes as prognostic markers of HIV-1 infection. Ann Internal Med 126:946, 1997.
16. Carpenter C, Fischl M, Hammer S, *et al.* Antiretroviral therapy for HIV infection in 1998: Updated recommendations of the International AIDS Society – USA panel. J Am Med Assoc 280:78, 1998.
17. Powderly W, Landay A, Lederman M. Recovery of the immune system with antiretroviral therapy: The end of opportunism? J Am Med Assoc 280:72, 1998.
18. Montaner J, Montessori V, Harrigan R, O'Shaughnessy M, Hogg R. Antiretroviral therapy: "The state of the art". Biomed Pharmacotherapy 53:63, 1999.
19. Schafer R, Vuitton D. Highly active antiretroviral therapy (HAART) for the treatment of infection with human immunodeficiency virus type 1. Biomed Pharmacotherapy 53:73, 1999.
20. Montaner J, Phillips P, Russell J. AIDS in the intensive care unit. In Hall J, Schmidt G, Wood L (eds). Principles of Critical Care. New York: McGraw-Hill, 1996: 773.
21. Casalino E, Mendoza-Sassi G, Wolff M, *et al.* Predictors of short- and long-term survival in HIV-infected patients admitted to the ICU. Chest 113:421, 1998.
22. Forrest D, Seminari E, Hogg R, *et al.* The incidence and spectrum of AIDS defining illnesses in persons treated with antiretroviral therapy. Clin Infect Dis 27:1379, 1998.

23. Schneider M, Borleffs J, Stolk R, Jaspers C, Hoepelman A. Discontinuation of prophylaxis for *Pneumocystis carinii* pneumonia in HIV-1 infected patients treated with highly active antiretroviral therapy. Lancet 353:201, 1999.
24. Montaner J, Zala C. The role of the laboratory in the diagnosis and management of AIDS-related *Pneumocystis carinii* pneumonia. Ballière's Clin Infect Dis 2:417, 1995.
25. Boldt M, Bai T. Utility of lactate dehydrogenase vs radiograph severity in the differential diagnosis of *Pneumocystis carinii* pneumonia. Chest 111:1187, 1997.
26. Raoof S, Rosen M, Khan F. Role of bronchoscopy in AIDS. Clinics in Chest Med 20:63, 1999.
27. Huang L, Hecht F, Stansell J, Montanti R, Hadley W, Hopewell P. Suspected *Pneumocystis carinii* pneumonia with a negative induced sputum examination: Is early bronchoscopy useful? Am J Resp Crit Care Med 151:1866, 1995.
28. De Gracia J, Miravitlles M, Mayordomo C, *et al.* Empiric treatments impair the diagnostic yield of BAL in HIV-positive patients. Chest 111:1180, 1997.
29. Baughman R, Dohn M, Shipley R, Buchsbaum J, Frame P. Increased *Pneumocystis carinii* recovery from the upper lobes in *Pneumocystis* pneumonia. Chest 103:426, 1993.
30. Agostini C, Adami F, Poulter L, *et al.* Role of bronchoalveolar lavage in predicting survival of patients with human immunodeficiency virus infection. Am J Resp Crit Care Med 156:1501, 1997.
31. Stringer J, Walzer P. Molecular biology and epidemiology of *Pneumocystis carinii* infection in AIDS. AIDS 10:561, 1996.
32. Levine S. *Pneumocystis carinii*. Clinics in Chest Med 17:665, 1996.
33. Walzer P. *Pneumocystis carinii*. In Mandell G, Bennett J, Dolin R (eds). Principles and Practice of Infectious Diseases. New York: Churchill Livingstone, 1996: 2475.
34. Keely S, Baughman R, Smulian A, Dohn M, Stringer J. Source of *Pneumocystis carinii* in recurrent episodes of pneumonia in AIDS patients. AIDS 10:881, 1996.
35. Meshnick S. Drug-resistant *Pneumocystis carinii*. Lancet 354:1318, 1999.
36. The National Institutes of Health-University of California Expert Panel for Corticosteroids as Adjunctive Therapy for Pneumocystis Pneumonia. Consensus statement on the use of corticosteroids as dajunctive therapy for *Pneumocystis* pneumonia in the acquired immunodeficiency syndrome. New Engl J Med 323:1500, 1990.
37. Benfield T, Prentø P, Junge J, Vestbo J, Lundgren J. Alveolar damage in AIDS-related *Pneumocystis carinii* pneumonia. Chest 111:1193, 1997.
38. Beck J. Pleural disease in patients with acquired immunodeficiency syndrome. Clinics in Chest Med 19:341, 1998.
39. Forrest D, Zala C, Djurdjev O, *et al.* Determinants of short and long term outcome in patients with respiratory failure due to AIDS-related *Pneumocystis carinii* pneumonia. Archives of Internal Med 159:741, 1999.
40. Cote R, Rosenblum M, Telzak E, *et al.* Disseminated *Pneumocystis carinii* infection causing extrapulmonary organ failure: Clinical, pathologic, and immunohistochemical analysis. Modern Pathology 3:25, 1990.
41. Klein J, Ducanson F, Lenox T, *et al.* Trimethoprim-sulfamethoxazole *versus* pentamidine for *Pneumocystis carinii* pneumonia in AIDS patients: Results of a large prospective randomized treatment trial. AIDS 6:301, 1992.
42. Kazanjian P, Locke A, Hossler P, *et al.* *Pneumocystis carinii* mutations associated with sulfa and sulfone prophylaxis failures in AIDS patients. AIDS 12:873, 1998.
43. Helweg-Larsen J, Benfield TL, Eugen-Olsen J, *et al.* Effects of mutations in *Pneumocystis carinii* dihydroperoate synthase gene on outcome of AIDS-associated P carinii pneumonia. Lancet 354:1347, 1999.
44. Montaner J, Lawson L, Levitt N, Belzberg A, Schechter M, Ruedy J. Corticosteroids prevent early deterioration in patients with moderately severe *Pneumocystis carinii* pneumonia and the acquired immunodeficiency syndrome (AIDS). Annals of Internal Med 113:14, 1990.
45. Guillemi S, Belzberg A, Lawson L, *et al.* Adjunctive corticosteroid therapy decreases lung permeability in patients with AIDS-related *Pneumocystis carinii* pneumonia Can Resp J 2:55, 1995.
46. Bozette S. Corticosteroids and other adjunctive agents. *Pneumocystis carinii* Pneumonia 633, 1993.
47. ACCP Consensus Conference. Mechanical ventilation. Chest 104:1833, 1993.
48. Hudson L. Protective ventilation for patients with acute respiratory distress syndrome. New Engl J Med 338:385, 1998.
49. Weg J, Anzueto A, Balk R, *et al.* The relation of pneumothorax and other air leaks to mortality in

the acute respiratory distress syndrome. New Engl J Med 338:341, 1998.

50. NIH ARDS Trials Network Study of Ventilator Management in ARDS. Meeting of the American Thoracic Society, San Diego, CA, April 1999.
51. Meduri G. Noninvasive positive-pressure ventilation in patients with acute respiratory failure. Clinics in Chest Med 17:513, 1996.
52. Forrest D, Djurdjev O, Zala C, *et al.* Validation of the modified multisystem organ failure score as a predictor of mortality in patients with AIDS-related *Pneumocystis carinii* pneumonia and respiratory failure. Chest in press, 1998.
53. Staikowsky F, Lafon B, Guidet B, Denis M, Mayaud C, Offenstadt G. Mechanical ventilation for *Pneumocystis carinii* pneumonia in patients with the acquired immunodeficiency syndrome. Is the prognosis really improved? Chest 104:756, 1993.
54. Schluger N. Issues in the treatment of active tuberculosis in human immunodeficiency virus-infected patients. Clin Infect Dis 28:130, 1999.
55. Havlir D, Barnes P. Tuberculosis in patients with human immunodeficiency virus infection. New Engl J Med 340:367, 1999.
56. Chin D, Hopewell P. Mycobacterial complications of HIV infection. Clinics in Chest Med 17:697, 1996.
57. Noskin G, Glassroth J. Bacterial pneumonia associated with HIV-1 infection. Clinics in Chest Med 17:713, 1996.
58. Rosen M. Overview of pulmonary complications. Clinics in Chest Med 17:621, 1996.
59. Moore R, Chaisson R. Natural history of opportunistic disease in an HIV-infected urban cohort. Annals of Internal Med 127:633, 1996.
60. Wallace J, Hansen N, Lavange L, *et al.* Respiratory disease trends in the pulmonary complications of HIV infection study cohort. Am J Resp Crit Care Med 155:72, 1997.
61. Schaffner A, Davis C, Schaffner T, *et al. In vitro* susceptibility to killing by neutrophil granulocytes discriminates between primary pathogenicity and opportunism. J Clin Invest 78:511, 1986.
62. Davies S, Sarosi G. Fungal pulmonary complications. Clinics in Chest Med 17:725, 1996.
63. Rosen M. Acquired immunodeficiency syndrome: Pulmonary complications and intensive care. In Rippe J, Irwin R, Fink M, Cerra F (eds). Intensive Care Medicine. Boston: Little, Brown and Company, 1996:874.
64. Wallace J. Viruses and other miscellaneous organisms. Clinics in Chest Med 17:745, 1996.
65. Polis M, Masur H. Cytomegalovirus infection in patients with HIV infection. In Merigan TCJ, Bartlett J, Bolognesi D (eds). Textbook of AIDS Medicine. Baltimore: Williams and Wilkins, 1999: 373.
66. Miles S. Kaposi's sarcoma and cloacogenic carcinoma: Virus-initiated malignancies. In Merigan TCJ, Bartlett J, Bolognesi D (eds). Textbook of AIDS Medicine. Baltimore: Williams and Wilkins, 1999: 421.
67. Price R. Neurologic complications of HIV-1 infection and AIDS. In Merigan TCJ, Bartlett J, Bolognesi D (eds). Textbook of AIDS Medicine. Baltimore: Williams and Wilkins, 1999: 477.
68. Fairchild P. Acquired immunodeficiency syndrome. In Rippe J, Irwin R, Fink M, Cerra F (eds). Intensive Care Medicine. Boston: Little, Brown and Company, 1996: 1186.
69. Cohen J, Raps E. Critical neurologic illness in the immunocompromised patient. Neurologic Clin N Am 13:659, 1995.
70. Denning D, Armstrong RW, Lewis B, *et al.* Elevated cerebrospinal fluid pressures in patients with cryptococcal meningitis and acquired immunodeficiency syndrome. Am J Med 91:267, 1991.
71. van der Horst CM, Saag M, Cloud GA, *et al.* Treatment of cryptococcal meningitis associated with the acquired immunodeficiency syndrome. N Eng J Med 337:15, 1997.
72. Fessler RD, Sobel J, Guyot L, *et al.* Management of elevated intracranial pressure in patients with cryptococcal meningitis. J Acquired Immune Deficiency Syndromes and Human Retrovirology 17:137, 1998.
73. National Working Group on Comprehensive Care for Persons with HIV Disease. Presenting symptoms: New or worsening headaches or CNS dysfunction in immunocompromised HIV-infected patients. In Tobin M, Chow F, Bowmer M, Bally G (eds). A Comprehensive Guide for the Care of Persons with HIV Disease. Mississauga: College of Family Physicians of Canada, 1996: 44.
74. Bourgoignie J, Diego J, Ortiz-Butcher C. Renal disease and AIDS. In Merigan TCJ, Bartlett J, Bolognesi D (eds). Textbook of AIDS Medicine. Baltimore: Williams and Wilkins 1999: 585.
75. Milei J, Grana D, Alonso GF, Matturi L, *et al.* Cardiac involvement in Acquired Immunodefi-

ciency Syndrome – A review to push action. Clinical Cardiology 21:465, 1998.
76. Cheitlin M. Cardiac involvement in the patient with AIDS. In Merigan TCJ, Bartlett J, Bolognesi D (eds). Textbook of AIDS Medicine. Baltimore: Williams and Wilkins, 1999: 601.
77. Lew E, Dietrich D, Poles M, Scholes J. Gastrointestinal emergencies in patients with AIDS. Critical Care Clinics 11:531, 1995.
78. Dietrich D, Poles M, Cappell M, Lew E. Gastrointestinal manifestations of HIV disease, including the peritoneum and mesentery. In Merigan TCJ, Bartlett J, Bolognesi D (eds). Textbook of AIDS Medicine. Baltimore: Williams and Wilkins, 1999: 537.
79. Greenspan J, Greenspan D. Oral manifestations of HIV infection and AIDS. In Merigan TCJ, Bartlett J, Bolognesi D (eds). Textbook of AIDS Medicine. Baltimore: Williams and Wilkins, 1999:521.
80. Winston J, Klotman M, Klotman P. HIV-associated nephropathy is a late, not early, manifestation of HIV-1 infection. Kidney Intl 55:1036, 1998.
81. Coyle T. Hematologic complications of human immunodeficiency virus infection and the acquired immunodeficiency syndrome. Medical Clin N Am 81:449, 1997.
82. Doweiko J. Hematologic manifestions of HIV infection. In Merigan TCJ, Bartlett J, Bolognesi D (eds). Textbook of AIDS Medicine. Baltimore: Williams and Wilkins, 1999: 611.
83. Cockerell C, Friedman-Kien A. Cutaneous manifestations of HIV infection. In Merigan TCJ, Bartlett J, Bolognesi D (eds). Textbook of AIDS Medicine. Baltimore: Williams and Wilkins, 1999: 499.
84. Sundar K, Suarez M, Banogon P, Shapiro J. Zidovudine-induced fatal lactic acidosis and hepatic failure in patients with acquired immunodeficiency syndrome: Report of two patients and review of the literature. Crit Care Med 25:1425, 1997.
85. Bissuel F, Bruneel F, Habersetzer F, *et al.* Fulminant hepatitis with severe lactic acidosis in HIV-infected patients on didanosine therapy. J Intern Med 235:367, 1994.
86. Lai K, Gang D, Zawacki J, Cooley T. Fulminant hepatic failure associated with 2'3'-dideoxyinosine (ddI). Ann Intern Med 115:283, 1991.
87. Lenzo N, Garas B, French M. Hepatic steatosis and lactic acidosis associated with stavudine treatment in an HIV patient: A case report [letter]. AIDS 11:1294, 1997.
88. Carr A, Smaras K, Burton S, *et al.* A syndrome of peripheral lipodystrophy, hyperlipidemia and insulin resistance in patients receiving HIV protease inhibitors. AIDS 12:F51, 1998.
89. Lee E, Walmsley S, Fantus I. New-onset diabetes mellitus associated with protease inhibitor therapy in an HIV-positive patient: case report and review. Can Med Assoc J 161:161, 1999.
90. Tsevat J, Sherman S, McElwee J, *et al.* The will to live among HIV-infected patients. Annals of Internal Med 131:194, 1999.
91. Lazard T, Retel O, Guidet B, Maury E, Valleron A-J, Offenstadt G. AIDS in a medical intensive care unit: Immediate prognosis and long-term survival. J Am Med Assoc 276:1240, 1996.
92. Forrest D, Schilder A, Montaner J. Critical care support of patients with AIDS-related *Pneumocystis carinii* pneumonia (PCP) and acute respiratory failure (ARF): A decision analysis. Am J Resp Crit Care Med 157:A237, 1998.
93. Blattner W, O'Brien T, Mueller N. Retroviruses – human immunodeficiency virus. In Evans A, Kaslow R (eds). Viral Infections of Humans: Epidemiology and Control. New York: Plenum, 1997: 721.

SECTION 2: USE OF ANTI-INFECTIVE THERAPY IN CRITICALLY ILL PATIENTS

M. Kollef

10. ANTI-FUNGAL THERAPY IN THE ICU

José-Artur Paiva

Introduction

Candidemia and systemic candidiasis were considered rare diseases until the 1950s; in 1964, only 48 cases of disseminated candidiasis were described. Endemic mycosis such as coccidiomycosis, blastomycosis and histoplasmosis, described in the early twentieth century, remained a medical curiosity for a long time.

Fungal diseases have become clinically important in the last three decades and Candida has emerged as one of the most important pathogens. In the 1970s the incidence of disseminated candidiasis was two cases per 1000 hospital discharges and at present is four cases per 1000 discharges. The NNIS study (USA) demonstrated that nosocomial fungal infection rate doubled from 2.0 to 3.8 infections per 1000 discharges from 1980 to 1990 [1]. The proportion of nosocomial fungal infections has risen from 6.4% to 10.4% over the same period and the highest rates were found in intensive care units, oncological, cardiac surgery and especially burn wards [2]. The EPIC study [3] showed that fungi were the fifth most frequent pathogen, after Enterobacteriaceae, *Staphylococcus aureus*, *Pseudomonas aeruginosa* and coagulase negative *Staphylococcus* and 17% of all intensive care unit (ICU) patients had deep fungal infections. Although the number may be overestimated as infection, 50% of the patients in whom fungi were isolated were receiving anti-fungals showing that the isolation was faced as clinically significant.

Candida spp. are the predominant cause of fungal infection in critically ill patients, accounting for 85.6% of fungal isolates in the NNIS survey and for 78% of all fungal infections in 1990 in the United States [1]. However the incidence of invasive aspergillosis has also increased in the last 20 years and other fungi like *Fusarium*, *Mucor*, *Trichosporum* and *Cryptococcus* are emerging as a significant problem.

Not only is the incidence increasing but also the attributable mortality of these infections is also marked, varying in different studies from 25 to 60% [4, 5] and an elegant study in a teaching hospital showed that the attributable mortality from nosocomial candidemia was 38% [6]. Morbidity is also marked, with a median length of stay longer than compared controls.

Anti-Fungal Agents

There are mainly four classes of anti-fungal agents: allylamines, flucytosine, azoles and polyene antibiotics. The anti-fungal effects of azoles, allylamines and polyene antibiotics are directed primarily against ergosterol and its synthesis [7], as ergosterol is the main sterol of the fungal cell membrane and has a fundamental function in cell proliferation (Figure 1). The allylamines like terbinafine and griseofulvin are primarily effective against dermatophyte infections, so they will not be dealt with in this chapter.

Flucytosine or 5-fluorocytosine is a synthetic fluorinated pyrimidine which inhibits fungal DNA and RNA protein synthesis. The enzyme cytosine permease transports it into a susceptible cell and the enzyme cytosine deaminase transforms it to either 5-fluoruracilo, which

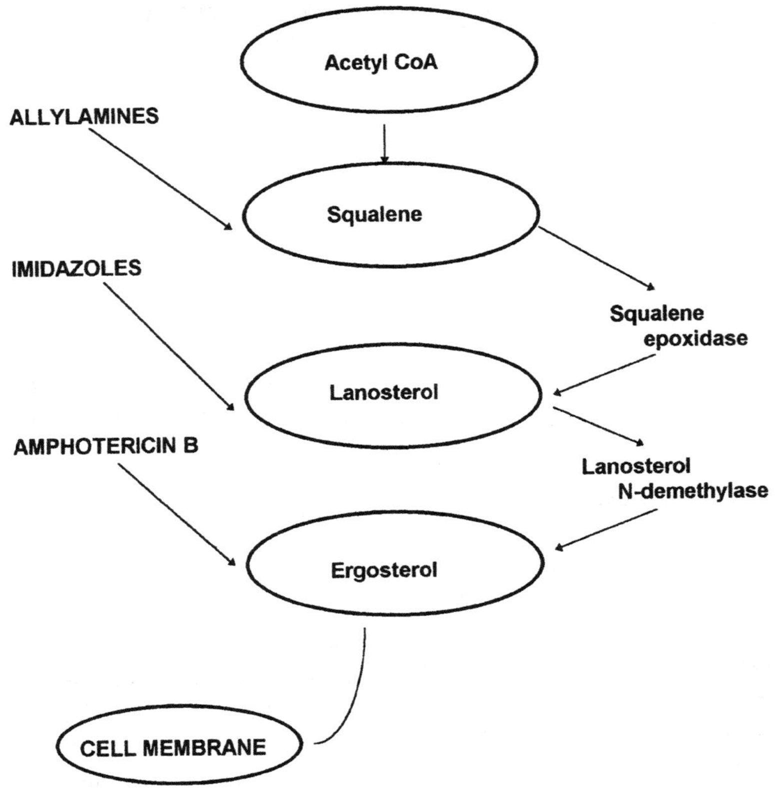

FIGURE 1. Action of the antifungal agents.

inhibits DNA synthesis, or to floxuridin, which inhibits thymidylate synthetase. Cytosine deaminase is present in fungal cells but not in human cells, although the intestinal flora can convert the parent compound into 5-fluoruracil [8–10].

Flucytosine is a fungistatic agent, with a narrow spectrum of activity – most *Candida* spp., *Cryptococcus neoformans* and some molds. Many fungi demonstrate primary or acquired resistance. Approximately 10% of *Candida albicans*, 20% of *Candida tropicalis* and 2% of *Cryptococcus neoformans* are resistant to flucytosine from the onset of treatment with MIC above 16 mg/l [11] and the development of resistance during treatment is common [12]. Therefore, it should not be used as monotherapy in *Candida* spp. infections. *Coccidioides immitis*, *Blastomyces dermatitidis* and *Pseudoallaescheria boydii* are resistant to flucytosine and *Aspergillus* spp. show variable susceptibility [13] and acquired resistance during treatment is frequent [12]. Flucytosine is used in combination with amphoterican B for systemic candidiasis and cryptococcosis, as synergism has been described between those two drugs [14–16] and this therapeutic combination is often well tolerated [17]. Nevertheless, there is no conclusive proof of benefit for this association. Indications for its use might be: (a) in neonates, because of the 45% incidence of meningitis; (b) in endophthalmitis, endocarditis, suppurative thrombophlebitis or meningitis; (c) in *Candida lusitanae* and *Torulopsis glabrata* infections; and (d) if the patient is critically ill and deteriorating. There have also been reports of successful treatment of candidiasis and cryptococcosis with flucytosine in combination with fluconazole or itraconazole, but further comparative trials are required before these combinations can be advocated [11, 18].

Flucytosine is well absorbed after oral administration and similar serum concentrations are obtained following oral and parenteral administration. Its half-life is 3 to 6 hours in patients with normal renal function and, as its protein binding is only 12%, it has a high penetration into organs, body fluids and cerebrospinal fluid [13] and tissue concentrations usually exceed 50% of simultaneous blood concentrations [19]. In adults with normal renal function, an oral dose of 25 mg/kg administered six-hourly results in peak serum levels of 30–80 mg/l at 1–2 hours [19, 20]. There is a slight accumulation of drug during the first four days of treatment and then peak concentrations remain constant. Most textbooks state that if renal function is normal, initial dose is 50–150 mg/kg given in four divided doses at six-hour intervals. If there is renal dysfunction, initial dose should be reduced to 25 mg/kg and subsequent doses and intervals adjusted to achieve peak serum concentrations of 70–80 mg/l and through of 30–40 mg/l (Table 1). However, these proposed doses are based on those needed to achieve penetration into the cerebrospinal fluid and flucytosine 25 mg/kg/day at 12 hour intervals should be adequate to maintain serum levels above MIC for most susceptible Candida [18, 21]. In small infants, as half-life is prolonged, intervals should be increased to 24 hours [20].

Main adverse effects consist of granulocytopenia and thrombocytopenia, rashes and gastrointestinal toxicity, namely nausea, vomiting and diarrhea; mild changes in liver function occur in around 10% of patients [19]. Bone marrow suppression occurs frequently in patients with AIDS and its use should be avoided in these patients. Myelotoxicity appears to be concentration dependent, although this adverse reaction may be due to the production of fluoruracil from enterobacillary flucytosine metabolism in the

TABLE 1. Doses and dose intervals of flucytosine according to renal function

Creatinine Cl. (ml/min)	Individual dose (mg/kg)	Dose interval (h)
>40	25.0–37.5	6
20–40	25.0–37.5	12
10–20	25.0–37.5	>24

gut, rather than to the parent compound [22]. The hematological and hepatic abnormalities usually resolve if treatment is discontinued, however liver necrosis has been rarely reported in patients receiving flucytosine as contributing directly to death. Due to its potentially teratogenic effects, it is contraindicated during pregnancy [10]. Serum creatinine must be monitored at least twice weekly and dosages appropriately adjusted and blood counts and liver function tests must also be performed regularly. Special caution must be taken when flucytosine is used with other nephrotoxic or myelosuppressive drugs. The use of this drug requires facilities for monitoring serum concentration [23], especially when it is used in association with amphotericin B or in patients with renal failure [20, 24]. Optimal and minimum serum concentrations for efficacy are not known, but toxicity occurs when blood levels exceed 100 mg/l for two or more weeks [10] or when it is used in combination with amphotericin B [10, 13, 25–27].

The azoles are classified as imidazoles (miconazole and ketoconazole) and triazoles (fluconazole and itraconazole). They inhibit ergosterol synthesis by inhibiting fungal cytochrome P450 enzymes, with accumulation of 14-alpha-methylsterols. Lanosterol 14-alpha-demethylase, the fungal cytochrome enzyme, is responsible for converting lanosterol to ergosterol, the principal sterol in fungal cell membranes [7, 28]. This demethylation step is dependent on the activation of cytochrome P450, a heme protein containing one molecule of protoporphyrin IX, which is the terminal oxidase of the hepatic microsomial oxidase system and has an important role in the synthesis and degradation of many substances. The interaction of azoles with the heme iron of the cytochrome P450 inhibits the cytochrome activation and the enzyme function with a consequent depletion of ergosterol; this depletion results in a breakdown of normal cellular function, increases cell membrane permeability and inhibits cell replication [29–33]. The triazoles have a greater affinity for fungal P450 – dependent enzymes than the imidazoles and thus exhibit greater anti-fungal activity and lower toxicity profile. We will discuss fluconazole and itraconazole and mention new azoles later.

The oral absorption of fluconazole is good, even almost complete, and, unlike itraconazole, is not altered by the presence of food or gastric acidity. Therefore, identical serum concentrations are attained after both oral and parenteral administration [34]. Peak plasma concentration is related to the dose, with a linear relationship [35], and occurs within 2 to 4 hours after oral administration [28]. After repeated dosing serum levels increase and a steady state is reached after about 14 days. Its protein binding is weak, about 12% of the drug, 80% is excreted by the kidney in unchanged active form and it has a prolonged half-life (20 to 30 hours) that allows once-daily dosing [36–38]. Therefore, dosages must be adjusted in renal failure and monitoring of serum levels is recommended, trying to maintain them at 6–20 mcg/ml [39]. The normal recommended dose should be given on day one, followed by a daily dose that should be reduced by 50% if the creatinine clearance is between 11 and 50 ml/min [20]. Dialysis removes 50% of the drug and a dose must be administered after each dialysis [40]. Fluconazole is widely and evenly distributed throughout the body [18] with constant levels achieved within one hour [41]. It penetrates well into cerebrospinal fluid, where drug concentration may reach 60 to 80% of the serum level [42, 43]. Bone is the place where concentrations are lowest and therefore higher doses should be used to treat bone fungal infections and also to treat muscle and central nervous system infections by *Cryptococcus neoformans*, *Coccidioidis immitis* and *Histoplasma capsulatum* [37, 44]. The dosage of fluconazole is, nevertheless, still a matter of debate: while the most widely used is 5 mg/kg/day, some centers prefer the use of a higher dose in the critically ill patient, namely 10 mg/kg/day. This question will be dealt with later in this chapter.

Fluconazole is a fungistatic agent active against most *Candida* species, *Cryptococcus neoformans*, *Coccidioides immitis*, *Histoplasma capsulatum*, *Paracoccidioidis brasiliensis*, *Sporothrix shenckii* and *Blastomyces dermatiditis* [28, 36]. It is ineffective against *Aspergillus* and *Mucor* species. *Torulopsis glabrata* is frequently resistant to fluconazole and it has virtually no activity against *Candida krusei* which has intrinsic resistance to the drug [45–47]. The widespread use of fluconazole in repeated low-dose courses as prophylaxis or therapy has resulted in acquired fungal resistance. Fluconazole-resistant strains of *Candida albicans* have become more and more common among patients with AIDS [48, 49] and more recently in non-HIV patients [50–52]. The SCOPE program showed that the level of resistance of Candida albicans to fluconazole was 9.6%, varying between 2.9% and 15.5% with geographical location [46].

Fluconazole is generally well tolerated. Nausea and vomiting are the most common side effects, but they seldom cause discontinuation of treatment [10, 36]. Elevation of hepatic enzymes occurs in a small percentage of individuals, but treatment should only be discontinued if there is symptomatic hepatitis or laboratory signs of persistent hepatic dysfunction, which are rare [10, 28, 53–55]. Stevens-Johnson syndrome has been described in AIDS or cancer patients, although a causal relationship has not been clearly established. The drug should be discontinued if bullous lesions or erythema multiform develop [20, 41]. Azoles interfere with the elimination of drugs metabolized by the hepatic cytochrome P450. The sedative effect of midazolan, the anticoagulant effect of warfarin, the hypoglycemic effect of sulfonylureas, the anticonvulsivant effect of phenytoin and carbamazepine as the effects of theophylline, cisapride and cyclosporine may be increased by the azoles; on the other hand rifampicin accelerates clearance of fluconazole [20, 41, 56, 57] (Table 2).

Itraconazole is a weak base and requires an acid environment for absorption. Absorption after oral administration is variable and incomplete and its hepatic excretion is complex, particularly in the critically ill patient [58]. Serum concentrations are markedly lower when gastric

TABLE 2. Drug interactions of anti-fungal agents

Anti-fungal	Drugs	Effect
Amphotericin B	Aminoglycosides	Nephrotoxicity
	Cyclosporin	Nephrotoxicity
	Corticosteroids	Hypokalemia/long QT
	Astemizole	Hypokalemia/long QT
	Terfenadine	Hypokalemia/long QT
	Digoxin	Arrythmia
Fluconazole and Itraconazole	Cisapride	Arrhythmia
	H 1 receptor antagonists	Arrhythmia
	Aminophiline	Arrhythmia
	Cyclosporin	Nephrotoxicity
	Lovastatin	Rhabdomyolisis
	Astemizole	Drug increased levels
	Carbamazepine	Drug increased levels
	Tacrolimus	Drug increased levels
	Triazolan	Drug increased levels
	Warfarin	Drug increased levels
Fluconazole	Sulphonylureas	Drug increased levels
	Phenytoin	Drug increased levels
	Rifampicin	Drug increased levels
	Rifabitin	Drug increased levels
	Midazolan	Drug increased levels
	Tacrolimus	Drug increased levels
	Saquinavir	Drug increased levels
Itraconazole (Itra)	Busulphan	Drug increased levels
	Calcium channel blocker	Drug increased levels
	Digoxin	Drug increased levels
	Midazolan	Drug increased levels
	Rifampicin	Drug increased levels
	Vincristin	Drug increased levels
	H2-receptor antagonists	Itra diminished absorption
	Proton pump inhibitors	Itra diminished absorption
	Sucralfate	Itra diminished absorption
	Rifampicin	Itra diminished levels
	Phenobarbitone	Itra diminished levels
	Phenytoin	Itra diminished levels

acid is reduced and capsules are used. Absorption is enhanced if we use liquid formulation or if we use an acid agent such a cola beverage with the capsules [20]. Unfortunately, it has only recently been approved for parenteral use. Doses used range from 200 to 400 mg per day. Peak plasma concentration after a 200 mg dose averages 0.3 mcg/ml and it is three to five times higher after 7 to 10 days of treatment. In other words, serum levels may take up to one week to reach therapeutic levels and that is why a load dose should be used and serum levels should be monitored, knowing that good levels are above 2 mcg/ml and ideal levels above 8 mcg/ml [59]. The half-life is dependent on the dose and duration of administration and varies from 15 to 42 hours [60]. 99% of the drug binds to protein [36] and, unlike fluconazole, it penetrates very poorly into cerebrospinal fluid [61], although tissue concentrations in the brain, kidney, liver, lung and skin are two to five times greater than in plasma [62]. It has the ability to reach high intracellular concentrations, particularly in the immune cells, namely the alveolar macrophages [63]. It is metabolized by the liver and excreted in the feces, therefore no drug adjustments are necessary in renal failure and dialysis does not remove the drug [10, 64]. Severe infections should be treated with a loading dose of 300 mg twice daily for 3 to 4 days, followed by 200 to 400 mg per day. Its use in critically ill patients is however hampered by the absence, until very recently, of a parenteral formulation [65].

Itraconazole is a fungistatic agent active against *Aspergillus* species [66]; European studies report response rates of 63–70% for aspergillosis and the response is better in pulmonary than in disseminated aspergillosis. It is also active against many *Candida* species and isolates that are resistant to fluconazole are not necessarily cross-resistant to itraconazole [67], such as is the case of some *Candida krusei* and *Torulopsis glabrata* [45]. However, strains of *Candida* spp. which are highly resistant to fluconazole often have reduced susceptibility to itraconazole and even the newer azoles, as the SCOPE program has shown [46, 68, 69].

Itraconazole is also well tolerated, but can cause nausea, vomiting, abdominal discomfort and epigastric pain, constipation, dizziness, pruritus and allergic rashes. These effects are usually self-limiting [20, 41]. Hypokalemia may occur after prolonged therapy and hepatic function should be monitored as plasma transaminase elevation may occur. At high doses, hypertension has been described [20, 41]. It is contraindicated in patients with known hypersensitivity to azole derivatives or with severe hepatic impairment and in pregnancy [20]. Drug interactions are similar to those described for fluconazole and are summarized in Table 2.

A word must be said concerning the investigational azoles. Three new triazoles are undergoing clinical trials – voriconazole, BMS 207 147 and SCH 56 592 – all with extended spectrum activity against yeasts and molds *in vitro*, namely *Aspergillus* spp. [45] and all have done well in animal models of infection [70, 71]. Voriconazole may be particularly useful in the treatment of infections caused by *Aspergillus terreus*, which is often refractory to conventional amphotericin B [72], and those caused by fluconazole-resistant Candida, such as *Candida krusei* [73].

Amphotericin B is a polyene naturally recovered from *Streptomyces nodosus* in 1953 and commercially available since 1956. It binds to ergosterol, the principal sterol in the membrane of susceptible fungal cells, causing impairment of membrane barrier function, loss of cell constituents, metabolic disruption and cell death. In addition to its membrane permeabilizing effects, the drug can cause oxidative damage to fungal cells [11, 74]. It has minimal cutaneous or mucosal absorption, namely minimal absorption from the gastrointestinal tract. After intravenous administration levels are proportional to the dose and rate of infusion. Peak serum concentrations are 1.2 and 2.4 mg/ml after intravenous administration of 0.5 and 1 mg per Kg, respectively, and the peak mean serum concentrations increase when the infusion rate is increased [75, 76]. Its metabolism is complex. Plasma initial half-life is 24 hours but elimination half-life reaches 15 days. After 12 hours, less than 10% remains in the blood; it is widely distributed in tissues, mainly to the liver (24–41%), lungs (2–6%), kidney (0.6–2%) and spleen (0.7–1.6%) and much less to adipose tissue or muscle. It is slowly degraded and plasma levels remain detectable 7 to 8 weeks after treatment is stopped and the drug has been detected for longer than one year in liver, kidney and spleen. Serum concentrations do not reflect tissue concentrations and serum and tissue concentrations have unclear relationships to either toxicity or efficacy – therefore measuring drug levels is rarely of clinical value [77]. Protein binding is high (90–95%), it enters serous cavities, but penetration into cerebrospinal fluid is poor [41]. Only a small part of the compound is eliminated through the kidneys and biliary tract, therefore renal or hepatic impairment have little effect on serum drug levels and dialysis does not modify blood levels [10]. As it is not a water-soluble compound, a carrier must be used for clinical use. In its conventional form, deoxycholate and a buffer are added to amphotericin B, producing a colloidal suspension dispersion suitable for intravenous administration when suspended in a 5% glucose solution [78].

Amphotericin B may be fungistatic or fungicidal, depending on the concentration obtained and the susceptibility of the fungus, but it has the widest spectrum of activity amongst all the anti-fungals, with fungicidal effect against *Candida* species, *Aspergillus* species, *Blastomyces dermatitidis*, *Coccidioides immitis*, *Cryptococcus neoformans*, *Histoplasma capsulatum*, *Paracoccidioides brasiliensis* and *Sporothrix schenckii*. It is effective in certain forms of mucormycosis, hyalophomycosis and phaeohyphomycosis, but often ineffective in pseudallescheriosis and trichosporonosis and some fusariosis. Treatment failure attributable to the development of amphotericin resistance is rare. *Candida lusitanae* is resistant to amphotericin B [79] and resistant strains of *Candida guilliermondii*, *Candida tropicalis* and *Candida krusei*, with alterations in the cell membrane, including reduced amounts of ergosterol, have been isolated during treatment, but overall emergence of resistance during treatment is rare [11, 12]. It has been the drug of choice for severe invasive fungal infections in the last thirty years due to its very broad fungicidal activity against *Candida* spp. and *Aspergillus* spp. [21, 80]. In clinical studies, response rates were 55% for *Aspergillus* spp., 55–65% for *Candida* spp. and 75% for *Cryptococcus neoformans* [6, 81]. *Candida* with higher MIC to amphotericin B are difficult to treat and one should aim for serum levels of 1–2.5 mcg/ml [12].

Adverse effects of amphotericin B deoxycholate may be divided into infusion-related or acute and dose-related or late (Table 3). The peak frequency of fever, rigors and other infusion-related reactions, caused by production of TNF and PgE by macrophages [82], occurs on the first to third day of therapy and subsequently declines, generally subsiding after one week of therapy even without treatment [83, 84]. Longer infusion times were associated with a reduction in the incidence of infusion-related toxicities. Normochromic, normocytic anemia accompanies most 2–3 week courses of amphotericin B, with a decrease in haematocrit by as much as 35%, occurring secondary to decreased production of erythropoietin rather than to diminished bone marrow production; this effect is reversible when the drug is discontinued [85]. Nephrotoxicity is the most significant toxic effect of amphotericin B administration and about 80% of the patients receiving the drug show some degree of renal impairment, although generally reversible, especially those submitted to a cumulative dose higher than 0.5–1 gr, with sodium depletion, older than 30 years old, with abnormal baseline renal function and under other nephrotoxic drugs [86]. It manifests as azotaemia, decreased urinary concentration ability, renal tubular acidosis, symptomatic hypokalemia or renal magnesium wasting [87]. Signs of nephrotoxicity usually occur within the

TABLE 3. Adverse effects of amphotericin B

Frequency	Dose-related	Infusion-related
Commom	Renal failure (30%) Kaliuria Magnesuria Anemia	Fever (30–90%) Rigors (30–75%) Nausea (4–60%) Vomiting Diarrhea
Uncommon	Bronchospasm Hypotension	Headache Thrombophlebitis Myalgia Arthralgia
Rare	Asystole Bradycardia Thrombocytopenia Neutropenia Malignant hyperthermia Ventricular fibrillation Acute liver failure Seizures Flushing/rash Hearing loss	

first four days of starting a course of treatment. An adequate assessment of patients before, during and after therapy may help reduce this toxicity [88]. Preventive measures consist of: avoiding salt depletion, use of concomitants antibiotics with sodium salts, loading with 0.9% saline prior to infusion of amphotericin B [87] and use of pentoxyfyline [89]. Monitoring for increased serum creatinine, hypokalemia and hypomagnesemia should occur daily during the first weeks of therapy. Nephrotoxicity is usually reversible by increasing sodium loading, reducing dose, increasing dosing interval with total dose reduction or temporarily suspending the treatment when serum creatinine reaches approximately 3 mg/dl. Recommendations for the prevention and management of nephrotoxicity are summarized in Table 4. Interactions of the drug are shown in Table 2.

Due to these adverse effects, the maximal tolerable dose of amphotericin B deoxycholate is usually 0.6–1.0 mg/kg/day. Although recent works suggest the efficacy of lower dose regimens of 0.3–0.7 mg/kg/day [90, 91], there is also the knowledge that the maximal tolerable doses may sometimes be suboptimal for clinical success. Pharmacy has tried to resolve this problem by combining amphotericin in lipid-based formulations to reduce the toxicity of the conventional compound, especially nephrotoxicity, as they do not contain deoxycholate which is responsible for direct tubular toxicity [92–96]. Three formulations have been developed that differ in the way amphotericin B interacts with the lipid and therefore have different properties, but all can be given at doses significantly higher than amphotericin deoxycholate with less side effects [97, 98]. The lipid compounds are less toxic, equally less nephrotoxic and with maximum tolerated doses higher than that of amphotericin B deoxycholate [24]. Not only is nephrotoxicity uncommon with the lipid compounds as renal function may be improved or stabilized when they are substituted [24, 99]. This is particularly important in critically ill patients that are susceptible to many other causes of renal failure, like trauma, sepsis, drugs, etc. Nevertheless, the doses recommended for

TABLE 4. Recommendations for the prevention and management of amphotericin B nephrotoxicity (adapted from [77])

Dose-test
- 1 mg Amphotericin B
- Infuse test dose over 10–30 minutes without premedication

Maintenance dose
- 250–1000 ml normal saline prior to infusion
- Infuse 0.5–1.0 mg/kg in 0.1 mg/ml D5%W
- Do not use solutions containing electrolytes
- Administer entire desired maintenance dose on first day
- *Circumstances for gradual dose escalation:*
  - test dose reaction
  - history of prior amphotericin tolerance
  - suboptimal cardiopulmonary function
  - renal impairment
  - indolent fungal disease
- *Options if creatinine increases:*
  - increase sodium loading
  - increase dosing interval with total dose reduction
  - temporary suppression of treatment (if serum creatinine ≥ 30 mg/l)

Duration
- Infuse daily dose over 1 hour if <0.9 mg/kg and Cr Cl < 25 mg/min
- Infuse daily dose over 2 hours if ≥1.0 mg/kg
- Infuse daily dose over 4–6 hours if Cr Cl > 25 ml/min or hyperkalemia

Medications
- Premedicate for first three doses or one week; if no reactions omit
  - Fever: hydrocortisone 25–50 mg i.v./infusate or acetaminophen, paracetamol or ibuprofen
  - Nausea: diphenydramine 25–50 mg p.o. or i.v.
- Add 1000 U heparin for infusion through peripheral line
- Meperidine 25–50 mg i.v. every 15 minutes × 3, as needed for rigors
- If rigors are predictable, add meperidine 20–30 minutes before infusion

the three formulations are different: amphotericin B lipid complex (Abelcet) 5 mg/kg/day, amphotericin B colloidal dispersion (Amphocil) 4 mg/kg/day and liposomal amphotericin B (Ambisome) 1–3 mg/kg/day. Remember that when equivalent doses are compared with conventional amphotericin B, concentrations in serum with lipid formulations are lower, probably because of accumulation in the liver and spleen [100]. In spite of the inexistence of a properly controlled trial comparing those formulations with the parent compound, preclinical and clinical studies suggest that lipid-based formulations are likely to be as effective as conventional amphotericin B [24] and their adverse events are the same but significantly rarer, especially nephrotoxicity. In addition, 40 to 60% of the patients in which fungal infection was refractory to amphotericin B deoxycholate may respond to lipid-based formulations.

The pharmacokinetics of the lipid-based amphotericin B are related to its molecular structures. Amphotericin B lipid-complex (Abelcet) is rapidly and significantly taken up by the reticuloendothelial system, resulting in lower plasma levels and higher tissue penetration, namely in the lungs, liver and spleen, than conventional amphotericin B; in other words it has a lower area under the curve and higher volume of distribution [94, 96, 101, 102]. The lower plasma levels partially justify the lower incidence of nephrotoxicity of this compound compared to the parent one [95]. Abelcet is well tolerated and infusion-related side effects, such as chills, fever, nausea and tremor, are the most frequent adverse events [99, 103].

Plasma levels of amphotericin B colloidal dispersion (Amphocil) are also lower than those of deoxycholate, but a fair proportion is rapidly taken up by phagocytosis by the liver, which acts as a reservoir that slowly releases the drug [104]. Lung tissue concentrations are lower than those of Abelcet [105]. The incidence of nephrotoxicity is also smaller than for deoxycholate [106] and the incidence of hepatic toxicity is also low [107]. The most frequent adverse events are infusion-related, namely fever and chills, with a frequency that justifies pre-medication [108, 109, 110].

The small size of the liposomal amphotericin B (Ambisome) molecule leads to a low reticuloendothelial uptake, low distribution into tissues and therefore higher plasma and area under the curve levels [93]. It is very well tolerated, with low nephrotoxicity and a very low incidence of infusion-related toxicities. The most frequent adverse effects are hypokalemia and an increase in liver enzymes [111]. A recent randomized, double-blind, multicenter trial showed that liposomal amphotericin B is as effective as conventional amphotericin B for empirical anti-fungal therapy in patients with fever and neutropenia and it is associated with fewer breakthrough fungal infections, less infusion-related toxicity and less nephrotoxicity [112].

The three lipid formulations have a reduced propensity for causing toxicity but, considering positive but limited efficacy data and cost, should be reserved for special situations that are discussed further below or for second line therapy [113]. They were shown to be as effective as the conventional compound, but there are no controlled, randomized studies available comparing the three preparations [102, 114] and the articles published addressing this issue reached no conclusion and lack consistency [115]. Johnson *et al.* [116] compared the *in vitro* activities of the three lipid-based amphotericin B formulations with the parent compound, using the National Committee for Clinical Laboratory Standards (NCCLS) methodology. Overall the lipid complex (Abelcet) showed similar or slightly greater *in vitro* activity against *Candida albicans*, *Torulopsis glabrata*, *Candida krusei*, *Cryptococcus neoformans* and *Aspergillus fumigatus* than conventional amphotericin B, while liposomal (Ambisome) and colloidal dispersion amphotericin B (Amphocil) were two to four times less active than the first two. Nevertheless, any extrapolation of *in vitro* studies to *in vivo* should not be done. without taking into account the different pharmacokinetics of the lipid preparations. Abelcet has a short plasma half-life and seems to reach higher levels than the other two lipid compounds and the conventional product, while Ambisome, in an animal model, seems to achieve significantly higher cerebral concentration than deoxycholate and the other two lipid formulations. The three formulas concentrate well in the liver and they all produce low renal concentrations of the drug [70].

The pneumocandins/echinocandins, water-soluble lipopeptides with broad-spectrum fungicidal activity *in vitro*, are undergoing phase II studies. They inhibit fungal glucan 1,3β – glucan synthase, an essential enzyme for biosynthesis of the fungal cell wall. They are fungicidal *in vitro* and clinical trials for efficacy are in progress [117].

Other anti-fungal strategies may also be useful. Immunomodulators may be important adjuncts for the therapy of invasive mycosis. This is not a surprise as it is well known that both adequate number and function of granulocytes and intact cell-mediated immunity are essential to a good outcome. In the prophylactic setting, the American Society of Clinical Oncology recommended that G-CSF and GM-CSF should be used in patients with more than a 40% chance of acquiring a fungal infection [118]. Another study showed that in non-neutropenic patients with acute traumatic brain injury and cerebral hemorrhage the prophylactic administration of G-CSF was associated with decreased risk of bacteremia, but did not alter the incidence of other nosocomial infections, length of stay or mortality in this patient group [119]. In the therapeutical setting, some *in vitro* studies have proven that G-CSF, GM-CSF and interferon gamma may augment anti-fungal response of the immune system and that interferon gamma may be better than the first two recombinant cytokines in its ability to improve immune function against fungi [120]. These agents may therefore be used in persistently neutropenic patients with proven severe fungal infection [121].

Therapy of Fungal Infections

Candida spp. causes the huge majority of fungal infections, approximately 85%. Other fungi, namely *Aspergillus*, *Mucor*, *Fusarium*, *Trichosporum* and *Cryptococcus* are also the cause of infection in the ICU, but usually in the immunocompromised patient [81].

Aspergillus is an important pathogen in the neutropenic patient and in all those receiving immunosuppressive treatment for cancer or transplantation. It may also cause disease in HIV-infected patients and in patients with chronic obstructive pulmonary disease, brochiectasis, lung carcinoma, sarcoid or tuberculosis or in patients that were submitted to long-term corticotherapy [19, 122–125]. Mucormycosis (zygomycosis) is seldom seen in normal patients, as the major risk factors are uncontrolled diabetes mellitus, other forms of metabolic acidosis, burns and malignant hematological disorders [11, 19]. *Fusarium* spp. are increasingly recognized as the cause of infection in neutropenic cancer patients and burn and trauma patients [19]. Disseminated trichosporonosis was reported in bone marrow and solid organ transplant, in neutropenic hematological oncological patients after chemotherapy and in AIDS patients; localized deep infections may occur in immunocompetent patients as a complication of cataract extraction, insertion of prosthetic heart valves, intravenous drug abuse, peritoneal dialysis and topical steroid treatment [19, 126]. *Pseudallescheria* infection may occur in patients with structural lung disease, immunosuppression and following trauma [19, 127]. *Cryptococcus neoformans* can cause disease in normal individuals, but a high proportion of human infections occur in compromised patients, especially in persons with impairment of T-cell-mediated immunological function, such as the HIV-patient [11, 19].

Table 5 describes the therapeutic strategies for non-Candida fungal infections. Amphotericin B is the drug of choice for all these infections, except Pseudallescheriosis and perhaps Trichosporonosis. In fact, amphotericin B resistant *Trichosporon beigelii* have been described [126] and *Pseudallescheria boydii* is often resistant to that drug [127]. However, the lipid formulations result in better tissue distribution in liver, spleen and lungs than deoxycholate and therefore may be active against infections where effective concentrations of amphotericin B are not readily achievable, such as those caused by *Aspergillus* spp., *Fusarium* spp. and *Mucorales* [128]. The dose of liposomal amphotericin B for invasive aspergillosis is still debatable. An EORTC study showed that doses of 1 mg/kg/day versus 4 mg/kg/day were equal in terms of clinical and radiological response or in survival rate, however the study included a small number of patients with proven cases [129].

Candida spp. are the cause of the vast majority of fungal infections in the ICU, but their diagnosis is usually very difficult. The gold standard of diagnosis is the presence of positive blood cultures and histological evidence from culture of tissue sample obtained at from least one internal organ, but most diagnoses are based in presumptive criteria and clinical suspicion is undoubtedly the key to diagnosis and to an adequate therapeutic decision. *Candida* genus includes more than 150 species and 11 of them

TABLE 5. Therapeutic strategies for non-*Candida* fungal infections in the ICU

Disease	Therapy	Alternative Therapy
Invasive acute aspergillosis	Ampho[a] 1.0–1.5 mg/kg/day or Ab[b] 5 mg/kg/day	Amb[c] ≥ 3–5 mg/kg/day or Amphocil 3–4 mg/kg/day or Itraco[d] 400–600 mg/day 4 days and then 200 mg bid
Cerebral aspergillosis	Amb ≥ 3–5 mg/kg/day	
Aspergillus Invasive sinusitis	Ampho 1 mg/kg/day or Amb 3–5 mg/kg/day	Itraco 400–600 mg/day
Cryptococcus meningitis	Ampho 0.7 mg/kg/day + Flucy[e] 37.5 mg/kg/day (4–6 w)	Fluco[f] 400–800 mg/day or Itraco 400 mg/day (6–8 w)
Cryptococcus meningitis in AIDS	Ampho 0.7 mg/kg/day + Flucy 100–150 mg/kg/day or Amb 5 mg/kg/day (6 w) (quicker response and less relapses)	Ampho 0.7 mg/kg/day (2 w) then Fluco 400 mg/day (8 w) then 200 mg/day or Fluco 800 mg/day
Pulmonary cryptococcosis	Ampho 0.3–0.6 mg/kg/day ± Flucy (4–6 w)	Fluco 400 mg/day (4–6 w)
Rhinocerebral, lung or cutaneous mucormycosis	Lipid Ampho ≥ 5 mg/kg/day (8 w) + Reversion predisposing conditions + agressive surgery	Ampho 1.0–1.5 mg/kg/day or Itraco
Fusariose	Lipid Ampho + correction of neutropenia	Ampho 1.0–1.5 mg/kg/day or Itraco
Trichosporonosis	Fluco 800–1200 mg/day + correction of neutropenia	Lipid Ampho
Pseudallescheria infection	Fluco 800–1200 mg/day + surgery, if possible	Itraco 200 mg bid or Miconazole 600 mg od

[a] Amphotericin B; [b] Abelcet; [c] Ambisome; [d] Itraconazole; [e] Flucytosine; [f] Fluconazole.

have already been isolated in the human. Although *Candida albicans* remains the most prevalent species, there has been a clear shift towards non-albicans species [46, 69, 130], namely *Candida tropicalis*, *Candida parapsilosis*, *Candida krusei* (particularly in the neutropenic patient) and *Torulopsis glabrata* (especially in patients with solid tumors). Six multicenter surveys showed that 42 to 50% of systemic fungal infections were caused by non-albicans species [69, 131–135]. SENTRY, epidemiology and fungal susceptibility program performed in the USA, Canada and South America, demonstrated that 47% of the candidemias were caused by non-albicans species and that *Candida parapsilosis*, *Torulopsis glabrata* and *Candida tropicalis* caused almost 40% [68]. A species very similar to albicans has also been described, first in oropharyngitis in HIV patients and more recently in HIV negative patients: *Candida dubliniensis* [136]. This increase in the incidence of non-albicans Candida species in intensive care units is in part due to the pressure caused by the frequent use of fluconazole [137–144]. This question has enormous clinical and therapeutic relevance as some species show some particularities. For instance, *Candida tropicalis* shows a higher invasive capacity as 50–60% of the colonized patients develop disseminated candidiasis; *Candida parapsilosis* is associated with total parenteral nutrition and with central venous catheter, infection by this species is often not preceded by colonization and it may be less susceptible to killing by amphotericin B; *Candida lusitanae* [145] may be resistant *ab initio* or easily develops resistance to amphotericin B and, less often, to fluconazole; *Torulopsis glabrata* is commonly resistant to fluconazole or resistance may emerge; *Candida krusei* is virtually always intrinsically resistant to this drug and *Candida dubliniensis* is sometimes but seldom resistant to fluconazole but susceptible to other azoles.

WHEN TO START ANTI-FUNGAL THERAPY?

As the diagnosis is difficult and usually presumptive, deciding when to start anti-fungal therapy is problematic and, given the high morbidity and mortality associated with fungal infections, the British Society of Antimicrobial Chemotherapy Working Party analyzed the four broad approaches to the use of antimicrobial therapy – prophylaxis, pre-emptive therapy, empirical therapy and definitive therapy – in terms of fungal infection [47].

Prophylaxis, the preventive therapy of a whole population regardless of individual risk factors, is not indicated in the ICU or in the surgical setting and concerns about the selection of less susceptible *Candida* spp. have limited this approach [21, 47]. Safran [145] showed that 22% of patients in a surgical ICU treated with fluconazole had secondary fungal infections frequently resistant to fluconazole and this finding was associated with a high mortality, namely 44% versus 9%. Even the use of anti-fungal agents, together with antibacterial agents, as oral nonabsorbable antimicrobials to decontaminate the gastrointestinal tract did not prove to result in any difference in survival in trauma patients and patients under prolonged mechanical ventilation [146, 147]. Nevertheless, although not recommended in the intensive care setting, prophylaxis may be beneficial in a subgroup of patients at high risk of infection [148], such as the neutropenic, the bone marrow transplant, the lung transplant with history of fungal infection and the fulminant liver failure or liver transplant recipient patient [80, 148]. Fluconazole is the drug of choice for all these cases and it should be used for the least time to prevent the selection of azole-resistant organisms. Although the value of anti-fungal prophylaxis in cancer patients as a whole did not prove to be of benefit [149], and a study in neutropenic leukemic patients outside the BMT setting has shown that fluconazole reduced the incidence of mucocutaneous candidiasis but not of hematogenously disseminated fungal infections [150], two recent studies showed that fluconazole 400 mg daily [151] and itraconazole oral solution [152] in patients receiving intensive cytotoxic therapy for acute leukemia or bone marrow transplantation were able to reduce the number of fungal infections and their mortality. Therefore, fluconazole 400 mg daily, either orally or intravenously, should be used as prophylaxis for bone marrow transplantation, both allogenic or high-risk autologous, while in neutropenic leukemic patients its use is still controversial and decisions should be made at each center on the basis of the fungal epidemiology [153], knowing that wherever and whenever the incidence of various forms of candidiasis is high its use is justifiable [154]. Selection of resistant species may be a problem [155], but such selection did not occur in several prospective, randomized studies involving neutropenic patients [150, 156]. In lung transplant recipients anti-fungal prophylaxis should be used for a minimum of 10 to 14 days after transplant and drugs with anti-Aspergillus activity should be preferred in centers where *Aspergillus* infections are frequent [148, 157]. Several studies showed that patients undergoing liver transplantation at high risk for fungal infections should receive fluconazole [158] and a retrospective review in the United Kingdom reported that the incidence of *Candida* infection and fungal infection mortality were decreased by the use of 100 mg/day of fluconazole [159].

Pre-emptive therapy is the treatment of individual patients thought to be at high risk of developing deep candidiasis, identified by clinical or laboratory markers, to prevent the disease. The British Working Party does not recommend this approach as there is no proof of its value [21, 47, 80], but they consider that patients at particular high-risk might be considered for this kind of therapy [47]. Some studies showed that subsets of critically ill patients in which the incidence of fungal infections is particularly high may benefit from the use of pre-emptive therapy. Such is the case of patients with extensive burns [160], patients on extracorporeal membrane oxygenation systems or on left ventricular assist devices [161, 162], patients with pancreatitis or those that have been submitted to gastrointestinal surgery [47]. A very recent randomized, prospective, double-blind, placebo-controlled study showed that fluconazole may prevent colonization and invasive intra-abdominal Candida infections in high-risk surgical patients [163].

Empirical therapy is the treatment of patients thought to have established deep candidiasis without microbiological, histological or serological confirmation. As fungal diagnosis is difficult, empirical therapy is and will continue to be necessary on some occasions. The Working Party proposed the following indications for empirical therapy: (a) clinically unstable or deteriorating premature neonate with skin breaks from which Candida has been grown or positive urine microscopy or culture for yeast was found; (b) candiduria in high-risk patient with deteriorating clinical status; (c) patients with prosthetic valve endocarditis likely to be due to *Candida*, even with negative blood cultures [47]. Some authors suggest that anti-candidal therapy should also be started in patients with peritonitis because of intestinal perforation below the duodenum, especially in cancer patients, immunosuppressed patients, when the perforation was not diagnosed for more than 24 hours, was hospital-acquired or occured in patients with unstable conditions, hepatic cirrhosis or pancreatitis or required a second unplanned abdominal operation [148]. Anti-fungal therapy is also frequently started empirically in cases of skin invasion in burn patients, candiduria in certain clinical settings defined in Table 6, two or more sites colonized by Candida in a high-risk patient and persistent fever unresponsive to broad-spectrum antibiotics in a high-risk patient.

TABLE 6. Candiduria plus any of these conditions should be considered high probability of invasive candidiasis and therefore a reason for anti-fungal therapy

Candiduria plus:
Piuria
Pseudo-hyphae in urine
Fever and signs of pyelonephritis
Tubular casts with *Candida*
Persistent candiduria even after changing urinary catheter
Candida tropicalis
Candida in other sites
Abdominal or urological surgery or procedure
Liver or renal transplant
Diabetes mellitus

Definitive therapy is the treatment of established deep candidiasis, which requires microbiological or histological evidence of fungal infection. The diagnosis of deep candidiasis is established by any of these: (a) at least one positive blood culture in an at risk patient or with acute clinical signs and symptoms compatible with the infection; (b) *Candida* isolated from any sterile site, except urine; (c) positive yeast microscopy from a sterile specimen; (d) histological evidence of yeast or mycelial forms in tissue from at risk patients [47].

Few are the cases in which anti-fungal therapy is started as definitive therapy. What usually happens in the intensive care setting is that you have to identify the patients at risk of developing fungal infection. The conditions associated with an increased risk [2, 164–166] are stated in Table 7. *Candida* colonization typically precedes infection with genotypically identical *Candida* strains. Thus *Candida* reservoir is clearly endogenous and colonization is an independent risk factor and also a prerequisite for *Candida* infection [167, 168]. Pittet *et al.* proposed the "Candida colonization index" to identify patients that should be put under early anti-

TABLE 7. Conditions associated with an increased risk of *Candida* infection

Immunosuppressive therapy
HIV infection
Malignancy
Major surgery, especially abdominal
Trauma
Burns
Malnutrition
Solid or bone marrow transplant
Neutropenia
Hepatic dysfunction
High severity score
Peritonitis
Acute pancreatitis
Advanced age
Broad-spectrum antibiotics (number and duration)
Total parenteral nutrition
Mechanical ventilation
Hemodyalisis
Invasive procedures
Long stay in ICU

fungal therapy [167]. The index is the ratio of the number of non-blood distinct sites colonized by *Candida* spp. to the total number of sites cultured and it was shown to predict the development of candidemia. A threshold of ≥0.5 accurately identified the infected patients. One must therefore maintain a high level of clinical suspicion for all these at risk patients in order to early identify patients with suspected fungal infection. In face of clinical suspicion, the following steps must be taken: (a) reassess risk factors for *Candida* infection; (b) assess the intensity of *Candida* colonization; (c) perform two sets of blood cultures per day in two consecutive days; (d) obtain cultures of all relevant specimens, according to the clinical scenario, namely respiratory specimens, urine, cerebrospinal fluid, wound, etc; (e) exclude other possible causes of fever; (f) perform chest teleradiography or chest CT scan if suspicion of fungal pneumonia; (g) assess sites of hematogenous dissemination: endophtalmitis (optic fundus examination) and septic thrombophlebitis.

WHICH ANTI-FUNGAL AGENT?

The choice of the anti-fungal for empiric therapy is based on the condition of the patient, namely his immune status and haemodynamic condition, and the species of Candida that are colonizing that specific patient or are more prevalent in that particular unit. In haemodynamically stable patients, not colonized by *Torulopsis glabrata* or *Candida krusei* and that were not previously treated with azoles and in units where these species are not prevalent, fluconazole may be used. If one of these conditions is not satisfied, amphotericin B should be preferred (Figure 2).

The choice of the anti-fungal agent for definitive therapy is based on the identity of the fungus and the condition of the patient (Figure 3). The currently available systemic antifungal agents useful in the intensive care setting are amphotericin B, amphotericin B lipid-preparations and fluconazole, while itraconazole and flucytosine are less often useful and utilized.

In the past, patients with candidemia thought to have a low risk of developing a disseminated candidiasis were left untreated. This was based on the belief that Candida was a "benign pathogen" and that candidemia was often transient, beliefs that were defended in the late 1960s [169, 170]. Clinical practice proved this strategy to be wrong and *Candida* spp. to be a serious pathogen with high morbidity and mortality. Our capacity to determine prognostic signs or to predict patients with candidemia that would progress to disseminated candidiasis is poor; in fact, retrospective studies have shown an error rate of around 30% in defining a population of candidemic patients who do not require treatment [171]. Besides, less toxic anti-fungals and ways of decreasing the toxicity of amphotericin B were developed. All this generated the clear consensus that all candidemia should and must be treated [172]. At least four studies [173–176] showed that, in stable non-neutropenic patients, fluconazole may be consid-

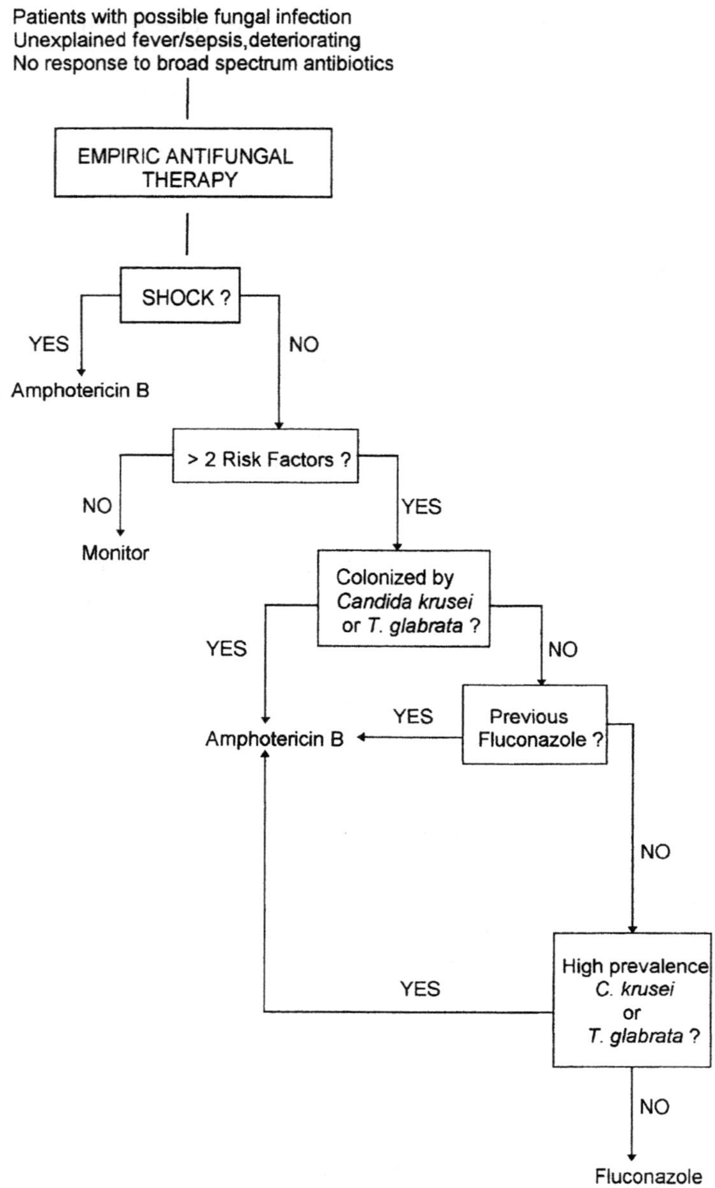

FIGURE 2. Algorithm for empiric antifungal therapy.

ered as an alternative to amphotericin B for first-line therapy of candidemia [148], unless it is caused by fluconazole-resistant yeasts like *Candida krusei* and often *Torulopsis glabrata* or it occurs in patients that have been previously or are at the moment under fluconazole or any other azole. Fluconazole showed the same efficacy but was significantly better tolerated and produced lower incidence of nephrotoxicity, namely in the Rex *et al.* study [176], the largest study of candidemia in non-neutropenic patients that compared fluconazole 400 mg per day with

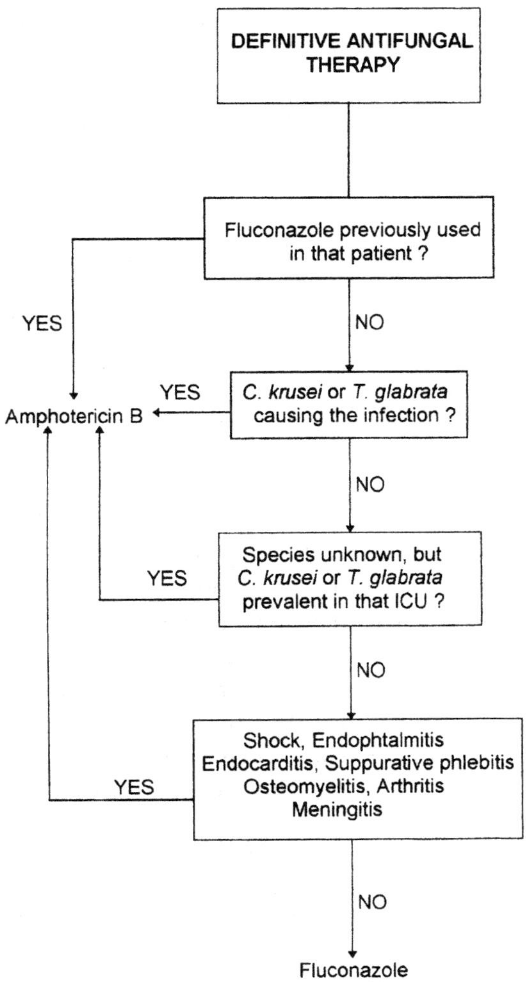

FIGURE 3. Algorithm for definitive antifungal therapy.

amphotericin B 0.6 mg/kg/day. Similar results were found in the neutropenic cancer patient [173]; side effects occurred in 5–12% for fluconazole and in 35–44% for amphotericin B. According to these results, fluconazole could be considered as the drug of choice for Candida infection, but this conclusion must be taken with caution as the number of non-albicans species, namely those intrinsically resistant and those with acquired resistance to fluconazole, are increasing [80, 133].

Fluconazole is clearly the best agent in two specific situations: infections caused by *Candida lusitanae* [177] and urinary tract candidiasis, due to its high urinary concentrations [47], while penetration of amphotericin B into the urine is poor. Candiduria is a frequent problem in the ICU, but the majority of cases do not require any treatment apart from catheter, and other urinary prosthetic materials, change [178, 179]; this measure is highly successful, 87 to 93% at 8 weeks, in clearing funguria [180]. Nevertheless, funguria may also be an early marker of disseminated infection in the critically ill patient [181] and a recent study documented that clinicians tend to react to any candiduria by prescribing anti-fungal therapy, either fluconazole or amphotericin B bladder irrigation or both [182]. Table 6 summarizes the conditions and situations in which we treat candiduria [183, 184], using catheter change and fluconazole 200–400 mg/day. If candiduria is persistent after this, we use irrigation with 5–10 mg of amphotericin B with an intravesical dwell time of 2 hours, once or twice daily for two days. Bladder irrigation is more effective when the drug concentration is 50 mg/l rather than 10 mg/l [185]. It has been compared with systemic fluconazole and shown to be equally effective for Candida cystitis [184, 186], but it is clearly more staff and time-consuming. Fluconazole may also be the preferred drug in oesophagitis, peritonitis, wound infection and pyelonephritis by *Candida*. There are, however, some doubts about the optimal dose of fluconazole, namely 5 mg/kg/day or 10 mg/kg/day. A study by Graninger *et al.* [187] showed higher cure rates when the higher dose was used: 83% versus 60%. Some authors recommend that treatment should be started with a higher dose, for instance 600–800 mg/day i.v., for three days and then followed by 400 mg/day i.v. or orally [21]. Although 5 mg/kg/day is the usual dose, at least patients on hemodiafiltration should receive a higher dose as the elimination rate of fluconazole by continuous veno-venous haemodyalisis depends on the combined dialysate/ultrafiltrate flow rate but is much higher than that achieved with continuous veno-venous haemofiltration or intermittent haemodyalisis [187–189]. A higher dose should also be used for catabolic patients and in children. In fact, fluconazole half-life in children is substantially shorter than in adults and therefore, because of the more rapid clearance [190, 191], life-threatening invasive candidiasis in children should be treated with a dosage of 6 mg/kg twice daily, assuming that renal function is normal. This dosing provides an area under the concentration versus time curve in children that approximates that in adults treated once daily. In infants, however, renal clearance of fluconazole is slower than in older children and therefore a dose of 5 mg/kg/day should be used [148]. A word for the fact that fluconazole has also been shown to be effective in the treatment of chronic disseminated candidiasis, even after prior amphotericin B therapy [192, 193] and that it can at least be useful for maintenance therapy after response to amphotericin B therapy. In the liver transplant setting, as the azoles, through their effect on hepatic microsomial function, inhibit the metabolism of cyclosporin and tacrolimus, doses of fluconazole should be limited to 200–400 mg/day and the safety and efficacy of these doses in this setting have been demonstrated, including in patients with severe allograft dysfunction [194, 195].

Amphotericin B should be preferred in any clinically unstable, deteriorating patient, in patients with high-grade candidemia or in patients with hematogenous deep-organ infections, like severe endophtalmitis, suppurative phlebitis, endocarditis, pericarditis, osteomyelitis and meningitis. It may be used alone or in association with flucytosine [18, 47, 80, 148, 196], but the use of this agent requires facilities for monitoring serum concentrations and seems to be only justified in patients with high-grade persistent fungaemia or perhaps with infection in sites where penetration of amphotericin B is far from ideal as vegetations, meninges and vitreous. In the case of endophtalmitis, amphotericin B i.v. is usually enough, but if lesions are expansive or close to the macula flucytosine should be added; consultation with an ophthalmologist is mandatory in all cases and in large, progressive or symptomatic lesions the use of 5 mg amphotericin B intra-vitreal and partial vitrectomy may be needed and even be sight-saving procedures. There are very few data on the efficacy of azole treatment for hematogenous candidal endophtalmitis, although its use is documented in 96 patients and 108 eyes with good response rate, about 90%, with 200–400 mg/day of fluconazole for 6–8 weeks [197] and some series also suggest its efficacy [198, 199]. However, two studies in animal models [200, 201] and one clinical study [202] have shown less satisfactory results.

The use of conventional amphotericin B is restricted by dose-limiting side effects, including infusion related symptoms and nephrotoxicity. The lipid formulations of amphotericin B are better tolerated. They should be used in patients who fail treatment with the conventional formulation – as 40 to 60% of the refractory patients may respond –, in patients who are intolerant to the parent compound, in patients with renal failure – creatinine clearance lower than 25 ml/min –, in patients receiving markedly nephrotoxic drugs and in patients infected by fungi with high MICs to amphotericin B, like *Mucorales*, *Fusarium* and some *Aspergillus*. These forms have, as we have stated before, higher therapeutic index, owing to reduced toxicity and to organ distribution, resulting in targeting the drug to the reticular endothelial system and sites of inflammation, such as liver, spleen and lung [203]. Although the clinical significance of the difference in the tissue distribution of the several compounds is not totally known, it seems to be an important determinant of treatment outcome. For instance, Abelcet obtains the highest concentration in the lung [204]. Recently a large study showed that patients with life-threatening mycosis were successfully treated with Abelcet 5 mg/kg/day, after failure of or intolerance to amphotericin B deoxycholate [99] and the same kind of results were obtained with Amphocil

(0.5–7.5 mg/kg/day) in patients with candidemia [205]. In a randomized, multicenter study in neutropenic patients with documented or suspected fungal infections, Ambisome 5 mg/kg/day was superior to amphotericin B 1 mg/kg/day in terms of efficacy and safety (114). Table 8 summarizes the therapies proposed for *Candida* infections in the critically ill patient.

Although *in vitro* studies indicated some antagonism between fluconazole and amphotericin B [206], this effect may not be relevant *in vivo* [207] and, although there are no definitive data to support combination therapy, it has been utilized by some in severely acutely ill patients with systemic mycosis and septic shock or even in transplant recipients [19]. A trial of fluconazole plus amphotericin B for candidemia in non-neutropenic patients is currently under way and until the combination has been adequately evaluated, it should be used with caution.

The American Society of Clinical Oncology and the European Organization for Research and Treatment of Cancer recommended the use of G-CSF and GM-CSF in patients with febrile neutropenia for whom expected incidence of infection is 40% or more and also in future chemotherapy cycles after a documented fungal febrile episode occurs in association with neutropenia during a prior chemotherapy cycle [118, 208]. The rationale for using immunomodulators in the treatment of systemic mycosis seems solid. Several *in vitro* and animal studies showed that interferon-gamma, colony-stimulating factors and various interleukins and interleukin-antagonists have a role in the treatment. Very few trials have been concluded in humans, however two studies recommend the use of granulocyte-colony stimulating factor (G-CSF) or granulocyte macrophage-colony stimulating factor (GM-CSF) for the treatment of proven persistent candidiasis in neutropenic

TABLE 8. Therapeutic strategies for *Candida* infection in the ICU

Infection	Agent of choice	Alternative
Candidemia	Amphotericin B 0.5–1 mg/kg/day or Fluconazole 400–600 mg/day	Lipid-based Amphotericin B
Endophtalmitis	Amphotericin B 1 mg/kg/day ± Flucytosine	Fluconazole 400–800 mg/day
Endocarditis	Amphotericin B 1 mg/kg/day ± Flucytosine	Fluconazole 400–800 mg/day or Ambisome 3 mg/kg/day
Meningitis	Amphotericin B 1 mg/kg/day ± Flucytosine	Fluconazole 400–800 mg/day
Suppurative phlebitis	Amphotericin B 0.5–1 mg/kg/day ± Flucytosine	Fluconazole 400–800 mg/day
Osteomyelitis/Arthritis	Amphotericin B 0.5–0.7 mg/kg/day	Fluconazole 400 mg/day
Pericarditis	Amphotericin B 0.5–0.7 mg/kg/day	Fluconazole 400 mg/day
Peritonitis and Intra-abdominal infection	Amphotericin B 0.5–0.7 mg/kg/day	Fluconazole 400–600 mg/day
Oesophagitis	Fluconazole 400 mg/day	Amphotericin B 0.5–0.7 mg/kg/day
Wound infection	Fluconazole 400 mg/day	Amphotericin B 0.5–0.7 mg/kg/day
Pyelonephritis	Fluconazole 400 mg/day	
Cystitis	Fluconazole 200–400 mg/day	

patients [121, 209] based on the fact that they may not only accelerate recovery from neutropenia but also enhance the activity of neutrophils against *Candida* [210, 211]. These recommendations were made, however, in the absence of any data from a proper clinical trial study and the use of cytokines as adjuncts to therapy has not proved to reduce mortality [148].

Non-pharmacological strategies are also fundamental for the success of the anti-fungal treatment. Fair amount of data shows that removal of intravenous catheters is essential for the therapy of candidemia and is associated with more rapid clearance of the bloodstream and probably with a reduction of mortality [171, 212–216]. Although some potential bias may be found in all these studies, they all point to the same conclusion. A post-hoc analysis of the Rex *et al.* study [133] is concordant with the same conclusion, showing that the removal of the catheter reduces the duration of candidemia from 5.5 to 4.2 days and in the Nguyen *et al.* study [175] mortality is reduced in around 20%. Generally, removal of prosthetic materials is essential for the cure of the *Candida* infection, namely urinary catheters in urinary tract infections and drains in peritonitis, that may also require peritoneal lavage. *Candida* suppurative phlebitis requires ressection of the vein or artery [217]. All patients with *Candida* endocarditis except neonates require valve replacement [218].

WHEN TO STOP ANTI-FUNGAL THERAPY?

The duration of therapy is also a matter of debate. For the most severe invasive mycosis it should be at least four weeks [47]. In severe forms, in very critically ill patients it should be even longer, around 8 weeks, although the intensity of dosing can often be decreased after the first two weeks of therapy [47]. For hematogenous candidiasis, immunosuppressed patients should be treated for at least 10 to 14 days and immunocompetent patients for at least 5 days after the disappearance of all symptoms and signs of infection [19]. In the neutropenic, it must be continued throughout the duration of neutropenia. In the case of endophtalmitis, therapy must be continued until at least 10 days after the ocular lesion has resolved [18]. The rate of visceral seeding following candidemia in solid organ transplant recipients is significantly higher than that for the general population, exceeding 50% at some centers, and therefore therapy must continue for at least 2 weeks after the last positive blood culture and clinical response has occurred [148].

Maintenance therapy is only indicated in patients with persistent presence of foreign material infected with Candida which cannot be removed, as vascular grafts, artificial joints or ventriculoperitoneal shunts. In the case of impossibility of removal, lifelong therapy with anti-fungal agent should be performed, usually with fluconazole 100–200 mg/day. If the agent is resistant to fluconazole, intermittent amphotericin B or itraconazole should be used, depending on susceptibility tests. However, patients with candidemia should be followed for at least three months after the initial episode, as most late complications occur during this period [219, 220].

Conclusions

The incidence of severe fungal infections has increased markedly in the last decade, especially in hospitalized critically ill patients and one of the reasons for this increase is, unarguably, the progress of medicine itself, both technologically and pharmacologically. The development of anti-fungal agents did not accompany the speed of augmentation of these infections and amphotericin B and fluconazole are still the most used anti-fungals in the intensive care setting. The increasing incidence and high attributable mortality raised the discussion about the use of prophylactic and pre-emptive anti-fungal therapy and the increasing and widespread use of these strategies is contributing to the selection of more resistant fungi.

Better diagnostic techniques are needed and until then we should reinforce the development of research about the identification of patients at high risk of fungal infection, so that a clear definition of an at risk population might produce a correct allocation of pre-emptive or empirical therapy. Equal reinforcement should be given for the research on new anti-fungals, with less toxicity and higher therapeutic index to overcome the emergence of resistant species.

References

1. Beck-Sague C, Jarvis WR. Secular trends in the epidemiology of nosocomial fungal infections in the United States, 1980–1990. J Infect Dis 167:1247, 1993.
2. Fridkin SK, Jarvis WR. Epidemilogy of nosocomial fungal infections. Clin Microbiol Rev 9:499, 1996.
3. Vincent JL, Bihari DJ, Suter PM, Bruining HA, White J, Nicolas-Chanoine M-H, Wolff M, Spencer RC, Hemmer MD. The prevalence of nosocomial infection in intensive care units in Europe (EPIC). JAMA 274:639, 1995.
4. Jarvis WR. Epidemiology of nosocomial fungal infections, with emphasis on *Candida* species. Clin Infect Dis 20:1526, 1995.
5. Pittet D. Nosocomial blood stream infections. In Wenzel RP (ed). Prevention and Control of Nosocomial Infections, 2nd edn. Baltimore Williams and Wilkins. 1993:512.
6. Wey SB, Motomi M, Pfaller MA, Woolson RF, Wenzel RP. Hospital acquired candidemia: the attributable mortality and excess length of stay. Arch Intern Med 148:2642, 1988.
7. Elewski BE. Mechanisms of action of systemic antifungal agents. J Am Acad Dermatol 28(5): S28, 1993.
8. Johnson E. Mycological activity of antifungal agents. In The management of fungal in the ICU. Vincent JL (ed). The Liposome Company, 1999:43.
9. Hoeprich PD. Chemotherapy for systemic mycosis. Prog Drug Res 33:317, 1989.
10. Terrell CL, Hughes CE. Antifungal agents used for deep-seated mycotic infections. Mayo Clin Proc 67:69, 1992.
11. Richardson MD, Warnock DW. Antifungal drugs. In Fungal infections – diagnosis and management. 2nd edn. Oxford Blackwell Science. 1997:21.
12. Iwata K. Drug resistance in human pathogenic fungi. Eur J Epidemiol 8:407, 1992.
13. Bennett JE. Flucytosine. Ann Int Med 86:319, 1977.
14. Benson JM, Nahata MC. Clinical use of systemic antifungal agents. Clin Pharm 7:424, 1988.
15. Medoff G, Comfort M, Kobayashi GS. Synergistic action of amphotericin B and 5-flucytosine against yeast-like organisms. Proc Soc Exp Biol Med 138:571, 1971.
16. Beggs WH, Andrews FA, Sarosi GA. Combined action of amphotericin B and 5-flucytosine on pathogenic yeasts susceptible to either drugs alone. Chemotherapy 27:247, 1981.
17. Francis P, Walsh TJ. Evolving role of flucytosine in immunocompromised patients: new insights into safety, pharmacokinetic and antifungal therapy. Clin Infect Dis 15:1003, 1992.
18. Anaissie E, Solomkin JS. Fungal infection. In Care of the surgical patient. Willmore DW, Cheung LY, Harken AH and American College of Surgeons (eds). New York Scientific American Medical 1994:1.
19. Hastings M, Wolff M. Current treatment of fungal infections in the ICU. In The management of fungal in the ICU. Vincent JL (ed). The Liposome Company, 1999:55.
20. Richardson MD, Kokki M. Therapeutic guidelines in systemic fungal infections. Current Medical Literature, London, 1998.
21. Vincent JL, Anaissie E, Bruining H, Demajo W, El-Ebiary M, Haber J, Hiramatsu I *et al.* Epidemiology, diagnosis and treatment of systemic *Candida* infection in surgical patients under intensive care. Int Care Med 24:206, 1998.
22. Schafer-Korting M. Pharmacokinetic optimization of oral antifungal therapy. Clin Pharmacokinet 25:329, 1993.
23. British Society for Antimicrobial Chemotherapy Working Party on Fungal Infections. Laboratory monitoring of antifungal chemotherapy. Lancet 35:1577, 1991.
24. Viscoli C, Castagnola E. Advantages and disadvantages of current therapy. In The management of fungal in the ICU. Vincent JL (ed). The Liposome Company:71, 1999.
25. Stamm AM, Diasio RB, Dismukes WE *et al.* Toxicity of amphotericin B plus flucytosine in 194 patients with cryptococcal meningitis. Am J Med 83:236, 1987.
26. Dellamonica P, Fournier JP, Garraffo R *et al.* Contribution à la surveillance des traitments comportant de la 5-fluocytosine. Pathol Biol (Paris) 33:642, 1985.

27. Bennett JE, Dismukes WE, Duma RJ *et al.* A comparison of amphotericin B alone and combined with flucytosine in the treatment of crytococcal meningitis. N Engl J Med 301:126, 1979.
28. Como JA, Dismukes WE. Oral azoles as systemic antifungal therapy. N Engl J Med 330:263, 1994.
29. Lavrijsen KLM, van Hout JMG, van Dick DMJ *et al.* Induction potential of fluconazole toward drug-metabolizing enzymes in rat. Amtimicrob Agents Chemother 34:402, 1990.
30. Joly V, Bolard J, Yeni P. *In vitro* models for studying toxicity of antifungal agents. Antimicrob Agents Chemother 36:1799, 1992.
31. vandenBossche H, Marichal P, Le Jeune L *et al.* Effects of itraconazole on cytochrome P450-dependent sterol 14-alpha-demethylation and reduction of 3-ketosteroids in *Crytococcus neoformans*. Antimicrob Agents Chemother 37(10): 2101, 1993.
32. Kramer KM, Tesquet D, Johnson AL, Johnston LH. Budding yeast RSI1/APC2, a novel gene necessary for initiation of anaphase, encodes an APC subunit. EMBO J 17:498, 1998.
33. Goa KL, Barradell LB. Fluconazole – an update of its pharmacodynamic, pharmacokinetic properties and therapeutic use in major superficial and systemic mycosis in immunocompromised patients. Drugs 50:658, 1995.
34. Blum RA, D' Andrea DT, Fiorentino BM *et al.* Increased gastric pH and the bioavailability of fluconazole and ketoconazole. Ann Int Med 114:755, 1991.
35. Anaissie EJ, Kontoyiannis DP, Huls C, Vartivarian SE, Karl C, Prince RA, Bosso J, Bodey GP. Safety, plasma concentrations and efficacy of high-dose fluconazole in invasive moulds infections. J Infect Dis 172:599, 1995.
36. Saag MS, Dismukes WE. Azole anti-fungal agents: emphasis on new triazoles. Antimicrob Agents Chemother 32(1):1, 1988.
37. Fischman AJ, Alpert NM, Livni E *et al.* Pharmacokinetics of 18 F-labeled fluconazole in healthy human subjects by positron emission tomography. Antimicrob Agents Chemother 37:1270, 1993.
38. Humphrey MJ, Jevons S, Tarbit MH. Pharmacokinetic evaluation of UK-49858, a metabolically stable triazole antifungal drug, in animals and humans. Antimicrob Agents Chemother 28:648, 1985.
39. Graybill JR. New antifungal agents. Eur J Clin Microbiol Infect Dis 8:402, 1989.
40. Toon S, Ross CE, Gokal R, Rowland M. An assessment of the effects of impaired renal function and hemodyalisis on the pharmacokinetics of fluconazole. Br J Clin Pharmacol 29:221, 1990.
41. Silvestri L, Mur Laffon D, Gullo A. Antifungal agents. In Infection control in the intensive care unit. van Saene HKF, Silvestri L, de la Cal MA (eds). Milano, Springer 1998:50.
42. Tucker RM, William PL, Arathon EG *et al.* Pharmacokinetics of fluconazole in cerebrospinal fluid and serum in human coccidioidal meningitis. Antimicrob Agents Chemother 32:369, 1988.
43. Arndt CAS, Walsh TJ, McCully CL *et al.* Fluconazole penetration into cerebrospinal fluid: implications for treating fungal infections of the central nervous system. J Infect Dis 157: 178, 1988.
44. Bery AJ, Rinaldi MG, Graybill JR. Use of high-dose fluconazole as salvage therapy for cryptococcal meningitis in patients with AIDS. Antimicrob Agents Chemother 36:690, 1992.
45. Nguyen MH, Yu CY. Voriconazole against fluconazole-susceptible and resistant *Candida* isolates: *in vitro* efficacy compared with that of itraconazole and ketoconazole. J Antimicrob Chemother 42:253, 1998.
46. Pfaller MA, Jones RN, Messer SA, Edmond MB, Wenzel RP. National surveillance of nosocomial bloodstream infections due to *Candida albicans*: frequency of occurrence and antifungal susceptibility in the SCOPE Program. Diagn Microbiol Infect Dis 31:327, 1998.
47. British Society for Antimicrobial Chemotherapy Working Party. Management of deep *Candida* infection in surgical and intensive care units. Intensive Care Med 20:522, 1994.
48. Sanglard D, Ischer F, Monod M, Bille J. Susceptibilities of *Candida albicans* multidrug transporter mutants to various antifungal agents and other metabolic inhibitors. Antimicrob Agents Chemother 40:2300, 1996.
49. Hernaez ML, Gil C, Pla J, Nombela C. Induced expression of the *Candida albicans* multidrug resistance gene CDR1 in response to fluconazole and other antifungals. Yeasts 14:517, 1998.
50. White MH, Bowden RA, Sandler ES *et al.* Randomized, double-blind clinical trial of amphotericin B colloidal dispersion versus amphotericin B in the empirical treatment of fever and neutropenia. Clin Infect Dis 271:296, 1998.

51. Marr KA, Lyons CN, Rustad T, Bowden RA, White TC. Rapid, transient fluconazole resistance in *Candida albicans* is associated with increased mRNA levels of CDR. Antimicrob Agents Chemother 42:2584, 1998.
52. Moran GP, Sanglard D, Donnelly SM, Shanley DB, Sullivan DJ, Coleman DC. Identification and expression of multidrug transporters responsible for fluconazole resistance in *Candida dubliniensis*. Antimicrob Agents Chemother 42:1819, 1998.
53. Bronstein JA, Gros P, Hernandez E, Larroque P, Molinie C. Fatal acute hepatitis necrosis due to dose-dependant fluconazole hepatotoxicity. Clin Infect Dis 25:1266, 1997.
54. Munoz P, Moreno S, Berenguer J *et al.* Fluconazole-related hepatotoxicity in patients with acquired immunodeficiency syndrome. Arch Intern Med 151:1020, 1991.
55. Hay RJ. Risk/benefit ratio of modern antifungal therapy: focus on hepatic reactions. J Am Acad Dermatol 29:S50, 1993.
56. Albengres E, Le Louet H, Tillement JP. Systemic antifungal agents. Drug interactions of clinical significance. Drug Saf 18:83, 1998.
57. Michalets EL. Update: clinically significant cytochrome P450 drug interactions. Pharmacotherapy 18:84, 1998.
58. Barone JA, Koh JA, Bierman RH *et al.* Food interaction and steady-state pharmacokinetics of itraconazole in healthy male volunteers. Antimicrob Agents Chemother 37:778, 1993.
59. Daneshmend TK, Warnock DW. Clinical pharmacokinetics of systemic anti-fungal drug. Clin Pharmacokinet 8:17, 1983.
60. Hardin TC, Graybill JR, Fetchick R *et al.* Pharmacokinetics of itraconazole following oral administration to normal volunteers. Antimicrob Agents Chemother 32:1310, 1998.
61. Perfect JR, Savani DV, Durack DT. Penetration of imidazoles and triazoles into cerebrospinal fluid of rabbits. J Antimicrob Chemother 16: 81, 1985.
62. van Cutsem J, van Gerven F, Janssen PA. Activity of orally, topically and parenterally administered itraconazole in the treatment of superficial and deep mycosis: animal models. Rev Infect Dis 9:S15, 1987.
63. Perfect JR, Savani DV, Durack DT. Uptake of itraconazole by alveolar macrophages. Antimicrob Agents Chemother 37:903, 1993.
64. Walsh TJ, Pizzo A. Treatment of systemic fungal infections: recent progress and current problems. Eur J Clin Microbiol Infect Dis 7: 460, 1988.
65. Denning DW, Lee JY, Hosteler JS *et al.* NIAID Mycosis Study Group: Multicenter trial of oral itraconazole therapy for invasive aspergillosis. Am J Med 97:135, 1994.
66. De Pauw BE, Meis JF. Progress in fighting systemic fungal infections in hematological neoplasia. Support Care Cancer 6:31, 1998.
67. Johnson EM, Davey KG, Szekely A, Warnock DW. Itraconazole susceptibilities of fluconazole susceptible and resistant isolates of five *Candida* species. J Antimicrob Chemother 36:787, 1995.
68. Pfaller MA, Jones RN, Doern GV, Sader HS, Hollis RJ, Messer SA. International surveillance of bloodstream infections due to *Candida* species: frequency of occurrence and antifungal susceptibilities of isolates collected in 1997 in the United States, Canada and South America for the SENTRY Program. The SENTRY Participant Group. J Clin Microbiol 36:1886, 1998.
69. Pfaller MA, Jones RN, Messer SA, Edmond MB, Wenzel RP. National surveillance of nosocomial bloodstream infections due to species of *Candida* other than *Candida albicans*: frequency of occurrence and antifungal susceptibility in the SCOPE Program. Diagn Microbiol Infect Dis 30:121, 1998.
70. Groll AH, Walsh TJ. Potential new antifungal agents. Curr Opin Infect Dis 10:449, 1997.
71. Marco F, Pfaller MA, Messer SA, Jones RN. Antifungal activity of a new triazole, voriconazole (UK-109 496), compared with three other antifungal agents tested against clinical isolates of filamentous fungi. Med Mycol 36: 433, 1998.
72. Sutton DA, Sanche SE, Revankar SG, Fothergill AW, Rinaldi MG. *In vitro* amphotericin B resistance in clinical isolates of *Aspergillus terreus*, with a head-to-head comparison to voriconazole. J Clin Microbiol 37:2343, 1998.
73. Ghannoum MA, Okogbole-Wonodi I, Bhat N, Sanati H. Antifungal activity of voriconazole (UK-109 496), fluconazole and amphotericin B against hematogenous *Candida krusei* infection in neutropenic guinea pig model. Chemother 11:34, 1999.
74. Kerridge D. Polyene macrolides antibiotics. In Aspergillus and aspergillosis. vandenBossche H, Mackenzie DWR, Cavenberg (eds). New York: Plenum Press, 147.
75. Fields BT Jr, Bates JH, Abernathy RS. Ampho-

tericin B serum concentrations during therapy. Applied Microbiology 19:955, 1970.
76. Atkinson AJ Jr, Bennett JE. Amphotericin B pharmacokinetics in humans. Antimicrob Agents Chemother 13:271, 1978.
77. van Burik JA, Bowden RA. Standard antifungal treatment, including role of alternative modalities to administer amphotericin B. In Meunier F (ed.) Invasive fungal infections in cancer patients. Bailliere's clinical infectious diseases. London, Bailliere Tindel, vol 2 (n°1); chap 5; 1995:89.
78. Brajtburg J, Powderly WG, Kobayashi GS, Medoff G. Amphotericin B delivery systems. Antimicrob Agents Chemother 34:381, 1990.
79. Bodey GP. Antifungal agents. In Bodey GP (ed.) Candidiasis: pathogenesis, diagnosis and treatment. New York: Raven Press, 1991:371.
80. Flanagan PG, Barnes RA. Fungal infections in the intensive care unit. J Hosp Infect 38:163, 1998.
81. Warnock DW. Fungal complications of transplantation: diagnosis, treatment and prevention. J Antimicrob Chemother 36:73, 1995.
82. Chia JKS, McManus EJ. *In vitro* tumour necrosis factor induction assay for analysis of febrile toxicity associated with amphotericin B preparations. Antimicrob Agents Chemother 34:906, 1990.
83. Grasela TH, Goodwin SD, Walawandu MK *et al.* Prospective surveillance of intravenous amphotericin B use patterns. Pharmacotherapy 10:341, 1990.
84. Gelfand JA, Kimball K, Burke JF, Dinarello CA. Amphotericin B treatment of human mononuclear cells *in vitro* results in secretion of tumour necrosis factor and interleukin-1. Clinical Research 36:456A, 1988.
85. Lin AC, Goldwasser E, Bernard EM, Chapman SW. Amphotericin B blunts erythropoietin response to anemia. J Infect Dis 161:348, 1990.
86. Gallis HA, Drew RH, Pickard WW. Amphotericin B: 30 years of clinical experience. Rev Infect Dis 12:308, 1990.
87. Branch RA. Prevention of amphotericin B-induced renal impairment: a review on the use of sodium supplementation. Arch Intern Med 148:2389, 1988.
88. Miano-Mason TM. Mechanisms and management of amphotericin B-induced nephrotoxicity. Cancer Pract 5:176, 1997.
89. Khoo SH, Bond J, Denning DW. Administering amphotericin B: a pratical approach. J Antimicrob Chemother 33:203, 1994.
90. Solomkin JS, Flohr A, Simmons RL. Candida infections in surgical patient. Dose requirements and toxicity of amphotericin B. Ann Surg 195:177, 1982.
91. Medoff G. Controversial areas of antifungal chemotherapy: short-course and combination therapy with amphotericin B. Rev Infect Dis 9:403, 1987.
92. Laenders AC, de Marie S. The use of lipid formulations of amphotericin B for systemic fungal infections. Leukemia 10:1570, 1996.
93. Mehta J. Do variations in molecular structure affect the clinical efficacy and safety of lipid-based amphotericin B preparations? Leuk Res 21:183, 1997.
94. Wingard JR. Efficacy of amphotericin B lipid complex injection (ABLC) in bone marrow transplant recipients with life-threatening systemic mycosis. BMT 19:343, 1997.
95. Luke RG, Boyle JA. Renal effects of amphotericin B lipid complex. Am J Kidney Dis 31: 780, 1998.
96. Rapp RP, Gubbins PO, Evans ME. Amphotericin B lipid complex. Ann Pharmacother 31:1174, 1997.
97. Tang CM, Bowler ICJW. Do the new lipid formulations of amphotericin B really work? Clin Micro Infect 16:98, 1997.
98. White MN, Bowden RA, Sandler ES *et al.* Randomized, double-blind clinical trial of amphotericin B colloidal dispersion versus amphotericin B in the empirical treatment of fever and neutropenia. Clin Infect Dis 27:296, 1998.
99. Walsh TJ, Hiemenz JW, Seibel NL *et al.* Amphotericin B lipid complex for invasive fungal infections: analysis of safety and efficacy in 556 cases. Clin Infect Dis 26:1383, 1998.
100. Garbino J, Pittet D. Candida infections in the intensive care unit. Clin Intensive Care 8:187, 1997.
101. Adedoyin A, Bernard JF, Swenson CE *et al.* Pharmacokinetic profile of Abelcet (amphotericin B lipid complex injection): combined experience from phase I and phase II studies. Antimicrob Agents Chemother 41:2201, 1997.
102. Anaissie EJ, White M, Uzon O *et al.* Amphotericin B lipid complex versus amphotericin B for the treatment of invasive candidiasis: a prospective randomized, multicenter trial. In Programs and abstracts of the 35th Interscience Conference on Antimicrobials Agents and Chemotherapy, 30: Abst. LM21, 1995.
103. Goff DA, Sierawski SJ. A clinical and economic

analysis of amphotericin B lipid complex (ABLC, Abelcet) vs amphotericin B. In Programs and abstracts 38th Interscience Conference on Antimicrobial Agents and Chemotherapy, 1998.

104. Fielding RM, Smith PC, Wang LH, Porter J, Guo LS. Comparative pharmacokinetics of amphotericin B after administration of a novel colloidal delivery system, ABCD, and a conventional formulation to rats. Antimicrob Agents Chemother 35:1208, 1991.

105. Taylor RL, Williams DM, Craven PC, Graybill JR, Drutz DJ, Magee WE. Amphotericin B in liposomes: a novel therapy for histoplasmosis. Am Rev Respir Dis 125:610, 1982.

106. Oppenheim BA, Herbrecht R, Kusne S. The safety and efficacy of amphotericin B colloidal dispersion in the treatment of invasive mycosis. Clin Infect Dis 21:1145, 1995.

107. Dupont B. Clinical efficacy of amphotericin B colloidal dispersion against infections caused by *Candida* spp. Chemotherapy 45 (Suppl 1):27, 1999.

108. Anaissie EJ, Mattiuzzi GN, Miller CB *et al.* Treatment of invasive fungal infections in renally impaired patients with amphotericin B colloidal dispersion. Antimicrob Agents Chemother 42:606, 1998.

109. Herbrecht R. Safety of amphotericin B colloidal dispersion. Eur J Clin Microb Infect Dis 16:74, 1997.

110. Gurwith M, Mamelok R, Pietrelli L, DuMond C. Renal sparing by amphotericin B colloidal dispersion: clinical experience in 572 patients. Chemotherapy 45 (Suppl 1):39, 1999.

111. Meunier F, Prentice HG, Ringden O. Liposomal amphotericin B (Ambisome): safety data from a phase II/III clinical trial. J Antimicrob Chemother 28:83, 1991.

112. Walsh TJ, Fingers RW, Arndt C, Hiemenz J, Schwartz C, Bondensterner D, Pappas P, Seibel N *et al.* Liposomal amphotericin B for empirical therapy in patients with persistent fever and neutropenia. National Institute of Allergy and infectious Diseases Mycosis Study Group. N Engl J Med 340:764, 1999.

113. Slain D. Lipid-based amphotericin B for the treatment of fungal infections. Pharmacotherapy 19:306, 1999.

114. Laenders ACA, Daenen S, Jansen RLH *et al.* Liposomal amphotericin B in the treatment of documented and suspected neutropenia-associated invasive fungal infections. Br J Haematol 103:205, 1998.

115. Clarck AD, Mackenreich S, Tansey PJ, Franklin JM, Chopra R. A comparative analysis of lipid-complexed and liposomal amphotericin B preparations in hematological oncology. Br J Haematol 103:198, 1998.

116. Johnson EM, Ojwang JO, Szekely A, Wallace TL, Warnock DW. Comparison of *in vitro* antifungal activities of free and liposome-encapsulated nystatin with three of four amphotericin B formulations. Antimicrob Agents Chemother 42:1412, 1998.

117. Zhanel GG, Karlowsky JA, Harding GA *et al.* *In vitro* activity of a new semisynthetic echinocandin, LY-303366, against systemic isolates of *Candida* spp., *Cryptococcus neoformans*, *Blastomyces dermatitidis* and *Aspergillus* spp. Antimicrob Agents Chemother 41:863, 1997.

118. American Society of Clinical Oncology. Recommendations for the use of hematopoietic colony-stimulating factors: evidence-based, clinical practice guidelines. J Clin Oncol 12: 2471, 1994.

119. Heard SO, Fink MP, Gamelli RL, Solomkin JS, Joshi M, Trask AL, Fabian TC, Hudson LD, Gerold KB, Logan ED. Effect of prophylactic administration of recombinant human granulocyte colony stimulating factor (filgrastin) on the frequency of nosocomial infections in patients with acute brain injury or cerebral hemorrhage. The filgrastin study group. Crit Care Med 26: 748, 1998.

120. Gaviria JM, van Burik JA, Dale DC, Root RK, Liles WC. Comparison of interferon gamma, granulocyte colony stimulating factor and granulocyte-macrophage colony stimulating factor for priming leukocyte mediated hyphal damage of opportunistic fungal pathogens. J Infect Dis 179:1038, 1999.

121. Freifeld A, Pizzo P. Colony-stimulating factors and neutropenia: intersection of data and clinical relevance. J Natl Cancer Inst 87:781, 1995.

122. Fisher BD, Armstrong D, Yu B, Gold JWM. Invasive aspergillosis: progress in early diagnosis and treatment. Am J Med 71:571, 1981.

123. Walsh TJ, Dixon DM. Nosocomial aspergillosis: environmental microbiology, hospital epidemiology, diagnosis and treatment. Eur J Epidemiol 5:131, 1989.

124. Wald A, Leisenring W, van Burik JA, Bowden RA. Epidemiology of *Aspergillus* infections in a large cohort of patients undergoing bone marrow transplantation. J Infect Dis 175:1459, 1997.

125. Rello J, Esandi ME, Mariscal D, Gallego M,

Domingo C, Valles J. Invasive pulmonary aspergillosis in patients with chronic obstructive pulmonary disease: report of eight cases and review. Clin Infect Dis 26:1473, 1998.

126. Walsh TJ, Melcher GP, Rinaldi MG *et al.* Trichosporum beigelii, an emerging pathogen resistant to amphotericin B. J Clin Microbiol 28:1616, 1990.
127. Lutwick LI, Galgiani JN, Johnson RH, Stevens DA. Visceral fungal infections due to pseudollascheria boydii (Allescheria boydii). *In vitro* drug sensitivity studies. Am J Med 61:632, 1976.
128. British Society for Antimicrobial Chemotherapy Working Party. Therapy of deep fungal infections in hematological malignancy. J Antimicrob Chemother 40:779, 1997.
129. Ellis M, Spence D, de Pauw B, Meunier F, Marinus A, Colette L, Sylvester R, Meis J, Boogaerts M, Selledag, Kcrmery V, von Sinner W, Mc Donald P, Doyen C, Vandeream B. An EORTC international multicenter randomized trial (EORTC number 19923) comparing two dosages of liposomal amphotericin B for treatment of invasive aspergillosis. Clin Infect Dis 27:1406, 1998.
130. Voss A, le Noble JL, Verduyn Lunel FM, Foudraine NA, Meis JF. Candidemia in intensive care unit patients: risk factors for mortality. Infection 25:8, 130.
131. Diaz E *et al.* Nosocomial candidemia risk factors. Intensive Care Med 24 (Suppl 1):S143, 1998.
132. Nguyen MH, Peacock JE Jr, Morris AJ *et al.* The changing face of candidemia: emergence of non-Candida albicans species and antifungal resistance. Am J Med 100:617, 1996.
133. Rex JH, Bennett JE, Sugar AM *et al.* Intravascular catheter exchange and duration of candidemia. NIAID Mycosis Study Group and the Candidemia Study Group. Clin Infect Dis 21:994, 1995.
134. Wingard JR. Importance of Candida species other than Candida albicans as pathogens in oncology patients. Clin Infect Dis 20:115, 1995.
135. Meunier F, Aoun M, Bitar N. Candidemia in immunocompromised patients. Clin Infect Dis 14:S120, 1992.
136. Kirkpatrik WR, Revanker SG, McAtee RK, Lopez-Ribot JL, Fothergill AW, McCarthy DI, Sanche SE, Canter RA, Rinaldi MG, Patterson TF. Detection of *Candida dubliniensis* in oropharyngeal samples from human immunodeficiency virus-infected patients in North America by Primary CHROMagar Candida screening and susceptibility testing of isolates. J Clin Microbiol 300:7, 1998.
137. Safran DB, Dawson E. The effect of empiric and prophylactic treatment with fluconazole on yeast isolates in a surgical trauma intensive care unit. Arch Surg 132:1184, 1997.
138. Blinkhorn RJ, Adelstein D, Spagnuolo PJ. Emergence of a new opportunistic pathogen, *Candida lusitanae.* J Clin Microbiol 27:236, 1989.
139. Warnock DW, Burke J, Cope NJ, Johnson EM, von Fraunhofer NA, Wiliams EW. Fluconazole resistance in *Candida glabrata*. Lancet II:1310, 1988.
140. Gleason TG, May AK, Caparelli D, Fan BM, Sawyer RG. Emerging evidence of selection of fluconazole-tolerant fungi in surgical intensive care units. Arch Surg 132:1197, 1997.
141. vandenBossche H, Marichal P, Odds FC, LeJeune L, Coene M-C. Characterization of an azole-resistant *Candida glabrata* isolate. Antimicrob Agents Chemother 36:2602, 1992.
142. Viscoli C, Girmenia C, Marinus A, Collette L, Martino P, Vandercam B, Doyen C, Lebean B, Spence D, Krcmery V, de Pauw B, Meunier F and the invasive fungal infection group of the EORTC. Candidemia in cancer patients: a prospective, multicenter surveillance study by the invasive fungal infection group (IFIG) of the European Organization for Research and treatment of Cancer (EORTC). Clin Infect Dis 28:1071, 1999.
143. Wingard JR, Merz WG, Rinaldi MG, Johnson TR, Karp JE, Saral R. Increase in *Candida krusei* infection among patients with BMT and neutropenia treated prophylatically with fluconazole. N Engl J Med 325:1274, 1991.
144. Seidenfeld SM, Cooper BH, Smith JW, Luby JP, Mackowiak PA. Amphotericin B tolerance: a characteristic of *Candida parapsilosis* not shared by other *Candida* species. J Infect Dis 147:116, 1983.
145. Merz WG. *Candida lusitanae*: frequency of recovery, colonization, infection and amphotericin B resistance. J Clin Microbiol 20:1194, 1984.
146. Gastinne H, Wolff M, Delatour F, Faurisson F, Chevret S. A controlled trial in intensive care units of selective decontamination of the digestive tract with nonabsorbable antibiotics. The French Study Group on selective decontamination of the digestive tract. N Engl J Med 326:594, 1992.

147. Quinio B, Albanese J, Bues-Charbit M, Viviand X, Martin C. Selective decontamination of the digestive tract in multiple trauma patients. A prospective, double-blind, randomized, placebo-controlled study. Chest 109:762, 1996.
148. Edwards JE Jr, Bodey GP, Bowden RA, Buchner T, de Pauw BF, Filler SG, Ghannoum MA, Glauser M *et al.* International Conference for the development of a consensus on the management and prevention of severe candidal infections. Clin Infect Dis 25:43, 1997.
149. Gotzsche PC, Johansen HK. Routine antifungal therapy in cancer patients. The Cochrane database of systematic reviews 4, 1998.
150. Winston DJ, Chandrasekar PH, Lazarus HM *et al.* Fluconazole prophylaxis of fungal infection in patients with acute leukemia: results of a randomized placebo-controlled, double-blind, multicenter trial. Ann Int Med 118:495, 1993.
151. Rotstein C, Bow EJ, Laverdiere M, Ioannou S, Carr D, Moghaddan N and the Canadian fluconazole prophylaxis for neutropenic cancer patients. Benefit base on purpose and intensity of cytotoxic therapy. Clin Infect Dis 28:331, 1999.
152. Menichetti F, DelFavero A, Martino P, Bucaneve G, Micozzi A, Girmenia C, Barbabietola G, Pagano L, Leoni P, Specchia G, Caiozzo A, Raimondi R, Mandelli F and the GIMENA infection program. Itraconazole oral solution as prophylaxis for fungal infections in neutropenic patients with hematological malignancies: a randomized, placebo-controlled, double-blind, multicenter trial. Clin Infect Dis 28:250, 1999.
153. Bohme A, Karthaus M, Hoelzer D. Antifungal prophylaxis in neutropenic patients with hematological malignancies: is there a real benefit? Chemotherapy 45:224, 1999.
154. British Society for Antimicrobial Chemotherapy Working Party. Antifungal prophylaxis in leukemia and transplantation. J Antimicrob Chemother 32:5, 1993.
155. Ellis ME, Clink H, Ernst P, Halins MA, Padmos A, Spence D *et al.* Controlled study of fluconazole in the prevention of fungal infections in neutropenic patients with hematological malignancies and bone marrow transplant recipients. Eur J Clin Microbiol Infect Dis 13:3, 1994.
156. Wingard JR. Importance of *Candida* species other than *Candida albicans* as pathogens in oncology patients. Clin Infect Dis 20:115, 1995.
157. Calvo V, Borro JM, Morales P, Morcillo A, Vicente R, Tarrazona V, Paris F. Antifungal prophylaxis during the early post-operative period of lung transplant. Valencia Lung Transplant Group. Chest 115:1301, 1999.
158. Collins LA, Samose MH, Robert MS *et al.* Risk factors for invasive fungal infections complicating orthotopic liver transplantation. J Infect Dis 170:644, 1994.
159. Kung N, Fisher N, Gunson B, Hastings M, Moltimer D. Fluconazole prophylaxis for high-risk liver transplant recipients. Lancet 345:1234, 1995.
160. Dubé MP, Heseltine PNR, Rinaldi MG, Evans S, Zawacki B. Fungemia and colonization with nystatin resistant *Candida rugosa* in a burn unit. Clin Infect Dis 18:77, 1994.
161. Burket JS, Bartlett RH, Hyde KV, Chenoweth CE. Nosocomial infections in adult patients undergoing extracorporeal membrane oxygenation. Clin Infect Dis 28:828, 1999.
162. Goldstein DJ, el-Amir NG, Ashton RCJ, Catanese K, Rose RA, Levin HR, Oz MC. Fungal infections in left ventricular assist device recipients. Incidence, prophylaxis and treatment. ASAID J 41:873, 1995.
163. Eggimann P, Francioli P, Bille J, Schneider R, Wu MM, Chapuis G, Chiolero R *et al.* Fluconazole prophylaxis prevents intra-abdominal candidiasis in high-risk surgical patients. Crit Care Med 27:1066, 1999.
164. Wenzel RP. Nosocomial candidemia: risk factors and attributable mortality. Clin Infect Dis 20:1531, 1995.
165. Wright WL, Wenzel RP. Nosocomial Candida. Epidemiology, transmission and prevention. Infect Dis Clin North Am 11:411, 1997.
166. Rello J, Diaz E. Epidemiology and aetiology of fungal infections in the ICU. In The management of fungal in the ICU, Vincent JL (ed). The Liposome Company; 1999:11.
167. Pittet D, Monod M, Suter PM, Frank E, Auckenthaler R. *Candida* colonization and subsequent infections in critically ill surgical patients. Ann Surg 230:751, 1994.
168. Petri MG, Konig J, Moecke HP *et al.* Epidemiology of invasive mycosis in ICU patients: a prospective multicenter study in 435 non-neutropenic patients. Intensive Care Med 23: 317, 1997.
169. Ellis CA, Spivack ML. The significance of candidemia. Ann Int Med 67:511, 1967.
170. Toala P, Schroeder SA, Daly AK, Finland M. *Candida* at Boston City Hospital. Clinical and epidemiological characteristics and susceptibil-

ity to eight antimicrobial agents. Arch Intern Med 126:983, 1970.

171. Fraser VJ, Jones M, Dunkel J, Storfer S, Medoff G, Dunagan WC. Candidemia in a tertiary care hospital: epidemiology, risk factors and predictors of mortality. Clin Infect Dis 15:414, 1992.

172. Edwards JE Jr. Invasive *Candida* infections – evolution of a fungal pathogen. N Engl J Med 324:1060, 1991.

173. Anaissie EJ, Darouiche RO, Abi-Said D *et al.* Management of invasive *Candida* infections: results of a prospective randomized, multicenter study of fluconazole versus amphotericin B and review of the literature. Clin Infect Dis 23:964, 1996.

174. Anaissie EJ, Vartivarian SE, Abi-Said D *et al.* Fluconazole versus amphotericin B in the treatment of hematogenous candidiasis: a matched cohort study. Am J Med 101:170, 1996.

175. Nguyen MH, Peacock JE Jr, Tanner DC *et al.* Therapeutic approaches in patients with candidemia. Evaluation in a multicenter prospective observational study. Arch Intern Med 155:2429, 1995.

176. Rex JH, Bennett JE, Sugar AM *et al.* A randomized trial comparing fluconazole and amphotericin B for the treatment of candidemia in patients with neutropenia. N Engl J Med 331:1325, 1994.

177. van't Wout JW. Fluconazole treatment of candidal infections caused by non-albicans *Candida* species. Eur J Clin Microbiol Infect Dis 15:238, 1996.

178. Ang BSP, Telenti A, King B, Steckelberg JM, Wilson WR. Candidemia from a urinary tract source: microbiological aspects and clinical significance. Clin Infect Dis 17:662, 1993.

179. Sobel JD. Management of asymptomatic candiduria. Int J Antimicrob Agents 11:285, 1999.

180. Potasman I, Castin A, Moskovitz B, Surg I, Natir O. Oral fluconazole for *Candida* urinary tract infection. Urol Int 59:252, 1997.

181. Nassoura Z, Ivatury RR, Simon RJ, Jabbour NN, Stahl WM. Candidemia as an early marker of disseminated infection in the critically surgical patient: the role of fluconazole therapy. J Trauma 35:290, 1993.

182. Ayeni O, Riederer KM, Wilson FM, Khabit R. Clinicians' reaction to positive urine culture for *Candida* organisms. Mycosis 42:215A, 1999.

183. Fisher JF, Newman CL, Sobel JD. Yeasts in the urine: solution for a budding problem. Clin Infect Dis 20:183, 1995.

184. Leu HS, Huang CT. Clearance of funguria with short-course antifungal regimens: prospective, randomized, controlled study. Clin Infect Dis 20:1152, 1995.

185. Nerbit SA, Katz LE, McClain BW, Murphy DP. Comparison of two concentrations of amphotericin B bladder irrigation in the treatment of funguria in patients with indwelling urinary catheters. Am J Health Syst Pharm 56:872, 1999.

186. Jacobs LG, Skidmore EA, Freeman K, Lipschultz D, Fox N. Oral fluconazole compared with bladder irrigation with amphotericin B for treatment of fungal urinary tract infections in elderly patients. Clin Infect Dis 20:30, 1996.

187. Graninger W, Presterie E, Schneeweiss B, Teleky B, Georgopoulos A. Treatment of *Candida albicans* fungaemia with fluconazole. J Infect 26:133, 1992.

188. Pittrow L, Penk A. Dosage adjustments of fluconazole during continuous renal replacement therapy (CAVH, CVVH, CAVHD, CVVHD). Mycosis 42:17, 1999.

189. Moody SB, Sveska KJ. Fluconazole dosing in renal impairment: a drug usage evaluation. Hosp Formul 28:499, 1993.

190. Lee JW, Seibel NL, Amantea M, Whitcomb P, Pizzo PA, Walsh TJ. Safety of pharmacokinetics of fluconazole in children with neoplastic diseases. J Pediatr 120:987, 1990.

191. Seay RE, Larson TA, Toscano JP, Bostrom BC, O'Leary MC, Udan DL. Pharmacokinetics of fluconazole in immunocompromised children with leukemia or other hematologic disease. Pharmacotherapy 15:52, 1995.

192. Kaufman CA, Bradley SF, Ross SC, Weber DR. Hepatosplenic candidiasis. Successful treatment with fluconazole. Am J Med 91:137, 1991.

193. Anaissie EJ, Bodey GP, Kantarjian H, David C, Barnett K, Bow E, Defelice R, Downs N, File T, Kram G, Potts D, Shelton M, Sugar A. Fluconazole therapy for chronic disseminated candidiasis in patients with leukemia and prior amphotericin B therapy. Am J Med 91:142, 1991.

194. Hadley S, Krchmer AW. Fungal infections in solid organ transplant recipients. Infect Dis Cli N Am 9:1045, 1995.

195. Hibberd PL, Rubin RH. Clinical aspects of fungal infection in organ transplant recipients. Clin Infect Dis 19 (Suppl 1):S33, 1994.

196. Pittet D, Anaissie E, Solomkin JS. When to start antifungal therapy in the non-neutropenic critically ill. In Vincent JL (ed), Yearbook of

Intensive Care and Emergency Medicine. Berlin: Springer-Verlag, 1996:964.
197. Penk A, Pittrow L. Status of fluconazole in the therapy of endogenous *Candida* endophtalmitis. Mycosis 41 (Suppl 2):41, 1998.
198. del Palacio A, Cuétara MS, Ferro M *et al.* Fluconazole in the management of endophtalmitis in disseminated candidiasis of heroin addicts. Mycosis 36:193, 1993.
199. Akler ME, Velland M, MvNealy DM, Walmsley SL, Gold WL. Use of fluconazole in the treatment of *Candida* endophtalmitis. Clin Infect Dis 20:657, 1995.
200. Filler SG, Cusllip MA, Mayer CL, Edwards JE Jr. Comparison of fluconazole and amphotericin B for the treatment of disseminated candidiasis and endophtalmitis in rabbits. Antimicrob Agents Chemother 35:288, 1991.
201. Savani DV, Perfect JR, Cobo LM, Durack DT. Penetration of new azole compounds into the eye and efficacy in experimental *Candida* endophtalmitis. Antimicrob Agents Chemother 31:6, 1987.
202. Nomura J, Ruskin J. Failure of therapy with fluconazole for *Candida* endophtalmitis. Clin Infect Dis 17:888, 1993.
203. Adler-Moore JP, Profitt RT. Development, characterization, efficacy and modes of action of (Ambisome), a unicellular liposomal formulation of amphotericin B. J Liposomal Res 3:429, 1993.
204. Wong-Beringer A, Jacobs RA, Guglielmo BJ. Lipid formulation of amphotericin B: clinical efficacy and toxicities. Clin Infect Dis 27:603, 1998.
205. Bowden RA, Cays M, Gooley T, Mamelok RD, vam Butik JA. Phase I study of amphotericin B colloidal dispersion for the treatment of invasive fungal infections after marrow transplant. J Infect Dis 173:1208, 1996.
206. Scheven M, Senf L. Quantitative determination of fluconazole-amphotericin B antagonism to *Candida albicans* by agar-diffusion. Mycosis 37:205, 1994.
207. Sugar AM, Hitchcock CA, Troke PF, Picard M. Combination therapy of murine invasive candidiasis with fluconazole and amphotericin B. Antimicrob Agents Chemother 19:598, 1995.
208. Boogaerts M, Cavalli F, Cortés-Funes H *et al.* Granulocyte growth factors: achieving a consensus. Ann Oncol 6: 237, 1995.
209. Mayordomo JI, Rivera F, Diaz-Puente MJ *et al.* Improving treatment of chemotherapy-induced neutropenic fever by administration of colony-stimulating factors. J Natl Cancer Inst 87:803, 1995.
210. Vecchiarelli A, Monari C, Baldelli F *et al.* Beneficial effect of recombinant human granulocyte colony-stimulating factor on fungicidal activity of polymorphonuclear leukocytes from patients with AIDS. J Infect Dis 171:1448, 1995.
211. Bober LA, Grace MJ, Pugliese-Sivo C *et al.* The effect of GM-CSF and G-CSF on human neutrophil function. Immunopharmacology 29:11, 1995.
212. Wey SB, Mori M, Pfaller MA, Woolson RF, Wenzel RP. Risk factors for hospital acquired candidemia: a matched case-control study. Arch Intern Med 149:2349, 1989.
213. Eppes SC, Troutman JL, Gutman LT. Outcome of treatment of candidemia in children whose central catheters were removed or retained. Pediatr Infect Dis J 8:99, 1989.
214. Dato VM, Dajani AS. Candidemia in children with central venous catheters: role of catheter removal and amphotericin B therapy. Pediatr Infect Dis J 9:309, 1990.
215. Lecciones JA, Lee JW, Navarro EE *et al.* Vascular catheter-associated fungemia in patients with cancer: analysis of 155 episodes. Clin Infect Dis 14:875, 1992.
216. Karabinis A, Hill C, Leclercq B, Tancrede C, Baume C, Baume D, Andremont A. Risk factors for candidemia in cancer patients: a case-control study. J Clin Microbiol 26:429, 1988.
217. Walsh TJ, Bustamente CI, Valahov D, Standiford HC. *Candida* suppurative peripheral thrombophlebitis: recognition, prevention and management. Infect Control 7:16, 1986.
218. Walsh TJ, Hutchins GM, Bulkley BH, Mendelsohn G. Fungal infections of the heart: analysis of 51 autopsy cases. Am J Card 45:357, 1980.
219. Donahue SP, Greven CM, Zurarleff JJ *et al.* Intraocular candidiasis in patients with candidemia: clinical implications derived from a prospective multicenter study. Ophtalmology 101:1302, 1994.
220. von Eiff M, Fahrenkamp A, Roos N, Fegeler W, van de Loo J. Hepatosplenic candidiasis – a late manifestation of *Candida* septicemia. Mycosis 33:283, 1990.

11. IMMUNOMODULATION IN SEPSIS

Steve Nelson, Carol M. Mason, Ping Zhang,
Warren R. Summer and Gregory J. Bagby

Introduction

The limitations of currently available therapies for sepsis are evidenced by the high, relatively fixed mortality rates associated with this disease despite advances in antibiotic therapy and critical care technology. If the various steps in the pathogenesis of sepsis are considered, beginning with tissue invasion by the offending pathogen and culminating in the pathophysiologic sequelae associated with the septic shock syndrome (Figure 1), it is clear that conventional therapy addresses only the initial and final stages of this process, i.e. antibiotics directed against the bacteria and supportive measures that attempt to compensate for failing organs. Few, if any standard approaches target key intermediate steps which likely play a critical role in the evolution of this disease process. In contrast, newer strategies are directed at these intermediate stages and are focused on the selective modification of the host immune response to the invading pathogen and/or its products (Figure 2).

Immunomodulation in non-human models of sepsis has, in general, poorly predicted clinical response in subsequent human trials. The potential explanations for the inability of preclinical studies to be predictive of outcomes in human sepsis trials are many, including species-specific immune responses, species differences in pharmacokinetics, lack of similarity between non-human models of sepsis and septic patients, the heterogeneity of the patient population studied, excessively high or low disease severity, and perhaps, most importantly, differences in the timing of the intervention. Pretreatment of humans with a biologic response modifier shortly before the onset of sepsis is generally not possible, and attempts to start treatment as early as possible after the onset of sepsis cannot approximate the early timing of interventions used in many animal models. With these limitations aside, recent human trials have shed considerable light on the pathogenesis of sepsis and as the complexities of the host pathogen interaction are further dissected, it is likely that the therapeutic benefits from these immunomodulators will be fully realized. In this chapter we will provide an overview of recent and ongoing investigations of these novel therapies.

Lipopolysaccharide Neutralization

Lipopolysaccharide (LPS), or endotoxin, is an integral component of the outer membrane of gram-negative bacteria. Current evidence suggests that LPS is the most important bacterial factor in the pathophysiology of sepsis and its sequelae [1]. Measurable levels of endotoxin have been found in 50–80% of patients with the sepsis syndrome and have been inversely correlated with survival in at least one study [2]. Furthermore, the pathogenic function of LPS makes it a prime target for new therapies that aim to neutralize the toxic properties of LPS, remove LPS from potential *in vivo* sites of action, inactivate functional LPS molecules, or prevent LPS interaction with receptors on susceptible host cells. However, efforts to block the innate immune response to LPS may also impair the host defense response to invading pathogens and thereby increase host susceptibility to infection.

Antibiotics. Antibiotics, the mainstay of current therapy, can have a significant influence on circulating endotoxin levels. It has been suggested that, under certain circumstances, shock might be precipitated in susceptible hosts by antibiotic-induced bacterial cell lysis which can lead to a sudden release of endotoxin from gram-negative bacteria [3, 4]. *In vitro* studies have demonstrated that endotoxin is released when bacteria are exposed to antibiotics [5–7]. Direct evidence that antibiotic therapy can promote endotoxin release *in vivo* has been provided by studies in rabbits infected with *Escherichia coli* [8]. Rokke *et al.* recently demonstrated that endotoxin is liberated during antibiotic therapy in a porcine sepsis model and that this release is associated with cardiac dysfunction [9]. It has also now been shown in patients undergoing antibiotic therapy for sepsis that endotoxin release can be induced following antibiotic administration and that this release is temporally associated with the onset of hypotension and an increase in plasma lactate.

Although results of animal and human studies support the hypothesis that endotoxin is liberated during antibiotic treatment of various gram-negative infections, appropriate antibiotic treatment significantly reduces mortality. Thus, the clinically relevant question is whether "equally effective" antibiotics differ in the amount of endotoxin release that they induce. Clearly, an effective antimicrobial agent that minimizes the release of endotoxin would be desirable. In general, the use of antibiotics acting upon the bacterial cell wall (such as B-lactam agents) tend to be associated with greater endotoxin release than those whose action leaves the cell wall intact [8]. It appears that aminoglycosides and imipenem have only a modest endotoxin liberating potential *in vitro*, whereas quinolones, penicillin and cephalosporins tend to liberate large amounts of endotoxin [10]. Such considerations in the selection of antibiotic therapy must be balanced by the fact that bacteriostatic drugs are not as effective as bactericidal drugs in decreasing the number of viable bacteria. There are also *in vitro* differences between the various B-lactam antibiotics which may relate to binding and inhibition of the different penicillin-binding proteins [11, 12]. Differences in binding have been proposed as a possible mechanism for a recent study showing that *E. coli* incubated in the presence of various B-lactams exhibit significant differences in the

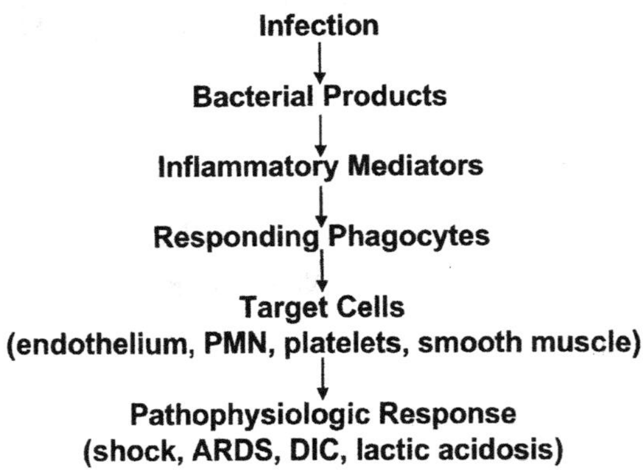

FIGURE 1. Pathophysiologic sequence of events during sepsis.

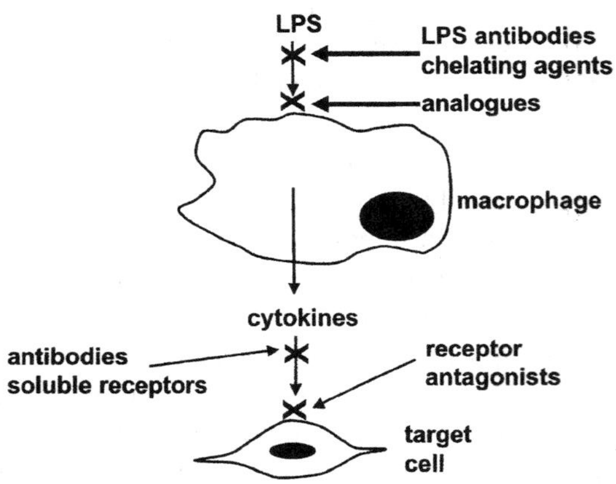

FIGURE 2. Possible sites for therapeutic intervention during sepsis.

release of tumor necrosis factor (TNF) from mononuclear cells stimulated by filtrates of these antibiotic-killed bacteria [13].

There have been relatively few trials evaluating the *in vivo* endotoxin-liberating potential of various antibiotics in humans. Prins *et al.* compared ceftazidime to imipenem in a prospective, randomized, double-blind trial in 30 patients with culture-proven, gram-negative urosepsis [14]. Only 23% of patients had detectable levels of endotoxemia at anytime during therapy. Although defervescence was faster in the imipenem-treated patients, there were no other clinical benefits and there was no statistical difference in endotoxin or cytokine levels over time.

It has even been suggested that a lower initial dose of antibiotics be administered in patients with presumed sepsis and/or that antibiotic treatment be delayed until the patient has been fluid resuscitated and hemodynamically stabilized. Alternatively, pretreatment of the patient with an antibody to LPS or a chelating agent (such as polymyxin B) prior to antibiotic administration has been proposed as a potentially effective strategy.

Antibodies to Endotoxin. Historically, immunization (active and passive) has proven effective against several bacterial infections. In general, this approach has been limited either to antitoxic immunity (e.g. tetanus toxoid) or to type-specific immunity (e.g. pneumococcus). The large number of species and serotypes responsible for gram-negative bacterial sepsis renders type-specific or passive immunization impractical for either the prevention or treatment of these infections.

The virtually identical composition of the core or lipid A regions of LPS from gram-negative bacteria suggest that epitopes common to all gram-negative bacteria would permit an antibody to these common antigens to neutralize the effects of endotoxin or to confer resistance to infection. The scientific rationale of utilizing such an antibody assumed that the antibody would avidly bind to lipid A, which is embedded deep within the bacterial membrane, and that it would subsequently neutralize the toxic effects of endotoxin. Two monoclonal IgM antibodies have been extensively evaluated in pre-clinical and clinical trials. HA-1A (Centoxin, HA-1A; Centocor, Malvern, PA) is derived from a human cell line and E5 (Xomen; Xoma, Berkeley, CA) is a murine antibody.

In vitro studies have questioned whether or not these antibodies can neutralize the toxic effects of endotoxin. For example, in a study by Warren *et al.* the addition of E5 or HA-1A to supernatants containing endotoxin failed to block macrophage activation and expression of proinflammatory cytokines [15]. Thus, the mode of action of these antibodies *in vivo* is unclear. It is important to note that the effects of HA-1A in animal models of sepsis have not been uniformly beneficial either. In a canine model of intra-abdominal sepsis, HA-1A significantly *decreased* survival from 57% to 15% [16].

Early reports of the use of anti-endotoxin antibodies in humans were encouraging but subsequent analyses and further investigation have tempered this enthusiasm. In 1991, Ziegler reported on the safety and efficacy of HA-1A in a prospective, randomized, placebo-controlled trial enrolling 543 patients with sepsis [17]. Overall survival was not improved, but a post hoc subset analysis of the 200 patients with gram-negative bacteremia showed reduced mortality in patients who had received HA-1A (49% for placebo vs 30% for HA-1A). A second large prospective trial of HA-1A was recently reported by McCloskey *et al.* [18]. Although 2199 patients with suspected gram-negative septic shock were enrolled, only 621 (28.2%) met all enrollment criteria, received treatment, and had confirmed gram-negative bacteremia. There was no 14 day survival benefit associated with HA-1A treatment in patients either without or with gram-negative bacteremia.

Similarly in the study by Greenman, 486 patients with presumptive gram-negative sepsis were administered E5 or placebo [19]. Again overall survival was not improved and again a post hoc analysis showed benefit in a subset of patients. Specifically, in patients with gram-negative sepsis who did not have refractory shock, 30 day survival was approximately two times greater in the E5 group compared to the placebo group. A second multicenter E5 trial enrolling 847 patients carefully restricted enrollment to patients with proven or suspected gram-negative infection without refractory shock, however no survival benefit for E5 was found when all treated patients were analyzed or when the 530 patients with documented gram-negative infection were analyzed separately [20].

It remains unclear as to whether passive immunization against gram-negative infection is a therapeutic option. Several studies using polyclonal antibody preparations have yielded positive results [21–23]. Prophylactic administration of unselected commercially available immunoglobulin has been shown to reduce the incidence of gram-negative sepsis in the first 100 days after bone marrow transplantation [24] and to reduce the number of infections after surgery for colorectal cancer in high risk patients [25]. In a study of 55 patients with gram-negative septic shock, where detection of endotoxemia was obligatory prior to inclusion in the trial, septic mortality was 4% in those patients receiving polyclonal, polyvalent immunoglobulin (IgG, IgM and IgA) containing high titers of anti-endotoxin antibodies vs 32% in the control group [26]. However, the methodology of this study has been questioned because randomization and treatment were unblinded, frequent interim analyses were performed and "septic mortality" was used in lieu of all cause mortality [27]. The mechanism by which polyclonal immunoglobins could effectively reduce morbidity and mortality due to gram-negative infection, where monoclonal immunoglobins have failed, remains unknown.

Bactericidal Permeability-Increasing Protein. The bactericidal permeability-increasing protein (BPI) of neutrophils is a potent cytotoxin, specific for gram-negative bacteria, that also inhibits endotoxin activity by binding to the lipid A region of LPS [28, 29]. It is a 55-kd cationic protein found in the granules of polymorphonuclear leukocytes (PMN). BPI is released into the phagocytic vacuole during phagocytosis where it binds to the surface of susceptible gram-negative bacteria, alters membrane permeability, and causes microbial death. BPI has also been shown to prevent neutrophil activation by LPS *in vitro* and to inhibit LPS-induced TNF production in whole blood [30]. Together with its potent antibacterial properties, these findings suggest that BPI may be able to down-regulate responses to LPS both by halting the proliferation of bacteria producing LPS and by directly binding LPS itself [31].

Desirable characteristics of an anti-endotoxin agent include specific and high affinity binding to lipopolysaccharide and the ability to prevent triggering of lipopolysaccharide-induced events. Interestingly, it has been shown that neither HA-1A or E5 monoclonal antibodies are as effective as BPI at binding or neutralizing endotoxin *in vitro* or *in vivo* (32). In a pneumonia model of gram-negative sepsis, the efficacy of a 23 kd recombinant N-terminal fragment of BPI ($rBPI_{23}$) was compared with that of E5 [33]. $rBPI_{23}$ conferred significantly greater protection from death than E5 (95% survival vs 20%, respectively) and enhanced the pulmonary and vascular clearance of the bacteria from the host. In other studies, our laboratory has shown that $rBPI_{23}$ inhibits lipopolysaccharide-induced TNF in the serum and lungs of rats [34].

BPI belongs to a family of endotoxin binding proteins that likely regulate the host response to endotoxin. BPI antagonizes the effects of endotoxin, whereas lipopolysaccharide binding protein (LBP) facilitates its actions [35]. LBP binds endotoxin and the resulting complex activates macrophages and neutrophils. Thus, BPI may compete with LBP for endotoxin in the infected host. This competition may be part of the normal mechanism for modulating the immune response to bacterial endotoxin.

BPI seems to be capable of neutralizing many of the biologic effects of endotoxin in humans.

In eight volunteers challenged with endotoxin, von der Mohlen *et al.* demonstrated that $rBPI_{23}$ enhances the clearance of endotoxin, attenuates the release of TNF, IL-6 and IL-10, and blunts the associated neutropenia and neutrophil degranulation [36].

Polymyxin. Polymyxin B is a cell wall active antibiotic that avidly binds to the lipid A moiety of LPS. After binding, LPS/polymyxin B particles are disintegrated into small fragments. This interaction attenuates many of the functional and toxic activities of LPS, including its ability to induce TNF and interleukin-1 (IL-1) secretion by macrophages, and to prime PMN for release of oxygen radicals [37–39]. Polymyxin B has also been shown to protect animals from various LPS-induced physiologic derangements and death related to *Hemophilus influenzae* and *E. coli* septicemia [40, 41]. A major limitation of polymyxin B's therapeutic potential is its toxicity. However, many of its anti-LPS properties are operational at concentrations that are relatively nontoxic. The clinical strategy of utilizing low-dose polymyxin B in combination with other antibiotics has yet to be explored.

Gentamicin, amikacin and tobramycin have also been shown to neutralize the effects of endotoxin, although to a lesser degree than polymyxin B. Interestingly, when amikacin or tobramycin was added to B-lactam antibiotics, bacterial lysis was accelerated, but endotoxin release and endotoxin-induced TNF production by macrophages or monocytes *in vitro* was reduced [10].

Lipid A Analogues. Lipid X is a monosaccharide biosynthetic precursor of lipid A, the major toxic moiety of endotoxin [42]. The structural similarities of lipid A and lipid X, combined with the substantially lower toxicity of lipid X, suggest that lipid X may serve as a competitive inhibitor (receptor antagonist) of lipid A, and therefore native LPS [43]. Lipid X has been shown to protect animals against LPS-induced lethality and block LPS-induced secretion of TNF by macrophages [44, 45].

Monophosphoryl (MPL) lipid A is another nontoxic derivative of lipid A. MPL has been shown to be up to 1000 times less toxic in animals than LPS [46]. MPL lipid A has been shown to significantly reduce mortality in animals given lethal challenges of *E. coli* [47]. The low toxicity of MPL was hypothesized to result from an inability to induce high levels of TNF *in vivo* in contrast to LPS or lipid A. However, it has been shown that both MPL and LPS, in fact, induce high levels of TNF, yet only LPS induces shock and death [48]. These findings suggest that other factors besides TNF are required for the lethal consequences of endotoxin.

Cytokine Antagonism

Tumor Necrosis Factor (TNF). Cytokines are potent polypeptide humoral and paracrine mediators that modulate the host defense response to invasive infections. TNF is a proximal pro-inflammatory mediator derived from mononuclear phagocytes that elicits a myriad of responses in the host. Immunoreactive TNF can be detected in the circulation of approximately one third of critically ill patients [49]. Waage *et al.* reported higher serum TNF activity in patients who subsequently died from meningococcal meningitis than in those who survived [50]. Since then, other investigators have also found that high circulating levels of TNF appear to correlate with the severity of illness, but this has not been uniformly observed [37, 50–55]. Moreover, Calandra *et al.* found severity of the underlying disease, patient age, documented bacteremia, urine output, and arterial pH to be more significant predictors of patients outcome than serum TNF levels [52].

To speculate that high TNF levels are causally related to the detrimental consequences of infections is tempting, but this conclusion cannot be drawn from elevated TNF levels alone. A number of studies conducted in both patients and animals demonstrate that high TNF levels are not by themselves sufficient to produce the full complement of adverse symptoms seen during overwhelming infections. For example, Feuerstein *et al.* found TNF levels reached their highest when sublethal doses of LPS were administered [56]. Also, as previously mentioned, both toxic and nontoxic forms of the lipid A component of LPS induce similar increases in TNF levels [48]. Furthermore, several investigators have increased serum TNF concentrations to levels typically seen in critically ill patients by administering purified recombinant human TNF or by injecting low doses of bacterial endotoxins under controlled conditions [57–60]. In these experiments, flu-like symptoms such as fever, chills, nausea, headache, tachycardia, increases in stress hormones, and hypermetabolism were observed, but a severe life-threatening state did not develop. Collectively, these findings suggest that other factors, such as the duration of the TNF response, the presence of synergistic mediators, or the site of infection (systemic versus localized) may be critical cofactors necessary to evoke a role for TNF-mediated mortality in sepsis.

In most instances, increases in serum TNF after experimental administration of bacteria or endotoxin are transient, which may explain why septic patients infrequently exhibit high levels of systemic TNF [54, 57, 61, 62]. Leroux-Roels and Oftner reported low but persistently detectable serum levels in 23 patients with sepsis [53]. The significance of this sustained elevation is unknown, but experimental studies suggest that continuous exposure of animals to TNF can have more severe consequences than does episodic exposure to this cytokine [63–65].

The consequences of passive immunization with antibodies directed against TNF offer the best means presently available for determining the role of TNF during severe infections. Pretreatment of animals with these antibodies protects them from lethal doses of LPS and from certain kinds of lethal bacterial and parasitic insults. Beutler *et al.* first demonstrated that passive immunization with anti-TNF serum rendered mice less sensitive to *E. coli* LPS [66]. Other laboratories, including our own, have substantiated this finding [61, 67, 68]. Such data provide compelling evidence that TNF elicited by endotoxin administration participates in the lethal consequences of sepsis. The detrimental role of TNF has been extended to lethal bacteremia by studies in baboons. Tracey *et al.* found that neutralizing monoclonal anti-TNF $F(ab')_2$ prevented death from a lethal intravenous challenge of live *E. coli* if administered 2 hours before the bacterial challenge [69]. An anti-TNF antibody used by Hinshaw *et al.* was similarly effective when administered to baboons up to 30 minutes after initiating a 2 hour infusion of bacteria [70].

One must be careful not to extend the relevance of these findings to all types of bacterial infections. A study conducted in our laboratory indicates that an intravenous injection of heat-killed *E. coli* produces a similar TNF response and percent lethality as does an equivalent dose of live bacteria. This implies that when large doses of bacteria are administered intravenously, their lethal effects are not dependent on their viability or proliferation, but instead are related to their inherent heat-stable chemical composition (LPS and other virulence factors). Thus, bacteremia produced by the rapid intravenous administration of microorganisms may more closely mimic LPS toxicity than a septic state in which bacterial proliferation is occurring and the infection is substantially compartmentalized.

Lethality from severe infections is not uniformly prevented by using antibodies against TNF. A lack of efficacy with anti-TNF antibodies has been reported in animals subjected to bacterial peritonitis. Evans *et al.* were unable to prevent mortality from cecal ligation and puncture by pretreating mice with a monoclonal antibody directed against murine TNF [67]. Their results are not particularly surprising because TNF was not detected in either the serum or the peritoneal cavity of mice subjected to this insult. We have also attempted to reduce the mortality induced by bacterial peritonitis in an *E. coli* fecal inoculum model without success [66]. In this case, low levels of TNF, that were completely neutralized by pretreatment with a goat anti-TNF immunoglobulin G, were detected in both the serum and the peritoneal cavity. Despite demonstrating that more than sufficient antibody was administered, mortality from gram-negative bacterial peritonitis was not abrogated in this model.

These data suggest that TNF is not an essential component in the cascade of events resulting in death during bacterial peritonitis. However, secreted TNF could potentially produce adverse effects within a microenvironment before being neutralized. Moreover, a cell-associated form of TNF that may be relatively inaccessible to administered anti-TNF has been identified [71]. Results to date indicate that this cell membrane-associated protein is biologically active and also serves as the precursor to the secreted form [72]. Keogh *et al.* found such a protein in the liver of rats 3 days after being subjected to thermal injury combined with topical application of *Pseudomonas aeruginosa* [73]. In an earlier experiment, these investigators were able to detect TNF in the circulation in only 18% of similarly treated animals [74].

Not only does anti-TNF therapy fail to protect animals against all forms of infections, in some cases using these antibodies may actually increase mortality. Mice infected with *Listeria monocytogenes* are adversely affected if pretreated with anti-TNF antibodies. Havell found spleen TNF levels to be increased between 1 to 3 days after intravenous inoculation with a sublethal dose of *Listeria* [75]. Treatment of infected mice on the first day with a monospecific anti-TNF immunoglobin resulted in an exponential growth of *Listeria* in both the liver and spleen and subsequent death within 3 days [75, 76]. Thus, the antibody converted a nonlethal infection into a lethal infection by neutralizing tissue expression of TNF. We have similarly reported that abrogation of the TNF response in animals infected with *P. aeruginosa* and other pathogens impairs critical aspects of host defense and results in heightened susceptibility to these microorganisms [77, 78].

Clinical trials utilizing anti-TNF antibodies have thus far failed to reduce the morbidity or mortality of human sepsis. Fisher *et al.* evaluated the safety, pharmacokinetics and clinical activity of murine monoclonal anti-TNF (CB0006, Celltech Inc.) in an open-label, dose-escalating trial in 80 patients with severe sepsis [79]. Interestingly, although the therapy was theoretically directed against circulating TNF, no biologically active TNF was detected in the plasma of any patient. Furthermore, the decline in the plasma levels of immunoreactive TNF after initiating therapy was independent of the dose of anti-TNF administered. Although no clinically important side-effects were identified, no clinically beneficial effects were observed either. In a subsequent trial (NORASEPT), Abraham *et al.* treated 971 patients with sepsis syndrome with either placebo or one of two doses of another murine monoclonal anti-TNF [80]. Twenty-eight day all cause mortality was not different among the anti-TNF and placebo groups. In a post hoc analysis, patients with shock treated with either of the two doses of active drug had a significantly better 3 day survival than the placebo group, although 28 day mortality was not improved. However, a second NORASEPT multicenter clinical trial testing the efficacy of anti-TNF in patients with septic shock failed to show any survival benefit [81].

Other investigators have focused on the use of monoclonal IgG anti-TNF $F(ab')_2$-fragments because these fragments are less immunogenic, have minimal interaction with Fc-receptors, and theoretically could provide better tissue penetration [82]. No survival benefit was demonstrated in a randomized, placebo-controlled, open label study of 122 patients with sepsis or septic shock. Subgroup analyses suggested potential benefit for patients with baseline serum IL-6 levels > 1000 pg/ml [82].

Recombinant, soluble human TNF receptors bind and neutralize circulating TNF with greater affinity than is possible utilizing monoclonal anti-TNF antibodies. Preclinical trials have demonstrated the ability of soluble TNF receptors to block TNF-mediated morbidity and mortality in animal models of endotoxemia [83]. However, a phase II clinical trial in 141 patients with sepsis syndrome using a synthetic 75 KDa soluble TNF receptor demonstrated a statistically significant increase in mortality in the active drug group [84]. One proposed mechanism for this paradoxical effect is decreased clearance of the receptor-ligand complex compared to unbound TNF. It has been hypothesized that this complex may later dissociate, in effect prolonging the action of TNF. Trials of a 55 KDa soluble TNF receptor have also shown no survival benefit [85].

Interleukin-1 (IL-1). IL-1 is another cytokine that shares proinflammatory properties with TNF and acts synergistically with TNF in various models to enhance tissue damage and death [86, 87]. Several lines of evidence implicate IL-1 in the development of sepsis. Serum IL-1 levels are frequently elevated in patients with sepsis and administration of low doses of IL-1 induces many of the signs and symptoms of sepsis [67, 88, 89]. In humans, IL-1 occurs in two forms: IL-1 alpha and IL-1 beta. It is *IL-1β* form that is usually elevated in sepsis (90). The actions of both forms are regulated by a plasma membrane glycoprotein receptor with broad distribution [91, 92]. At least one IL-1 receptor antagonist (IL-1ra) occurs naturally and was originally discovered in the urine of patients with monocytic leukemia [93]. IL-1ra is a 26-kd protein produced by monocytes [94]. Recombinant technology has produced a nonglycosylated form of IL-1ra which blocks the action of IL-1 and seems to have no detectable agonist activity [95]. When dosing was started immediately before injection of endotoxin in rabbits, IL-1ra increased survival from 20% to 90% [96]. When injected prior to a continuous infusion of live *E. coli*, IL-1ra improved survival and hemodynamics, and reduced the severity of lactic acidemia in baboons [97].

The results of a phase II, open-label, placebo-controlled multicenter trial of IL-1ra in 99 patients with sepsis syndrome was reported by Fisher *et al.* [98]. A statistically significant, dose-dependent reduction in mortality was observed with active drug treatment (from 44% in the placebo group to 16% in the highest dose IL-1ra group). Furthermore, there was a significant, dose-related rate of improvement in severity of illness (APACHE II) over the 3 days of study drug infusion. Subsequently, a double-blind, randomized, controlled trial using high-dose IL-1ra in 893 patients with sepsis syndrome failed to demonstrate a significant reduction in mortality [99]. Post hoc analyses suggested a beneficial drug effect in more severely ill patients (those with a predicted mortality ≥24%). A third phase III trial which limited enrollment to patients with a high predicted mortality was initiated but was subsequently discontinued after an interim analysis showed that a statistically significant reduction in mortality was not likely to be observed.

Other Anti-Inflammatory Therapies

Non-Steroidal Anti-Inflammatory Drugs (NSAIDS). Cyclooxygenase derived metabolites of arachidonic acid, especially thromboxane-A_2 and prostacyclin, are elevated in septic patients [100]. Inhibition of cyclooxygenase with NSAIDS has been shown to prevent or reverse many of the pathophysiologic manifestations of sepsis in animal models [101, 102]. Preliminary studies in small cohorts of septic patients had suggested that ibuprofen, a reversible cyclooxygenase inhibitor, could improve gas exchange and reverse hypotension. Recently, a prospective, randomized, placebo-controlled study of 455 patients with sepsis syndrome was completed [103]. Results showed improvement in temperature, heart rate, minute ventilation, oxygen consumption, and arterial lactate in the ibuprofen group, but no change in the development of shock, the acute respiratory distress syndrome

(ARDS) or mortality when compared to the placebo group.

Steroids. No pharmacologic treatment in sepsis has been as extensively studied as glucocorticoids. Preclinical data have been overwhelmingly positive, especially when steroids are administered prior to the septic challenge. A recent metanalysis of nine randomized, controlled clinical trials not only showed no benefit to steroid administration but suggested a trend towards increased mortality in steroid-treated patients [104]. However, recent studies suggest that "stress" doses of glucocorticoids over an extended period of time may be of benefit in patients with septic shock [105].

Other Inflammatory Mediator Antagonists. Platelet activating factor (PAF) is released early following septic challenge in animal models and plasma levels of PAF are elevated in humans with sepsis [106]. A fundamental role of PAF appears to be the amplification of the production of TNF and IL-1. Antagonizing PAF can reduce morbidity and mortality in animals after LPS challenge [107, 108]. In a preliminary report of 262 patients with severe gram-negative sepsis, treatment with a PAF antagonist (ginkgolide B, BN 52021) conferred no statistically significant 28 day survival benefit compared to placebo (49% for placebo vs 58% for BN 52021) [109], however, in a subgroup analysis of patients with documented gram-negative infection, mortality was reduced 42% compared to control. Fifty-three European centers have recently completed a phase III study of 608 patients, 70% of whom had documented gram-negative infection, and 76% of whom had shock. Mortality was not significantly different between the two groups (53% in the active drug group and 51% in the placebo group) [106].

Bradykinin is a potent pro-inflammatory vasodilator that is thought to contribute to hypotension and vascular permeability associated with sepsis. Antagonism of bradykinin improves outcomes after experimental gram-negative infection [110]. However, a 3 day infusion of a bradykinin antagonist (CP027) in 500 patients with presumed sepsis showed no statistically significant effect on mortality [111].

Pro-Inflammatory Strategies

To date, investigative approaches have not met with clear success in clinical trials. Indeed, attempts at down-regulating the inflammatory response through the administration of anti-cytokines and similar agents have, in some cases, even suggested an adverse effect. Thus, attention has turned to strategies that amplify rather than suppress the host defense response. Evidence indicates that the underlying condition of the host is the primary determinant of response to therapy and survival in patients with severe infections. The implication is that when sepsis develops, key elements in the normal host defense apparatus fail or are inadequate. Perhaps, the host defense system during sepsis should be considered one more of multiple failing organ systems. If this is true, then clearly approaches that employ an anti-inflammatory intervention may only further compromise the remaining vestiges of the host's immune defense system. Therefore, restoration or amplification of selective components of the host defense system may be an appropriate strategy for the septic patients who is, in fact, an immunocompromised host. One experimental approach to accomplish this is through the use of granulocyte colony-stimulating factor (G-CSF) to upregulate the host's neutrophil response to invading pathogens.

Granulocyte Colony-Stimulating Factor (G-CSF). Colony-stimulating factors (CSFs) are acidic glycoproteins that are required for the proliferation and differentiation of hematopoietic progenitor cells [112]. Of this cytokine family, which includes granulocyte-macrophage colony-stimulating factor (GM-CSF), macrophage colony-stimulating factor (M-CSF), interleukin-3, and granulocyte colony-stimulating factor (G-CSF), it is G-CSF that plays a vital role in maintaining the normal blood PMN count and in determining the neutrophil's response in both inflammatory and infectious diseases. Native human G-CSF is a protein of 174 amino acids encoded by a single gene located on chromosome 17q [113].

G-CSF is found in all major organs at concentrations higher than those present in the circulation, and production rates of this factor can be rapidly elevated after exposure to an appropriate stimulus [114]. Bacterial products and/or secondary inflammatory mediators induced by an infection are known to be potent stimuli for the production of G-CSF [115]. TNF and IL-1 – two of the early pro-inflammatory cytokines induced by endotoxin – are known to activate human endothelial cells [116, 117], fibroblasts [118, 119], mononuclear phagocytes [120, 121], and bone marrow stromal cells [122, 123] to increase G-CSF mRNA expression in these cells and promote secretion of active G-CSF. Since these are the cells that are most likely to initially encounter invading microorganisms, this mechanism is highly efficient in initiating a rapid host response to augment the number and/or function of PMN. We have determined plasma G-CSF activity in rats challenged intravenously with 10^6 colony-forming units (CFU) of live *E. coli*. G-CSF levels rose abruptly following the bacterial challenge, peaked between 5 and 6 hours, and returned to baseline values by 8 hours [124].

In studies of healthy human volunteers, serum G-CSF concentrations are typically <30 pg/ml [125]. Circulating G-CSF levels rise promptly as an acute phase response to endotoxin injections and in various infectious diseases. In patients with acute bacterial infections, reported G-CSF concentrations ranged between 30–3200 pg/ml [125]. In this study, there was no relationship between the circulating level of G-CSF and the peripheral white blood cell count in these patients. In the recovery phase, G-CSF concentrations returned to those typically found in uninfected volunteers. It is important to note that – like those of other cytokines – serum G-CSF concentrations may not directly reflect local tissue content during infections.

In addition to its important role in the regulation of granulopoiesis, G-CSF also significantly modulates the function and activity of developing and mature neutrophils. In response to tissue infection, neutrophils must initially migrate to the site of an invading pathogen and then effectively destroy the pathogen via their microbicidal mechanisms. Recent investigations have demonstrated effects of G-CSF both *in vitro* and *in vivo* on a variety of the physiological properties of neutrophils. G-CSF has many effects which can be compared with those induced by other cytokines, such as GM-CSF and interferon-gamma, which also have potential therapeutic applications in the management of clinical infectious diseases. *In vitro*, G-CSF enhances neutrophil cheactaxis at low concentrations and inhibits neutrophil cheactaxis at high concentrations [126–128]. This biphasic dose response serves to attract and then immobilize neutrophils at sites of inflammation or infection. *In vitro*, G-CSF stimulates chemotaxis, phagocytic activity of normal neutrophils, enhances the microbicidal activity of normal neutrophils against bacterial pathogens, and primes neutrophils for the respiratory burst [128–130].

In summary, G-CSF induces significant alterations in both the number and the biological activities of neutrophils, which may augment host defenses to invading microorganisms. This potentially beneficial modulation of neutrophil functional activity renders G-CSF an attractive candidate for biological immunotherapy in patients with clinical infections.

In a well-established model of sepsis involving cecal ligation and puncture in mice, G-CSF was highly efficacious in increasing the survival rate when administered either before or at the time of cecal ligation and puncture [131]. Furthermore, the combination of gentamicin and G-CSF resulted in a survival rate higher than among untreated control mice and that among mice receiving G-CSF alone. In a similar rat model, neutrophils were recovered 24 hours following cecal ligation and puncture, and their functional status was evaluated [132]. Neutrophils from control animals exhibited suppressed chemotaxis and depressed superoxide production. Administration of G-CSF immediately following the cecal ligation and puncture restored both the depressed chemotaxis and the superoxide production to levels equal to or greater than those of normal uninfected controls.

Eichacker *et al.* studied the cardiopulmonary effects of G-CSF in a canine model of bacterial sepsis [133]. G-CSF (high dose – 5 µg/kg, low dose – 0.1 µg/kg) or placebo was administered for nine days before and until 3 days after intraperitoneal placement of an *E. coli* infected blood clot. High dose G-CSF increased the mean peripheral neutrophil count prior to clot implantation by approximately 5-fold compared to the low dose G-CSF and control groups. Survival was significantly greater in the high dose G-CSF group than in the low dose G-CSF and control groups. High dose G-CSF improved cardiovascular function, as evidenced by an increased left ventricular ejection fraction and mean arterial blood pressure compared with the other two study groups. High dose G-CSF decreased mean serum endotoxin and TNF levels and lowered blood bacteria counts. Thus, G-CSF, which increased the number of peripheral neutrophils before and during peritonitis and septic shock in this canine model, enhanced host defense, reduced cytokine levels, and improved cardiovascular function and survival. It is of interest that in this same model system, these investigators previously had shown that the monoclonal antibody to endotoxin, HA-1A, did not lower circulating endotoxin levels and resulted in an increased mortality compared to control animals [16].

Smith *et al.* studied the effect of G-CSF in a rabbit model of gram-negative pneumonia and sepsis [134]. Rabbits were transtracheally inoculated with *Pasteurella multocida* and treated 24 hours later with penicillin G and either G-CSF or placebo once daily for 5 days. In these animals, sepsis-induced leukopenia was a predictor of significantly improved survival with G-CSF therapy (57% versus 39% in controls). Interestingly, the majority of the survival benefit occurred within the first 24 hours of G-CSF treatment which was prior to the onset of peripheral leukocytosis.

While neutrophils are a key component of the host's defenses against invading pathogens, they have also been implicated as mediators of tissue damage in a variety of inflammatory disorders such as the adult respiratory distress syndrome (ARDS) and ischemic reperfusion injury of various organs. Because G-CSF enhances both the adhesion of neutrophils to endothelial cell surfaces and the release of superoxide anion in response to various stimuli, it is possible that administration of G-CSF under certain conditions could lead to inadvertent tissue damage and subsequent organ dysfunction.

Three investigations of the effects of prior treatment with G-CSF on responses to endotoxin have recently been published. Fink *et al.* showed that G-CSF-induced neutrophilia did not adversely affect the pulmonary and hemodynamic responses of pigs to intravenous endotoxin [135]. In a sheep model of endotoxin-induced lung injury, pretreatment of G-CSF, resulting in a 4-fold increase in circulating neutrophils, did not exacerbate this injury [136]. In a guinea pig model, Kanazawa *et al.* showed that pretreatment with G-CSF actually decreased endotoxin-induced pulmonary edema and alveolar capillary protein leakage [137]. In a canine model, pretreatment with G-CSF improved survival from bacterial sepsis and did not precipitate lung injury [133].

While the results of these studies should be viewed cautiously with regard to their significance for the clinical arena, they do suggest that the beneficial effect of G-CSF-induced neutrophilia on antimicrobial host defenses can be explored safely in infected patients.

On the basis of these preclinical studies, several clinical trials have recently been completed studying the effect of G-CSF in nonneutropenic patients with pneumonia. The first trial was phase I study of 30 nonneutropenic patients hospitalized with community-acquired pneumonia (CAP) [138]. All patients received intravenous antibiotics in addition to G-CSF (75–300 μg) subcutaneously daily for a maximum of 10 days. Overall, the median change in the absolute neutrophil count from baseline was approximately 200% and the peak was achieved by day four of G-CSF administration. Aside from mild bone pain, no adverse pulmonary or systemic side effects occurred that were attributable to G-CSF.

A phase III, double-blind, placebo-controlled trial of recombinant human G-CSF (Filgrastim) for the treatment of hospitalized patients with CAP has recently been concluded [139]. This was a multicenter trial involving 756 patients enrolled in 71 centers in the United States, Canada, and Australia. Participants in this study were randomized to receive 300 μg/day G-CSF (376 patients) or placebo (370 patients) in addition to conventional antibiotic therapy. Treatment duration was up to 10 days and the length of the study observation period was 28 days or until death. The primary objectives of this study were to determine safety and the effect of G-CSF on time to resolution of morbidity (TRM) [140]. TRM was defined as an index of several clinical variables which are useful in determining if a patient with pneumonia is benefitting from therapy. In this study, in order to reach TRM a patient had to have either an improved or stable chest radiograph, resolve their tachypnea, become afebrile, and improve or normalize their oxygenation. Mortality was low (6%) in this study and length of stay was only 7 days. Both variables were unaffected by G-CSF treatment. Similarly, TRM was four days in each treatment group. In the intent-to-treat analysis, G-CSF did increase blood neutrophils three-fold, significantly accelerated radiological resolution of pneumonia, and reduced serious complications (i.e. ARDS and disseminated intravascular coagulation [DIC]). Post hoc analyses showed that these benefits were more pronounced in patients with multilobar (> two lobes) pneumonia. In this study, there were 261 patients with multilobar pneumonia (G-CSF, n = 138; placebo, n = 123) and 28% of these patients were admitted to an ICU at study entry. G-CSF administration was safe and well-tolerated in this study.

G-CSF has also been studied in the treatment of patients with pneumonia and severe sepsis [140]. Eighteen patients were randomized in a 2:1 ratio to G-CSF (300 μg/day intravenously) or placebo for a maximum of 5 days in addition to standard therapy. Inclusion criteria included a chest radiograph compatible with pneumonia, a respiratory pathogen on gram stain or culture, fever, tachycardia, tachypnea or need for mechanical ventilation, and either hypotension despite volume resuscitation requiring vasopressors or, in the absence of shock, two end organ dysfunctions (metabolic acidosis, ARDS, acute renal failure, DIC). Three of 12 G-CSF treated patients and four of six placebo treated patients died. Septic shock resolved in 9 of 10 G-CSF treated patients and none of four placebo treated patients. ARDS resolved in two of five G-CSF treated patients and one of four placebo treated patients. G-CSF was well tolerated in these septic patients.

Based on the favorable trends seen in these studies, additional trials in patients with multilobar pneumonia and in patients with severe pneumonia and sepsis were initiated and recently completed. The primary endpoint in the study of G-CSF in patients with multilobar pneumonia was a reduction in the development of organ dysfunction (ARDS, DIC, acute renal failure, shock). A reduction in mortality was the primary efficacy endpoint in the pneumonia/sepsis trial. Although these studies are undergoing continuing analyses, the primary endpoint in both trials was not significantly different for the G-CSF and placebo treatment groups.

Why have these trials failed, as of yet, to show a clear clinical benefit? Several possibilities include the timing of the intervention, the selection of the appropriate patient population, the dose and duration of therapy, and the type and site of infection. Furthermore, it is unclear if the potential benefits of G-CSF therapy are due solely to an increase in the number of neutrophils or also result from enhancing the function of these effector cells or modulating their interactions with other immunocompetent cells. It is simplistic to assume that all patients with a variety of comorbidities and pathogens presenting at different stages of their disease will respond to G-CSF therapy in a predictable and uniform fashion. We need to increase our understanding of how underlying illnesses and their attendant therapies disrupt normal host defense mechanisms if we are to develop effective cytokine-based therapies. Also, the choice of antibiotic therapy may be of importance when using cytokines as adjuvant therapy. The therapeutic efficacy of certain antibiotics is affected by the number of blood neutrophils present at the time of infection and G-CSF has also been reported to increase the uptake of certain antibiotics by neutrophils [141–142]. As G-CSF has been shown in animal models to increase the number of neutrophils that are delivered to an infected tissue site, one could potentially optimize therapy by "targeting" antibiotic delivery to an infected site by choosing an appropriate antibiotic in combination with G-CSF. This would be particularly useful in parts of the body where adequate antibiotic concentrations might be difficult to achieve and/or if the patient is infected with a relatively resistant pathogen. In addition, the primary focus of recent clinical trials with G-CSF has been on the treatment of infected patients, while the majority of preclinical studies showing benefit have administered G-CSF before the infectious challenge.

Conclusion

The care and management of the septic patient represents a formidable challenge to the physician. As long as the basic underlying host defense defects in these patients remain elusive, the clinician's approach will remain reactive and empirical. Further knowledge of the underlying pathophysiology of sepsis and its sequelae will undoubtedly provide innovative approaches to both the prevention and the early and effective treatment of this disease. However, the more we learn, the more we realize how extraordinarily complex the host defense system is. The complexity of this system makes it unlikely that any one agent will prove to be efficacious in a majority of patients. Furthermore, information is needed on how best to titrate these agents in an individual patient. Most likely, the development of a multi-modal approach, including components of immune modulation and immune restoration, is needed to improve the multiple aberrations in the host defense system induced by sepsis.

References

1. Young L, Proctor R, Beutler B, *et al.* University of California/Davis interdepartmental conference on gram-negative septicemia. Rev Infect Dis 13:666, 1991.
2. Casey L, Balk R, Bone R. Plasma cytokine and endotoxin levels correlate with survival in patients with sepsis syndrome. Ann Intern Med 119:771, 1993.
3. Hopkin B. Too-rapid destruction of gram-negative organisms. Lancet 2:603, 1977.
4. Hopkin B. A nasty shock from antibiotics. Lancet 2:594, 1985.
5. Cohen J, McConnell J. Antibiotic induced endotoxin release. Lancet 2:1069, 1985.
6. Cohen J, McConnell J. Release of endotoxin from bacteria exposed to ciprofloxacin and its prevention with polymyxin. B. Eur J Clin Microbiol 5:13, 1986.
7. McConnell J, Cohen J. Release of endotoxin from *Escherichia coli* by quinolones. J Antimicrob Chemother 18:765, 1986.
8. Shenep J, Barton R, Morgan K. Role of antibiotic class in the rate of liberation of endotoxin during the therapy for experimental gram-negative bacterial sepsis. J Infect Dis 151:1012, 1985.
9. Rokke O, Revhaug A, Osterud B, *et al.* Increased plasma levels of endotoxin and corresponding changes in circulatory performance in a porcine sepsis model: the effect of antibiotic administration. Prog Clin Biol Res 272:247, 1988.

10. Prins J, van Deventer S, Kuijper E, *et al.* Clinical relevance of antibiotic-induced endotoxin release. Antimicrob Chemother 38:1211, 1988.
11. Dofferhoff A, Nijland J, deVries-Hospers H, *et al.* Effects of different types and combinations of antimicrobial agents on endotoxin release from gram-negative bacteria: an *in vitro* and *in vivo* study. Scand J Infect Dis 23:745, 1991.
12. Neu H. Relation of structural properties of beta-lactam antibiotics to antibacterial activity. Am J Med 79 (Suppl 2A):2, 1985.
13. Simon D, Koenig G, Trenholme G. Differences in release of tumor necrosis factor from THP-1 cells stimulated by filtrates of antibiotic-killed *Escherichia coli*. J Infect Dis 164:800, 1991.
14. Prins J, van Agtmael M, Kuijper E, *et al.* Antibiotic-induced endotoxin release in patients with gram-negative urosepsis: a double-blind study comparing imipenem and ceftazidime. J Infect Dis 172:886, 1995.
15. Warren H, Amato S, Fitting C, *et al.* Assessment of ability of murine and human anti-lipid A monoclonal antibodies to bind and neutralize lipopolysaccharide. J Exp Med 177:89, 1993.
16. Quezado Z, Natanson C, Alling D, *et al.* A controlled trial of HA-1A in a canine model of gram-negative septic shock. JAMA 269:2221, 1993.
17. Ziegler E. Treatment of gram-negative bacteremia and septic shock with HA-1A human monoclonal antibody against endotoxin. N Engl J Med 324:429, 1991.
18. McCloskey R, Straube R, Sanders C, *et al.* Treatment of septic shock with human monoclonal antibody HA-1A: a randomized, double-blind, placebo-controlled trial. Ann Intern Med 121:1, 1994.
19. Greenman R. A controlled clinical trial of E5 murine monoclonal IgM antibody to endotoxin in the treatment of gram-negative sepsis. JAMA 266:1097, 1991.
20. Bone R, Balk R, Fein A, *et al.* A second large controlled clinical study of E5, a monoclonal antibody to endotoxin: results of a prospective, multicenter, randomized, controlled trial. Crit Care Med 23:994, 1995.
21. Ziegler E, McCutchan J, Fierer J, *et al.* Treatment of gram-negative bacteremia and shock with human antiserum to a mutant *Escherichia coli*. N Engl J Med 307:1225, 1982.
22. Baumgartner J, Glauser M, McCutchan J, *et al.* Prevention of gram-negative shock and death in surgical patients by antibody to endotoxin core glycolipid. Lancet 2:59, 1985.
23. Glinz W, Grob P, Nydegge RU, *et al.* Polyvalent immunoglobulins for prophylaxis of bacterial infections in patients following multiple trauma. A randomized, placebo-controlled study. Intensive Care Med 11:288, 1985.
24. Sullivan K, Kopecky K, Jocom J, *et al.* Immunomodulatory and antimicrobial efficacy of intravenous immunoglobulin in bone marrow transplantation. N Engl J Med 323:705, 1990.
25. Cafiero F, Gipponi M, Bonalumi U, *et al.* Prophylaxis of infection with intravenous immunoglobulins plus antibiotic for patients at risk for sepsis undergoing surgery for colorectal cancer: results of a randomized, multicenter clinical trial. Surgery 112:24, 1992.
26. Schedel I, Dreikhausen U, Nentwig B, *et al.* Treatment of gram-negative septic shock with an immunoglobulin preparation: a prospective, randomized clinical trial. Crit Care Med 19:1104, 1991.
27. Wortel C, Dellinger R. Treatment of gram-negative septic shock with an immunoglobulin preparation: a prospective, randomized clinical trial. Crit Care Med 21:163, 1993.
28. Schumann R, Leong S, Flaggs G, *et al.* Structure and function of lipopolysaccharide binding protein. Science 249:1429, 1990.
29. Tobias P, Mathison J, Ulevitch R. A family of lipopolysaccharide binding proteins involved in responses to Gram-negative sepsis. J Biol Chem 263:13479, 1988.
30. Ooi C, Weiss J, Doerfler M, *et al.* Endotoxin-neutralizing properties of the 25 kD N-terminal fragment and a newly isolated 30 kD C-terminal fragment of the 55–60 kD bactericidal/permeability-increasing protein of human neutrophils. J Exp Med 174:649, 1991.
31. Weiss J, Elsbach P, Olsson I, *et al.* Purification and characterization of a potent bactericidal and membrane active protein from the granules of human polymorphonuclear leukocytes. J Biol Chem 253:2664, 1978.
32. Marra M, Thornton M, Snable J, *et al.* Endotoxin-binding and neutralizing properties of recombinant bactericidal/permeability-increasing protein and monoclonal antibodies HA-1A and E5. Crit Care Med 22:559, 1994.
33. Kelly C, Cech A, Argenteanu M, *et al.* Role of bactericidal permeability-increasing protein in the treatment of gram-negative pneumonia. Surgery 114:140, 1993.

34. Summer R, Summer W, Mason C, *et al.* Bactericidal/permeability-increasing protein inhibits lipopolysaccharide-induced tumor necrosis factor in serum and lung. J Invest Med 44:78A, 1996.
35. Kohn F, Ammons W, Horwitz A, *et al.* Protective effect of a recombinant amino-terminal fragment of bactericidal/permeability-increasing protein in experimental endotoxemia. J Infect Dis 168:1307, 1993.
36. von der Mohlen M, Kimmings A, Wedel N, *et al.* Inhibition of endotoxin-induced cytokine release and neutrophil activation in humans by use of recombinant bactericidal permeability-increasing protein. J Infect Dis 172:144, 1995.
37. Damas P, Reuter A, Gysen P, *et al.* Tumor necrosis factor and interleukin-1 serum levels during severe sepsis in humans. Crit Care Med 17:975, 1989.
38. Craig W, Turner J, Kunin C. Prevention of the generalized Shwartzman reaction and endotoxin lethality by polymyxin B localized in tissues. Infect Immun 10:287, 1974.
39. Stokes D, Shenep J, Fishman M, *et al.* Polymyxin B prevents lipopolysaccharide induced release of tumor necrosis factor-α from alveolar macrophages. J Infect Dis 160:52, 1989.
40. Walterspiel J, Kaplan S, Mason EJ. Protective effect of subinhibitory polymyxin B alone and in combination with ampicillin for overwhelming *Haemophilus influenzae* type B infection in the infant rat: evidence for *in vivo* and *in vitro* release of free endotoxin after ampicillin treatment. Pediatr Res 20:237, 1986.
41. Flynn P, Shenep J, Stokes D, *et al.* Polymyxin B moderates acidosis and hypotension in established, experimental gram-negative septicemia. J Infect Dis 156:706, 1987.
42. Takayama K, Qureshi N, Mascagni P, *et al.* Fatty acyl derivatives of glucosamine-1-phosphate in *Escherichia coli* and their relation to lipid A. J Biol Chem 258:7379, 1983.
43. Raetz C. The enzymatic synthesis of lipid A: molecular structure and biologic function of monosaccharide precursors. Rev Infect Dis 6:463, 1984.
44. Proctor R, Will J, Burhop K, *et al.* Protection of mice against lethal endotoxemia by a lipid A precursor. Infect Immun 52:905, 1986.
45. Danner R, Joiner K, Parrillo J. Inhibition of endotoxin-induced priming of human neutrophils by lipid X and 3 aza-lipid X. J Clin Invest 80:605, 1987.
46. Takayama K, Qureshi N, Ribi E, *et al.* Separation and characterization of toxic and nontoxic forms of lipid A. Rev Infect Dis 6:439, 1984.
47. Chase J, Kubey W, Dulek M, *et al.* Effect of monophosphoryl lipid A on host resistance to bacterial infection. Infect Immun 53:711, 1986.
48. Kiener P, Marek F, Rodgers G, *et al.* Induction of tumor necrosis factor, IFN-γ, and acute lethality in mice by toxic and non-toxic forms of lipid A. J Immunol 141:870, 1988.
49. Waage A, Espevik T, Lamvik J. Detection of tumor necrosis factor-like cytotoxicity in serum from patients with septicaemia, but not from untreated cancer patients. Scand J Immunol 24:739, 1986.
50. Waage A, Halstensen A, Espevik T. Association between tumor necrosis factor in serum and fatal outcome in patients with meningococcal disease. Lancet 1:355, 1987.
51. Cannon J, Tompkins R, Gelfand J, *et al.* Circulating interleukin-1 and tumor necrosis factor in septic shock and experimental endotoxin fever. J Infect Dis 161:79, 1990.
52. Calandra T, Baumgartner J-D, Grau G, *et al.* Prognostic values of tumor necrosis factor/cachectin, interleukin-1, interferon-alpha, and interferon-gamma in the serum of patients with septic shock. J Infect Dis 161:982, 1990.
53. Leroux-Roels G, Oftner F. Tumor necrosis factor in sepsis. JAMA 263:1494, 1990.
54. Marks J, Marks C, Luce J, *et al.* Plasma tumor necrosis factor in patients with septic shock: mortality rate, incidence of adult respiratory distress syndrome, and effects of methylprednisolone administration. Am Rev Respir Dis 141:94, 1990.
55. DeGroote M, Martin M, Densen P, *et al.* Plasma tumor necrosis factor levels in patients with presumed sepsis: results in those treated with antilipid A antibody vs placebo. JAMA 262:249, 1989.
56. Feuerstein G, Hallenbeck J, Vanatta B, *et al.* Effect of gram-negative endotoxin on levels of serum corticosterone, TNF-alpha, circulating blood cells, and survival of rats. Circ Shock 30:265, 1990.
57. Michie H, Manogue K, Spriggs D, *et al.* Detection of circulating tumor necrosis factor after endotoxin administration. N Engl J Med 318:1481, 1988.
58. Michie H, Spriggs D, Manogue K, *et al.* Tumor necrosis factor and endotoxin induce similar

metabolic responses in human beings. Surgery 104:280, 1988.

59. Hesse D, Tracey K, Fong Y, *et al.* Cytokine appearance in human endotoxemia and primate bacteremia. Surg Gynecol Obstet 166:147, 1988.
60. Fong Y, Marano M, Moldawer L, *et al.* The acute splanchnic and peripheral tissue metabolic response to endotoxin in humans. J Clin Invest 85:1896, 1990.
61. Mathison J, Wolfson E, Ulevitch R. Participation of tumor necrosis factor in the mediation of gram negative bacterial lipopolysaccharide-induced injury in rabbits. J Clin Invest 81: 1925, 1988.
62. Nelson S, Bagby G, Bainton B, *et al.* Compartmentalization of intraalveolar and systemic lipopolysaccharide-induced tumor necrosis factor and the pulmonary inflammatory response. J Infect Dis 159:189, 1989.
63. Darling G, Fraker D, Jensen J, *et al.* Cachectic effects of recombinant human tumor necrosis factor in rats. Cancer Res 50:4008, 1990.
64. Michie H, Sherman M, Spriggs D, *et al.* Chronic TNF infusion causes anorexia but not accelerated nitrogen loss. Ann Surg 209:19, 1989.
65. Mullen B, Harris R, Patton J, *et al.* Recombinant tumor necrosis factor chronically administered in rats: lack of cachectic effect. Proc Soc Exp Biol Med 193:318, 1990.
66. Beutler B, Milsark I, Cerami A. Passive immunization against cachectin/tumor necrosis factor protects mice from lethal effect of endotoxin. Science 229:869, 1985.
67. Evans G, Snyder Y, Butler L, *et al.* Differential expression of interleukin-1 and tumor necrosis factor in murine septic shock models. Circ Shock 29:279, 1989.
68. Bagby G, Plessala K, Wilson L, *et al.* Divergent efficacy of anti-TNF-α antibody in intravascular and peritonitis models of sepsis. J Infect Dis 163:83, 1991.
69. Tracey K, Fong Y, Hesse D, *et al.* Anti-cachectin/TNF monoclonal antibodies prevent septic shock during lethal bacteraemia. Nature 330:662, 1987.
70. Hinshaw L, Tekamp-Olson P, Chang A, *et al.* Survival of primates in LD 100 septic shock following therapy with antibody to tumor necrosis factor (TNF-α). Circ Shock 30:279, 1990.
71. Chensue S, Remick D, Shmyr-Forsch C, *et al.* Immunohistochemical demonstration of cytoplasmic and membrane-associated tumor necrosis factor in murine macrophages. Am J Pathol 133:564, 1988.
72. Kriegler M, Perez C, DeFay K, *et al.* A novel form of TNF/cachectin is a cell surface cytotoxic transmembrane protein: ramifications for the complex physiology of TNF. Cell 53:45, 1988.
73. Keogh C, Fong Y, Marano M, *et al.* Identification of a novel tumor necrosis factor/cachectin from the livers of burned and infected rats. Arch Surg 125:79, 1990.
74. Marano M, Moldawer L, Fong Y, *et al.* Cachectin/TNF production in experimental burns and Pseudomonas infection. Arch Surg 123:1383, 1988.
75. Havell E. Evidence that tumor necrosis factor has an important role in antibacterial resistance. J Immunol 143:2894, 1989.
76. Havell E. Production of tumor necrosis factor during murine listeriosis. J Immunol 139: 4225, 1987.
77. Nelson S, Bagby G, Summer W. Anti-tumor necrosis factor-alpha antibody suppresses pulmonary antibacterial defenses. Am Rev Respir Dis 143:A393, 1991.
78. Adams L, Mason C, Kolls J, *et al.* Exacerbation of acute and chronic murine tuberculosis by administration of a tumor necrosis factor receptor-expressing adenovirus. J Infect Dis 171:400, 1995.
79. Fisher C Jr, Opal S, Dhainaut J, *et al.* Influence of an anti-tumor necrosis factor monoclonal antibody on cytokine levels in patients with sepsis. Crit Care Med 21:318, 1993.
80. Abraham E, Wunderink R, Silverman H, *et al.* Efficacy and safety of monoclonal antibody to human tumor necrosis factor alpha in patients with sepsis syndrome. A randomized, controlled, double-blind, multicenter clinical trial. JAMA 273:934, 1995.
81. Abraham E, Anzueto A, Gutierrez G, *et al.* Double-blind randomized controlled trial of monoclonal antibody to human tumour necrosis factor in treatment of septic shock. Lancet 351:929, 1998.
82. Reinhart K, Wiegand-Lohnert C, Grimminger F, *et al.* Assessment of the safety and efficacy of the monoclonal anti-tumor necrosis factor antibody fragment, MAK 195F, in patients with sepsis and septic shock: a multicenter, randomized placebo-controlled, dose-ranging study. Crit Care Med 24:733, 1996.
83. Mohler K, Torrance D, Smith C, *et al.* Soluble tumor necrosis factor (TNF) receptors are effective therapeutic agents in lethal endotoxemia

and function as both TNF carriers and TNF antagonists. J Immunol 151:1548, 1993.
84. Agosti J, Fisher J, Opal S, *et al.* Treatment of patients with sepsis syndrome with soluble TNF receptor (STNFr). 34th Interscience Conference on Antimicrobial Agents and Chemotherapy: 65, 1994.
85. Baumgartner JD, Calandra T. Treatment in sepsis. Past and future avenues. Drugs 57:127, 1999.
86. Dinarello C, Cannon J, Wolff S, *et al.* Tumor necrosis factor (cachectin) is an endogenous pyrogen and induces production of interleukin 1. J Exp Med 163:1433, 1986.
87. Okusawa S, Gelfand J, Ikejima T, *et al.* Interleukin 1 induces a shock like state in rabbits. Synergism with tumor necrosis factor and the effect of cyclooxygenase inhibition. J Clin Invest 81:1162, 1988.
88. Casey L, Balk R, Bone R. Cytokines in patients with the sepsis syndrome. The Second International Congress on the Immune Consequences of Trauma, Shock, and Sepsis: Mechanisms and Therapeutic Approaches. Munich, Germany, 1991.
89. Zuckerman S, Shelhaas J, Butler L. Differential regulation of lipopolysaccharide-induced interleukin-1 and tumor necrosis factor synthesis: effects of endogenous glucocorticoids and the role of the pituitary-adrenal axis. Eur J Immunol 19:301, 1989.
90. Dinarello C, Cannon J, Wolff S. New concepts on the pathogenesis of fever. Rev Infect Dis 10:168, 1988.
91. Dower S, Kronheim S, March C, *et al.* Detection and characterization of high-affinity plasma membrane receptors of human interleukin-1. J Exp Med 162:501, 1985.
92. Dower S, Kronheim S, Hopp T, *et al.* The cell surface receptors for interleukin-1 alpha and interleukin-1 beta are identical. Nature 324: 266, 1986.
93. Balavoine J, deRochemonteix B, Williamson K, *et al.* Prostaglandin E2 and collagenase production by fibroblasts and synovial cells is regulated by urine-derived human interleukin-1 and inhibitor(s). J Clin Invest 78:1120, 1986.
94. Mazzei G, Seckinger P, Dayer J, *et al.* Purification and characterization of a 26-kDa competitive inhibitor of interleukin-1. Eur J Immunol 20:683, 1990.
95. Hannum C, Wilcox C, Arend W, *et al.* Interleukin-1 receptor antagonist activity of a human interleukin-1 inhibitor. Nature 343:336, 1990.
96. Ohlsson K, Bjork P, Bergenfeldt M, *et al.* An interleukin-1 receptor antagonist (IL-1ra) blocks effect of IL-1 beta in the rabbit, rat and mouse and reduces the mortality in endotoxin shock. The Second International Congress on the Immune Consequences of Trauma, Shock, and Sepsis: Mechanisms and Therapeutic Approaches. Munich, Germany, 1991.
97. Fischer E, Marano M, vanZee K, *et al.* IL-1 receptor blockade attenuates the hemodynamic and metabolic consequences of lethal. *E. coli* septic shock. The Second International Congress on the Immune Consequences of Trauma, Shock, and Sepsis: Mechanisms and Therapeutic Approaches. Munich, Germany, 1991.
98. Fisher CJ, Slotman G, Opal S, *et al.* Initial evaluation of human recombinant interleukin-1 receptor antagonist in the treatment of sepsis syndrome: a randomized open-label, placebo-controlled multicenter trial. Crit Care Med 22:12, 1994.
99. Fisher CJ, Dhainaut J, Pribble J. A study to evaluate the safety and efficacy of human recombinant interleukin-1 receptor antagonist in the treatment of patients with sepsis syndrome. Clin Intensive Care 4:8S, 1993.
100. Bernard G, Reines H, Halushka P, *et al.* Prostacyclin and thromboxane A2 formation is increased in human sepsis syndrome. Effects of cyclooxygenase inhibition. Am Rev Respir Dis 144:1095, 1991.
101. Gnidec A, Sibbald W, Cheung H, *et al.* Ibuprofen reduces the progression of permeability edema in an animal model of hyperdynamic sepsis. J Appl Physiol 65:1024, 1988.
102. Kopolovic R, Thrailkill K, Martin D, *et al.* Effects of ibuprofen on a porcine model of acute respiratory failure. J Surg Res 36:300, 1984.
103. Bernard GR, Wheeler AP, Russell JA, *et al.* The effects of ibuprofen on the physiology and survival of patients with sepsis. N Engl J Med 236:912, 1997.
104. Cronin L, Cook D, Carlet J, *et al.* Corticosteroid treatment for sepsis: a critical appraisal and meta-analysis of the literature. Crit Care Med 23:1430, 1995.
105. Briegel J, Forst H, Haller M, *et al.* Stress doses of hydrocortisone reverse hyperdynamic septic shock: a prospective, randomized, double-blind, single-center study. Crit Care Med 27:723, 1999.

106. Guinot P. Clinical experience with platelet-activating factor antagonists. Past, present, and near future. Clin Rev Allergy 12:397, 1994.
107. Ruggiero V, Chiapparino C, Manganello S, *et al.* Beneficial effects of a novel platelet-activating factor receptor antagonist, ST 899, on endotoxin-induced shock in mice. Shock 2:275, 1994.
108. Abu-Zidan F, Walther S, Lennquist S. Modulation of lung injury by platelet-activating factor antagonism in nonhypotensive porcine endotoxemia. Circ Shock 44:148, 1994.
109. Dhainaut J, Tenaillon A, Le Tulzo Y, *et al.* Platelet-activating factor receptor antagonist BN52021 in the treatment of severe sepsis; a randomized, double-blind, placebo-controlled, multicenter clinical trial. Crit Care Med 22: 1720, 1994.
110. Ridings P, Blocher C, Fisher B, *et al.* Beneficial effects of a bradykinin antagonist in a model of gram-negative sepsis. J Trauma 39:81, 1995.
111. Cortech I. Phase II Bradycor trial does not show clinically meaningful reduction of 28-day mortality in sepsis. Cortech News Release, 1994.
112. Weisbart R, Gasson J, Golde D. Colony-stimulating factors and host defense. Ann Intern Med 110:297, 1989.
113. Demetri G, Griffin J. Granulocyte colony-stimulating factor and its receptor. Blood 78:2791, 1991.
114. Sheridan J, Metcalf D. Studies on the bone marrow colony stimulating factor (CSF): relation of tissue CSF to serum CSF. J Cell Physiol 80:129, 1972.
115. Metcalf D. Sources and biology of regulatory factors active on mouse myeloid leukemic cells. J Cell Physiol Suppl 1:175, 1982.
116. Seelentag W, Mermod J, Montesano R, *et al.* Additive effects of interleukin-1 and tumor necrosis factor-α on the accumulation of the three granulocyte and macrophage colony-stimulating factor mRNAs in human endothelial cells. EMBO J 6:2261, 1987.
117. Zsebo K, Yuschenkoff V, Schiffer S, *et al.* Vascular endothelial cells and granulopoiesis: interleukin-1 stimulates release of G-CSF and GM-CSF. Blood 73:99, 1988.
118. Koeffler H, Gasson J, Ranyard J, *et al.* Recombinant human TNF-α stimulates production of granulocyte colony-stimulating factor. Blood 70:55, 1987.
119. Yang Y, Tsai S, Wong G, *et al.* Interleukin-1 regulation of hematopoietic growth factor production by human stromal fibroblasts. J Cell Physiol 134:292, 1988.
120. Metcalf D, Nicola N. Synthesis by mouse peritoneal cells of G-CSF, the differentiation inducer for myeoid leukemia cells: stimulation by endotoxin, M-CSF, and multi-CSF. Leuk Res 9:35, 1985.
121. Rambaldi A, Young D, Griffin J. Expression of the M-CSF (CSF-1) gene by human monocytes. Blood 69:1409, 1987.
122. Fibbe W, van Damme J, Billiau A, *et al.* Interleukin-1 induces human marrow stromal cells in long-term culture to produce granulocyte colony-stimulating factor and macrophage colony-stimulating factor. Blood 71:430, 1988.
123. Rennick D, Yang G, Gemmell L, *et al.* Control of hemopoiesis by a bone marrow stromal cell clone: Lipopolysaccharide and interleukin-1-inducible production of colony-stimulating factors GM-CSF and G-CSF. Blood 69:682, 1987.
124. Nelson S, Bagby G, Mason C, *et al.* Ethanol suppresses *Escherichia coli*-induced plasma granulocyte colony-stimulating factor. Am J Respir Crit Care Med 151:A14, 1995.
125. Kawakami M, Tsutsumi H, Kumakawa T, *et al.* Levels of serum granulocyte colony-stimulating factor in patients with infections. Blood 76:1962, 1990.
126. Wang J, Chen Z, Colella S, *et al.* Chemotactic activity of recombinant human granulocyte colony-stimulating factor. Blood 72:1456, 1988.
127. Wang J, Colella S, Allavena P, *et al.* Chemotactic activity of human recombinant granulocyte-macrophage colony-stimulating factor. Immunology 60:439, 1987.
128. Weisbart RH, Golde DW. Physiology of granulocyte and macrophage colony-stimulating factors in host defense. Hematol Oncol Clin North Am 3:401, 1989.
129. Ogle JD, Noel JG, Sramkoski RM, *et al.* The effects of cytokines, platelet-activating factor, and arachidonate metabolites on C3b receptor (CR1, CD35) expression and phagocytosis by neutrophils. Cytokine 2:447, 1990.
130. Roilides E, Walsh T, Pizzo P, *et al.* Granulocyte colony-stimulating factor enhances the phagocytic and bactericidal activity of normal and defective human neutrophils. J Infect Dis 163:579, 1991.
131. O'Reilly M, Silver G, Greenhalgh G, *et al.* Treatment of intra-abdominal infection with

granulocyte colony-stimulating factor. J Trauma 33:679, 1992.

132. Goya T, Torisu M, Doi F, *et al.* Effects of granulocyte colony-stimulating factor and monobactam antibiotics (aztreonam) on neutrophil functions in sepsis. Clin Immunol Immunopath 69:278, 1993.

133. Eichacker P, Waisman Y, Natanson C, *et al.* Cardiopulmonary effects of granulocyte colony-stimulating factor in a canine model of bacterial sepsis. J Appl Physiol 77:2366, 1994.

134. Smith W, Sumnicht G, Sharpe R, *et al.* Granulocyte colony-stimulating factor versus placebo in addition to penicillin G in a randomized blinded study of gram-negative pneumonia sepsis: analysis of survival and multisystem organ failure. Blood 86:1301, 1995.

135. Fink M, O'Sullivan B, Menconi M, *et al.* Effect of granulocyte colony-stimulating factor on systemic and pulmonary responses to endotoxin in pigs. J Trauma 34:571, 1993.

136. Koizumi T, Kubo K, Shinozaki S, *et al.* Granulocyte colony-stimulating factor does not exacerbate endotoxin-induced lung injury in sheep. Am Rev Respir Dis 148:132, 1993.

137. Kanazawa M, Ishizaka A, Hasegawa N, *et al.* Granulocyte colony-stimulating factor does not enhance endotoxin-induced acute lung injury in guinea pigs. Am Rev Respir Dis 145:1030, 1992.

138. deBoisblanc B, Summer W, Mason C, *et al.* Phase 1 study of granulocyte colony stimulating factor (G-CSF) in community acquired pneumonia. Am Rev Respir Dis 147:A204, 1993.

139. Nelson S, Farkas S, Fotheringham N, *et al.* Filgrastim in the treatment of hospitalized patients with community-acquired pneumonia (CAP). Am J Respir Crit Care Med 153:A535, 1996.

140. Wunderink R, Leeper K, Schein R, *et al.* Clinical response to filgrastim (G-CSF) in severe pneumonia with severe sepsis. Am J Respir Crit Care Med 153:A123, 1996.

141. Yasuda H, Ajiki Y, Shomozato T, Kasahara M, Kawada H, Iwata M, Shimizu K. Therapeutic efficacy of granulocyte colonystimulating factor alone and in combination with antibiotics against *Pseudomonas aeruginosa* infections in mice. Infect Immun 58:2502–2509, 1990.

142. McKenna PH, Nelson S, Andresen J. Filgrastim (rhuGCSF) enhances ciprofloxacin uptake and bactericidal activity of human neutrophils *in vitro* (abstract). Am J Respir Crit Care Med 153S:A535, 1996.

12. USING INFORMATION SYSTEMS TECHNOLOGY TO IMPROVE ANTIBIOTIC PRESCRIBING

Thomas C. Bailey, S. Troy McMullin and Janette Coble

Abstract

The selection of antimicrobial agents in the hospital setting is still a largely manual task and, therefore, fraught with the potential for error. This includes the choice of agents, dosage regimens, and monitoring for response and toxicity. The authors describe current and future strategies to use information technology to improve the process of antimicrobial selection, avoid dosing errors and contraindicated drug combinations.

Introduction

Physicians have been anticipating the impact of computers in medicine since the 1970s. However, much of the research in this area has been both exciting and disappointing. From the earliest work with protocol-based computer reminders to the latest publications describing the impact of locally developed, non-exportable expert systems, the advantages of these systems have been limited to a small percentage of patients. For decades, researchers have pointed to the imperfectability of man as a major obstacle in achieving optimal health care [1]. Yet in reality, we are entering the new millennium with very few hospitals, physicians, or patients realizing the full potential of information systems technology.

Predictable factors such as lack of funding and patient confidentiality have often come in direct conflict with the pursuit of improved decision-making and error prevention. The Institute of Medicine estimates that at least 44,000 and perhaps as many as 98,000 Americans die each year as the result of medical errors. Medication errors, occurring in or out of the hospital, account for over 7000 deaths annually [2]. Not all medication errors result in an adverse drug event, and not all adverse drug events are the result of errors. However, preventable adverse drug events in hospitals are frequent, occurring in approximately two per cent of hospital admissions [2]. The rate of preventable adverse drug events in the intensive care unit (ICU) may be even higher, and often involve inappropriate antibiotic selection, dosing, or drug combinations [3–5]. In addition to causing morbidity and mortality, these events are also costly, resulting in an estimated $2 billion in direct hospital costs annually in the United States [2, 6].

Improving Selection

Inappropriate empiric antibiotic treatment is a strong predictor of mortality in critically ill patients. Unfortunately, physicians in the ICU seldom have access to current data regarding local prevalence of pathogens and local antibiotic

Gram-Positive Cocci 1998 Full-House	# Strains	# Strains Tested	Oxacillin	Tetracycline	Clindamycin	Nitrofurantion	Erythromycin	Ciprofloxacin	Trimeth/Sulfa	Gentamicin	Penicillin	Ceftriaxone	Cefepime	Ampicillin	High Level Strep	High Level Gent	Vancomycin
Staph aureus	2705	1885	65		69		53	60	89	87	5						100
Staph species not aureus	4264	656	35		68		32	50	52	80	10						100
E. faecalis	248	215		50		98		14						100	71	70	98
Strep. pneumoniae	154	109					90				69	87	77				
E. faecium	122	102		66		26		3						19	32	66	48

FIGURE 1. The "Whole House Antibiogram" showing frequent pathogens and their susceptibility patterns.

resistance patterns to guide their empiric antibiotic selections. Instead, physicians are forced to rely upon their perceptions. In 20–50% of patients with severe infections, empiric antibiotic selection by physicians results in inadequate coverage for the isolated pathogen. In another 15–25% of cases, the initial antibiotic regimen provides overly broad coverage [7]. Improving physicians' access to historical infection-related information to guide their antibiotic choices is an important goal.

Antibiograms. A frequent means to disseminate rudimentary information regarding common pathogens and their susceptibility patterns is the "whole house antibiogram" (Figure 1). While this a good start to providing necessary information for antibiotic selection, these antibiograms have several shortcomings. First, microbial flora and antibiotic susceptibilities vary within the hospital, with more resistant species seen in the intensive care setting [8]. Second, pathogens vary by the site of infection. Third, pathogens and susceptibilities differ for community-acquired and nosocomial infections. Finally, the patterns of these infectious agents vary over time. The whole house antibiogram cannot reflect this level of complexity.

Decision support. Displaying antibiogram data should take these variables into account. As shown in Figure 2, microbiological data can include pathogen frequency, susceptibility by functional area within the hospital, and site of infection, stratified by community-acquired and nosocomial origin. Decision support systems may also contain important patient-specific clinical information such as known allergies, previous therapeutic failures, or the presence of neutropenia, sickle cell anemia, cystic fibrosis, and other conditions that may alter the potential pool of pathogens. Providing physicians with this type of decision support to guide them through the process of choosing an antibiotic has been shown to improve antibiotic selection, control antibiotic costs, and slow the emergence of resistance [9–11]. In addition, such strategies are more likely than administrative measures to preserve physician autonomy and satisfaction in the control of prescribing practices. While published data involve highly complex technological approaches, providing this sort of information through lower technology solutions might also be expected to achieve some of these goals. This is worthy of further study.

Improving Dosing

Adverse drug events involving antibiotics constitute a significant proportion of preventable

A	B	C	D	E	F	G	H	I	J	K	L	M	N	O	P	Q
GRAM POSITIVE COCCI, Ward: 83ICU, Nosocomial_Only, 10/1/98-9/30/99	#STRAINS	OXACILLIN	TETRACYCLINE	CLINDAMYCIN	NITROFURANTION	ERYTHROMYCIN	CIPROFLOXACIN	TRIMETH	GENTAMICIN	PENICILLIN	CEFTRIAXONE	CEFEPIME	AMPICILLIN	HIGH_LEVEL_STREP	HIGH_LEVEL_GENT	VANCOMYCIN
Staph aureus	13	15		31		23	15	69	75	8						100
Staph species not aureus	105	14		54		7	36	50	88	0						100
E. faecalis	14		46		92		15						100	62	27	100
E. faecium	17		35		53		0						0	0	67	24
Strep. pneumoniae	0															
Strep. group A	0															

Gram Positive - Blood / Gram Positive- Respiratory / Gram Positive-Urine

FIGURE 2. An example of a "Unit Specific Antibiogram", in this case showing nosocomially acquired pathogens from respiratory specimens over a defined period of time from a specific ICU.

events, the most common of which are dosing errors due to altered drug metabolism or elimination. Many critically ill patients will suffer hepatic or renal insults during their stay in the ICU, necessitating antibiotic dosage adjustments. Other patients may have increased dosing requirements over time as they recover from hepatic or renal dysfunction. Even the most astute physician may inadvertently disregard this important aspect of antibiotic therapy in a patient with a complex and critical illness. Automated clinical information systems have an important role in detecting dosing errors, and they have been shown to improve physicians' prescribing practice [3].

Non-integrated information systems. Standard commercial software coupled with freestanding pharmacy dispensing systems usually provides simple dose range checking, flagging those orders that exceed certain preset maximums. While these packages can be useful for catching egregious errors, such as those that involve improper units (e.g., milligrams vs micrograms), they suffer a number of shortcomings. If they are not integrated with other hospital information systems, they cannot provide tailored recommendations that include important factors such as the patient's age, weight, renal function, hepatic function, or site of infection. Furthermore, they usually do not catch under-dosing errors, which result in suboptimal therapy and encourage the development of antibiotic resistance. Most of these systems are proprietary, and therefore do not permit users to customize the rule base for local practice variations or to delete rules that are trivial. As a result, the flags from these systems are both insensitive and non-specific, and they are very likely to be ignored by the busy hospital pharmacist or physician, even when correct.

Integrated information systems. Systems that have access to pertinent patient information to guide dosing decisions will be more sensitive and specific than their non-integrated counterparts. Commercial software exists for both pharmacy dispensing systems and for physician order entry, but for the most part these are immature products that have not become mainstream. Currently, physician order entry is available in fewer than 10% of American hospitals. Even in most of these hospitals, direct entry by physicians accounts for fewer than 25% of the inpatient medication orders [12]. Clearly, improvements in this area are needed. Software that requires the physician to manually enter patient information that should be available electronically represents a distraction from the patient care process rather than adding value to that process. Furthermore, lack of standardization in healthcare information means that a system that may work well in one locale may not work well in another. Solutions to these problems are potentially very expensive to develop and maintain.

Avoiding Adverse Drug Combinations

Critically ill patients are usually treated with multiple medications, often prescribed by multiple physicians. As the number of medications with which patients are treated increases, so does the risk of an adverse drug interaction [5]. Serious drug interactions in the ICU may occur through pharmacodynamic (e.g., theophylline antagonizing the effects of adenosine, haloperidol increasing the arrhythmogenic potential of procainamide) or pharmacokinetic mechanisms (e.g., rifampin decreasing chloramphenicol blood concentrations, dalfopristin-quinupristin increasing cyclosporin blood concentrations).

Once again, commercial drug interaction software packages often fall short of their goal to prevent these interactions. Some do not distinguish trivial from significant interactions resulting in poor specificity of drug order flags, overwhelming the user. Most do not allow the knowledge base to be customized. Finally, the capacity to detect newly recognized drug interactions must await software upgrade availability, and inevitable delays in installation.

One example of an important drug interaction in the intensive care setting is the use of cisapride, a gastrointestinal promotility agent, in combination with an azole anti-fungal agent or macrolide antibiotic. These drugs, when used in combination, may result in fatal cardiac dysrhythmias, particularly Torsade de Pointes. Because of the poor specificity of drug interaction detection software, clinicians must be alert to the possibility that the dispensing pharmacist may not detect these potentially dangerous combinations. In one study, 3–9% of patients receiving cisapride also received one of these contraindicated medications during their hospital stay [4]. This rate of contraindicated drug use with cisapride is similar to that still occurring with terfenadine, nearly five years after the initial warnings about this drug were issued. Subtler potential adverse drug effects such as augmentation of neuromuscular blockade by aminoglycosides or worsening of myasthenia may also be ignored by the dispensing pharmacist because of lack of access to clinical information about the patient.

Computerized drug interaction screening software should incorporate a "forcing function" to prevent pharmacists from processing an order for a contraindicated medication. In the absence of such a blocking mechanism, these systems should include a safety net function that could send a second notice on potentially life-threatening drug interactions that have slipped through the system or been overridden during order processing. This method of detecting performance lapses has been shown to decrease the rate of potentially dangerous drug combinations

[4]. An ideal computerized drug interaction screening system would also allow its users to restrict the list of interactions to those associated with clinically significant adverse outcomes.

Synchronous versus Asynchronous Decision Support

Synchronous decision support. A strong case can be made for "front-end" physician order entry systems that guide the prescribing physician to make the appropriate antibiotic selection, choose the appropriate dosage regimen (avoiding both under dosing and over dosing), and prevent potential adverse drug combinations [10, 13, 14]. However, such systems must be integrated with sources of important clinical data, raise flags only when clinically important to do so, be fast and intuitive to use, and be economically feasible to implement. Furthermore, these systems must be able to detect dosing errors that occur as a result of changes in a patient's renal function after the original order has been written, and have a means to notify the responsible physician at a time that is appropriate. Few, if any, commercially available systems satisfy all of these conditions.

Asynchronous decision support. An alternative strategy is to use software to screen orders after the fact, notifying the physician only when a potential problem is detected. Such a strategy requires an integrated clinical database coupled with a knowledge-based expert system that issues clinical alerts when potential problems are detected. The participation of pharmacists on daily work rounds is an effective means of preventing adverse drug events [15]. At our institution, clinical pharmacists handle expert system alerts as part of their daily workflow. While the efficiency of physician order entry to prevent the problem at the source is potentially lost, the physician is not forced to interact with a computer 100% of the time for the few inappropriate orders that require attention. Instead, the strategy can be to filter such potential problem orders through a clinical pharmacist, who can then exercise judgment as to their urgency and importance. Under our current system, approximately 8% of orders that are screened result in a clinical alert that is routed to a clinical pharmacist. The clinical pharmacists agree with approximately 50% of these alerts and bring them to the attention of the responsible physician, who in turn agrees to change the order approximately 75% of the time. Thus, approximately 3% of orders screened are changed as a result of this process. Such a system can serve as a safety net to catch problem orders that slip through a suboptimal front-end screening system. In addition, such systems are inherently poised to detect dosing errors that occur after the original order was written as a result of changes in renal function. We have shown that such systems, while acting on the "back-end", can result in learning that improves the front-end process of choosing dosing regimens (Figure 3) and avoiding contraindicated drug combinations (Figure 4). Commercial systems also exist to detect mismatches between the antibiotic regimen and the bacterial drug susceptibility from patients' cultures. With improvements in messaging technology and notification modalities, the ability exists to make such back-end screening processes nearly real time, making the choice between front-end and back-end screening strategies less obvious.

Barriers to Implementation

Many barriers exist to the implementation of automated solutions to the problem of improving antibiotic prescribing, some of which have already been discussed. The major barrier is the fragmentation of information in multiple, distributed legacy information systems in the form of data that is not coded and not standardized. This barrier makes it prohibitively expensive for many institutions and for commercial software companies to build software solutions that can be scaled across multiple institutions. In the meantime, healthcare institutions are faced with difficult choices regarding front-end or back-end

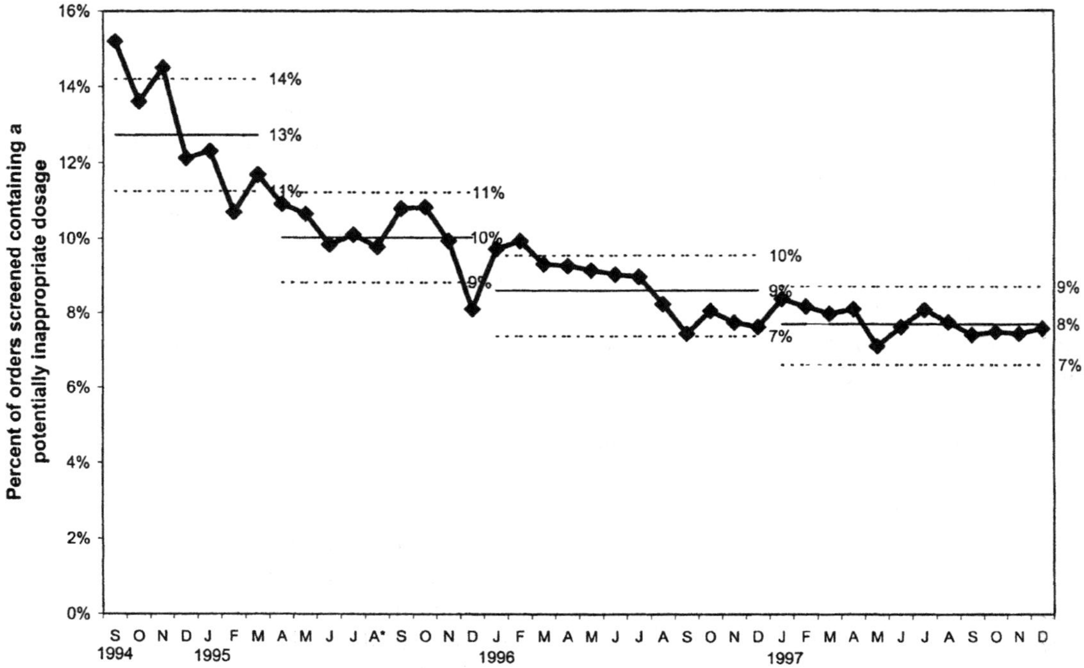

FIGURE 3. Improvement in dosing regimens after implementing an asynchronous decision support tool.

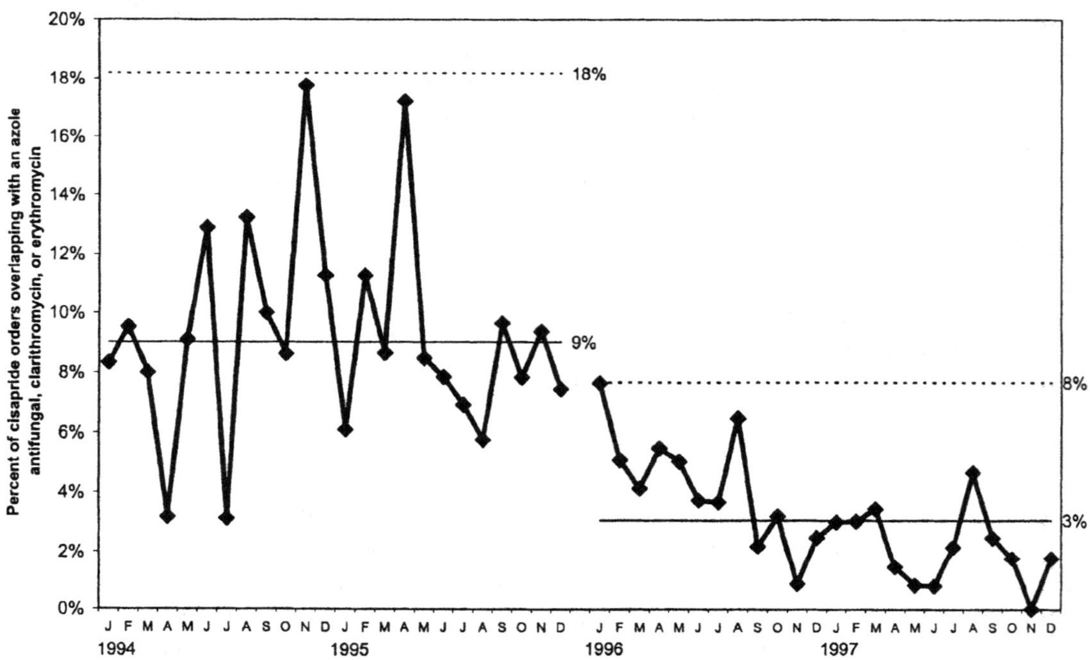

FIGURE 4. Reduction in contraindicated drug combinations after implementing an asynchronous decision support tool.

decision support, and either settling for what is currently available or striving for what we know is possible. We have chosen to build our own industry standard clinical database using currently available database software. Once this was done, our institution was poised to build our own decision support software or accept a commercial package. Because of the shortcomings of currently available commercial software, we have chosen to do the former. However, justifying the labor-intensive tasks of building and maintaining a clinical database and writing and maintaining custom software is a constant struggle. It is difficult to quantitate the return on investment of software tools that make previously impossible tasks possible, or those that avoid errors before they occur. In an environment where every dollar spent is scrutinized, and where the demand for technical expertise in other industries is high, employee turnover is high and institutional memory is short. We are buoyed on by the enthusiasm of our colleagues and by the knowledge that we are doing the right thing for our patients.

Conclusions

Improving antibiotic and other pharmaceutical prescribing is technically feasible but commercial solutions are currently suboptimal. For antibiotic selection, optimizing the current standard antibiogram to provide more useful information for the hospital setting will be a major advance. Automated matching of individual patient antibiotic regimens against their culture and susceptibility data is currently possible but not widely utilized. For dosing, automating the process of screening dosage regimens requires an integrated clinical database and constant monitoring beyond the initial drug order to be optimally effective. To avoid contraindicated drug combinations, a back-end safety net is necessary to catch those combinations that slip through the front-end screening process. Barriers to implementation exist, none of which is insurmountable.

References

1. McDonald CJ. Protocol-based computer reminders, the quality of care and the non-perfectability of man. New England Journal of Medicine. 295:1351, 1976.
2. Kohn L, Corrigan J, Donaldson M (eds). To err is human: building a safer health system. Committee on Quality of Health Care in America. Institute Of Medicine. Washington, D.C.; National Academy Press, 1999.
3. McMullin ST, Reichley RM, Watson LA, Steib SA, Frisse ME, Bailey TC. Experience with advanced technologies that reduce medication errors. In Proceedings, Enhancing Patient Safety and Reducing Errors in Health Care. National Patient Safety Foundation of the American Medical Association, 1999:132.
4. McMullin ST, Reichley RM, Watson LA, Steib SA, Frisse ME, Bailey TC. Impact of a Web-based clinical information system on cisapride drug interactions and patient safety. Arch Intern Med 159:2077, 1999.
5. Cullen DJ, Sweitzer BJ, Bates DW, Burdick E, Edmondson A, Leape LL. Preventable adverse drug events in hospitalized patients: a comparative study of intensive care and general care units. Critical Care Medicine 25:1289, 1997.
6. Bates DW, Spell N, Cullen DJ, Burdick E, Laird N, Petersen LA, Small SD, Sweitzer BJ, Leape LL. The costs of adverse drug events in hospitalized patients. JAMA 277:307, 1997.
7. Leibovici L, Gitelman V, Yehezkelli Y, Poznanski O, Milo G, *et al.* Improving antibiotic empirical antibiotic treatment: prospective, nonintervention testing of a decision support system. J Intern Med 242:395, 1997.
8. Kaufman D, Haas CE, Edinger R, Hollick G. Antibiotic susceptibility in the surgical intensive care unit compared with the hospital-wide antibiogram. Archives of Surgery 133:1041, 1998.
9. Pestotnik SL, Classen DC, Evans RS, Burke JP. Implementing antibiotic practice guidelines through computer-assisted decision support: clinical and financial outcomes. Ann Intern Med 124:884, 1996.
10. Evans RS, Pestotnik SL, Classen DC, Clemmer TP, Weaver LK, Orme JF Jr, Lloyd JF, Burke JP. A computer-assisted management program for antibiotics and other antiinfective agents. New England J Med 338:232, 1998.
11. Pestotnik SL, Evans RS, Burke JP, Gardner RM, Classen DC. Therapeutic antibiotic monitoring:

surveillance using a computerized expert system. American J Med 88:43, 1990.

12. Ringold DJ, Santell JP, Schneider PJ, Arenberg S. ASHP national survey of pharmacy practice in acute care settings: prescribing and transcribing-1998. Am J Health-Syst Pharm 56:142, 1999.
13. Bates DW, Teich JM, Lee J, Seger D, Kuperman GJ, Ma'Luf N, Boyle D, Leape L. The impact of computerized physician order entry on medication error prevention. J American Med Informatics Association 6:313, 1999.
14. Bates DW, Leape LL, Cullen DJ, Laird N, Petersen LA, Teich JM, Burdick E, Hickey M, Kleefield S, Shea B, Vander Vliet M, Seger DL. Effect of computerized physician order entry and a team intervention on prevention of serious medication errors. JAMA 280:1311, 1998.
15. Leape LL, Cullen DJ, Dempsey Clapp M, Burdick E, Demonaco HJ *et al.* Pharmacist participation on physician rounds and adverse drug events in the intensive care unit. JAMA 282:267, 1999.

13. USE OF ANTIBIOTICS IN PREGNANT PATIENTS IN THE ICU

Josep-E. Baños and Magí Farré

Infections and Critical Care in Obstetric Patients

The critically sick pregnant patient challenges the intensive care physician. Several features, such physiological changes associated with pregnancy, specific obstetric diseases and the presence of the fetus greatly complicate the assessment and treatment of these patients [1]. Several studies have analyzed obstetric admissions to the intensive care unit ICU [1–10]. They conclude that less than 1% of deliveries is referred to the ICU, mainly by preeclampsia, and maternal mortality may be highly variable (from 0 in the study of Lapinsky *et al.* [1] to 20% in Collop and Sahn's study [6]). Bacterial infections were a significant, although not highly prevalent, cause of sickness in these critically ill patients.

Infectious diseases are not uncommon during pregnancy and postpartum period [11, 12]. Severe infections are much less common and fortunately very few pregnant women with infectious diseases should be cared for at the ICU setting (see Correa *et al.*, in this book). Although pneumonia, pyelonephritis and abortion-related infections may be life-threatening, many patients may be treated in regular wards and only severe infections in high risk patients require critical care. However, it has been shown that infections may account for the 24% of all referral diagnoses [5]. The main causes were sepsis and pneumonia [5, 13, 14].

The characteristics of septic shock in pregnant women have been described in detail by several authors [13–15]. Main causes that predispose to septic shock include pyelonephritis, chorioamnionitis, Stevens-Johnson syndrome, premature rupture of membranes, necrotizing fasciitis, septic abortion and endometritis. Microorganisms that may cause septic shock are mainly Gram-negative bacteria, usually *Escherichia coli*, but anaerobes, such as *Bacteroides fragilis*, and Gram-positive can also be seen [14].

General Considerations on the Use of Antibiotics in Pregnant Patients

Pregnancy always complicates drug treatment. Any drug may be harmful to the mother and also the fetus and, accordingly, no pharmacological therapy must be initiated unless a clear benefit is expected. Nonetheless, the benefit risk-index advises active treatment in ICU patients. From the pharmacological point of view, antibiotics are relatively safe drugs when used in pregnant patients with severe infections. Many current antibiotics have been used for at least thirty years and most of them seems to be free of significant teratogenic effects, at least in animals. They are given in short courses so their adverse effects are rather predictable, but some appreciation of the balance of risks in more serious cases is also needed. However, the understandable reluctance of physicians and pharmaceutical companies to study drugs in pregnant women greatly limits the scientific evidence of the effectiveness and safety of all drugs, and also antibiotics, in pregnancy. Three aspects deserve special attention when antibiotic use in pregnant women is considered: the first relates to pharmacokinetic changes induced by pregnancy, the second to potential toxicity to mother and fetus, and the third refers to the effectiveness of antibiotic regimes in obstetric infections.

Pregnancy may change the way in which women handle antimicrobial agents and therefore some quantitative changes on treatment effects may appear. Most pregnancy-induced effects are of a pharmacokinetic nature. In general, low maternal concentrations have been found after administration of antimicrobials, such as penicillins, cephalosporins, aminoglycosides and erythromycin [16]. The main implications of these findings refer to dosage. For instance, a moderate increase in the dosage of penicillins has been recommended [17]. As a rule, full doses should be used to treat infections in pregnancy and, therefore, treatment regimes should assure that the patient is receiving her right dose. Thus, measurement of blood levels may be needed in some cases when drug pharmacokinetics are influenced by pregnancy. The reason is two-fold: first, to assure the correct dosage according to the patient; second, to avoid unnecessary high blood levels that may be toxic both in the mother and the fetus [11]. Also, the length of treatment should be established by the specific disease and not by the consideration that the patient is pregnant.

In spite of the assertions made in previous paragraphs, a troublesome aspect of antibiotic treatment is its theoretical ability to harm the maternal-fetal unit. Major studies which indicate an association of antibiotic exposure in pregnancy and congenital malformations are lacking [18]. Certain drugs should be avoided as toxicity may be expected in the pregnant woman herself, the fetus, or the neonate. Aminoglycosides, tetracyclines, chloramphenicol and fluoroquinolones must be used with special care in pregnancy [11]. Most authors recognize that tetracyclines and aminoglycosides may have some teratogenic effects [18, 19]. Moreover, tetracyclines may have an increased risk of toxicity in the pregnant woman [19]. In turn, neonates may be damaged by sulfonamides and chloramphenicol. The withdrawal of these antibiotic drugs is mandatory when the treatment of minor infections by otherwise drug sensitive bacteria is considered. Nonetheless, these principles may be questioned when severe infection by resistant microorganisms appears.

Antibiotics are used in pregnancy to treat various specific infections related to pregnancy *per se* (chorioamnionitis), for infections unrelated but complicating pregnancy (pneumonia, bacterial endocarditis) and for conditions which if untreated would affect adversely the outcome of pregnancy (asymptomatic bacteriuria). Urinary and respiratory tract infections rank high in pregnant women [11]. Clinical trials showing efficacy of antibiotics in pregnant women are scarce if compared with other areas of drug therapy. This paucity of studies is so important that some textbooks rely in the experience or the personal opinion of the authors [12]. Hence, this chapter will avoid any reference to the specific therapeutics of infections seen in the ICU and will only consider the first two topics described earlier, i.e. the pharmacokinetic changes induced by pregnancy and the safety of antibiotic drugs in the mother and the fetus.

In conclusion, the treatment of maternal infections should follow the general principles of pharmacological therapy in pregnant women. Moreover, drug efficacy ranks first in ICU patients, although safety of embryo or fetus should always be considered. Antibiotics must be chosen by susceptibility studies or, more often, by empirical evaluation of the most likely group of microorganisms and their most probable antibiotic susceptibility. Only when this aspect has been considered, must embryonic or fetal safety concerns arise [17].

Pregnancy Related Pharmacokinetic Changes of Clinical Relevance

Drug pharmacokinetics is mainly affected by pregnancy in two ways. The first are the progressive changes in maternal physiology during pregnancy which are most evident during the third trimester and immediate postpartum. These changes affect the absorption, distribution, metabolism and elimination of some drugs. The second factor is related to the placental-fetal unit/compartment and modifies the amount of drug crossing the placenta, the fraction metabolised by the placenta and the distribution and elimination of the drug by the fetus [20].

ABSORPTION

The gastrointestinal tract physiology is altered by pregnancy as showed by a delay in both gastric and intestinal motilities. The increases of plasma progesterone levels during pregnancy seem to be responsible for a 30–50% increase in gastric and intestinal emptying time. Decreased gastric acid secretion (40% less than in non-pregnant women) and peptic activity, and an increase in mucus secretion convey an increase in gastric pH. This could influence the ionization of weak acids and bases and may result in unpredictable absorption of orally administered drugs. However, the final consequences of these changes are probably of minor importance.

Increased cardiac output during pregnancy increases blood flow to other organs and tissues. Thus, drugs given by the intramuscular route may be more rapidly absorbed. The increase in the pulmonary blood flow could favor alveolar uptake of drugs administered by inhalation [21].

DISTRIBUTION

The plasma volume expands by approximately 50%, starting around the sixth week of pregnancy and reaching a plateau at 30 to 34 weeks of gestation, therefore the volume of distribution of some drugs may be altered. The total mean increase in body water is from 7 to 8.5 liters, most of which is extracellular, distributed to the placenta, fetus and amniotic fluid (60%) and maternal tissues (40%). This increase in the apparent volume of distribution can diminish maternal peak serum drug concentrations (Cmax) of many drugs. Those drugs that are mainly distributed in water compartments and having a relatively small distribution volume (Vd) will show the most important decrease in Cmax. In consequence, increased drug dosage requirements would be needed to reach similar plasma concentrations [22]. Moreover, body fat increases by an average of 25% during pregnancy and therefore plasma concentration of drugs which mainly distribute to fat tissues decrease [17].

The plasma volume expands faster than albumin production, creating a physiological dilutional hypoalbuminaemia, with a decreasing binding capacity. The free fraction of highly protein-bound drugs increases. This increase in free fraction may lead to a decrease in total drug concentration, because more drug is available to be metabolized by hepatic enzymes or cleared from the body. The unbound concentrations can more easily penetrate tissues and may have a greater effect than expected from total serum drug concentrations. The direct determination of free-drug concentration in critical patients is recommended [17, 21].

HEPATIC METABOLISM

The elevated progesterone and estrogen concentrations observed in pregnancy appear to activate hepatic microsomal enzymes. This increased hepatic activity can accelerate the biotransformation of the parent drug to active and inactive metabolites. If the drug is being transformed into less active or inactive products, an increased dose of the parent drug or a decreased dosing interval may be necessary. On the other hand, the elimination of other drugs could be reduced by competitive inhibition of microsomal oxidases by progesterone and estradiol. The importance of these changes should be considered for each drug and no general rule can be applied [17, 21].

RENAL ELIMINATION

Renal blood flow and glomerular filtration rate can increase by up to 50% by the fourth month of pregnancy. The consequence of renal changes is an increase of clearance of substances that are mainly eliminated unchanged by renal route. For example, the clearance of ampicillin doubles during pregnancy. An increased dose or a shortened dosing interval may be needed to achieve desired steady-state concentrations [17, 21].

TRANSPLACENTAL PASSAGE OF DRUGS

Drugs can move bidirectionally across the placenta as a consequence of passive diffusion. Drugs that cross the placenta more easily include small molecules (with low molecular weight), lipophilic substances, and those with a large free fraction or low protein binding. The placenta increases its surface area and thins with advancing pregnancy, and this increase is proportional to age and fetal weight. The main effect is an enhancement of transplacental diffusion from the mother to the fetus. The fetal plasma pH is slightly more acidic than the maternal and therefore weak bases can be concentrated in the fetus (ion trapping) [20].

The placenta and the fetus are able to metabolize drugs. However, most enzymatic processes are immature in fetus, and then its contribution to drug elimination is only marginal. The equilibrium of maternal-fetal drug concentrations depends of the physicochemical properties of the drug. The time to reach similar maximal concentrations in both sides of the placenta is delayed in the fetus side [20].

The overall effect of the above mentioned pharmacokinetic changes is the decrease in 10 to 50% of drug concentrations during late pregnancy compared to non-pregnant females. In the early postpartum period, pharmacokinetics remains similar to those seen during the third trimester of pregnancy – despite the removal of the placenta and fetus. The therapeutic implications of these changes should be kept in mind during the postpartum period.

Antibiotics and Pregnancy

The body of scientific evidence that justifies and guides the rational use of antibiotics in pregnancy is scarce and incomplete. There are justified reasons for this limited number of clinical studies but, as a consequence, many pharmacological treatments in pregnancy are empirically based and often clinical personal experience is the main criteria to make a choice. Taking into account these considerations, we will review the main clinical studies that have centered on evaluating the use of antibiotics in pregnancy. A brief consideration of some commonly used drugs of each group follows. A detailed review of the general use of antibiotics in pregnancy can be found elsewhere [12, 14, 17, 20, 21, 23].

PENICILLINS

In general, β-lactams should be considered as probably safe in pregnancy [19]. No adverse effects must be expected in the first trimester but their ability to cross the placental barrier may result in allergy and the possibility that the fetus may be sensitized can not be ruled out [11]. Although little information is available to have full evidence of these assertions, experience gained in the last 50 years did not suggest increased toxicity. In a collaborative project, in 3546 women who took penicillin derivatives in the first trimester of pregnancy no teratogenic effects were seen [24, 25]. However, unconditional confidence in new drugs, even if they are from the same β-lactam group, is not recommended.

Several pharmacokinetic studies of penicillins have been performed in pregnant women [23, 26–29]. These studies have shown that the serum levels of these drugs are lower and their renal clearance is higher during pregnancy when data were compared with non-pregnant women. Most penicillins cross the placenta but drugs with high protein binding (oxacillin, cloxacillin, dicloxacillin, nafcillin) have a lower ability to cross the placental barrier resulting in lower fetal tissue and amniotic fluid levels. In contrast, poorly bound penicillins (ampicillin, amoxicillin, methicillin) cross better and achieve concentrations in amniotic fluid 0.5–1 times that of maternal plasma concentration [20].

Penicillin G (benzylpenicillin) has been used to treat maternal infections for many years. It crosses the placenta quickly and reaches the fetal circulation and amniotic fluid [30]. At term, maternal serum and amniotic fluid concentrations were equal 60–90 min after intravenous injection and continuous infusions of penicillin G produced similar concentrations in maternal serum, cord serum, and amniotic fluid [31]. Nathan *et al.* [32] have analyzed the pharmacokinetic properties of benzathine penicillin G (benzathine benzylpenicillin) to treat syphilis in pregnant women in the week prior to delivery. Drug concentrations in maternal and fetal tissues gave a wide variability, so the authors recommended caution when treating pregnant women at this stage by the risk that altered pharmacokinetics may affect drug efficacy. A study analyzing the pharmacokinetics of penicillin V (phenoxymethylpenicillin) during the last two trimesters of pregnancy showed that faster elimination rates of the drug from the plasma of the pregnant patients compared with non-pregnant women [33].

Regarding the potential of penicillin G to cause birth defects, two studies have analyzed this possibility. In a controlled study, penicillin G was given to pregnant women in the first trimester for a total of 107 weeks. No differences were seen in the incidence of congenital abnormalities between treated and control groups [34]. In a retrospective study, the Collaborative Perinatal Project, 7171 exposures to penicillin G were recorded at anytime during the pregnancy, 3546 in the first trimester [25]. No evidence was found linking penicillin G and birth defects. Therefore, the probability that penicillin G is teratogenic is very low [23]. The same conclusions may apply to penicillin V [23, 25].

Several authors have studied the pharmacokinetic properties of ampicillin in pregnant women [23, 25]. Plasma levels of ampicillin are lower in women during pregnancy than in non-pregnant patients and this fact is observed across the pregnancy [23]. It seems that pregnant women will require higher doses of ampicillin to achieve comparable plasmatic levels [36]. In a recent study [37] ampicillin pharmacokinetics were compared during and after the pregnancy in the same women. It was shown that pregnancy significantly increased the elimination rate constant, decreased the area under the curve (AUC) by 20% and increased the total body clearance. This antibiotic rapidly crosses the placenta and drug levels exceeding the minimum inhibitory concentrations for most of microorganisms causing intrauterine infections can be found in fetal blood and amniotic fluid [38]. The drug was given intravenously to women of 15–40 weeks of gestation. When given by infusion to patients at term, the cord to maternal ratios increased with time and approached unity within two hours. Cord concentrations were greater than 5 mg/l for at least four hours. Amniotic fluid levels can be detected in 90 minutes reaching 20% of maternal serum peak in 8 hours.

Ampicillin has been extensively used in the last half of pregnancy to prevent maternal or fetus infections at risk pregnancies like, for instance, premature rupture of membranes [39]. Although it has been linked to congenital heart disease [40], other studies have concluded that it is unlikely that ampicillin is teratogenic [23, 25]. Bacampicillin, a pro-drug of ampicillin, has been poorly studied in pregnant women but there is no available data linking bacampicillin and birth defects [23].

Amoxicillin has been extensively used to treat bacteriuria in pregnancy [41] and no birth defect linking amoxicillin has been published [23, 25]. Amoxicillin has been administered orally to patients at term [42]. Blood amoxicillin concentrations peaked 4.5 hours after administration in the mother and also in the fetus, and then rapidly decayed. Therefore, it would appear that amoxicillin transfers across the placenta completely.

Several studies have described the use of amoxicillin and clavulanic acid for various infections in pregnant women. No adverse effects in the fetus or in the newborn linked to the combination has been observed [23]. Several studies have analyzed the pharmacokinetics of amoxicillin and clavulanic acid in pregnant women [43, 44]. Both drugs cross the placenta quickly and maternal serum and umbilical cord peak levels occur at two hours with a fetal: maternal ratio of 0.56. The combination has been used in the treatment of infections in pregnancy and no adverse effects have been seen in the fetus or in the newborn [45], although it has been suggested to avoid its routine use until more evidence is available [11].

The antistaphylococcal penicillins dicloxacillin and oxacillin cross the placenta and drug levels, although low due to the high maternal protein binding, can be found in fetal circulation and amniotic fluid [46–48]. Meticillin rapidly crosses the placenta into the fetal circulation and amniotic fluid. When infused in pregnant women, they reached similar concentrations in fetal and maternal sera within 30 minutes, and equilibration occurred within one hour [49]. No evidence has been found linking congenital defects and dicloxacillin, cloxacillin, meticillin, nafcillin or oxacillin and these drugs should probably be considered non-teratogenic [23, 25].

The carboxypenicillins (carbenicillin, its derivative carbenicillin indanyl, and ticarcillin) are used by their antipseudomonal activity. As other penicillins, these drugs are probably safe. There is limited information on the effects of these drugs on pregnancy and therefore they should be reserved to treat serious infections by susceptible bacteria. Carbenicillin crosses the placenta and distributes to fetal tissues but concentrations in amniotic fluid are only a tenth of maternal peak concentrations [49, 50]. Ticarcillin crosses the placenta rapidly and significant drug levels can be found in amniotic fluid and in fetal circulation [51]. No adverse effects on fetus have been described associated with both carboxypenicillins [23, 25].

The general considerations suggested for carboxypenicillins also apply to ureidopenicillins. Piperacillin, a piperazine derivative of ampicillin, has been used in the last weeks of pregnancy to delay delivery in women with premature rupture of the membranes [52]. When given during pregnancy, piperacillin rapidly crosses the placenta but fetal: maternal serum level ratio is low [53, 54]. Bourget *et al.* [55] have studied the pharmacokinetics of the intermittent administration of piperacillin-tazobactam in pregnant women. The kinetic behavior of both drugs was almost identical with an increase in the distribution volume and clearance of the combination, probably by a notable decrease in area under the curve concentrations. The maternal blood levels were at four hours less than the MIC of the target organism. Therefore, the authors suggest that a continuous infusion is a better option than intermittent administration. Following this assumption, piperacillin-tazobactam should be infused at an hourly rate of 8 mg/min. The transplacental transfer was significant but not complete and penetrated poorly the amniotic fluid [56]. There is no evidence that piperacillin may cause birth defects [23]. The Cmax values after administration of piperacillin were lower in the pregnant women than in non-pregnant women whereas the total clearance was faster in pregnant women [54]. Azlocillin has also been studied after intravenous administration in late pregnancy [57]. Concentrations equilibrated between the maternal and fetal compartments 2–3 hours after administration. This drug penetrated the amniotic fluid and reached concentrations similar to serum maternal concentrations [20].

CEPHALOSPORINS

This group includes a high number of compounds that may be administered by oral and/or parenteral route. They are classified in a rather arbitrary way in first, second, third and fourth generation cephalosporins and this criterion follows the differences in their antibacterial activity. Cephalosporins may be considered as probably safe, but uncertainty with the newer compounds is a consequence of the lack of information available. Some injectable cephalosporins are a reasonable choice for treatment of infections in critically ill patients. It has been suggested that some cephalosporins, such cefamandole, might interfere with vitamin K metabolism and should be avoided [11].

As it happens with penicillins, maternal serum concentrations of cephalosporins are also reduced because of increased renal clearance associated with pregnancy and, therefore, an increase in dosage should be considered [58]. This consideration has special importance when bactericidal concentrations must be achieved, as it happens in severe infections. Pharmacokinetic data obtained with cephalosporins showed that maternal serum levels are only a fraction of those obtained in the absence of pregnancy. First generation cephalosporins do not cross the placenta easily and the fetal serum concentrations rarely exceed 10% of maternal concentrations [59]. The mean serum concentration of cefalexin, cephalotin and cefazolin are all considerably lower in pregnant women when compared with non-pregnant women [21]. Second- and third-generation cephalosporins do a little better at this point but fetal concentrations are still significantly below maternal levels. An exception to this rule is ceftizoxime [60]. However, transplacental transfer of cephalosporins is also fairly rapid and adequate bactericidal levels are reached in fetal structures [20].

There is no clinical evidence that cephalosporins as a group are teratogenic [12]. Some animal studies have revealed potential adverse fetal effects with cephalosporins containing the N-methylthiotetrazole side chain [61]. Some generation second and third cephalosporins have such side chains (i.e. cefamandole and cefoperazone). These reasons have been invoked by some authors to suggest the theoretical advantage of drugs devoid of N-methylthiotetrazole side chain when indicated during pregnancy [61].

OTHER β-LACTAMS ANTIBIOTICS

Imipenem, meropenem and aztreonam are other β-lactam antibiotics that may be used in severe infections. Some other β-lactams compounds devoid of antibiotic activity are the β-lactamase inhibitors, such as clavulanic acid (potassium clavulanate), sulbactam and tazobactam. Clavulanic acid and tazobactam have been considered when amoxicillin and piperacillin have been previously reviewed.

Imipenem-cilastatin crosses the placenta to the fetus and their pharmacokinetics during pregnancy have been evaluated [62]. It was shown that after a single dose, plasma concentration in pregnant women was significantly lower than in non-pregnant women, both in early and late pregnancy, and clearance from plasma was faster. Peak amniotic fluid : maternal blood ratios for imipenem-cilastatin was approximately 0.30 and 0.45, respectively [63]. Although no clinical reports describing the use of this antibiotic in the first trimester are available, it seems to be a safe and effective agent during the perinatal period [23]. No reports have been located that describe the use of meropenem in human pregnancy [23].

After a single 1 g intravenous dose of aztreonam, detectable concentrations of the antibiotic in fetal serum and amniotic fluid were found. No reports describing the therapeutic use of the antibiotic in human pregnancy have been located [23].

AMINOGLYCOSIDES

Serum concentrations of aminoglycosides decrease during pregnancy. The half-life of these drugs is shorter and total body clearance is increased. Aminoglycosides distribute primarily into extracellular water, the increased extracellular fluid during pregnancy increases the volume of distribution, and, as a consequence, the serum concentrations are lower. Aminoglycosides are also eliminated by the kidney via glomerular filtration, and the increased renal clearance observed in pregnancy contributes to a shorter half-life. Therefore, patients may have increased dosage requirements. Therapeutic drug monitoring, including peak and trough serum concentrations, is needed to ensure adequate dosage [12].

The aminoglycosides cross the placenta and concentrations in fetal plasma are lower than those reached in the mother. The penetration of aminoglycosides in amniotic fluid is low (30% of maternal serum concentrations), but considerable concentrations of aminoglycosides have been found in fetal renal tissues. The potential ototoxicity is the major concern of its use during pregnancy but kanamycin seems to be the only aminoglycoside able to produce clear ototoxicity during pregnancy. Some cases of eighth cranial nerve damage and hearing loss have been reported after *in utero* exposition to kanamycin [23].

Streptomycin crosses the placenta rapidly and obtains concentrations in amniotic fluid and placenta lower than 50% of maternal blood. The use of streptomycin to treat tuberculosis during pregnancy seems safe but there are a few cases of eighth cranial nerve damage in newborns exposed to streptomycin. This ototoxicity included cochlear or vestibular effects. Although the incidence is probably low, this drug is not recommended during pregnancy [23].

During pregnancy, gentamicin plasma concentrations are lower than in non-pregnant women and could be subtherapeutic for some infections, therefore requiring a dose increase. Gentamicin rapidly crosses the placenta and maximal cord levels are 34–44% of maternal serum concentrations, and peak 1–2 hours after intramuscular administration. Ammniotic fluid concentration is maximal 8 hours after treatment. Ototoxicity has not been reported after its use during pregnancy [64].

Tobramycin and amikacin cross the placenta and distribute in most fetal tissues except brain. The highest fetal concentrations are observed in kidney and urine. Cord concentrations at term were 33–50% of maternal serum levels [65]. No reports linking the use of tobramycin or amikacin and congenital defects have been located. As with other aminoglycosides, possible ototoxicity and nephrotoxicity are major concerns when used during pregnancy [11].

VANCOMYCIN

Vancomycin crosses the placenta and reaches fetal concentrations that are sufficient to treat chorioamnionitis. This antibiotic seems to accumulate in amniotic fluid after repeated administration. The cord concentrations are about 76% of maternal serum levels [66]. Vancomycin administration during pregnancy has been related to the induction of fetal bradycardia. There is one report describing ototoxicity in newborns exposed *in utero* to the drug. The loss of hearing was recovered after 3–12 months. The renal function of newborns exposed to vancomycin was normal suggesting the lack of nephrotoxicity [67].

MACROLIDES

Erythromycin has been used during pregnancy for the treatment of mycoplasma infections. Erythromycin concentrations during pregnancy show a high variability and it crosses the placenta although the concentrations are very low [68]. Erythromycin does not have adverse effects on the fetus and neonate, but erythromycin estolate can induce hepatotoxicity in pregnant women. Around 10% of patients treated with this salt during the second trimester of pregnancy have elevated hepatic transaminases. Therefore, erythromycin estolate is contraindicated during pregnancy [69, 70].

Spiramycin is used in some countries as the treatment of choice for primary toxoplasmosis in pregnant women. Spiramycin crosses the placenta, and the cord: maternal ratio is approximately 0.5. Moreover, the concentrations in the placenta are 2–4 times higher than those achieved in plasma. The drug has not been related to fetal harm or teratogenesis [23].

There are some case reports of possible teratogenic effects of clarithromycin. Although evidence is scarce, the drug is not recommended during pregnancy at present [23].

The safety of azithromycin during pregnancy has not been fully established, although no reports of congenital defects have been reported. Azithromycin has been used as a single-dose therapy for chlamydial infections during pregnancy [12].

NITROFURANTOIN

Nitrofurantoin crosses the placenta and may induce fetal haemolytic anaemia in glucose-6-phosphate dehydrogenase in deficient fetuses. Its use has not been associated with congenital defects [23, 71].

SULFONAMIDES AND TRIMETHOPRIM

Sulfonamides are teratogenic in some animal species, but most studies have found no association in humans and it is currently believed that sulfonamides do not seem to have teratogenic risk [12]. Sulfonamides can displace bilirrubin from its albumin binding sites and therefore induce hyperbilirrubinemia. This increase could theoretically cause kernicterus in neonates and, thus, sulfonamides should be avoided in the third trimester of pregnancy and also in neonates [17]. Sulfonamides cross the placenta and fetal concentrations are 70–90% of maternal at 2–3 hours after administration.

Trimethoprim is mainly used in combination with sulfamethoxazole (cotrimoxazole). Both substances cross the placenta and reach concentrations in fetal and amniotic fluid similar to those found in maternal plasma. An increased risk of cardiovascular malformations has been suggested in a study where a sample of 2296 neonates exposed to cotrimoxazole during the first trimester of pregnancy [23].

TETRACYCLINES

Tetracyclines penetrate poorly in amniotic fluid and concentrations of tetracycline were lower in cord serum in comparison to maternal blood during labor [18]. Tetracyclines can produce adverse effects on fetal teeth and bones, maternal liver toxicity, and congenital defects. Tetracyclines cause yellow discoloration of bone and teeth if administered during the period of development of these tissues. The mechanism implies the deposition of the drug in the calcifying bones and teeth. An association between tetracycline use during pregnancy and liver toxicity has been reported. The toxicity included azotemia, jaundice and acute fatty degeneration. Tetracycline administration has been associated to the appearance of hypospadias, inguinal hernia, hypoplasia of limb and clubfoot. Therefore, all tetracyclines are contraindicated during pregnancy [17, 23].

LINCOSAMIDES

Plasma concentrations of clindamycin in pregnancy are similar to those in non-pregnant. Clindamycin crosses the placenta and achieves cord levels approximately 50% of the maternal. The maternal : placenta concentrations ratio is 1 and fetal concentrations are in the therapeutic range [72]. No reports linking the use of clindamycin with congenital defects have been located. Lincomycin crosses the placenta achieving cord levels about 25% of the maternal serum levels. No effects on the newborn have been observed.

METRONIDAZOLE

Metronidazole crosses the placenta with a cord : maternal plasma ratio of 1. The use of metronidazole in pregnancy is controversial. Metronidazole is mutagenic and carcinogenic in bacteria and animals. Several studies have described the safety of metronidazole in pregnancy. In a series of 1020 women who received metronidazole during the first trimester for treatment of vaginitis, no birth defects attributable to the drug were observed [73]. Similar results have been reported after the analysis of pregnancy outcomes of 1307 women who received metronidazole between 30 days before and 120 days after the onset of their last normal menstrual period. The use of metronidazole was not associated with an increased risk of congenital malformations [74]. However, concerns remain and have led to advice against its use in pregnancy.

The manufacturer considers metronidazole to be contraindicated to treat trichomoniasis during the first trimester of pregnancy. It may be used during the second and third trimester if other alternative therapies have failed [23].

CHLORAMPHENICOL

Chloramphenicol crosses the placenta and serum cord concentrations ranged from 30–106% of maternal levels. No reports linking the use of chloramphenicol and congenital defects have been located. Chloramphenicol is metabolized by glucuronoconjugation. In newborns and premature neonates, the immaturity of this metabolic pathway produce high plasma concentrations of the drug that has been associated with the appearance of the "gray baby syndrome". Therefore, the drug should be avoided at term or during third trimester but some authors even consider that chloramphenicol is contraindicated during all pregnancy [12, 23].

FOSFOMYCIN

In pregnant women (28–32 weeks) given a 3 g single oral dose of fosfomycin, the maximal blood concentrations were lower than those observed in non-pregnant women (20.5 µg/ml at 2 hours). Fosfomycin crosses the placenta slowly and achieves a concentration in cord and fetal blood 50% lower than that in maternal blood. Fosfomycin has been safely used during all trimesters of pregnancy, and no teratogenic effects have been reported [23].

RIFAMPICIN

Rifampicin has been used to treat both bacterial infections and tuberculosis. As other antimycobacterial agents, it crosses the placenta and reaches high levels in fetal plasma. The cord: maternal concentration ratio has ranged from 0.12 to 0.33. The risk for fetal malformations is lower than leaving tuberculosis untreated [23].

FLUOROQUINOLONES AND QUINOLONES

Fluoroquinolones are widely used to treat severe infections that require hospitalization. Flouroquinolones have a high affinity for cartilage and studies in laboratory animals have demonstrated arthropathy of weight-bearing joints after the administration of fluoroquinolones in animal youth and during pregnancy.

Although there are some cases of arthropaty in children treated with quinolones during pregnancy or childhood, the epidemiological evidence seems to indicate a low risk of congenital malformations. The analysis of human surveys seems to indicate that the frequency of congenital anomalies was not increased above background during the first trimester exposure to fluoroquinolones [75]. A recent study following 200 pregnant women exposed to fluoroquinolones (norfloxacin, ciprofloxacin and ofloxacin) have shown a similar rate of major congenital defects than observed in a control group (2.2% vs 2.6% respectively). There was no clinically significant musculoskeletal dysfunction in children exposed to fluoroquinolones *in utero* [76]. However, quinolones are contraindicated during pregnancy and until adolescence and the only accepted use is treatment of lung infections in children with cystic fibrosis.

In pregnant women receiving ciprofloxacin (200 mg i.v. every 12 hours), serum concentrations were much lower than those found in non-pregnant patients. This is probably related to an increased renal excretion [77]. Ciprofloxacin crosses the placenta slowly, and its amniotic concentration was approximately 57% of that obtained in plasma [77].

In the case of pefloxacin, a quinolone mainly eliminated by the hepatic route, plasma concentrations were similar in pregnant and non-pregnant women. Concentrations of pefloxacin in amniotic fluid are lower than those observed in plasma (70%) [77].

Ofloxacin was administered to 20 pregnant women (19–25 weeks gestation). Serum and amniotic fluid concentrations were determinated 6, 10 and 24 hours after dosing (two doses 400 mg i.v. every 12 hours). Maternal blood levels at these times were 0.68, 0.21 and 0.07 µg/ml whereas amniotic fluid levels were 0.25, 0.15, 0.13 µg/ml [77], respectively.

Levofloxacin is a new marketed fluoroquinolone. In terms of chemical structure, it is one of the two optical isomers of ofloxacin. Its pharmacokinetic properties should be similar to those of ofloxacin.

References

1. Lapinsky SE, Kruczynski K, Seaward GR, Farine D, Grossman RF. Critical care management of the obstetric patient. Can J Anaesth 44:325, 1997.
2. Graham SG, Luxton MC. The requirement for intensive care support for the pregnant population. Anaesthesia 44:581, 1989.
3. Kirshon B, Hinkley CM, Cotton DB, Miller J. Maternal mortality in a maternal-fetal medicine intensive care unit. J Reprod Med 35:25, 1990.
4. Mabie WC, Sibai BM. Treatment in an obstetric intensive care unit. Am J Obstet Gynecol 162:1, 1990.
5. Kilpatrick SJ, Matthay MA. Obstetric patients requiring critical care. A five-year review. Chest 101:1407, 1992.
6. Collop NA, Sahn SA. Critical illness in pregnancy. An analysis of 20 patients admitted to a medical intensive care unit. Chest 103:1548, 1993.
7. Monaco TJ Jr, Spielman FJ, Katz VL. Pregnant patients in the intensive care unit: a descriptive analysis. South Med J 86:414, 1993.
8. Lewinsohn G, Herman A, Leonov Y, Klinowski E. Critically ill obstetrical patients: outcome and predictability. Crit Care Med 22:1412, 1994.
9. Bouvier-Colle MH, Salanave B, Ancel PY, Varnoux N, Fernández H, Papiernik E, Breart G, Benhamou D, Boutroy P, Caillier I, Dumoulin M, Fournet P, Elhassani M, Puech F, Poutot C. Obstetric patients treated in intensive care units and maternal mortality. Regional teams for the survey. Eur J Obstet Gynecol Reprod Biol 65:121, 1996.
10. El-Solh AA, Grant BJB. A comparison of severity of illness scoring systems for critically ill obstetrical patients. Am J Resp Crit Care Med 153:A362, 1996.
11. Wise R. Antibiotics. In Rubin P (ed). Prescribing in pregnancy. 2nd edn, London: BMJ Pub Group, 1995:29.
12. Gilstrap LC, Little BB. Antimicrobial agents during pregnancy. In Gilstrap LC, Little BB (eds). Drugs and pregnancy 2nd edn, New York: Chapman and Hall, 1999:45.
13. Lee W, Clark SL, Cotton DB, Gonik B, Phelan J, Faro S, Giebel R. Septic shock during pregnancy. Am J Obstet Gynecol 159:410, 1988.
14. Gallagher MW, Repke JT, Goldstein PJ. Pharmacologic approach to the critically ill obstetric patient. In Chernow B (ed). The pharmacologic approach to the critically ill patient. Baltimore: William and Wilkins, 1994:847.
15. Mabie WC, Barton JR, Sibai B. Septic shock in pregnancy. Obstet Gynecol 90:553, 1997.
16. Hamod KA, Khouzami VA. Antibiotics in pregnancy. In Nyebil JR (ed). Drug use in pregnancy. 2nd edn, Philadelphia: Lea and Fabiger, 1988:29.
17. Theis JGW, Koren G. Maternal and fetal clinical pharmacology. In En Speight TM, Holford HG (eds). Avery's drug treatment. 4th edn, Auckland: Adis, 1997:75.
18. Folb PI, Dukes MNG. Drug safety in pregnancy. Amsterdam: Elsevier, 1993.
19. Ho JL, Barza M. Chemotherapy of infection. In Gleicher N (ed). Principles of medical therapy in pregnancy. New York: Plenum Med. Book Co., 1985:406.
20. Pacifici GM, Nottoli R. Placental transfer of drugs administered to the mother. Clin Pharmacokinet 28:235, 1995.
21. Loebstein R, Lalkin A, Koren G. Pharmacokinetic changes during pregnancy and their clinical relevance. Clin Pharmacokinet 33:328, 1997.
22. Rubin PC. Prescribing in pregnancy. General principles. BMJ 293:1415, 1986.
23. Briggs GG, Freeman RK, Yaffe SJ. Drugs in pregnancy and lactation, 5th edn. Baltimore: William and Wilkins, 1998.
24. Kullander K, Kallen B. A prospective study of drugs and pregnancy. Acta Obstet Gynecol Scand 55:287, 1976.
25. Heinonen OP, Slone D, Shapiro S. Birth defects and drugs in pregnancy. Littleton: Publishing Sciences Group, 1977.
26. Kunin CM. Clinical pharmacology of the new penicillins. I. The importance of serum protein binding in determining antimicrobial activity and concentration in serum. Clin Pharmacol Ther 7:166, 1966.
27. MacAulay MA, Berg SA, Charles D. Placental transfer of dicloxacillin at term. Am J Obstet Gynecol 102:1162, 1968.
28. Philipson A. Pharmacokinetics of ampicillins during pregnancy. J Infect Dis 136:370, 1975.
29. Philipson A. Pharmacokinetics of antibiotics in pregnancy and labour. Clin Pharmacokinet 4:297, 1979.
30. Wasz-Hockert O, Nummi S, Vuopala S, Jarvinen P. Transplacental passage of azidocillin, ampicillin and penicillin G during early and late

pregnancy. Acta Paediatr Scand (Suppl) 206:109, 1970.

31. Woltz J, Zintel H. The transmission of penicillin to amniotic fluid and fetal blood in the human. Am J Obstet Gynecol 49:663, 1945.
32. Nathan L, Bawdon RE, Sidawi JE, Stettler RW, McIntire DM, Wendel GD Jr. Penicillin levels following the administration of benzathine penicillin G in pregnancy. Obstet Gynecol 82:338, 1993.
33. Heikkilä AM, Erkkola RV. The need for adjustment of dosage regimen of penicillin V during pregnancy. Obstet Gynecol 81:919, 1993.
34. Ravid R, Toaff R. On the possible teratogenicity of antibiotic drugs administered during pregnancy – a prospective study. In Klinberg M, Abramovici A, Chemki J (eds). Drugs and fetal development. New York: Plenum, 1972:105.
35. Noschel VH, Peiker G, Schroder S, Meinhold P, Muller B. Untersuchungren zur pharmakokinetik von antibiotika und sulfanilamiden in der schwangerschaft und unter der geburt. Zentralbl Gynakol 104:1514, 1982.
36. Kraybill EN, Chaney NE, McCarthy LR. Transplacental ampicillin: inhibitory concentrations in neonatal serum. Am J Obstet Gynecol 138:793, 1980.
37. Chamberlain A, White S, Bawdon R, Thomas S, Larsen B. Pharmacokinetics of ampicillin and sulbactam in pregnancy. Am J Obstet Gynecol 168:667, 1993.
38. MacAulay MA, Abou-Sabe M, Charles D. Placental transfer of ampicillin. Am J Obstet Gynecol 96:943, 1966.
39. Morales WJ, Angel JL, O'Brien WF, Knuppel RA. Use of ampicillin and corticosteroids in premature rupture of membranes: a randomized study. Obstet Gynecol 173:721, 1989.
40. Zierler S. Maternal drugs and congenital heart disease. Obstet Gynecol 65:155, 1985.
41. Jakobi P, Neiger R, Merzbach D, Paldi E. Single-dose antimicrobial therapy in the treatment of asymptomatic bacteriuria in pregnancy. Am J Obstet Gynecol 156:1148, 1987.
42. Bergogne-Berenzin E, Lambert-Zechovsky N, Rouvillois JL. Etude du passage transplacentaire des beta-lactamines. J Gynecol Obstet Biol Reprod (Paris) 8:359–364, 1979.
43. Matsuda S. Augmentin treatment in obstetrics and gynaecology. In Leigh DA, Robinson OPW (eds). Augmentin: Proceedings of an international symposium. Montreux, Switzerland. July 1981. Excerpta Medica 1982:179.
44. Takase Z, Shirafuji H, Uchida M. Clinical and laboratory studies on BRL25000 (clavulanic acid-amoxicillin) in the field of obstetrics and gynecology. Chemotherapy (Tokyo) 30 (Suppl 2):538, 1982.
45. Pedler SJ, Bint AJ. Comparative study of amoxicillin-clavulanic acid and cephalexin in the treatment of bacteriuria during pregnancy. Antimicrob Agents Chemother 27:508, 1985.
46. Prigot A, Froix C, Rubin E. Absorption, diffusion, and excretion of new penicillin, oxacillin. Antimicrob Agents Chemother 2:402, 1962.
47. Depp R, Kind A, Kirby W, Johnson W. Transplacental passage of methicillin and dicloxacillin into the fetus and amniotic fluid. Am J Obstet Gynecol 107:1054, 1970.
48. MacAulay M, Molloy W, Charles D. Placental transfer of methicillin. Am J Obstet Gynecol 115:58, 1973.
49. Biro L, Ivan E, Elek E, Arr M. Data on the tissue concentration of antibiotics in man. Tissue concentrations of semi-synthetic penicillins in the fetus. Int Z Pharmakol Ther Toxikol 4:321, 1970.
50. Elek E, Ivan E, Arr M. Passage of penicillins from mother to fetus in umans. Int J Clin Pharmacol Ther Toxicol 6:223, 1972.
51. Cho N, Nakayama T, Vehara K, Kunii K. Laboratory and clinical evaluation of ticarcillin in the field of obstetrics and gynecology. Chemotherapy (Tokyo) 25:2911, 1977.
52. Lockwood CJ, Costigan K, Ghidini A, Wein R, Cetrulo C, Alvarez M, Berkowitz L. Double-blind, placebo-controlled trial of piperacillin sodium in preterm membrane rupture. Am J Obstet Gynecol 169:970, 1993.
53. Brown CEL, Christmas JT, Bawdon RE. Placental transfer of cefazolin and piperacillin in pregnancies remote from term complicated by Rh isoimmunization. Am J Obstet Gynecol 163:938, 1990.
54. Heikkilä A, Erkola R. Pharmacokinetics of piperacillin during pregnancy. J Antimicrob Chemother 28:419, 1991.
55. Bourget P, Sertin A, Lesne-Hulin A, Fernández H, Ville Y, Van Peborgh P. Influence of pregnancy on the pharmacokinetic behaviour and the transplacental transfer of the piperacillin-tazobactam. Eur J Obstet Gynecol Reprod Biol 76:21, 1998.
56. Brown CEL, Christmas JT, Bawdon RE. Placental transfer of cefazolin and piperacillin in pregnancies remote from term complicated by Rh

isoimmunization. Am J Obstet Gynecol 162: 549–554, 1990.
57. Voigt R, Schroder S, Peiker G. Pharmacokinetic studies of azlocillin and piperacillin during late pregnancy. Chemotherapy 31:417–424, 1995.
58. Chow AW, Jewesson PJ. Pharmacokinetics and safety of antimicrobials agents during pregnancy. Rev Infect Dis 7:287, 1985.
59. Graham JE, Oshiro BT, Blanco JD. Limited spectrum (first generation) cephalosporins. Obstet Gynecol Clin North Amer 19:449, 1992.
60. Eriksen NL, Blanco JD. Extended-spectrum (second- and third-generation) cephalosporins. Obstet Gynecol Clin North Amer 19:461, 1992.
61. Martens MG. Cephalosporins. Obstet Gynecol Clin North Amer 16:291, 1989.
62. Heikkilä A, Renkonen O-V, Erkkola R. Pharmacokinetics and transplacental passage of imipenem during pregnancy. Antimicrob Agents Chemother 36:2652, 1992.
63. Hirabayashi K, Okada E. Pharmacokinetic and clinical studies of imipenem/cilstatin sodium in the perinatal period. Jpn J Antibiot 11:1797, 1988.
64. Graham JM, Blanco JD, Oshiro BT, Magee KP. Gentamicin levels in pregnant women with pyelonephritis. Am J Perinatol 11:40, 1994.
65. Fernández H, Bourget P, Deluis C. Fetal levels of tobramycin following maternal administration. Obstet Gynecol 76:992, 1990.
66. Bourget P, Fernandez H, Delouis C, Ribou F. Transplacental passage of vancomycin during the second trimester of pregnancy. Obstet Gynecol 78:908, 1991.
67. Reyes MP, Ostrea EM, Cabinian AE, Schamit C, Rintelmann W. Vancomycin during pregnancy: does it cause hearing loss or nephrotoxicity in the infant? Am J Obstet Gynecol 161:977, 1989.
68. Philipson A, Sabaath LD, Charles D. Erythromycin absorption and elimination in pregnant women. Clin Pharmacol Ther 19:68, 1976.
69. McDormack WM, George H, Donner A, Kodgis LF, Albert S, Lowe EW, Kass EH. Hepatotoxicity of erythromycin estolate during pregnancy. Antimicrob Agents Chemother 12:630, 1977.
70. Garland SM, O'Reilly MA. The risks and benefits of antimicrobial therapy in pregnancy. Drug Saf 13:188, 1995.
71. Ben David S, Einarson T, Ben David Y, Nulman I, Pastuszak A, Koren G. The safety of nitrofurantoin during the first trimester of pregnancy: meta-analysis. Fundamen Clin Pharmacol 9:503, 1995.
72. Philipson A, Sabaath LD, Charles D. Transplacental passage of erythromycin and clindamycin. N Engl J Med 288:1219, 1973.
73. Rosa FW, Baum C, Shaw M. Pregnancy outcomes after first trimester vaginitis drug therapy. Obstet Gynecol 82:348, 1993.
74. Piper JM, Mitchelm EF, Ray WA. Prenatal use of metronidazole and birth defects: no association. Obstet Gynecol 82:348, 1993.
75. Schaefer C, Amoura-Elefant E, Vial T, Omory A, Garbis H, Robert E, Rodríguez-Pinilla E, Pexiedir T, Prapas N, Merlob P. Pregnancy outcome after prenatal quinolone exposure. Evaluation of a case registry of the European Network of Teratology Information Services (ENTIS). Eur J Gynecol Reprod Biol 69:83, 1996.
76. Loebstein R, Addis A, Ho E, Andreou R, Sage S, Donnenfeld AE, Schick B, Bonati M, Moretti M, Lalkin A, Pastuszak A, Koren G. Pregnancy outcome following gestational exposure to fluoroquinolone: a multicenter prospective controlled study. Antimicrob Agents Chemother 42:1336, 1998.
77. Giamarellou H, Kolohythas E, Petrikkos G, Gazis J, Aravantinos D, Sfikakis P. Pharmacokinetics of three newer quinolones in pregnant and lactating women. Am J Med 87 (Suppl 5A):49S, 1989.

14. PHARMACOKINETICS OF ANTIBIOTICS IN SERIOUSLY INFECTIOUS PATIENTS

Miguel Angel Campanero Martínez, José Ramón Azanza Perea, Emilio García Quetglas, and Belén Sádaba Díaz de Rada

The infectious patient in a critical situation can present several series of alterations which can be considered to be of great importance, not only because of the need to adopt multiple therapeutical measures, but also because some of the processes that regulate the disposition of a drug in the human organism (absorption, distribution, metabolism and elimination) can become significantly modified. Hemodynamic alterations, an impaired renal function, respiratory insufficiency, hepatic dysfunction, dysproteinemia, are typical examples of almost constant situations in seriously infectious patients.

Modification of the pharmacokinetic profile of any drug can have serious consequences. It is possible that a slower elimination of a drug can result in its accumulation, with the corresponding toxicity risk. Another possibility is that the concentration reached could be a value which is less than that needed to obtain its pharmacological effect.

All of these effects are considered undesirable consequences for any of the drugs that a patient may need, but the situation can be especially complex if the drug affected is one of the antibiotics that the patient needs for treating his infectious disease. In order to determine the inherent problems affecting these types of situations, it is absolutely indispensable to prescribe an adequate antibiotic treatment adapted to the characteristics of each patient. Therefore, in a text such as this one, there should be a chapter which specifically describes the modifications of the pharmacokinetic profile of the antibiotics in the seriously infectious patient.

Previous Considerations

Pharmacokinetic studies, in a quantitative manner, are those processes which govern the temporary evolution of a drug in the human organism: absorption, distribution, metabolism and excretion, through the application of mathematical models adapted to experimental data: blood (generally serum or plasma) and urine concentrations. The pharmacokinetic parameters thus obtained permit characterization of the drug disposition, meaning its evolution in the human organism, although it does not permit an exact estimation of its evolution in the place of action. In Table 1, summarized information is collected regarding the principal pharmacokinetic parameters of the antibiotics obtained in patients with different types of situations which occur frequently in the critical patient.

Pharmacokinetic Characteristics in the Critical Patient

ADMINISTRATION AND ABSORPTION ROUTE

In the treatment of the seriously infectious patient it is important to reach therapeutic concentrations of antibiotics in the systemic circulation quickly and, more specifically, in the place

TABLE 1. Pharmacokinetic values for antimicrobials in non-critically ill and critically ill patients

Drug	PB (%)	V_{ss} (L/kg) Not critical	Critical	Renal	Hepatic	$t^1/_2\beta$ (h) Not critical	Critical	Renal	Hepatic	CL (ml/min/kg) Not critical	Critical	Renal	Hepátic	Ae (% dose)
Aminoglycosides														
Amikacin [8, 14, 46, 52]	4	0.25	0.36–27.9	0.21–0.5		2.3	29.7	1.1–2.2 17–150		1.17		0.3 0.6		98
Gentamicin [8, 14, 51]	10	0.25	0.14–0.67	↔		1.1–69.3	1.2–17.8	20–60		1.52	0.05–3.35	0.3		90
β-Lactams														
Cefazolin [11]	90	0.14		↑	↔	1.8		47–70	↓	0.95		↓	↔	80
Cefotaxime [16]	36	0.23	0.22–0.56			1.1	4.48	15	↔	3.7	16	0.2	↔	55
Cefotetan [12]	85	0.14		↔		3.6		13–25		0.53		↓		67
Ceftazidime [7]	21	0.23	0.35	↔		1.6	1.6–6.0	13–25		1.92	1.0	0.3		84
Cefpirone [11]	10	0.29		↔		2.0		9.2						85
Ceftriaxone [16, 39, 42]	90	0.16		↔	↑	7.3	5.3–13.7	12–24	↑	0.24		0.03	↓	49
Aztreonam [13]	56	0.16		↔	↑	1.7		6–8	↔	1.3		0.1	↑	68
Imipenem [49]	20	0.23	0.36	↑		0.9	1.7	2–4		2.9	3.6	0.3–1.5		69
Piperacillin [54]	30	0.18		↔		0.9		3–5		3.83		0.3	↓	71
Ticarcillin [13]	65	0.21				1.2		11–16		1.6		0.1	↓	77
Tazobactam [54]	22	0.21				1.0		7					↓	80
Clavulanic acid	22	0.21		↔		0.9		3.5		3.6		0.3		43
Phenicols														
Chloramphenicol [2]	53	0.94			↔	4.0		3–7	↑	2.4		0.2	↓	25

Glycopeptides														
Teicoplanin [24]	90	1.0		1.0		40–60	99	62–289		11.4		0.07	↓	77
Vancomycin [17, 25]	30	0.39		↔		5.6		200–250		1.57		0.2		79
Macrolides														
Azithromycin [40]	7–5031				↔	40		↔	↔	9		↔	↔	12
Erythromycin [18]	84	0.78		↑		1.6		5.5	↑	9.1		0.06		12
Lincosamides														
Clindamycin [27]	94	1.1		↔		2.9		4	↑	4.7		0.03	↓	13
Quinolones														
Ciprofloxacin [4, 32]	40	1.8	1.1–1.5			4.1	↑	8–609	↔	6.0	5.54	0.2	↔	65
Ofloxacin [15, 34]	25	1.8	↑			5.7	↑	15–60		3.5	↓	0.3		64
Sulfamides														
Sulfamethoxazole [5]	62	0.21	0.5	↑		10.1	15.5	20–50		0.32	0.4	0.1		14
Trimethoprim [5, 30]	37	1.6	1.6	↔		10	10.9	20–49		1.0	1.88	0.2		63
Tetracyclines														
Doxycycline [29]	88	0.75 (V_z)					16	18–25		0.53		↔		41
Tetracycline [29]	65	1.5				10.6		57–108	↑	1.67		↓	↓	58
Others														
Metronidazole [56, 57]	11	0.74		↔	↔	8.5		7–21	↑	1.3		0.3		10
Rifampin [45]	89	0.97				3.5		9.2	↑	3.5		0.04		7

Abbreviations: Ae = % dose excreted unchanged in urine; CL = plasmatic clearance; PB = protein binding; $t^{1}/_{2}\beta$ terminal half-life; V_{ss} = volume of distribution at steady state; V_z = volume of distribution in the terminal phase; ↑ = increased; ↓ = decreased; ↔ = no altered.

where the infection is located. Consequently, the administration route of the drug is very important. The rapid intravenous injection and intravenous infusion through peripheral veins are the two administration routes often used in this type of situation. Exceptionally, the administration of the antibiotic through an additional type of route or the use of another process may be of interest. Administration by oral route (with the exception of those cases in which the objective is the eradication of microorganisms in the gastrointestinal tract) does not seem adequate in any case. At least two facts should be considered: on the one hand, this route only allows the administration of reduced doses (always under 1 gr), and on the other, the process of absorption implies a good gastrointestinal performance, very infrequent in the critical patient, resulting in an erratic absorption process [1]. The alteration of the absorption can consist of modifications in the speed with which the drug is released from the pharmaceutical form, and/or in the percentage of the drug that remains in a nonionized form. Therefore, the process of absorption of the antibiotics can be affected in its quantity as well as in its speed [2].

Another factor of importance lies in the difficulty of administering drugs by oral route in patients that usually require the utilization of a probe-nasogastric tube. The need of altering the pharmaceutical form to make administration possible and the coincidence in this type of patients with enteral nutrition are two inconveniences that can notably alter the absorption of antibiotics [3]. Sulfametoxazole and trimethoprim are two of the exceptions because their bioavailability not only remains unchanged but can even be enhanced when either one is administered through a nasogastric tube in patients infected with HIV and which present a respiratory depression [4, 5].

Administration by rectal route does not present interest in these situations and administration through intramuscular injection is formally dissuaded in infectious patients in critical situations, in relationship with the modifications of the absorption due to the hemodynamic situation and/or the disorders of the microvascularization [1].

Inhalation through the respiratory tract can also be used for antibiotic administration, because this measures can be adapted in order to obtain enhanced antibiotic concentrations in the bronchial secretions. This route is usually used for the administration of aminoglycosides, polypeptides and some antifungals; however, a significant absorption of these drugs is not observed in any of the cases. Nevertheless, it must be kept in mind that the therapeutic efficiency of this administration route has not been demonstrated in an evident manner [6, 7].

Finally, it is not uncommon to appeal to antibiotic administration by topical route in systems of anatomical or pathological cavities irrigation. This administration system is usually chosen when the antiobiotic treatment administered through more conventional processes fails. The experiences are anecdotal and therefore, the information available does not permit assurance of an effective or innocuous result. Nevertheless, there are some important exceptions, such as the intrathecal administration of aminoglycosides in the treatment of meningitis caused by *P. aeruginosa* or *Acinetobacter* [8, 9] or that of vancomycin used for treating some meningeal infections.

DISTRIBUTION

Modification of drug distribution in the seriously infectious patient is related to changes in the plasma protein concentrations, the volume of the corporal fluids, and the alteration of the permeability of some barriers.

Plasmatic Proteins. The critically infectious patient is characterized by a presentation of albumin concentrations which are lower than those observed in healthy subjects, a result of hepatic or renal disease or due to contribution deficiency [10]. Consequently, the free fraction of drugs that are bound preferably to albumin is greater. The repercussion of these alterations depends on the volume of distribution and on the elimination pathway used by each drug. In infectious patients with renal impairment, there are functional alterations of the albumin, acidosis and uremia, in addition to presenting hypoalbuminemia. These changes significantly affect the percentage of drug bound to plasma proteins.

The modifications in plasma protein concentration have clinical repercussions on the antibiotics that present a small volume of distribution (<0.15 l/kg), and which circulate in the blood bound to proteins in great proportion (>80%). The reduction in plasma proteins will produce an increase in the fraction of drug not bound to proteins, free fraction, resulting in a greater distribution capacity of the drug. This is the situation for some cephalosporines (ceftriaxone, cefonicid, cefazolin) [11] and isoxazolylpenicillins (cloxacillin and oxacillin) [12]. Furthermore, and although these drugs have a very large volume of distribution, the reduction of plasma protein concentration also increases the tissue diffusion capacity of roxithromycin, doxycycline and rifampin [13].

Furthermore, an increase in free-drug percentage enhances drug plasma clearance with restrictive elimination, through slow renal excretion or low hepatic fraction of extraction. In the first case, antibiotics which are eliminated preferably by glomerular filtration and highly bound to plasma proteins, such as cefonicid or ceftriaxone, are found [11]. In the other case, clindamycin can be found, a drug bounded to plasma proteins in 94% and with a low rate of hepatic extraction: 0.23 [13].

The critical patient can also present an increase in the concentration of acid α_1-glycoprotein and consequently, those drugs which preferably bind to this protein, such as erythromycin, can present significant decreases in their free fraction. Nevertheless, this fact does not seem to have special significance because this drug presents a large volume of distribution.

Volume of Corporal Water. In some seriously infectious patients, modifications are often observed in the physiology of the cardiovascular system. It is typical to observe a reduction of the cardiac output and generalized vasoconstriction. As a direct consequence, fluid retention is produced which in turn, results in an increase of the volume of corporal water. In this situation the volume of distribution of any drug enhances, which implies that the plasma concentration reached with the same dose results in lower concentration than that expected.

The use of mechanical ventilation can cause increases in the volume of distribution of drugs in patients that present cardiac failure and respiratory insufficiency. This situation has been described with aminoglycosides [14], and with some quinolones as ofloxacin [15]. The cause of this alteration is an increase of intrathoracic pressure, which produces activation of the homeostatic mechanisms that increase the volume of corporal water.

Alteration of the Permeability of the Barriers. The presence of an infectious process can alter the membrane permeability, permitting diffusion of antibiotics to those tissues in which this is normally limited; such as the hematoencephalic barrier. Under normal conditions, this barrier usually blocks an adequate peuetration of numerous autibiotics into the subarachnoid space and from reaching effective concentrations in the cerebrospinal fluid. Alteration of the hematoencephalic barrier as the result of an infection can increase the permeability by approximately five times for some antibiotics, such as the betalactams, (penicillins and cephalosporines) and some glycopeptides. Thus, concentrations of ceftriaxone and cefotaxime in the cerebrospinal fluid of patients with inflamed meningeal are five times higher to those observed in normal subjects [16]. The concentration of vancomycin in cerebrospinal fluid reaches values between 7 and 20% of that detected in plasma in patients with meningitis [17].

ELIMINATION

Elimination is the pharmacokinetic process most altered in patients with a seriously infectious process. The alterations in the elimination of the drugs can affect the metabolism and/or renal excretion.

Metabolism. The hepatic dysfunction is an alteration whose presence is greater than 54% in the infectious patients who are found in a critical state [18]. This alteration can produce modifications in the pharmacokinetics of antibiotics that are eliminated through hepatic metabolism. The alterations in the elimination of these drugs are directly related to two circumstances: the decrease of the hepatic blood flow and/or the decrease of the enzymatic activity of the hepatic microsomal system.

The hepatic blood flow can experience considerable variations in the seriously infectious patient. It has been estimated that the value of the hepatic blood flow can be reduced by two thirds in patients in a state of septic shock [19]. Hepatic cirrhosis can also cause a reduction in the hepatic blood flow as a result of structural alterations present. Therefore, those drugs with a high hepatic extraction rate (>0.7), in which the hepatic clearance depends on hepatic blood flow, will present lower values of plasma clearance. This situation corresponds to some macrolides, such as dirythromycin [20].

The hepatic metabolism is a catabolic process mediated by two types of reactions: the phase II reactions (conjugation with glucuronide, sulfates and gluthation) and the oxidation reactions or phase I, catalyzed through isoenzymes of the hepatic microsomal system. Recently, it has been demonstrated that the catabolic activity of the hepatic microsomal system suffers a reduction in seriously infectious patients [21]. This reduction is caused by a decrease in the synthesis processes of the isoezymes that catalyze the oxidation reactions. It is possible that some endotoxins could produce the inactivation of some isoenzymes [22].

A decrease of the catabolic activity of the hepatic microsomal system produces alterations in the pharmacokinetic parameters of antibiotics that present a low rate of hepatic extraction (less than 0.3). In this group of antibiotics, the plasma clearance value depends on the intrinsic metabolic capacity of the liver, more specifically, on the enzymatic activity of the hepatic microsome, and on the degree of union to plasma proteins. If these drugs have a high affinity to proteins (>80%), an increase in the free fraction which is secondary to the hepatic disease becomes present, and an increase in clearance would also result. If drugs present restrictive clearance depending on the union to proteins, this increase in the hepatic elimination can not be produced due to the hepatocellular injury; therefore, the repercussion of the hepatic disease on the clearance of these drugs is variable, depending on the balance that is established between the greater free fraction and the metabolic capacity of the liver.

If the drugs are bound to plasma proteins by a small degree (<30%), they are not affected by the modifications in the albumin, and therefore, the clearance depends only on the alterations on the hepatocellular function.

These facts result in the alteration, to a greater or lesser degree, of the hepatic clearance (depending on the microsomal system) of some penicillins, glycopeptides, macrolides, fluoroquinolones, sulfamides, chloramphenicol, isoniacid or rifampin. Drugs such as cefotaxime, cephoperazone and ceftriaxone can also experience alterations in their biological disposition as a result of the decrease in hepatic clearance [12, 23]; the same occurs with teicoplanin [24] and vancomycin [25]. Nevertheless, these alterations do not imply a need to adjust the dose, because these drugs are considered to be eliminated as unchanged drug by renal route in an important proportion. However, clindamycin [27], rifampin and rifabutin [31] are drugs with low renal elimination. Therefore, it may be necessary to re-adjust the dose, because the decrease of hepatic clearance could result in an increase in plasma concentration of these antibiotics in the organism, reaching toxic values.

Furthermore, in the case of clindamycin, an antibiotic with a low extraction fraction and highly bound to proteins (greater than 70%), a clearance value similar to or even higher than that which is customary can be presented, because the hepatic dysfunction produces hypoalbuminemia, hyperbilirubinemia and a decrease of the acid α_1-glycoprotein which combined together, produce an increase in the volume of distribution of this drug as the free fraction increases (caused by hypoproteinemia and displacement by bilirubin).

The slowness of the conjugation reactions, glucuronization and acetylation in the critically infectious patient also has consequences in the disposition of some antibiotics. The clearance value of chloramphenicol [26], doxycycline [28], tetracycline [29], sulfamethoxazole [30] and isoniacid [31] experience a decrease in these patients as a result of a reduction in the processes of glucuronidation and acetylation. However, the sulfonation of ciprofloxacin is not altered. In the case of chloramphenicol, doxycycline and tetracycline, it is necessary to re-adjust the dose, because these are drugs with a low hepatic extraction rate and consequently, a decrease of the phase I reactions implies an increase of the plasma concentration of these antibiotics in the organism.

The bioavailability of antibiotics that experience an important first pass effect shows modifications in patients with hepatic dysfunction when the drug is administered by oral route. In this case, a significant increase in the bioavailability, resulting from the decrease of the hepatic first pass effect, is observed. The plasma concentrations of some macrolides and quinolones after administration by oral route can be increased with respect to that observed in patients with a normal hepatic function. The bioavailability of ciprofloxacin, pefloxacin and ofloxacin in critically infectious patients with hepatic dysfunction is similar to and even higher than that observed in mild patients [32–34].

Finally, if given a severe hepatic dysfunction, it must be taken into account that the organism presents other metabolic systems which are different to the hepatic one, located in the lung and in the gastrointestinal tract. These systems are of small relevance given the hepatic activity is normal, but can be of great significance in the case of severe hepatic dysfunction [35].

Hepatic disease can increase the terminal half-life of antibiotics by reduction of hepatic clearance, or by an increase in the volume of distribution as a result of the decrease in the binding to proteins. Consequently, this situation leads to the presence of plasma concentrations lower than expected but longer lasting. Furthermore, it must be taken into consideration that in addition to these abnormalities, those conditioned by the probable associated renal impairment will also be added.

Biliar Excretion. Generally, it can be said that biliar excretion of the antibiotics is not usually altered in the hepatic hepatocellular disease. Nevertheless, there are exceptions. Rifampin is an antibiotic excreted by bile in high proportion and presents enterohepatic circulation. The presence of cholestasis may produce an increase in the concentrations of this antibiotic, reaching toxic concentrations [36]. Possibly, the same consideration should be made for the antibiotics with important biliar excretion (Table 2).

TABLE 2. Biliar excretion of antibiotics

Bilis/serum ratio >4	bilis/serum ratio = 1–4	bilis/serum ratio <1
Rifampin	Metronidazole	Aminoglycosides
Macrolides	Chloramphenicol	Vancomycin
Doxycycline	Piperacillin	Sulfamides
Tetracycline	Mezlocillin	
Ceftriaxone	Ticarcillin	
Cefoperazone	Imipenem	
Cefoxitin	Azthreonam	
Cefamandole		
Clindamycin	Quinolones	
	Trimethoprim	

Renal Excretion. It has already been stated that infectious patients with renal insufficiency present functional alterations of the albumin, acidosis, uremia and hypoalbuminemia. Therefore, drugs with acidicfunctional groups and higher plasma protein biuding may require a dose re-adjustment. This is the case of some cephalosporines, such as cephazoline and ceftriaxone [38, 39], doxycycline, penicillin G and some sulfamides [28, 30].

Renal insufficiency does not affect the binding of drugs of basic character (azythromycin [40], acid α_1-glucoprotein and lipoproteins whose levels may even be increased in chronic renal insufficiency. As stated earlier, the antibiotics that bind preferably to this type of protein show high volumes of distribution; therefore, the decrease in free fraction does not produce alterations in the pharmacokinetic parameters.

A decrease of renal function, extremely frequent in seriously infectious patients, produces important alterations in the pharmacokinetics of the antibiotics that are eliminated by this route and indirectly, can have repercussions in the distribution of antibiotics that do not use this route of elimination.

Renal insufficiency leads to an increase in the volume of corporal water, which produces an increase in the volume of distribution of the antibiotics.

Furthermore, it is necessary to keep in mind that the metabolites of many drugs are excreted through urine. Therefore, renal insufficiency can be expected to produce an increase of the concentration in the organism of some antibiotics and different metabolites. Although it is not common in the case of antibiotics, some of these metabolites may be active and even present a pharmacological activity which is higher than that of its parent drug. Therefore, their accumulation can be very dangerous. It is more frequent for the metabolite to present characteristics of toxicity. This is the case of sulfadiazine and sulfamide, which present an active metabolite, acetyl sulfadiazine, whose accumulation increases the intensity of the adverse reactions related to this drug [41].

Renal insufficiency has repercussions in the hepatic metabolism of the antibiotics. A decrease of the metabolic activity has been observed in drugs that present reduction reactions, acetylation and in those which are catalyzed via the plasma esterases. Nevertheless, the repercussions of these alterations are minimal. Drugs that are catalyzed through oxidative, glucuronization, sulfatation and O-metilation processes do not suffer consequences [42].

Logically, renal insufficiency mainly affects the elimination of antibiotics that are excreted preferably through the urine in unchanged form, whether or not they are eliminated by glomerular filtration or tubular secretion, and whether or not tubular reabsorption is produced.

The excretion of drugs which are eliminated exclusively by glomerular filtration is significantly reduced in infectious patients with renal insufficiency, as a result of the decrease in the number of nephrons and of alteration of the permeability of its membranes. The terminal half-life of aminoglycosides can be increased 10 times, making it necessary to re-adjust the dose as well as the dosing interval [43].

The excretion of antibiotics that are eliminated by tubular secretion is also slower. The acidity of urine is the factor which is responsible for this alteration, because tubular secretion is a process that depends on the pKa of the drug and on the pH of urine. Therefore, in drugs with acid character and with a pKa between 3.0 and 7.5, renal secretion will experience a reduction, while in drugs with basic character and a pKa between 5.0 and 11.3, the opposite effect will be observed. The great majority of antibiotics that are eliminated by tubular secretion, such as cephalosporines, penicillins and sulfamides, have an acid character. Therefore, their elimination will be slower. Some of these drugs combine this excretion mechanism with that of glomerular filtration, as is the case of penicillins and cephalosporines (with the exception of ceftriaxone, cefoperazone, ceforanide and ceftazidime)

[44], or with that of tubular reabsorption, such as occurs with sulfamides [37].

The influence of renal insufficiency is particularly intense in the case where the drug is nephrotoxic, such as with the aminoglycosides [37]. In this group of drugs, the reduction of the renal function leads to an increase in the toxicity of the drug, because the drug accumulates at the renal level. This is also true in the case of vancomycin, a glycopeptide excreted preferably by glomerular filtration and whose terminal half-life is increased by up to 40 times in the case of renal insufficiency [25].

Renal insufficiency also has repercussions in the pharmacokinetics of drugs that are preferably eliminated by a metabolic route when high doses are administered, because in this case, the renal excretion can participate as a route of elimination for the drug. This is the case of rifampin, whose terminal half-life is reduced to half when it is administered in high doses (900 mg) [45].

Frequently, patients with renal insufficiency are submitted to dialysis. In this case, the concentrations of the drug in the organism can be altered, making it necessary to administer a supplementary dose of the same drug after the dialysis session in order to replace that which has been eliminated. For an antibiotic to be dialyzable, its molecular weight must be low, it should be soluble in water, bind poorly to plasma proteins and/or have a small volume of distribution. Such is the case for: aminoglycosides [46, 47], carbapenems such as imipenem, azthreonam [48, 49], and cephalosporines, with the exception of those which present a high degree of binding to plasma proteins (ceftriaxone and cephoperazone) [50]. These drugs experience reductions of 27–50% in their plasma concentrations [51, 52]. In other cases, the percentages are lower, such as occurs with the penicillins; therefore, it is not necessary to provide a supplementary dose [53]. Glycopeptides are not easily dialyzable drugs, with the exception of vancomycin, in the case of the hemodiafiltration. In a patient undergoing hemodialysis, the dose of vancomycin is administered every 5–7 days, while in the case of continuous hemodiafiltration, it is necessary to administer it every 2–3 days.

Groups of Antibiotics

Any conclusions which could be drawn up to now are of little practical interest. The implications of vital risk situations are so numerous that they can hardly be estimated except on an individual patient basis. Nevertheless, a description of each one of the principal groups of antibiotics is included in this chapter, and the principal pharmacokinetic alterations are expressed in Table 3.

BETALACTAMS

Betalactams are characterized by their elimination, which is mainly by renal route, although a significant percentage of metabolism exists in some, such as cephalosporines and the ureidopenicillins. The binding to plasma proteins is relevant only in the case of the isoxazolylpenicillins, ceftriaxone, cefonicid and cefazolin. This results in an increase in the volume of distribution of these drugs as well as in the hepatic or renal clearance, given that both systems operate in an adequate way. In the case of renal or hepatic insufficiency, elimination will be compromised and the accumulation of the free drug will be important. Nevertheless, due to the limited distribution and good tolerance that this group of antibiotics normally presents, the pharmacokinetic modifications of the corporal water or of the free fraction do not imply significant alterations. Only the limitation of the renal function or the need of purification through different techniques requires a modification of the dosage in most of the drugs in this group.

AMINOGLYCOSIDES

Aminoglycosides are characterized by their limited distribution and their renal elimination through glomerular filtration, presenting a low proportion of the antibiotics bound to plasma proteins. Usually, the modifications in critical

TABLE 3. Physiopathological changes related to serious disease and their effects on the different processes of the disposition of drugs

Pharmacokinetics	Changes related to serious disease	Secondary pharmacokinetic changes
Absorption	↓ gastrointestinal motility and gastric emptying delay or hypermotility	↓ absorption speed of some drugs
	↓ intestinal blood flow	↓ bioavailability
	↓ intramuscular blood flow	↓ bioavailability by intramuscular injection
Distribution	↑ total corporal water	↑ volume of distribution of the majority of the drugs
	↓ proteins and plasma albumin	↑ free or active fraction of the drugs bound to albumin
	↑ α_1-glycoprotein	↓ free fraction of the drugs bound to α_1-glycoprotein
	tissues perfusion alteration	tissue diffusion modification
	modification of the hematoencephalic barrier	
Metabolism	↓ mass and number of hepatic cells	↓ metabolism of some drugs (low extraction rate)
	↓ hepatic blood flow	↓ metabolism of drugs with a high extraction rate
	↓ oxidative (CYP 450) and conjugation capacity	↑ bioavailability of drugs with an important first-pass effect
Renal elimination	↓ renal blood flow	↓ renal elimination of drugs
	↓ glomerular filtration (creatinine clearance)	
	↓ tubular secretion	

patients imply an increase in the volume of distribution and an important deterioration in the elimination of the drug, making it necessary to space the administration intervals greatly. All of these drugs are eliminated through hemodialysis, requiring administration of supplements after each session. It is possible to monitor the plasma concentrations of these drugs, thereby greatly aiding optimization of the posology.

MACROLIDES

Macrolides are antibiotics with an important volume of distribution, reaching high concentrations at an intracellular level, although they do not cross the hematoencephalic barrier. This kind of antibiotics preferably bind to the α_1-glycoprotein. In seriously infectious patients, these drugs are highly bound to plasma proteins, although without much repercussion on plasma or tissue concentrations. Macrolides can present pharmacokinetic modifications in the case of hepatic dysfunction, because they are metabolized through microsomal hepatic enzymes, CYP3A4, upon which some of the components of this group can act, modifying the catabolism speed of other drugs. Some of the metabolites which are excreted by renal route, such as clarithromycin, present activity and therefore, in the case of renal insufficiency, some important pharmacokinetic modifications can be found.

GLYCOPEPTIDES

At present, there are two glycopeptides, drugs of preferably renal elimination and differing from each other in the aspect of protein binding (higher in the case of teicoplanin), which conditions a slower elimination speed. The modifications in the corporal water and in the renal function require adjustments in the posology, which can be determined with the aid of plasma concentration monitorization. A certain degree of metabolism of these drugs exists, although not in a significant enough proportion so as to require important posology adjustments. Hemodiafiltration eliminates 25–35% of vancomycin, while hemodialysis hardly clears any of this drug.

PHENICOLS

Phenicols are drugs of high distribution and hepatic elimination (as in the case of chloramphenicol), through oxidation in the CYP3A4 isoenzyme as well as through glucuronization. The metabolites produced are eliminated to a large extent by renal route. In critical patients, the kinetic modifications can produce accumulation of chloramphenicol, a drug whose toxicity is largely concentration-dependent, thereby requiring special care when handling it.

LINCOSAMIDES

Clindamycin is a drug with a large distribution (although it does not cross the hematoencephalic barrier), whose elimination is produced in the liver, with a low hepatic extraction. Due to its high binding to proteins, the hepatic modifications reduce the drug clearance only if a decrease in the intrinsic metabolic capacity occurs, regardless of whether or not flow is produced. If there are no hepatic alterations, the clearance of the drug is enhanced, resulting from a higher free fraction. It scarcely dialyzes.

FLUORQUINOLONES

The group of fluorquinolones presents great heterogeneity in its pharmacokinetic characteristics, especially with regard to its absorption and elimination. The bioavailability of some of the drugs of this group can be increased as a result of hepatic alterations that reduce the first pass effect. With regard to distribution, all of the drugs in this group present high volumes of distribution. Therefore, pharmacokinetic modifications will depend on the alterations in the process of elimination. In the case of alterations in renal elimination, ofloxacin and levofloxacin will be the drugs most affected. In the case of hepatic route, ciprofloxacin will be the most affected. It is important to consider that, although the fluorquinolones are not drugs that are bound to plasma proteins in a high proportion, the modifications of the corporal water can increase the volume of distribution and favor the neurological toxicity.

SULFAMIDES AND TRIMETHOPRIM

The principal pharmacokinetic modifications of sulfamides and trimethoprim are related to the alterations in the renal function, because both are compounds with a high volume of distribution. Therefore, in critical patients, elimination is clearly compromised, including that of some of the active metabolites, as is the case of sulfadiazine, which may increase the nephrotoxic or medullary potential.

TETRACYCLINES

The kinetics of tetracyclines are modified by both renal and hepatic alterations, depending on the different components of the group. The metabolism depends fundamentally on conjugation reactions, this being the most important elimination route in the cases of doxicyclin and minocycline. The modifications of the corporal water and plasma albumin can greatly alter doxycycline and demeclocyclin. These are drugs with an important biliar excretion, a fact that must be taken into account if any modifications are present at this level.

RIFAMICINS

Kinetic modifications in seriously infectious patients can be important because rifamicins are drugs which highly bind to plasma proteins and are eliminated by both the renal and hepatic routes; although these are the principal elimination routes, the biliar excretion and the possibility of enterohepatic circulation should not be forgotten.

METRONIDAZOLE

Ten per cent of metronidazole and its active metabolite are eliminated by renal route, although the most important kinetic modifications are related to modifications in biliar excretion.

Conclusions

In daily clinical practice, it can be very difficult to estimate the consequences which the alterations of the seriously infectious patient would have on the pharmacokinetic characteristics of an antibiotic. The information available in most cases is incomplete and therefore, insufficient. Moreover, it is quite complicated to set up quantitative pharmacokinetic models that can facilitate posology adjustment of the drugs when patients present many of the alterations that can modify the pharmacokinetic behavior. Therefore, the actual tendencies propose the necessity to perform an adjustment of the posology with relation to plasma concentrations of the antibiotic. This routine method, in the case of drugs with a narrow therapeutic margin (aminoglycosides and vancomycin) may be strictly necessary in these types of situations.

References

1. Bush LM, Levison ME. Antibiotic selection and pharmacokinetics in the critically ill. Crit Care Clin 4:299, 1987.
2. Mann HJ, Fuhs DW, Cerra FB. Pharmacokinetics and pharmacodynamics in critically ill patients. World J Surg 11:210, 1987.
3. Jellet LB, Heazlewood VJ. Pharmacokinetics in acute illness. Med J Aust 153:534, 1990.
4. Healy DP, Brodbeck MC, Clendening CE. Ciprofloxacin absorption is impaired in patients given enteral feedings orally and via gastrostomy and jefunostomy tubes. Antimicrob Agents Chemother 40:6, 1996.
5. Chin TW, Vandenbroucke A, Fong IW. Pharmacokinetics of trimethroprim-sulfamethoxazole in critically ill and non-critically ill AIDS patients. Antimicrob Agents Chemother 39:28, 1995.
6. Kleinschmidt R, Rommelsheim K, Exner M, *et al.* The effectiveness of intratracheal antibiotic administration: clinical, microbiologic and pharmacologic results. Anasth Intensivther Noft Med 24:143, 1989.
7. Bressolle F, De la Coussaye JE, Ayoub R, *et al.* Endotracheal and aerosol administrations of ceftazidime in patients with nosocomial pneumonia: pharmacokinetics and absolute bioavailability. Antimicrob Agents Chemother 36: 1404, 1992.
8. Kaiser AB, Mc Gee ZA. Aminoglycoside therapy of gram-negative bacillary meningitis. N Engl J Med 293:1215, 1975.
9. Scheld WM. Theoretical and practical considerations of antibiotic therapy for bacterial meningitis. Pediatr Infect Dis 4:74, 1985.
10. Boucher BA, Glifton GD. In Williams, Williams (eds). Textbook of therapeutics: drug and disease management, 1823–1840. London, 1996.
11. Yuk-Choi HJ, Nightingale CH, Williams Jr TW. Considerations in dosage selection for third generation cephalosporins. Clin Pharmacokinet 22:132, 1992.
12. Van Dalen R, Vree TB. Pharmacokinetics of antibiotics in critically ill patients. Intens Care Med 16 (Suppl. 3):S235, 1990.
13. Reynolds JEF (ed). Martindale: the extra pharmacopoeia. London: The Pharmaceutical Press, 1996.
14. Watling SM, Dasta JF. Aminoglycoside dosing considerations in intensive care unit patients. Ann Pharmacother 27:351, 1993.
15. Martin C, Lambert D, Bruguerolle B, *et al.* Ofloxacin pharmacokinetics in mechanically ventilated patients. Antimicrob Agents Chemother 35:1582, 1991.
16. Nau R, Prange HW, Muth P, *et al.* Passage of cefotaxime and ceftriaxone into cerebrospinal fluid of patients with uninflamed meninges. Antimicrob Agents Chemother 37:1518, 1993.
17. Luer MS, Hatton J. Vancomycin administration into the cerebrospinal fluid: a review. Ann Pharmacother 27:912.
18. Hawker F. The critically ill patient with abnormal liver function tests. In Park GR (ed). The liver. London: WB Saunders Co Ltd, 1993:286.
19. Macnab MS, Macrae DJ, Guy E, *et al.* Profound reduction in morphine clearance and liver blood flow in shock. Intens Care Med 12:366, 1986.
20. La Breque D, Johlin F, Janda R, Shreves T, Gereats D, De Sante K, Cerimele B, Lanier T, Sides G. Pharmacokinetics of diritromycin in patients with impaired hepatic function. J Antimicrob Chemother 32:741, 1993.
21. Park GR, Pichard L, Tinel M, *et al.* What changes drug metabolism in critically ill patients: two preliminary studies in isolated human hepatocytes. Anesthesia 49:188, 1994.
22. Muller CM, Scierka A, Stiller RL, *et al.* Nitric oxide mediates hepatic cytochrome P450 dysfunction induced by endotoxin. Anesthesiology 84:1435, 1996.
23. Stockel K, Koup JR. Pharmacokinetics of ceftriaxone in patients with renal and liver insufficiency and correlations with a physiologie nonlinear protein binding model. Am J Med 77:26, 1984.

24. Brogden RN, Peters DH. Teicoplanin: a reappraisal of its antimicrobial activity, pharmacokinetic properties and therapeutics efficacy. Drugs 47:823, 1994.
25. Leader WG, Chandler MH, Castiglia M. Pharmacokinetic optimisation of vancomycin therapy. Clin Pharmacokinet 28:327, 1995.
26. Ambrose PJ. Clinical pharmacokinetics of chloramphenicol and chloramphenicol succinate. Clin Pharmacokinet 9:222, 1984.
27. Mann HJ, Townsend RJ, Fuhs DW, *et al.* Decreased hepatic clearance of clindamycin in critically ill patients with sepsis. Clin Pharm 6:154, 1987.
28. Benet LZ, Zech K. Pharmacokinetics: a relevant factor for the choice of a drug? Aliment Pharmacol Ther 8 (Suppl. 1):25, 1994.
29. Raghuram TC, Krishnaswamy K. Pharmacokinetics of tetracycline in nutritional edema. Chemotherapy 28:428, 1982.
30. Hess MM, Boucher BA, Laizure SC, *et al.* Trimethoprim sulfamethoxazole pharmacokinetics in trauma patients. Pharmacotherapy 13:602, 1993.
31. Israili ZH, Rogers CM, el-Attar H. Pharmacokinetics of antituberculosis drugs in patients. J Clin Pharmacol 27:78, 1987.
32. Buijk SLCE, Vanden Berg MFQ, Mouton JW, *et al.* Bioavailability of ciprofloxacin after multiple oral and intravenous doses in intensive care patients with gram negative intra-abdominal infections. Intens Care Med 22 (Suppl. 3):S391, 1996.
33. Bressolle I, Goncalves F, Gouby A, *et al.* Pefloxacin clinical pharmacokinetics. Clin Pharmacokinet 27:418, 1994.
34. Lamp KC, Bailey EM, Rybac MJ. Ofloxacin clinical pharmacokinetics (review). Clin Pharmacokinet 22:32, 1992.
35. Power BM, Millar A, Van Heerden PV, Ileet KF. Pharmacokinetics of drugs used in critically ill adults. Clin Pharmacokinet 24:25, 1998.
36. St Peter WL, Redic-Kill KA, Halstenson CE. Clinical pharmacokinetics of antibiotics in patients with impaired renal function. Clin Pharmacokinet 22:169, 1992.
37. Elston AC, Bayliss MK, Park GR. Effect of renal failure on drug metabolism by the liver. Br J Anaesth 71:282.
38. Dasta JF, Armstrong DK. Variability in aminoglycoside pharmacokinetics in critically ill surgical patients. Crit Care Med 16:327, 1988.
39. Heinemeyer G, Link J, Weber W, *et al.* Clearance of ceftriaxone in critical care patients with acute renal failure. Intens Care Med 16:448, 1990.
40. Mazzei T, Surrenti C, Novelli A, *et al.* Pharmacokinetics of Azithromycin in patients with renal impaired renal function. J Antimicrobial Chemotherapy 31 (Suppl. E):57, 1993.
41. Adam WR, Dawborn JK. Urinary excretion and plasma levels of sulphonamides in patients with renal impairment. Australasian Annals of Medicine 19:250, 1970.
42. Losno García R, Santivanez V, Battilana CA. Single-dose pharmacokinetics of ceftriaxone in patients with end-stage renal disease and hemodialysis. Chemotherapy 34:261, 1989.
43. Miglioli PA, Merlo F, Campanile F, *et al.* Effects of cardiopulmonary bypass on teicoplanin serum disposition. Int J Clin Pharmacol Res 15:23, 1995.
44. Bergan T. Pharmacokinetic properties of the cephalosporins. Drugs 34 (Suppl. 2):89, 1987.
45. Chandler MH, Toler SM, Rapp RP, *et al.* Multiple-dose pharmacokinetics of concurrent oral ciprofloxacin and rifampicin therapy in elderly patients. Antimicrob Agents Chemother 34:442, 1995.
46. Kihara M, Ikeda Y, Takagi N, *et al.* Pharmacokinetic of single-dose intravenous amikacin in critically ill patients undergoing slow hemodialysis. Intens Care Med 21:348, 1995.
47. Santre C, Leroy O, Simin M, *et al.* Pharmacokinetics of vancomycin during continuous hemodiafiltration. Intens Care Med 19:347, 1993.
48. Kihara M, Ikeda Y, Shibata K, *et al.* Pharmacokinetic profiles of intravenous imipenem/cilastatin during slow hemodialysis in critically ill patients. Clin Nephrol 42:193, 1994.
49. Vos MC, Vincent HH, Yzerman EP. Clearance of imipenem/cilastatin in acute renal failure patients treated by continuous hemodiafiltration (CAVHD). Intens Care Med 18:282, 1992. Fish DN, Bainbridge JL, Peloquin CA. Variable disposition of ciprofloxacin in critically ill patients undergoing continuous arteriovenous hemodiafiltration. Pharmacotherapy 15:236, 1995.
50. Davies SP, Lacey LF, Kox WJ, *et al.* Pharmacokinetics of cefuroxime and ceftazidime in patients with acute renal failure treated by continuous arteriovenous haemodialysis. Nephrol Dialysis Transplant 6:971, 1991.
51. Ernest D, Cutler DJ. Gentamicin clearance during continuous arteriovenous hemodiafiltration. Crit Care Med 20:586, 1992.

52. Armstrong DK, Hodgman T, Visconti JA, *et al.* Hemodialysis of amikacin in critically ill patients. Crit Care Med 16:517, 1988.
53. Scheltz M, Ferdinande P, Van den Berghe G, *et al.* Pharmacokinetics of continuous renal replacement therapy. Intens Care Med 21:612, 1995.
54. Sorgel F, Kinzig M. Pharmacokinetic characteristics of piperacillin/tazobactam. Intens Care Med 20 (Suppl. 3):S14, 1994.
55. Forrest A, Nix DE, Ballow CH, *et al.* Pharmacokinetics of intravenous ciprofloxacin in seriously ill patient. Antimicrob Agents Chemother 37:1073, 1993.
56. Lau AH, Lam NP, Piscitelli SC, *et al.* Clinical pharmacokinetic of metronidazole and other nitromidazole anti-infectives. Clin Pharmacokinet 23:328, 1992.
57. Ljungberg B, Nilsson-Ehle I, Ursing B. Metronidazole: pharmacokinetic observations in severely ill patients. J Antimicrob Chemother 14:275, 1984.
58. Triginer C, Izquierdo I, Fernández R, *et al.* Gentamicin volume of distribution in critically ill septic patients. Intens Care Med 16:303, 1990.

15. ANTIMICROBIAL PROPHYLAXIS IN THE INTENSIVE CARE UNIT

Ina S. Petersen, Dominique L. Monnet and Ole B. Jepsen

Introduction

The strategies used to prevent infections can be characterized as primary, secondary, or tertiary, depending primarily on the respective position of the preventive action and exposure to the pathogen [1]. Immunization is a classic example of primary prevention, in which the host is protected against infection before exposure to the pathogen. Antimicrobial prophylaxis is another type of primary prevention since antimicrobials are also given before exposure to microorganisms, for example before incision in patients undergoing a surgical procedure.

It is important to realize that antimicrobial prophylaxis is different from empirical antibiotic treatment. In the case of prophylaxis, antimicrobials are given before relevant clinical signs of infection are present. The term "empirical" indicates that the treatment is initiated on the basis of clinical signs of infection such as fever, hypotension, meningeal signs, sputum production, dysuria, etc, and this before identification and susceptibility results from relevant microbiological samples are available. A further description of empirical antimicrobial treatment is beyond the scope of this chapter. Similarly, documented antimicrobial therapy, which is based on available microbiological results, is not covered in the present chapter that focuses on the various aspects of antimicrobial prophylaxis in the intensive care unit (ICU).

Consumption of antimicrobials in ICU patients is abundant, often exceeding 100 Defined Daily Doses (DDD, as defined by WHO) per 100 patient days [2–4]. Even though antimicrobial courses are most frequently initiated as empirical treatment or documented therapy, prophylaxis represents a substantial fraction of ICU antimicrobial use. For example, it represented 13% of all indications for prescription of antimicrobials in a Duth ICU in 1994 [5]. In 1996, a study in four Danish ICUs showed that antimicrobials were prescribed for prophylaxis in 18% (span: 11–75%) of all patient days with antimicrobials [4]. Such large differences among ICUs were explained by the systematic use of a specific prophylactic regimen aiming at the selective decontamination of the digestive tract (SDD) in one of the ICUs. SDD represents the best known and one of the most debated types of antimicrobial prophylaxis applied to ICU patients. However, antimicrobial prophylaxis in the ICU is also applied to specific patient groups such as patients undergoing certain surgical interventions [6, 7], patients with severe immune deficiencies [8, 9] or some transplant patients [10, 11].

Selective Decontamination of the Digestive Tract (SDD)

DEFINITION OF SDD

The SDD regimen was introduced in 1983 by van Saene *et al.* [12] and its use was first reported in 1984 by Stoutenbeek *et al.* in a group of patients with multiple trauma [13]. The full

SDD protocol includes the following four elements: 1) a high standard of hygiene in the ICU, 2) the administration of a parenteral antibiotic, often cefotaxime sodium, during the first four days following admission of the patient in the ICU, 3) the topical application of antibiotics which are not absorbed systemically, often polymyxin, tobramycin and amphotericin B, applied throughout the stay in the ICU as a paste in the oral cavity and as a solution through a nasogastric tube to the stomach, 4) regular surveillance samples of the patient's throat and rectum to monitor the emergence of resistant microorganisms [14].

The theory behind the SDD regimen is that all ICU infections are of either exogenous, primary endogenous or secondary endogenous nature, depending on the pathogenic mechanisms [15]. Exogenous infections are caused by microorganisms, not carried by the patient at admission but acquired by the patient during the ICU stay. These infections may occur throughout the patients' stay in the ICU and can only be prevented by a high standard of hygiene – the first element in the SDD regimen. Primary endogenous infections generally occur within the first four days in the ICU. They are caused by microorganisms that do not relate to the ICU ecology, but are carried by the patient on ICU admission. These infections are described to be prevented by the parenteral antibiotic given to the patient the first days after admission – the second element in the SDD regimen. Secondary endogenous infections are caused by microorganisms not carried by the patient on admission, but acquired during stay in the ICU in the oropharynx and gut, followed by colonization and subsequent infections of the internal organs. These infections are prevented by the local antibiotic treatment of the throat and gut – the third element in the SDD regimen. Surveillance samples represent the last element in the SDD regimen and are performed to detect carriage of potentially pathogenic microorganisms, to monitor compliance and efficacy of the treatment and to detect emergence of resistant strains [16]. Although proper application of the SDD protocol should include these four components as originally described, a regimen which did not include the parenteral antibiotic component has been used to prevent infections in liver transplant patients [17], and, as a preoperative prophylaxis beginning 48 hours before the surgery, in patients undergoing oesophagal resection [18]. The complete SDD regimen includes antibiotics that eliminate or reduce the amount of aerobic bacteria in the gastrointestinal tract, while retaining the anaerobic flora. This is based on studies on mice and monkeys which showed that, if this anaerobic flora remains in the gastrointestinal tract, colonization with aerobic and fungal flora is less likely to occur [19, 20]. The complete SDD regimen is presented by van Saene *et al.* as active against 14 microorganisms commonly responsible for pneumonia and other infections in ICU patients, i.e. *Streptococcus pneumoniae*, *Haemophilus influenzae*, *Moraxella catarrhalis*, *Escherichia coli*, *Candida albicans*, methicillin-susceptible *Staphylococcus aureus*, *Klebsiella* spp., *Proteus* spp., *Morganella* spp., *Enterobacter* spp., *Citrobacter* spp., *Serratia* spp., *Acinetobacter* spp. and *Pseudomonas* spp. The SDD regimen is not active against *Streptococcus viridans*, *Enterococcus* spp., coagulase-negative staphylococci, anaerobes and methicillin-resistant *Staphylococcus* aureus (MRSA) [16]. If the patient carries MRSA at ICU admission, control measures such as patient isolation, skin decontamination, addition of oral vancomycin to the drug regimen, and withdrawal of SDD should be considered [21].

SDD IN MECHANICALLY VENTILATED PATIENTS

When compared to non-ventilated patients, mechanically ventilated patients are at a notoriously increased risk of infection, especially of the respiratory tract [22, 23], and this even after control for severity of illness [24]. SDD has especially been investigated as a strategy to prevent respiratory tract and other infections in mechanically ventilated patients. However, although the

SDD regimen is the best evaluated intervention in the history of intensive care, with more than 40 controlled trials, several reviews and at least six meta-analyses [25–35], its application is still controversial and it is not routinely used in most ICUs.

Several diverging points of view have been debated. First, despite the fact that in almost all studies the rate of respiratory tract infections was significantly reduced by 25–75% with SDD, the effect on mortality was more ambiguous, with a reported effect ranging from 50% higher mortality among treated patients in a study on 49 patients [36] to a 40% reduction in mortality in a study on 91 patients [37]. In a recent meta-analysis of randomized controlled trials with pooled data from unselected ICU patients [27], a significant reduction in mortality (odds ratio (OR) 0.80, confidence interval (CI) 0.69–0.93) was shown for patients receiving the complete SDD regimen. When only topical antibiotics were used, this meta-analysis showed no significant reduction in mortality (OR 1.01), even though these topical antibiotics had an effect on the rate of respiratory tract infections (OR 0.56, CI 0.46–0.68). This observation clearly questions the size of the contribution of respiratory tract infections to mortality in mechanically ventilated critical ill patients. While some studies on the outcome of nosocomial pneumonia in mechanically ventilated patients have shown no excess in mortality in patients with ventilator-associated pneumonia [38, 39], at least two studies by Fagon *et al.* have shown an excess in mortality [40, 41].

Secondly, since heterogeneous patient populations have been analyzed in most studies on SDD, it might be that the beneficial effect of SDD is only connected to some specific patient characteristics, whereas patients without these characteristics do not gain from SDD. This possibility is addressed later in this chapter.

Thirdly, van Saene *et al.* reported that in some of the randomized and placebo-controlled studies of SDD with negative conclusions, the applied regimen differed from the original full SDD protocol [16]. For example, one or several of the four elements in the protocol were omitted or the reported infections were caused by microorganisms which were not covered by the regimen.

Fourth, the cost of SDD has been opposed to its routine application. Four randomized studies reporting on the cost per survivor found that this measure was lower in patients receiving SDD than in patients who did not; a result which has been attributed to a lower incidence of infections, a lower use of antibiotics and blood products and a higher proportion of survivors [42]. Although intensive care is expensive and the cost of SDD might only represent a small fraction of the costs of ICU patient care, cost-effectiveness analysis in an ICU is problematic because of the difficulty to quantify the relative contribution of a single intervention such as SDD [43]. Besides the cost of prophylactic antibiotics and the additional workload connected to their use, implementation of the full SDD regimen requires a high level of hygiene and a consistent microbiological surveillance in the ICU. These two components are costly but essential, and their absence has been advocated as a reason for emergence of antimicrobial-resistant microorganisms and failure of SDD to prevent infection and death. Emerging antimicrobial resistance represents a final diverging point view and is discussed later in this chapter.

SDD IN OTHER GROUPS OF PATIENTS

Most studies dealing with SDD are based on heterogeneous populations of surgical and medical ICU patients. The only common important criteria of inclusion in many of these studies is mechanical ventilation during the ICU stay. The effects of SDD on subgroups of ICU patients have only been analyzed in a few meta-analyses. In a recent meta-analysis, Nathens and Marshall showed a lower mortality in critically-ill surgical patients treated with SDD (OR 0.7, CI 0.52–0.93), while SDD had no effect on the mortality of critically-ill medical patients [32].

In 1996, another meta-analysis showed a similar lower mortality in patients with high mortality risks at study entry [44]. In 1992, a third meta-analysis showed a trend toward decreased mortality for cardio-thoracic surgery patients, trauma patients, and patients with relatively long ICU stays and mid-range mortality risks at study entry [45]

Burn patients [46] and patients undergoing oesophagal resection [18] have been shown to benefit from SDD in terms of reduced rates of infection. In 1996, Quinio *et al.* showed that SDD resulted in lower bronchopneumonia but not lower mortality rates in multiple trauma patients [47]. In this study, the parenteral component of the full SDD regimen was not included. Finally, Bion *et al.* showed that patients undergoing elective liver transplantation who received SDD had lower rates of pulmonary infection and colonization; however, SDD had no effect on endotoxemia or development of organ system failure [48].

It has only seldom been shown that subgroups of medical ICU patients gain from the SDD regimen. In 1997, Luiten *et al.* showed that patients with severe acute pancreatitis receiving SDD had less gram-negative pancreatic infections and a lower mortality [49]. In 1996, Rolando *et al.* concluded that parenteral antibiotics were effective in reducing infections in patients with acute liver failure; however, use of SDD did not bring any additional benefit [50]. In myelosuppressed patients, oral treatment with ciprofloxacin was found to be equally effective in reducing rates of bacterial infections as an antibiotic modulation of the gut flora with the combination of neomycin, polymyxin B and nalidixic acid [51]. In 1989, Vollaard *et al.* demonstrated the value of an SDD regimen associating oral norfloxacin and amphotericin B to prevent catheter-associated UTIs [52]. Finally, systematic application of the topical component of SDD to patients admitted for more than 48 hours has been shown to provide some help in the control of outbreaks of multi-resistant *Enterobacteriaceae* [53, 54].

EMERGENCE OF ANTIMICROBIAL RESISTANCE AND SDD

After decades of use of antimicrobials, it is commonly admitted that overuse of these drugs leads to emergence of resistance. A recent European study showed that ICUs which routinely used SDD had an antimicrobial consumption two to three times higher than other ICUs [55]. As a consequence of extensive use of antimicrobials for SDD, one would expect a high frequency of infections due to resistant microorganisms. Numerous studies have reported on an increase in colonization by microorganisms resistant to the SDD regimen, or rebound colonization, due to emergence of resistance in gram-negative bacteia and overgrowth of gram-positive cocci not covered by SDD, or on an increase in infections due to microorganisms resistant to the SDD regimen [27, 33, 56–71]. An intriguing observation is that studies reporting an increase in infections due to resistant microorganisms following SDD seem to be less frequent than reports of emergence of resistance in only colonizing microorganisms. This may only be due to the necessary delay needed between the increase in resistance in colonization sites, then the increase in infection sites; a hypothesis which could be investigated by long-term surveillance of both colonization and infections in ICUs using SDD. However, for the promoters of SDD, the reasons for this observation can be found in the SDD protocol, i.e. the combination of short-term systemic plus long-term non-absorbable antibiotics (as opposed to systemic antibotics only), a high standard of hygiene to prevent cross-transmission of resistant-microorganisms, and surveillance cultures to monitor emergence of resistance which requires prompt implementation of control measures and modification of the composition of the topical antibiotic regimen [42]. For example, when surveillance samples of throat or rectum detect MRSA carriage, control measures, including patient isolation and skin decontamination, and addition of oral vancomycin to the topical regimen should be introduced, if necessary with the withdrawal of SDD [21, 72].

It might be that, if applied properly, SDD does not lead to an increase in infections due to resistant microorganisms. Additionally, in at least two cases, SDD has been shown to reduce gram-negative colonization rates not only in the patients who received SDD but also in patients from the same ICU who did not (control group), suggesting that SDD contributes to a decrease in the overall burden of potential pathogens in an ICU [53, 73].

Unfortunately, proper application of SDD is complex and hospital hygiene might not be optimal in all ICUs. One could therefore imagine another scenario in which, because SDD often leads to colonization by resistant microorganisms, poor hygiene practices could result in transmission of these microorganisms to other patients in the same ICU. Now that the clinical benefits of SDD have been demonstrated, studies should focus on ecological consequences, not only at the patient level but also for whole groups of patients. For example, we need studies comparing long-term trends in antibiotic resistance and hospital hygiene in a large group of ICUs which used or did not use SDD during the past years. Studies should also focus on hospitalization units that frequently admit patients transferred from ICUs using SDD. It is possible that, because of lower standards of hygiene in other hospitalization units, resistance emerges outside of the ICU from patients that benefited from SDD during a previous ICU stay. Finally, future studies should aim at investigating patterns of infection, including resistance patterns, as middle- and long-term ecological consequences in those patients who benefited from SDD.

SHOULD WE RECOMMEND USE OF SDD IN ICU PATIENTS?

It is by now certain that the SDD regimen prevents infections, especially lower respiratory tract infections. Additionally, recent meta-analyses have also shown that SDD also helps in reducing mortality in mechanically ventilated ICU patients; although this effect is much less marked than on infections. Both effects seem to be connected with specific groups of patients, such as mechanically ventilated critically ill surgical or trauma patients, with involvement of thorax or abdomen, but without "end stage" of severe underlying diseases, or severe and advanced dysfunction of multiple organs, and SDD should probably be applied in priority to those patients. Unfortunately, there are still areas of uncertainty concerning the application of SDD. We still do not know whether the full SDD regimen is cost-effective, and what are the real consequences of SDD on antimicrobial resistance. Concerns about additional costs and risk of emergence of antimicrobial-resistant bacterial isolates are probably the reasons why it is only used in a limited number of ICUs. If we follow the principles of evidence-based medicine, we should now apply SDD to the categories of patients in which SDD has been proven useful to prevent infection and death. However, this should be done with extreme caution after considering possible drawbacks such as additional costs and emergence of antimicrobial resistance. One should also pay attention to apply the fully SDD regimen, i.e. including a high level of hospital hygiene and regular colonization surveillance samples, and that SDD is applied in a proper fashion. For example, if SDD is used in trauma patients, it should be initiated as soon as possible after trauma. In surgical patients, SDD should be initiated in due time before the surgical procedure, as should be the case for other surgical antibiotic prophylaxis regimens.

Other Antimicrobial Prophylaxis in ICU Patients

ROUTINE PROPHYLAXIS WITH SYSTEMIC ANTIMICROBIALS IN ICU PATIENTS

A randomized prospective study conducted in the 1970s in an ICU in Austria showed that prophylaxis using systemic penicillin G plus ampicillin did not reduce the infection or mortality rate in ICU patients [74, 75]. When they found that most infections were caused by microorganisms that were resistant to the antibiotics used, the authors changed the prophylaxis regimen to a combination of cefazolin and gentamicin which resulted in an outbreak of *Serratia marcescens* infections. In 1989, a multicenter placebo-controlled randomized study showed that prophylaxis using penicillin G or cefoxitin did not prevent early onset pneumonia or death in ICU patients [76]. Although our experience shows that routine prophylaxis using only systemic antimicrobials in most patients might still be used in some Eastern European ICUs [77], this study clearly demonstrates this practice, if still in use, must be abandoned.

Routine anti-fungal prophylaxis has been proposed to prevent yeast colonization and sepsis in non-transplant/non-burned critically ill surgical and trauma patients. In a randomized controlled study, Savino *et al.* showed that independent risk factors for yeast colonization and sepsis were treatment with three or more antibiotics, an APACHE II score higher than 10 and ventilatory support for more than 48 hours, confirming that overuse of antibiotics contributes to an increase in yeast infections [78]. Additionally, patients receiving either clotrimazole, ketoconazole or nystatin prophylaxis had a significantly lower rate of yeast colonization, but not yeast sepsis, when compared to controls who did not receive an anti-fungal [78]. In the absence of proof that routine anti-fungal prophylaxis prevents yeast sepsis and reduces mortality and because of the possible emergence of anti-fungal-resistant yeast isolates [79], this practice should be avoided.

PROPHYLAXIS IN ICU PATIENTS WITH A CENTRAL VENOUS CATHETER

Antibiotic prophylaxis at insertion of a central venous catheter is not recommended on the basis of available data [80]. Although because of a limited number of samples, the possibility of a beneficial effect cannot be ruled out, three studies using either vancomycin [81] or teicoplanin [82, 83] failed to demonstrate a reduction of the incidence of early catheter-related infections. Addition of vancomycin or a combination of vancomycin and ciprofloxacin to catheter flush or total parenteral nutrition solutions has been shown to reduce the incidence of catheter-related infections in neonates [84, 85] and immunocompromised patients [86, 87]. However, prolonged administration of vancomycin has been associated with reduced vancomycin susceptibility in staphylococcal isolates and colonization with vancomycin-resistant enterococci, and the Centers for Disease Control and Prevention guidelines recommend against prophylactic use of vancomycin [88]. Therefore, as advocated by Mermel, "prevention of intravascular catheter-related infections should not involve vancomycin or other therapeutic agents" "efforts should be focused on interventions that are not likely to encourage the emergence of antimicrobial resistance, such as maximal barrier precautions" [80].

PROPHYLAXIS IN ICU PATIENTS WITH A URINARY CATHETER

Antimicrobial solutions for irrigation of the bladder have been proposed to prevent catheter-associated urinary tract infections (UTIs). A well designed study by Warren *et al.* was unable to show any benefit of a neomycin-polymixin irrigant and found that more resistant microorganisms were responsible for infections in patients receiving this type of prophylaxis [89]. Additionally, the method used for these irrigations had the disadvantage of necessitating a break in the closed drainage system. Local application of anti-microbials has also been proposed to reduce meatal colonization and prevent catheter-associated UTIs. A study by Classen *et al.* showed that a mixture of polymyxin B, neomycin and gramicidin applied as a cream for meatal care in patients catheterized more than two days did not significantly reduce acquired bacteriuria and could therefore not be recommended in all patients [90]. In this study, use of any systemic anti-microbial during catheterization and before bacteriuria was shown to have a slight preventive effect against development of bacteriuria. Indeed, since the 1970s, several studies have shown that systemic anti-microbials administered either at catheter insertion [91] or during the whole catheterization period, could decrease the occurrence of UTIs in catheterized patients; however, this preventive effect disappeared after approximately one week when patients were at increased risk for colonization and infection with resistant microorganisms [92]. A more recent double-blind placebo-controlled randomized trial showed that ciprofloxacin was effective at preventing bacteriuria and symptomatic urinary tract infections in patients who required up to 14 days drainage [93]. This regimen did not result in the emergence of ciprofloxacin resistance among normally susceptible gram-negative bacteria. However, there was a marked change in the distribution of microorganisms isolated from urine samples of patients receiving ciprofloxacin which were virtually only gram-positive bacteria. Additionally, ciprofloxacin-resistant alpha-haemolytic streptococci and *Staphylococcus epidermidis* were isolated from faeces and urine samples from these patients.

Recurrent UTIs are a common complication in patients with spinal cord injury or neuropathic bladder who require long-term catherization. In these patients, long-term indwelling catherization results in recurrent UTIs, which has not been shown to be prevented by antibiotic prophylaxis [94]. Other methods such as intermittent catheterization are preferred for bladder emptying. A study by Gribble and Puterman showed that antibiotic prophylaxis using trimethoprim-sulfamethoxazole prevented bacteriuria and symptomatic UTI in patients on intermittent catheterization [95]. However, these authors mentioned that adverse reactions attributable to trimethoprim-sulfamethoxazole and emergence of resistance may limit the usefulness of this practice. Biering-Sørensen *et al.* showed that low-dose, long-term ciprofloxacin prevented in patients with spinal cord injury and bladder dysfunction [96]; however, only seven of the 21 patients enrolled in their study used clean intermittent self-catheterization. Finally, one should consider the cost of anti-microbial prophylaxis. In a cost-benefit analysis published in 1989, Platt *et al.* found that use of a sealed junction catheter was less expensive than oral antibiotic prophylaxis and therefore did not recommend routine use of the latter to prevent catheter-associated urinary tract infections [97]. In view of the risks, side-effects and costs of anti-microbial prophylaxis, it seems that, as for central venous catheters, prevention of infections associated with urinary catheters still mainly relies on proper use of catheters and good hospital hygiene practices.

PROPHYLAXIS IN ICU PATIENTS WITH ALTERED IMMUNE DEFENCE

ICU patients with immunodeficiencies have a fundamental increased risk of infection when compared to otherwise similar ICU patients without immunodeficiencies. Depending on the character and the extent of the immunodeficiency, some microorganisms are more likely to be pathogenic. When lymphocyte T cells are affected causing a cell-mediated immunodeficiency, as in acquired immunodeficiency syndrome (AIDS), infections caused by *Pneumocystic carinii*, *Cryptococcus neoformans*, *Mycobacterium* spp., cytomegalovirus (CMV) and herpes simplex virus (HSV) are frequently diagnosed. In the case of a lack of lymphocyte B cells and decrease in humoral immunity, patients have an increased susceptibility to encapsulated bacteria: *Haemophilus influenzae* and *Streptococcus pneumoniae*, and to infections due to with *Giardia lamblia*, *Campylobacter* spp., and enteroviruses. Patients with neutrophil immunological disorders have an increased risk of infections due to gram-negative bacteria such as *Pseudomonas* spp., *Serratia marcescens* and *Klebsiella* spp., to *Staphylococcus* spp., fungi such as *Candida* spp., or *Aspergillus* spp., and viruses such as HSV, varicella-zoster virus or CMV.

In case of fever or other signs of infection in ICU patients with severe immunodeficiency, initiation of empirical antibiotic treatment covering all likely pathogens and sampling of relevant microbiological specimens should be a promptly initiated. However, systemic antibiotic prophylaxis has been shown to prevent infections in specific categories of immunocompromised ICU patients. In neutropenic patients, several studies have investigated prophylaxis of bacterial infections using fluoroquinolones, trimethoprim/sulfamethoxazole or vancomycin. It seems like a prophylaxis regimen with a fluoroquinolone has some beneficial effect, although it generally results in an increased prevalence of gram-positive infections [98–102]. The combination of a fluoroquinolone and another antibiotic aimed at the prophylaxis of gram-positive bacteremia (penicillin, macrolides or vancomycin) has been shown to be effective in reducing the frequency of bacteremia due to streptococcal species and other gram-positive bacteria [103, 104].

Pulmonary infections by *Pneumocystic carinii* (PCP) are a feared complication in patients with deficiency in the cellular immunity. Administration of prophylactic trimetroprim-sulfamethoxazole prevents PCP infections in patients with low levels of CD4 lymphocytes [8, 9]. Prophylactic administration of clarithromycin or azithromycin has been shown to prevent infections due to the *Mycobacterium avium* complex in AIDS patients [105, 106]. For neutropenic patients, as for patients in induction therapy for bone marrow allografting, prophylaxis using acyclovir and ganciclovir is used for the prevention of HSV and CMV infections, respectively [107, 108]. In cancer patients undergoing therapy for metastatic malignancies and in patients undergoing marrow transplantation, a decreased frequency of fungal infections were found in patients receiving fluconazole prophylaxis [109, 110]. In 1995, a review of the literature on anti-microbial prophylaxis in bone marrow transplantation concluded that since survival benefit has not always been demonstrated, toxicity and cost-effectiveness of the prophylactic strategies should be critically evaluated [111]. In addition, emergence of resistance and infections due to resistant microorganisms have been observed in immunocompromised patients receiving anti-microbial prophylaxis [112] and this point should also be considered.

PROPHYLAXIS IN PATIENTS WITH ACUTE NECROTIZING PANCREATITIS

Schwarz *et al.* showed that patients suffering acute necrotizing pancreatitis who received prophylaxis with ofloxacin and metronidazole had an improved clinical course as measured by repeated APACHE II scores; however prophylaxis did not prevent bacterial infections of the necrotic pancreas [113]. Inversely, Pederzoli *et al.* showed that prophylaxis using imipenem in patients with acute necrotizing pancreatitis resulted in a decreased incidence of pancreatic sepsis [114].

PROPHYLAXIS IN CIRRHOTIC PATIENTS

A meta-analysis showed an overall decrease in mortality in cirrhotic patients with gastro-intestinal bleeding [115]. In cirrhotic ICU patients with a high risk of infection, i.e. Child-Pugh's class C and/or rebleeding, systemic antibiotic prophylaxis with a combination of ciprofloxacin and amoxicillin-clavulanate from the day of admission to three days after cessation of the hemorrhage was effective to prevent bacterial infections [116]. Unfortunately, at least two studies have shown an association between either prior or long-term norfloxacin prophylaxis in cirrhotic patients and emergence of quinolone resistance in colonizing microorganisms [117, 118]; an observation which precludes routine use of antibiotic prophylaxis in cirrhotic patients.

PROPHYLAXIS IN TRAUMA PATIENTS

The role of prophylactic antibiotics for tube thoracostomy in chest trauma patients has been evaluated in a meta-analysis [119], and since then in at least two clinical trials [120, 121].

Both the meta-analysis and the two following trials showed that patients receiving prophylactic antibiotics while undergoing tube thoracostomy for trauma had a reduced incidence of infectious complications as compared to patients receiving placebo. Studies have also been performed in other kinds of trauma patients i.e. head injury [122, 123], or penetrating injuries of the chest [124] or the abdomen [125] and suggest that antibiotic prophylaxis plays a role in the management of penetrating injuries of the truncus and of certain fractures of the skull.

PROPHYLAXIS IN ICU SURGICAL PATIENTS, INCLUDING LIVER TRANSPLANT PATIENTS

Patients admitted to an ICU after a surgical procedure often receive one or several doses of antibiotics as the remaining part of the perioperative prophylaxis regimen. Although these patients are severe enough to be admitted in an ICU, prophylaxis beyond what is indicated in the local surgical antibiotic prophylaxis guidelines is not justified and the guidelines should be strictly applied. For specific procedures such as liver transplant, antibiotic prophylaxis is often extended to 2–5 days after the intervention and often includes a cephalosporin and a broad-spectrum penicillin; although regimens vary among centres [126].

Recently, Eggimann *et al.* showed that fluconazole prophylaxis prevents colonization and invasive intra-abdominal *Candida* infections in surgical patients with recurrent gastrointestinal perforations and anastomotic leakages [127]. However, these authors warned of the possibility of emergence of non-*C. albicans* species with reduced susceptibility to azole anti-fungals with liberal use of fluconazole and advised strictly restricting fluconazole prophylaxis to those patients who have prospectively been identified as having a high risk of developing candidiasis.

PROPHYLAXIS IN PATIENTS UNDERGOING TRANSESOPHAGEAL ECHOCARDIOGRAPHY

Transesophageal echocardiography can induce transient bacteremia. Although the need for antibiotic prophylaxis has been questioned for patients undergoing this procedure, results of a prospective study in ICU patients showed that this practice is not justified [128].

Conclusion

Over the past few decades, various antimicrobial prophylaxis regimens have shown their effectiveness to prevent infections, and sometimes death, in specific categories of ICU patients. Antimicrobial prophylaxis should only be used in these categories of ICU patients for which effectiveness has been clearly demonstrated. If the decision is made to apply antimicrobial prophylaxis, one should be aware that the advantages for the individual patient are often counterbalanced by potential ecological risks, such as emergence of antimicrobial resistance, that affect not only the patients who receive prophylaxis but often the whole group of patients hospitalized in the same ICU. Other risks, such as, for example, the consequences of the spread outside of the ICU of these emerging resistant microorganisms in patients who received prophylaxis, have not been evaluated and cannot be ruled out. Finally, cost-effectiveness analysis of interventions is difficult in the ICU setting and complex antimicrobial prophylaxis regimens such as the full SDD regimen, including a high level of hygiene and regular samples for surveillance of colonization, cannot definitely be accepted as cost-effective. In this context, the decision to apply antimicrobial prophylaxis to ICU patients should be examined with caution after a thorough consideration of these risks and costs.

References

1. Osterholm MT, Hedberg CW, MacDonald KL. Epidemiology of infectious diseases. In Mandell GL, Bennett JE, Dolin R (eds). Mandell, Douglas and Bennett's principles and practice of infectious diseases. New York: Churchill Livingstone, 1995:158.

2. WHO Collaborating Centre for Drug Statistics Methodology. Anatomical therapeutic chemical (ATC) classification index – including defined daily doses (DDD) for plain substances. Oslo, Norway: WHO Collaborating Centre for Drug Statistics Methodology, 1995:74.
3. Friis H. Antibiotic consumption in defined daily dosage (DDD) – advantages and disadvantages. Ugeskr Læger 148:2565, 1986.
4. Petersen IS, Hesselbjerg L, Jørgensen L, Renstrup J, Barnung S, Schierbeck J, *et al.* High antibiotic consumption in Danish intensive care units? APMIS 107:989, 1999.
5. Bergmans DCJJ, Bonten MJM, Gaillard CA, van Tiel FH, van der Geest S, de Leeuw PW, *et al.* Indications for antibiotic use in ICU patients: a one-year prospective surveillance. J Antimicrob Chemother 39:527, 1997.
6. Baum ML, Anish DS, Chalmers TC, Sacks HS, Smith H, Fagerstrom RM. A survey of clinical trials of antibiotic prophylaxis in colon surgery: evidence against further use of no-treatment controls. N Engl J Med 305:795, 1981.
7. Kreter B, Woods M. Antibiotic prophylaxis for cardiothoracic operations. Meta-analysis of thirty years of clinical trials. J Thorac Cardiovasc Surg 104:590, 1992.
8. Center for Disease Control and Prevention. Recommendations for prophylaxis against *Pneumocystis carinii* pneumonia for adults and adolescents infected with human immunodeficiency virus. Morb Mortal Wkly Rep 41(RR-4):1, 1992.
9. Kovacs JA, Masur H. Prophylaxis for *Pneumocystis carinii* pneumonia in patients infected with human immunodeficiency virus. Clin Infect Dis 14:1005, 1992.
10. Fox BC, Sollinger HW, Belzer FO, Maki DG. A prospective, randomized, double-blind study of trimetroprim-sulfamethoxazole for prophylaxis of infection in renal transplantation: clinical efficacy, absorption of trimethoprim-sulfamethoxazole, effects on the microflora, and the cost-benefit of prophylaxis. Am J Med 89:255, 1990.
11. Winston DJ, Ho WG, Nakao SL, Gale RP, Champlin RE. Norfloxacin versus vancomycin/polymyxin for prevention of infections in granulocytopenic patients. Am J Med 80:884, 1986.
12. van Saene HKF, Stoutenbeek CP, Miranda DR, Zandstra DF. A novel approach to infection control in the intensive care unit. Acta Anaesthiol Belg 34:193, 1983.
13. Stoutenbeek CP, van Saene HKF, Miranda DR, Zandstra DF. The effect of selective decontamination of the digestive tract on colonization and infection rate in mutiple trauma patients. Intensive Care Med 10:185, 1984.
14. van Saene HKF, Alcock SR, Rommes JH, Baxby D, Percival A. Impact of SDD on ICU ecology. Intensive Care Med 20:459, 1994.
15. Baxby D, van Saene HKF, Stoutenbeek CP, Zandstra DF. Selective decontamination of the digestive tract: 13 years on, what it is and what it is not. Intensive Care Med 22:699, 1996.
16. van Saene HKF, Nunn AJ, Stoutenbeek CP. Selective decontamination of the digestive tract in intensive care patients. Br J Hosp Med 54:558, 1995.
17. Wiesner RH, Hermans PE, Rakela J, Washington JA, Perkins JD, DiCecco S, *et al.* Selective bowel decontamination to decrease gram-negative aerobic bacterial and *Candida* colonization and prevent infection after orthotopic liver transplantation. Transplantation 45:570, 1989.
18. Tetteroo GWM, Wagenvoort JHT, Castelein A, Tilanus HW, Ince C, Bruining HA. Selective decontamination to reduce gram-negative colonisation and infections after oesophagal resection. Lancet 335:704, 1990.
19. van der Waaij D, Berghuis-de Vries JM, Lekkerkerk-van der Wees JEC. Colonization resistance of the digestive tract in conventional and antibiotic treated mice. J Hyg (Camb) 69:405, 1971.
20. van der Waaij D, Berghuis-de Vries JM. Selective elimination of enterobacteriaceae species from the digestive tract in mice and monkeys. J Hyg (Camb) 72:205, 1974.
21. Rogers CJ, van Saene HK, Suter PM, Horner R, Orme ML. Infection control in critically ill patients: effects of selective decontamination of the digestive tract. Am J Hosp Pham 51:631, 1994.
22. Center for Disease Control and Prevention. Guidelines for prevention of nosocomial pneumonia. Morb Mortal Wkly Rep 46(RR-1):1, 1997.
23. Cunnion KM, Weber DJ, Broadhead WE, Hanson LC, Pieper CF, Rutala WA. Risk factors for nosocomial pneumonia: comparing adult critical-care populations. Am J Respir Crit Care Med 153:158, 1996.
24. Chevret S, Hemmer M, Carlet J, Langer M, the European Cooperative Group on Nosocomial Pneumonia. Incidence and risk factors of pneu-

monia acquired in intensive care units. Results from a multicenter prospective study on 996 patients. Intensive Care Med 19:256, 1993.

25. Brun-Buisson C, Legrand P. Can topical and nonabsorbable antimicrobials prevent cross-transmission of resistant strains in ICUs? Infect Control Hosp Epidemiol 15:447, 1994.
26. Cockerill FR. Indications for selective decontamination of the digestive tract. Semin Respir Infect 8:300, 1993.
27. D'Amico R, Pifferi S, Leonetti C, Torri V, Tinazzi A, Liberati A. Effectiveness of antibiotic prophylaxis in critically ill adult patients: systematic review of randomised controlled trials. BMJ 316:1275, 1998.
28. Donnelly JP. Selective decontamination of the digestive tract and its role in antimicrobial prophylaxis. J Antimicrob Chemother 31:813, 1993.
29. Heyland DK, Cook DJ, Jaeschke R, Griffith L, Lee HN, Guyatt GH. Selective decontamination of the digestive tract. An overview. Chest 105:1221, 1994.
30. Hurley JC. Prophylaxis with enteral antibiotics in ventilated patients: selective decontamination or selective cross-infection? Antimicrob Agents Chemother 39:941, 1995.
31. Kollef MH. The role of selective digestive tract decontamination on mortality and respiratory tract infections. A meta-analysis. Chest 105: 1101, 1995.
32. Nathens AB, Marshall JC. Selective decontamination of the digestive tract in surgical patients: a systematic review of the evidence. Arch Surg 134:170, 1999.
33. Saunders GL, Hammond JMJ, Potgieter PD, Plumb HA, Forder AA. Microbiological surveillance during selective decontamination of the digestive tract (SDD). J Antimicrob Chemother 34:529, 1994.
34. Selective decontamination of the digestive tract trialists' collaborative group. Meta-analysis of randomised controlled trials of selective decontamination of the digestive tract. BMJ 307:525, 1993.
35. Vandenbroucke-Grauls CMLE, Vandenbroucke JP. Effect of selective decontamination of the digestive tract on respiratory tract infections and mortality in the intensive care unit. Lancet 338:859, 1991.
36. Finch RG, Tomlinson P, Holliday M, Sole K, Stack C, Rocker G. Selective decontamination of the digestive tract (SDD) in the prevention of secondary sepsis in a medical/surgical intensive care unit. Abstracts of the 17th International Congress of Chemotherapy, Berlin, no. 0471, 1991.
37. Jacobs S, Foweraker JE, Roberts SE. Effectiveness of selective decontamination of the digestive tract (SDD) in an ICU with a policy encouraging a low gastric pH. Clin Intensive Med 3:52, 1992.
38. Rello J, Quintana E, Ausina V, Castella J, Luquin M, Net A, *et al.* Incidence, etiology, and outcome of nosocomial pneumonia in mechanically ventilated patients. Chest 100:439, 1991.
39. Leu HS, Kaiser DL, Mori M, Woolson RF, Wenzel RP. Hospital-acquired pneumonia. Attributable mortality and morbidity. Am J Epidemiol 129:1258, 1989.
40. Fagon J-Y, Novara A, Stephan F, Girou E, Safar M. Mortality attributable to nosocomial infections in the ICU. Infect Control Hosp Epidemiol 15:428, 1994.
41. Fagon J-Y, Chastre J, Vuagnat A, Trouillet J-L, Novara A, Gibert C. Nosocomial pneumonia and mortality among patients in intensive care units. JAMA 275:866, 1996.
42. Silvestri L, Mannucci F, van Saene HKF. Selective decontamination of the digestive tract: a life saver. J Hosp Infect 45:185, 2000.
43. Liberati A, D'Amico R, Pifferi S, Telaro E. Antibiotic prophylaxis in intensive care units: meta-analyses versus clinical practice. Intensive Care Med 26:S38, 2000.
44. Sun X, Wagner DP, Knaus WA. Does selective decontamination of the digestive tract reduce mortality for severely ill patients? Crit Care Med 24:753, 1996.
45. Occhipinti DJ, Itokazu G, Danziger LH. Selective decontamination of the digestive tract as an infection-control measure in intensive care unit patients. Pharmacotherapy 12(6 Pt 2):50S, 1992.
46. Mackie DP, van Hertum WAJ, Schumburg T, Kuijper EC, Knape P. Prevention of infection in burns: preliminary experience with selective decontamination of the digestive tract in patients with extensive injuries. J Trauma 32: 570, 1992.
47. Quinio B, Albanèse J, Bues-Charbit M, Viviand X, Martin C. Selective decontamination of the digestive tract in multiple trauma patients. A prospective double-blind, randomized, placebo-controlled study. Chest 109:765, 1996.
48. Bion JF, Badger I, Crosby H, Hutchings P, Kong K-L, Baker J, *et al.* Selective decontamination of the digestive tract reduces gram-

negative pulmonary colonization but not systemic endotoxemia in patients undergoing elective liver transplantation. Crit Care Med 22:40, 1994.

49. Luiten EJT, Hop WCJ, Lange JF, Bruining HA. Differential prognosis of gram-negative versus gram-positive infected and sterile pancreatic necrosis: results of a randomized trial in patients with severe acute pancreatitis treated with adjuvant selective decontamination. Clin Infect Dis 25:811, 1997.
50. Rolando N, Wade JJ, Stangou A, Gimson AES, Wendon J, Philpott-Howard J, *et al.* Prospective study comparing the efficacy of prophylactic parenteral antimicrobials, with or without enteral decontamination, in patients with acute liver failure. Liver Transpl Surg 2:8, 1996.
51. Jansen J, Cromer M, Akard L, Black JR, Wheat LJ, Allen SD. Infection prevention in severely myelosuppressed patients: a comparison between ciprofloxacin and a regimen of selective antibiotic modulation of the intestinal flora. Am J Med 96:335, 1994.
52. Vollaard EJ, Clasener HAL, Zambon JV, Joosten HJM, van Griethuysen AJA. Prevention of catheter-associated Gram-negative bacilluria with norfloxacin by selective decontamination of the bowel and high urinary concentration. J Antimicrob Chemother 23:915, 1989.
53. Brun-Buisson C, Legrand P, Rauss A, Richard C, Montravers F, Besbes M, *et al.* Intestinal decontamination for control of nosocomial multiresistant gram-negative bacilli. Study of an outbreak in an intensive care unit. Ann Intern Med 110:873, 1989.
54. Taylor ME, Oppenheim BA. Selective decontamination of the gastrointestinal tract as an infection control measure. J Hosp Infect 17: 271, 1991.
55. Monnet DL, Suetens C, Jepsen OB, Burman LG, Carsauw H, Gastmeier P, *et al.* Overall antimicrobial use and control strategies in intensive care units from 6 European countries [abstract P-S2-03]. In On-Site Program of the 4th Decennial International Conference in Nosocomial and Healthcare-Associated Infections, Atlanta, Georgia, March 5–9, 2000, 107.
56. Abele-Horn M, Dauber A, Bauernfeind A, Russwurm W, Seyfarth-Metzger I, Gleich P, *et al.* Decrease in nosocomial pneumonia in ventilated patients by selective oropharyngeal decontamination (SDD). Intensive Care Med 23:187, 1997.
57. Bonten MJM, Gaillard CA, van Tiel FH, van der Geest S, Stobberingh EE. Colonization and infection with *Enterococcus faecalis* in intensive care units: the role of antimicrobial agents. Antimicrob Agents Chemother 39:2783, 1995.
58. Bonten MJM, van Tiel FH, van der Geest S, Smeets HGW, Stobberingh EE, Gaillard CA. Topical antimicrobial prophylaxis of nosocomial pneumonia in mechanically ventilated patients. Microbiological observations. Infection 21:137, 1993.
59. Daschner F. Emergence of resistance during selective decontamination of the digestive tract. Eur J Clin Microbiol Infect Dis 11:1, 1992.
60. Duncan RA, Steger KA, Craven DE. Selective decontamination of the digestive tract: risks outweigh benefits for intensive care unit patients. Seminars in Respiratory Infections 8:308, 1993.
61. Cockerill FR III, Muller SR, Anhalt JP, Marsh HM, Farnell MB, Mucha P, *et al.* Prevention of infection in critically ill patients by selective decontamination of the digestive tract. Ann Intern Med 11:545, 1992.
62. Ferrer M, Torres A, Gonzalez J, Puig de la Bellacasa J, el-Ebiary M, Roca M, *et al.* Utility of selective digestive decontamination in mechanically ventilated patients. Ann Intern Med 120:389, 1994.
63. Gastinne H, Wolff M, Delatour F, Faurisson F, Chevret S, the French Study Group on Selective Decontamination of the Digestive Tract. A controlled trial in intensive care units of selective decontamination of the digestive tract with nonabsorbable antibiotics. N Engl J Med 326: 594, 1992.
64. Hammond JMJ, Potgieter PD. Long-term effects of selective decontamination on antimicrobial resistance. Crit Care Med 23:637, 1995.
65. Hammond JMJ, Potgieter PD, Saunders GL, Forder AA. Double-blind study of selective decontamination of the digestive tract in intensive care. Lancet 340:5, 1995.
66. Lingnau W, Berger J, Javorsky F, Fille M, Allerberger F, Benzer H. Changing bacterial ecology during a five year period of selective intestinal decontamination. J Hosp Infect 39: 195, 1998.
67. Nardi G, Valentinis U, Proietti A, De Monte A, Di Silvestre A, Muzzi R, *et al.* Epidemiological impact of prolonged systematic use of topical SDD on bacterial colonization of the tracheobronchial tree and antibiotic resistance. Intensive Care Med 19:273, 1993.

68. Nau R, Ruchel R, Mergerian H, Wegener U, Winkelmann T, Prange HW. Emergence of antibiotic-resistant bacteria during selective decontamination of the digestive tract. J Antimicrob Chemother 25:881, 1990.
69. Rocha LA, Martin MJ, Pita S, Paz J, Seco C, Margusino L, *et al.* Prevention of nosocomial infection in critically ill patients by selective decontamination of the digestive tract. A randomized, double blind, placebo-controlled study. Intensive Care Med 18:398, 1992.
70. Tetteroo GWM, Wagenvoort JHT, Bruining HA. Bacteriology of selective decontamination: efficacy and rebound colonization. J Antimicrob Chemother 34:139, 1994.
71. Winter R, Humphreys H, Pick A, MacGowan AP, Willatts SM, Speller DC. A controlled trial of selective decontamination of the digestive tract in intensive care and its effect on nosocomial infection. J Antimicrob Chemother 30:73, 1992.
72. van Saene HKF, Unertl KE, Alcock SR, Stoutenbeek CP, Hart CA. Emergence of antibiotic resistance during selective digestive decontamination? J Hosp Infect 24:158, 1993.
73. Bonten MJM, Gaillard CA, Johanson WG Jr, van Tiel FH, Smeets HGW, van der Geest S, *et al.* Colonization in patients receiving and not receiving topical antimicrobial prophylaxis. Am J Respir Crit Care Med 150:1332, 1994.
74. von Rotter M, Pichler H, Wewalka G, Lackner F, Coraim F. Routinemäßige Chemoprophylaxe bei Intensivpatienten. Anaesthesiol Reanim 4:175, 1979.
75. Wewalka G, Koller W, Rotter M, Lackner F, Coraim F, Pichler H. Der Patient als Keimquelle in der Intensivpflegestation. Einfluß von Antibiotika und trachealer Intubation. Infection 4:204, 1976.
76. Mandelli M, Mosconi P, Langer M, Cigada M, Intensive Care Unit Group of Infection Control. Prevention of pneumonia in an intensive care unit: a randomized multicenter clinical trial. Crit Care Med 17:501, 1989.
77. Monnet DL, Burman L, Carsauw H, Gastmeier P, Jurkuvenas V, Sainz A, *et al.* European Strategy for Antibiotic Prophylaxis: preliminary report on a 3-month pilot phase in 6 countries [abstract S25 06]. In Program and Abstracts of the 5th International Conference on the Prevention of Infection, Nice, France, May 6–7, 1998: 80.
78. Savino JA, Agarwal N, Wry P, Policastro A, Cerabona T, Austria L. Routine prophylactic antifungal agents (clotrimazole, ketoconazole, and nystatin) in nontransplant/nonburned critically ill surgical and trauma patients. J Trauma 36:20, 1994.
79. Safran DB, Dawson E. The effect of empiric and prophylactic treatment with fluconazole on yeats isolates in a surgical trauma intensive care unit. Arch Surg 132:1184, 1997.
80. Mermel LA. Prevention of intravascular catheter-related infections. Ann Intern Med 132:391, 2000.
81. McKee R, Dunsmuir R, Whitby M, Garden OJ. Does antibiotic prophylaxis at the time of catheter insertion reduce the incidence of catheter-related sepsis in intravenous nutrition? J Hosp Infect 6:419, 1985.
82. Ljungman P, Hägglund H, Björkstrand B, Lönnqvist B, Ringdén O. Peroperative teicoplanin for prevention of gram-positive infections in neutropenic patients with indwelling central venous catheters: a randomized, controlled study. Support Care Cancer 5:485, 1997.
83. Pellizzer G, Nicolin R, D'Emilio A, Figoli G, Bragagnolo L, Merlo F, *et al.* Teicoplanin (T) prophylaxis in tunneled central venous catheter (TCVC). In Abstracts of the 35th Interscience Conference on Antimicrobial Agents and Chemotherapy, 17–20 September 1995, San Francisco, CA. Washington, DC: American Society for Microbiology; 1995:273.
84. Spafford PS, Sinkin RA, Cox C, Reubens L, Powell KR. Prevention of central venous catheter-related coagulase-negative staphylococcal sepsis in neonates. J Pediatr 125:259, 1994.
85. Ocete E, Ruiz-Extremera A, Goicoechea A, Lozano A, Robles C, Rey ML, *et al.* Low-dosage prophylactic vancomycin in central-venous catheter for neonates. Early Hum Dev 53:S181, 1998.
86. Barriga FJ, Varas M, Potin M, Sapunar F, Rojo H, Martinez A, *et al.* Efficacy of a vancomycin solution to prevent bacteremia associated with an indwelling central venous catheter in neutropenic and non-neutropenic patients. Med Pediatr Oncol 28:196, 1997.
87. Henrickson KJ, Axtell RA, Hoover SM, Kuhn SM, Pritchett J, Kehl SC, *et al.* Prevention of central venous catheter-related infections and thrombotic events in immunocompromised children by the use of vancomycin/ciprofloxacin/heparin flush solution: a randomized, multicenter, double-blind trial. J Clin Oncol 18:1269, 2000.

88. Hospital Infection Control Practices Advisory Committee (HICPAC). Recommendations for preventing the spread of vancomycin resistance. Infect Control Hosp Epidemiol 16:105, 1995.
89. Warren JW, Platt R, Thomas RJ, Rosner B, Kass EH. Antibiotic irrigation and catheter-associated urinary-tract infections. New Engl J Med 299:570, 1978.
90. Classen DC, Larsen RA, Burke JP, Alling DW, Stevens LE. Daily meatal care for prevention of catheter-associated bacteriuria: results using frequent applications of polyantibiotic cream. Infect Control Hosp Epidemiol 12:157, 1991.
91. Mountokalakis T, Skounakis M, Tselentis J. Short-term versus prolonged systemic antibiotic prophylaxis in patients treated with indwelling catheters. J Urol 134:506, 1985.
92. Stamm WE. Nosocomial urinary tract infections. In Bennett JV, Brachman PS (eds). Hospital Infections. Boston (MS): Little Brown, 1991:597.
93. van der Wall E, Verkooyen RP, Mintjes-de Groot J, Oostinga J, van Dijk A, Hustinx WNM, *et al.* Prophylactic ciprofloxacin for catheter-associated urinary-tract infection. Lancet 339:946, 1992.
94. Warren JW. Catheter-associated urinary tract infections. Inf Dis Clin North Am 1:823, 1987.
95. Gribble MJ, Puterman ML. Prophylaxis of urinary tract infection in persons with recent spinal cord injury: a prospective, randomised, double-blind, placebo-controlled study of trimethoprim-sulfamethoxazole. Am J Med 95:141, 1993.
96. Biering-Sørensen F, Høiby N, Nordenbo A, Ravnborg M, Bruun B, Rahm V. Ciprofloxacin as prophylaxis for urinary tract infection: prospective, randomized, cross-over, placebo-controlled study in patients with spinal cord lesion. J Urol 151:105, 1994.
97. Platt R, Polk F, Murdock B, Rosner B. Prevention of catheter-associated urinary tract infection: a cost-benefit analysis. Infect Control Hosp Epidemiol 10:60, 1989.
98. Nagatomo A, Watanabe K, Kunikane H, Okamoto H, Kunitoh H. A randomized controlled trial of sulfamethoxazole/trimethoprim plus norfloxacin versus sulfamethoxazole/trimethoprim alone for the prophylaxis of bacterial infection during chemotherapy for lung cancer. Lung Cancer 19:121, 1998.
99. Winston DJ, Ho WG, Bruckner DA, Gale RP, Champlin RE. Ofloxacin versus vancomycin/polymyxin for prevention of infections in granulocytopenic patients. Am J Med 88:36, 1990.
100. Kern W, Kurrle E. Ofloxacin versus trimethoprim-sulfamethoxazole for prevention of infection in patients with acute leukemia and granulocytopenia. Infection 19:73, 1991.
101. Fanci R, Leoni F, Bosi A, Guidi S, Ciolli S, Longo G, *et al.* Chemoprophylaxis of bacterial infections in granulocytopenic patients with ciprofloxacin vs ciprofloxacin plus amoxicillin. J Chemother 5:119, 1993.
102. Del Favero A, Menichetti F. The new fluorinated quinolones for antimicrobial prophylaxis in neutropenic cancer patients. Eur J Cancer 29A(Suppl 1):S2, 1993.
103. International Antimicrobial Therapy Cooperative Group of the European Organization for Research and Treatment of Cancer. Reduction of fever and streptococcal bacteremia in granulocytopenic patients with cancer. A trial of penicillin V or placebo combined with pefloxacin. JAMA 272:1183, 1994.
104. Cruciani M, Rampazzo R, Melena M, Lazzarini L, Todeschini G, Messori A, *et al.* Prophylaxis with fluoroquinolones for bacterial infections in neutropenic patients: a meta-analysis. Clin Infect Dis 23:795, 1996.
105. Pierce M, Crampton S, Henry D, Heifets L, LaMarca A, Montecalvo M, *et al.* A randomized trial of clarithromycin as prophylaxis against disseminated *Mycobacterium avium* complex infection in patients with advanced acquired immunodeficiency syndrome. N Engl J Med 335:384, 1996.
106. Young LS. Treatment and prophylaxis of *Mycobacterium avium* complex. Int J STD AIDS 7(Suppl 1):23, 1996.
107. Rubin RH, Ferraro MJ. Understanding and diagnosing infectious complications in the immunocompromised host. Current issues and trends. Hematol Oncol Clin North Am 7:795, 1993.
108. Schmidt GM, Horak DA, Niland JC, Duncan SR, Forman SJ, Zaia JA. A randomized, controlled trial of prophylactic ganciclovir for cytomegalovirus pulmonary infection in recipients of allogenic bone marrow transplant. N Engl J Med 324:1005, 1991.
109. Bodey GP, Samonis G, Rolston K. Prophylaxis of candidiasis in cancer patients. Semin Oncol 17(3 Suppl 6):24, 1990.
110. Slavin MA, Osborne B, Adams R, Levenstein MJ, Schoch HG, Feldman AR, *et al.* Efficacy and safety of fluconazole prophylaxis for fungal

infections after marrow transplantation – a prospective, randomized, double-blind study. J Infect Dis 171:1545, 1995.

111. Momin F, Chandrasekar PH. Antimicrobial prophylaxis in bone marrow transplantation. Ann Intern Med 123:205, 1995.
112. Dejace P, Klastersky J. Emergence of resistance as a consequence of antimicrobial prophylaxis in immunocompromised patients. Scand J Infect Dis Suppl 49:165, 1986.
113. Schwarz M, Isenmann R, Meyer H, Berger HG. Antibiotic use in necrotizing pancreatitis. Results of a controlled study. Dtsch Med Wochenschr 122:356, 1997.
114. Pederzoli P, Bassi C, Vesentini S, Campedelli A. A randomized multicenter clinical trial of antibiotic prophylaxis of septic complications in acute necrotizing pancreatitis with imipenem. Surg Gynecol Obstet 176:480, 1993.
115. Bernard B, Grange JD, Khac EN, Amiot X, Opolon P, Poynard T. Antibiotic prophylaxis for the prevention of bacterial infections in cirrhotic patients with gastrointestinal bleeding: a meta-analysis. Hepatology 29:1655.
116. Pauwels A, Mostefa-Kara N, Debenes B, Degoutte E, Lévy V-G. Systemic antibiotic prophylaxis after gastrointestinal hemorrhage in cirrhotic patients with a high risk of infection. Hepatology 24:802, 1996.
117. Aparicio JR, Such J, Pascual S, Arroyo A, Plazas J, Girona E, *et al.* Development of quinolone-resistant strains of *Escherichia coli* in stools of patients with cirrhosis undergoing norfloxacin prophylaxis: clinical consequences. J Hepatol 31:277, 1999.
118. Dupeyron C, Mangeney N, Sedrati L, Campillo B, Fouet P, Leluan G. Rapid emergence of quinolone resistance in cirrhotic patients treated with norfloxacin to prevent spontaneous bacterial peritonitis. Antimicrob Agents Chemother 38:340, 1994.
119. Fallon WF Jr, Wears RL. Prophylactic antibiotics for the prevention of infectious complications including empyema following tube thoracostomy for trauma: results of meta-analysis. J Trauma 33:110, 1992.
120. Cant PJ, Smyth S, Smart DO. Antibiotic prophylaxis is indicated for chest stab wounds requiring closed tube thoracostomy. Br J Surg 80:464, 1993.
121. Gonzalez RP, Holevar MR. Role of prophylactic antibiotics for tube thoracostomy in chest trauma. Am Surg 64:617, 1998.
122. Demetriades D, Charalambides D, Lakhoo M, Pantanowitz D. Role of prophylactic antibiotics in open and basilar fractures of the skull: a randomized study. Injury 23:377, 1992.
123. Dunn LT, Foy PM. Anticonvulsant and antibiotic prophylaxis in head injury. Ann R Coll Surg Engl 76:147, 1994.
124. Demetriades D, Breckon V, Breckon C, Kakoyiannis S, Psaras G, Lakhoo M, *et al.* Antibiotic prophylaxis in penetrating injuries of the chest. Ann R Coll Surg Engl 73:348, 1991.
125. Demetriades D, Lakhoo M, Pezikis A, Charalambides D, Pantanowitz D, Sofianos C. Short-course antibiotic prophylaxis in penetrating abdominal injuries: ceftriaxone versus cefoxitin. Injury 22:20, 1991.
126. Kramer DJ, Selby R, Fung JJ. Intensive care of liver transplant recipients. In Shoemaker WC, Ayres SM, Grenvik A, Holbrook PR (eds). 3rd edn. Textbook of critical care. Philadelphia: Saunders, 1993:1638.
127. Eggimann P, Francioli P, Bille J, Schneider R, Wu M-M, Chapuis G, *et al.* Fluconazole prophylaxis prevents intra-abdominal candidiasis in high-risk surgical patients. Crit Care Med 27:1066, 1999.
128. Mentec H, Vignon P, Terré S, Cholley B, Roupie E, Legrand P, *et al.* Frequency of bacteremia associated with transesophageal echocardiography in intensive care unit patients: a prospective study of 139 patients. Crit Care Med 23:1194, 1995.

16. PRESCRIPTION OF ANTIMICROBIAL AGENTS IN PATIENTS UNDERGOING CONTINUOUS RENAL REPLACEMENT THERAPY

M. Schetz and C. Verwaest

Introduction

Acute renal failure (ARF) is a frequent complication (10–30%) in critically ill patients, that is mostly part of a multi-organ dysfunction syndrome (MODS). Continuous renal replacement therapy (CRRT) is becoming the central component of the supportive care of these patients, especially in Europe and Australia, and appears to be superior to intermittent hemodialysis (IHD) in patients with hemodynamic instability, extracellular volume overload, cerebral oedema and hypercatabolism [1]. Sepsis is an important contributor to the pathogenesis of ARF [2] and most patients on CRRT are treated with antibiotics. Correct dosing of these antibiotics is of the utmost importance. Subtherapeutic levels may result in treatment failure and in the emergence of bacterial resistance [3, 4]. On the other hand, critically ill patients have a limited physiologic reserve in several organ systems and badly tolerate toxic effects. CRRT indiscriminately removes all solutes that circulate in plasma water including drugs. The design of a rational antibiotic dosage regimen in patients treated with CRRT should take into account this extracorporeal elimination. In this chapter, the principles of pharmacokinetics and general guidelines for drug dosage adjustment during CRRT are discussed, followed by their application to antimicrobials frequently used in intensive care medicine. Several reviews on drug removal during CRRT have recently been published [5–8].

Pharmacokinetics in Critically Ill Patients

Even in healthy humans, a large interindividual variability of pharmacokinetic parameters, unexplained by disease or measurable patient characteristics, is observed [9]. In critically ill patients, cardiocirculatory, pulmonary, hepatic, renal or gastrointestinal failure may cause important deviations from anticipated pharmacokinetics [reviewed in 10–15]. The simultaneous failure of several organs and the instability of organ functions increase the degree of uncertainty about the fate of a drug in these patients. Delivering proper drug doses, optimal adaptation of dosing schedules to altered organ function and correctly utilising therapeutic drug monitoring requires an understanding of the meaning of pharmacokinetic parameters [13, 16, 17].

BIOAVAILABILITY (F)

Bioavailability is defined as the percentage of an administered drug that reaches the systemic circulation [16, 17]. Since in critically ill patients the majority of the antibiotics are administered through the intravenous route, giving rapid and reliable 100% bioavailability, this pharmacokinetic parameter is mostly not an issue.

VOLUME OF DISTRIBUTION (VD)

Volume of distribution is a measure of the extent to which a drug is distributed throughout the body [13, 16, 17]. The ability of a drug to cross cell membranes and to penetrate into body tissue depends on its degree of ionization at physiologic pH, lipid solubility, molecular weight and protein binding. Plasma protein binding, tissue binding and total body water are the most important determinants of Vd. Drugs highly bound to certain tissues have a large distribution volume, whereas drugs highly bound to plasma proteins have a distribution volume approaching plasma volume. The volume of distribution is a conceptual volume referring to the volume the drug would occupy if the body were a single homogenous compartment with drug concentration equal to the plasma concentration. It relates the plasma concentration of a drug to the amount of drug present in the body at any given time and may be used to calculate the loading dose required to reach a target concentration.

$$\text{Vd} = \text{Amount in the body}/\text{plasma concentration}$$

$$\text{Loading dose} = V_d \times \text{target concentration}$$

Alterations of the volume of distribution may be related to changes of extracellular fluid volume caused by blood loss, fluid shifts, fluid resuscitation, capillary leak, ascites, oedema, vomiting, diarrhoea etc or to changes of the concentration and/or characteristics of binding proteins (malnutrition, acute phase response) or of the factors that govern intercompartmental transfer [10]. Circulatory failure may induce changes in Vd because of the lack of distribution to organs with decreased blood flow [16]. Important changes in the Vd of several antibiotics, including aminoglycosides [18–21], sulfamethoxazole [22], aztreonam [23, 24], vancomycin [25], imipenem [23] and ceftazidime [26], have been described in critical illness. By removal of fluid, the CRRT itself may induce alterations of Vd.

PROTEIN BINDING (PB)

Proteinbinding determines the free fraction of a drug and hence the amount that is distributed, pharmacologically active at the tissue receptor sites, metabolised and excreted. Acidic and neutral drugs tend to bind to albumin, whereas basic drugs bind more commonly to alpha-1-acid glycoprotein. Protein binding is altered by acidosis, by hypoalbuminemia due to increased capillary permeability and decreased hepatic synthesis, and by raised levels of alpha-1-acid glycoprotein, that is an acute phase reactant. Protein binding is also affected by an increased body temperature and by the presence of displacing substances such as organic acids retained in uremia, free fatty acids that may increase after heparin administration, bilirubin or other drugs [10, 16, 17, 27]. A reduction of protein binding may lead to misinterpretation of the results of therapeutic drug monitoring. Most assays do not distinguish free from bound drug. A decreased protein binding may therefore result in a decreased total drug concentration, whereas the free (active) drug concentration is maintained [16, 28].

CLEARANCE (CL)

Clearance measures the intrinsic ability of the body to eliminate a drug from the blood or plasma and is defined as the volume that can be cleared of the drug in unit time. Renal elimination is the resultant of glomerular filtration, tubular secretion and tubular reabsorption. Metabolic clearance usually represents hepatic biotransformation although some drugs undergo substantial extrahepatic metabolism. Hepatic clearance depends on three parameters: hepatic blood flow, the unbound drug fraction and intrinsic clearance or theoretical maximal clearance reflecting enzymatic activity [16, 17]. Impaired hepatic blood flow decreases the clearance of drugs with significant hepatic extraction

[12, 16]. Hepatic enzyme activity is influenced by hypoxemia, inflammatory mediators, hepatocellular damage, other drugs, hormones, stress, fever and age [12]. Renal failure may also alter the metabolic transformation of drugs in both liver and kidney [29, 30].

Clearance only applies to substances with first order kinetics, which means that a constant fraction of the substance is eliminated per unit time, or the rate of decrease of the plasma concentration depends on the concentration at time $t(C_t)$ and the elimination rate constant k: $dC/dt = k \times C_t$. First order kinetics apply to most drugs. Total body clearance is the sum of all regional clearances (renal, metabolic and biliary clearance) and may be defined by the following equations, where AUC represents the area under the concentration versus time curve [16, 17].

$$Cl = \text{Dose}/\text{AUC}$$

$$Cl = \text{Rate of elimination}/\text{plasma concentration}$$

$$Cl = \text{Dosing rate}/\text{steady state concentration}$$

In clinical practice clearance is used to calculate the maintenance dose at steady state using the following formula, where C_p is the desired plasma concentration and τ the dosing interval.

$$\text{Maintenance dose} = Cl \times C_p \times \tau$$

ELIMINATION HALF LIFE ($T_{1/2}$)

Half life ($T_{1/2}$) is the term most commonly used to express the duration of action of a drug: it is the time it takes for the plasma concentration of a drug to diminish by 50% after distribution equilibrium has been attained [16]. The elimination half life reflects the elimination rate constant (k) and is defined by the equation:

$$T_{1/2} = 0.693/k$$

The most important use of $T_{1/2}$ is to predict how long it takes for a dosing regimen to achieve a steady-state concentration i.e. after four to five half lives if no loading dose has been administered. If $T_{1/2}$ changes by disease, a new steady-state is reached after another four or five half lives. Clearance and Vd are the fundamental pharmacokinetic parameters that contribute to what is clinically observed: the rate of decline of drug concentration and effect. The elimination half life is a dependent variable, its magnitude being directly related to Vd (determining the concentration presented to the clearing organ) and inversely to Cl. $T_{1/2}$ can be derived by the following equation:

$$T_{1/2} = 0.693 \times V/Cl$$

Factors Affecting Drug Removal by Continuous Renal Replacement Therapy

PRESENCE IN PLASMA WATER: PB, VD, RBC PARTITIONING

Only a water-soluble unbound drug present in plasma water can be removed through the artificial kidney membrane. Protein binding and volume of distribution are therefore important determinants of a drug's extracorporeal removal since they govern the fraction that is presented to the membrane. Even if extracorporeal clearance is high, drugs with large Vd are eliminated slowly, because the reservoir is large and thus the plasma level low. Intracellular partition in RBC, as has been described for ethambutol, also renders the drug inaccessible for extracorporeal removal. An increased hematocrit reduces the elimination of these drugs [31]. The continuous character of CRRT reduces the impact of Vd or RBC partition on extracorporeal drug removal because of the continuous reequilibration between the different body compartments.

DRUG MEMBRANE INTERACTIONS

Drug membrane interactions may result from drug charge and the Gibbs-Donnan effect, where negatively charged proteins along the membrane result in retention of cationic drugs. Drug adsorption to the membrane has also been

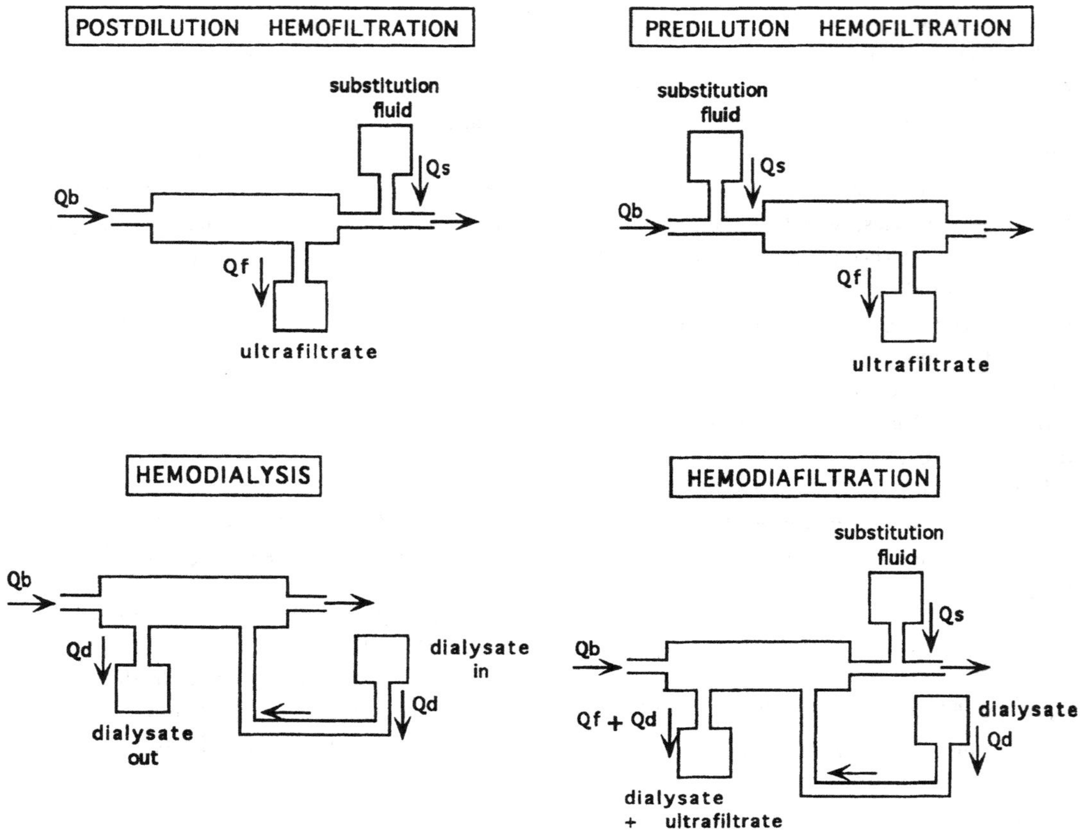

FIGURE 1. Different modalities of CRRT. Qb = blood flow; Qs = substitution flow rate; Qf = filtration rate; Qd = dialysate flow rate.

described and depends on the properties of both the drug and the artificial membrane. The most important interaction that has been described is the relatively large adsorption of aminoglycosides to the AN69 membrane [32–35]. Since drug adsorption is mostly a saturable phenomenon, it is only relevant during the first hours after a new filter has been started. It is not clear if adsorbed drugs can return to the circulation later on.

MECHANISM OF SOLUTE TRANSFER: DIFFUSION OR CONVECTION

Hemofiltration: Convection. During continuous hemofiltration solute transport is based on convection, where solutes are carried along with plasma water that is driven through the membrane by a pressure gradient. Blood purification is achieved by infusion of a substitution fluid containing water, electrolytes and a buffer (Figure 1). The ultrafiltrate contains plasma water and all dissolved solutes with molecular size below the membrane pore size or cut-off. For most hemofiltration membranes this cut-off is around 30,000 dalton and hence far above the molecular weight of almost all drugs. Convective removal of drugs present in plasma water is therefore independent of molecular weight and only determined by the ultrafiltration rate (Qf), that in turn depends on membrane hydraulic permeability (K_f), membrane surface area

(A) and transmembrane pressure (TMP) [27, 36–38].

$$Qf = K_f \times A \times TMP$$

The capacity of a drug to pass the membrane by convection is mathematically expressed in the sieving coefficient (S), that is defined as the relationship between drug concentration in the ultrafiltrate and in the plasma [36, 38]. The main determinant of the sieving coefficient is protein binding and, in the absence of important drug-membrane interactions, the free fraction (1-PB) is a good approximation [7]. Convective clearance (Cl_f) is determined by multiplying the filtration rate with the sieving coefficient.

$$S = C_f / C_p \approx (1 - PB)$$
C_f = drug concentration in filtrate

C_p = drug concentration in plasma
$$Cl_f = Q_f \times S \approx Q_f \times (1 - PB)$$

The above equations only apply to postdilution hemofiltration, where the substitution fluid is administered after the filter. In predilution hemofiltration, where the substitution fluid is infused prior to entry into the filter (Figure 1), the patient's blood is diluted, lowering the solute concentration in the filter compared with the plasma concentration. In this setting the sieving coefficient, and hence also the clearance, is decreased by a factor determined by the ratio between blood flow (Q_b) and the combined blood flow and substitution rate (Q_s) [8]:

$$Cl_{f_{predilution}} = Q_f \times (1 - PB) \times (Q_b / Q_b + Q_s)$$

Hemodialysis: Diffusion. Solute removal in hemodialysis is based on diffusion driven by a concentration gradient between blood and dialysate (Figure 1). Diffusion is a size limited process: drugs with low molecular weight diffuse with greater ease than those with large molecular weight. Most drugs fall in the low to middle molecular weight category (<1,000 dalton).

TABLE 1. Factors determining sieving coefficient (S) and dialysate saturation (S_d)

	S	S_d
Molecular weight	–	++
Protein binding	++++	++++
Drug-membrane interactions	+	+
Membrane thickness	–	+
Membrane pore size	–	+
Dialysate/blood flow	–	+

Diffusive solute removal also depends on membrane characteristics being easier through thin membranes and membranes with high porosity (high flux membranes) [37]. Dialysis membranes can be divided in two categories: cellulosic membranes (cuprophane, cellulose (di)(tri)acetate, hemophane) are made of natural polymers, are usually thin and have small pores, whereas synthetic membranes (polysulfone, polyamide, polymethylmethacrylate, polyacrylonitrile), that are commonly used in continuous renal replacement therapy, are thicker but have a higher porosity [39].

The capacity of a drug to diffuse through the membrane and to saturate the dialysate is mathematically expressed in the dialysate saturation (S_d) [5]. Dialysate saturation is derived in the same way as the sieving coefficient by dividing dialysate concentration (C_d) by plasma concentration (C_p). Table 1 summarizes the factors determining S and S_d. The main determinant of S_d is protein binding. However, in contrast to the sieving coefficient, S_d also depends on drug molecular weight, on the nature of the membrane (thickness and pore size) and on the ratio of dialysate and blood flow, the latter determining the time available for diffusion and being especially important for larger solutes, that require more time to diffuse and saturate the dialysate. During continuous dialysis, the countercurrent dialysate flow (Q_d) (10–30 ml/min) is considerably smaller than the blood flow (Q_b) (100–200 ml/min) enabling complete equilibration between blood and dialysate, at least for small solutes with easy diffusion. This results in an S_d of small drugs approaching the free fraction (1-PB). Diffusive clearance (Cl_d) of these small drugs is determined by multiplying the dialysate flow with the dialysate saturation and the product of Q_d with the free fraction is a good approximation.

$$S_d = C_d / C_p \approx (1 - PB)$$

C_d = drug concentration in dialysate

C_p = drug concentration in plasma

$$Cl_d = Q_d \times S_d \approx Q_d \times (1 - PB)$$

However, for larger drugs and higher dialysate flow rate, the saturation of the dialysate will be incomplete and the calculated clearances will overestimate the real clearance [5, 6, 40, 41].

Hemodiafiltration: Diffusion + Convection. Continuous hemodiafiltration combines diffusion and convection (Figure 1). For small unbound solutes such as urea and creatinine, diffusive and convective clearances have been shown to be additive [42]. On the assumption that this also applies to drugs, the hemodiafiltration clearance (Cl_{df}) can be calculated from the filtration rate (Q_f), the dialysate flow rate (Q_d) and the protein binding:

$$Cl_{df} = Q_f \times S + Q_d \times S_d \approx Q_f \times (1 - PB) + Q_d \times (1 - PB)$$

Interactions between diffusive and convective solute transfer, however, increase the complexity of kinetics in hemodiafiltration [27, 37]. Admixture of the ultrafiltrate and the dialysate may diminish the concentration gradient, and hence the diffusive clearance of small solutes. Diffusive removal on the other hand lowers the plasma concentration and decreases the amount removed by convection. Ignoring these interactions mostly results in an overestimation of the combined clearance.

THE CONCEPT OF FRACTIONAL EXTRACORPOREAL CLEARANCE (Fr_{EC})

Whether extracorporeal drug clearance is clinically important and thus requires dosage adaptation depends on the fractional extracorporeal clearance (Fr_{EC}) [5]. Fr_{EC} relates the extracorporeal clearance (Cl_{EC}) to the total body clearance, or the sum of all regional clearances, comprising renal (Cl_R), non-renal (Cl_{NR}) and extracorporeal clearance.

$$Fr_{EC} = Cl_{EC} / Cl_{EC} + Cl_R + Cl_{NR}$$

It is generally accepted that a regional clearance, whether extracorporeal or in an individual organ, is only clinically important if its contribution to total body clearance or Fr_{EC} exceeds 25% [5–7, 27, 43].

Table 2 illustrates the impact of Cl_{NR} on the Fr_{EC} of five antibiotics with different kinetics. The total clearance, with absolute and relative renal and non-renal contribution, are data from the literature [44] and represent values in healthy volunteers. The Cl_{EC} of a renal replace-

TABLE 2. The influence of Cl_{NR} on Fr_{EC} (see text for comments). Cl_T = total clearance, Cl_R = renal clearance, Cl_{NR} = non-renal clearance, DA_{anuria} = dosage adaptation required for renal failure, Cl_{EC} = extracroporaeal clearance, Fr_{EC} = extracorporeal clearance fraction, DA_{CRRT} = dosage adaptation required for CRRT

	Cl_T	Cl_R (%)	Cl_{NR} (%)	DA_{anuria}	Cl_{EC} (Cl_{cr} = 25)	Fr_{EC}	DA_{CRRT}
Pefloxacin	150	15 (10)	135 (90)	no	20	0.13	no
Ciprofoxacin	600	450 (75)	150 (25)	yes	17.5	0.1	no
Cefotaxime	322	193 (60)	129 (40)	yes	15	0.1	no
Aztreonam	80	60 (75)	20 (25)	yes	11	0.35	yes
Temocillin	44	35 (80)	9 (20)	yes	6.25	0.41	yes
Tobramycin	90	81 (90)	9 (10)	yes	23.7	0.72	yes

TABLE 3. The influence of the operational characteristics of CRRT on Fr_{EC} (see text for comments). CAVH = continuous arteriovenous hemofiltration, HVCVVH = high volume continuous venovenous hemofiltration, Q_f = filtration rate, Fr_{EC} = extracorporeal clearance fraction

	CAVH Q_f = 500 ml/h	HVCVVH Q_f = 3000 ml/h
Vancomycin	Fr_{EC} = 0.23	Fr_{EC} = 0.65
Piperacillin	Fr_{EC} = 0.12	Fr_{EC} = 0.45
Ofloxacin	Fr_{EC} = 0.17	Fr_{EC} = 0.56

ment therapy with a creatinine clearance of 25 ml/min is calculated with the above mentioned formulas assuming normal protein binding. The calculation of the Fr_{EC} assumes that the patient is anuric and has a normal Cl_{NR}. Pefloxacin has an almost exclusive Cl_{NR} (90%) which, despite a substantial Cl_{EC}, results in a low Fr_{EC} and neither renal failure nor extracorporeal elimination will require dosage adjustment. For ciprofloxacin, cefotaxime, aztreonam and temocillin the renal contribution to total body clearance is important and demands a substantial dose reduction in anuric patients. However, the application of the extracorporeal epuration technique does not require dosage adaptation for ciprofloxacin and cefotaxime, because the absolute Cl_{NR} of these drugs is high resulting in a low Fr_{EC} (Table 2).

Table 3 illustrates the impact of the operational characteristics of the CRRT on the fractional extracorporeal clearance. The Fr_{EC} of vancomycin, piperacillin or ofoxacin with a low clearance technique such as continuous arteriovenous hemofiltration (CAVH) with filtration rate of 500 ml/h is low, excluding the need for dosage adaptation. High volume continuous venovenous hemofiltration (HVCVVH), that has been suggested to be beneficial in septic patients [45], has a filtration rate of at least 3 l/h. With this treatment the extracorporeal elimination of vancomycin, piperacillin and ofloxacin contributes substantially to total body clearance and indeed requires dosage adaptation (Table 3).

The concept of Fr_{EC} explains why no dosage adaptation is required for drugs with low extracorporeal clearance, either resulting from a high PB or from a low Q_f or Q_d. Extracorporeal elimination should also not be taken into account for drugs with a high non-renal clearance or in patients with a high residual renal clearance (as might be the case when hemofiltration is applied for non-renal indications [1].

Approaches to Drug Dosage Adjustment During CRRT

THE LOADING DOSE

The achievement of therapeutic plasma levels with maintenance doses takes four to five half lives, which may be greatly prolonged in renal failure and thus delay effective therapy. Administration of a loading dose, especially of antibiotics, is therefore primordial in infected critically ill patients with absent renal function. The loading dose only depends on the volume of distribution and the required target concentration, and should not be adapted neither for renal failure nor for extracorporeal elimination, except when their influence on Vd is substantial.

ADAPTATION OF MAINTENANCE DOSE TO REDUCED RENAL FUNCTION

Subsequent maintenance doses have to be adapted to the reduced renal clearance. Extensive literature is available on this subject [43, 46–50]. The application of these literature data should take into account the impact of critical illness on pharmacokinetics.

ADAPTATION OF MAINTENANCE DOSE TO EXTRACORPOREAL ELIMINATION IF $Fr_{EC} > 0.25$

A) A first approach to drug dosage adjustment during CRRT is to consult the *literature*. However, the available clinical studies mostly have very small patient numbers. Moreover, intensive care patients on renal replacement therapy represent a very heterogeneous population, with great variability in underlying pathophysiology (and pharmacokinetics), and the operational characteristics of renal replacement therapy may differ considerably from one center to another. Extrapolations from literature data to the individual situation may therefore induce significant errors and should only be applied if the patient characteristics and the CRRT characteristics are comparable.

B) A second approach to determine the maintenance dose is based on the patient's *total creatinine clearance* (Cl_{creat}), being the sum of the extracorporeal Cl_{creat} and the residual endogenous Cl_{creat}. Extracorporeal Cl_{creat} equals the filtration rate (Q_f) for continuous hemofiltration, it equals the dialysate flow rate (Q_d) for continuous hemodialysis and the sum of Q_f and Q_d for hemodiafiltration. In this approach patients on CRRT receive drug dosages that are recommended for patients with comparable endogenous Cl_{creat} [51]. It may perform well for a lot of drugs. On the other hand, it starts with the assumption that renal drug clearance is a linear function of creatinine clearance ($Cl_{drug} = Cl_{NR} + a \times Cl_{creat}$), and that this relation is the same in the extracorporeal and natural kidney. However, for drugs with tubular secretion or reabsorption, the relationship between endogenous drug and creatinine clearance is not linear and different from the relationship between the extracorporeal drug and creatinine clearance. For drugs with important tubular reabsorption, dosage adaptation based on Cl_{creat} will underestimate the extracorporeal contribution. This is illustrated by the case of fluconazole, that, after glomerular filtration, undergoes substantial tubular reabsorption resulting in an endogenous renal clearance that is much lower than the endogenous creatinine clearance. However, in the extracorporeal circuit, fluconazole is only filtered resulting in a much higher ratio of fluconazole to creatinine clearance. This explains why the fluconazole clearance during continuous hemofiltration may approach values that have been reported in healthy volunteers and why normal doses of fluconazole are required in CRRT patients [52–55].

For drugs with tubular secretion, e.g. some beta-lactams or acyclovir, the effect of hemofiltration on drug elimination will be overestimated, because hemofiltration only replaces the filtration part of their elimination. On the other hand, Cl_{creat} generally overestimates GFR because creatinine is also eliminated by tubular secretion and, in addition, intestinal secretion of drugs can compensate for the missing tubular secretion (the so-called Lauterbach effect), which may compensate or minimize the error of overestimation [51].

C) A third approach relies on the determination of *extracorporeal drug clearance* and the extracorporeal clearance fraction Fr_{EC} with the previously mentioned formulas. If Fr_{EC} exceeds 0.25, dosage adjustment is required and two methods are available: either augmentation of the anuric dose (D_{anuria}) or shortening of the anuric dosing interval (τ_{anuria}) [5].

$$D = D_{anuria} / (1 - Fr_{EC})$$

$$\tau = \tau_{anuria} \times (1 - Fr_{EC})$$

The choice for either of these methods will depend on the pharmacodynamic properties of the drug e.g. for antibiotics with concentration-dependent killing and a post-antibiotic effect, such as aminoglycosides, the first method (an increase of the maintenance dose) is preferred, whereas for antibiotics with time-dependent killing, that require plasma level exceeding the MIC for at least 50% of the time, such as beta-lactams, the second approach (a shorter dosing interval) is probably optimal [3, 4, 56, 57].

D) For drugs with a narrow therapeutic index, *monitoring of serum levels* is essential, because the above mentioned formulas assume the absence of drug membrane interactions and normal non-renal pharmacokinetics. Adjustment to the desired serum level can be done with the following formula, again assuming that the distribution volume is normal and therefore requiring repetitive control of blood levels:

dose = (desired − present level) × V_d × BW

E) For drugs with little dose-related toxicity it is advisable to risk overdose rather than subtherapeutic levels.

F) Drugs whose pharmacodynamic effect is easy to monitor, can be administered according to their *clinical effect*. This applies to analgesics and sedatives and to most cardiovascular drugs, but unfortunately not to antimicrobial agents.

Elimination of Antibiotics by CRRT

AMINOGLYCOSIDES

Aminoglycosides are potent antibiotics that, despite their toxicity, are widely used in life-threatening infections. Aminoglycosides have a low Vd and thus high plasma levels, a low PB and an almost negligible non-renal clearance, resulting in a high Fr_{EC} and hence significant extracorporeal removal with CRRT [5, 6]. Adsorption of aminoglycosides to the AN69 membrane further complicates their pharmacokinetics [32–35]. *In vitro* experiments have shown the adsorption of 10 to 20 mg tobramycin [35]. The clinical importance of this adsorption remains to be determined.

Pharmacodynamically, aminoglycosides are characterized by a strong concentration-dependent bactericidal activity and a significant post-antibiotic effect against Gram-negative bacilli [3, 4, 57]. High peak concentrations of 8 to 12 times the minimal inhibitory concentration (MIC) are required for therapeutic efficacy [3, 56], whereas toxicity seems to be related to high trough concentrations [11]. A single high daily dose is thought to be associated with less toxicity and is probably at least as efficacious [58–60]. In patients with renal failure the total dose will have to be reduced, and corresponding high peak levels may not be achieved, unless by prolonging the dosage interval to 48 h or more. It is, however, not clear if extending the dosing interval to more than 24 h is safe [57]. In patients on CRRT, extracorporeal aminoglycoside removal may help to attain acceptable trough levels, allowing to advance subsequent doses and bactericidal peak levels.

Based on the previously mentioned formulas, and assuming an extracorporeal treatment with creatinine clearance of 25 ml/min, the anuric dose of aminoglycosides should be augmented with a factor 6 to 12 (Table 4). Literature data on the removal of aminoglycosides with CRRT are limited to case reports or very small patient series [61–66]. They mostly confirm the high sieving coefficient and significant extracorporeal removal. The variability of aminoglycoside pharmacokinetics in critically ill patients [18–21], the eventual adsorption to the membrane and the narrow therapeutic range necessitate frequent monitoring of serum levels. In the determination of an optimal dosing regimen, not only the pharmacokinetic data but also the severity of the infection, the susceptibility (MIC) of the pathogen and the patient's clinical condition are important. With the advent of newer potent antibiotics, it is even questionable if the use of aminoglycosides in the setting of sepsis with acute renal failure should still be considered.

FLUOROQUINOLONES

Although most quinolones have low protein binding, their high total body clearance with important non-renal contribution [46, 47] explains why the extracorporeal removal during CRRT is insignificant [5, 6]. An exception is ofloxacin that, because of a lower non-renal clearance, requires dosage adaptation. Since fluoroquinolones are concentration-dependent antibiotics with post-antibiotic effect against Gram-negative bacteria [3, 4, 67], an increase of the anuric dose is preferred over a shortening of the dosing interval. Theoretically, the dose of ofloxacin should be increased with 65% for a technique with extracorporeal creatinine clearance of 25 ml/min (Table 4).

Clinical studies on the elimination of ofloxacin during CRRT are lacking. An *in vitro*

TABLE 4. The correction factor that should be applied to the anuric dose (D_{anuria} or the anuric dosing interval (t_{anuria}) of some antimicrobials requiring dosage adaptation during CRRT (assuming an extracorporeal creatinin clearance of 25 ml/min, normal protein binding and normal non-renal clearance that are taken from [44] except if stated otherwise)

Drug	$t = t_{anuria} \times$	Drug	$D = D_{anuria} \times$	$t = t_{anuria} \times$
Ampicillin	× 0.65	ofloxacin [46]	× 1.65	
Amoxicillin	× 0.55	amikacin	× 12.5	
Azlocillin	× 0.75	gentamicin	× 7.1	
Piperacillin	× 0.7	tobramycin	× 7.1	
Ticarcillin	× 0.55	netilmycin	× 5.9	
Temocillin	× 0.6	trimethoprim	× 1.3	× 0.8
Cefuroxime	× 0.2	SMTX	× 1.5	× 0.65
Cefamandole	× 0.5	flucytosine	× 20	× 0.05
Ceftazidime	× 0.5	fluconazole	× 6.6	× 0.15
Cefepime	× 0.55	ganciclovir	× 1.8	× 0.55
Meropenem [107]	× 0.6			
Aztreonam [47]	× 0.75			
Vancomycin	× 0.5			
Teicoplanin [46]	× 0.7			

study by Journois *et al.* demonstrated important sieving of pefloxacin with an AN69 membrane [68]. However, *in vitro* studies do not take into account the endogenous clearance and therefore do not allow to make conclusions about required dosage adaptations. The extracorporeal removal of ciprofloxacin has been shown to be 6–7% of the total body clearance and therefore does not require dosage adaptation [69, 70].

BETA-LACTAMS

The extracorporeal elimination of penicillins and cephalosporins is difficult to discuss as a group, because they have a variable degree of protein binding and a variable non-renal elimination [5, 6]. Penicillinase-resistant penicillins such as dicloxacillin and oxacillin have a high protein binding and therefore do not require dosage adaptation during CRRT. Clinical studies have shown insignificant elimination of piperacillin [71] and ceftriaxone [72]. The reported Fr_{EC} is 0.29 for piperacillin [73], between 0.13 and 0.5 (depending on the liver function) for mezlocillin [74], between 0.34 and 0.63 for cefuroxime [75, 76], 0.53 for ceftazidime [76] and 0.72 for cefepime [77]. Several authors have reported a ceftriaxone sieving coefficient of approximately 0.7, which far exceeds the free fraction in healthy volunteers. This finding is difficult to explain but could suggest a considerable decrease of protein binding or a contribution of the Gibbs-Donan effect [7, 78–80]. Van de Wetering *et al.* demonstrated that the administration of the fixed combination piperacillin-tazobactam during CVVH in anuric patients results in some accumulation of tazobactam [81].

Since penicillins as well as cephalosporins are time-dependent antibiotics, requiring a plasma level exceeding the MIC for at least 50% of the time, dosage adaptation is preferentially realized by shortening the dosing interval [3, 4, 57]. Table 4 shows the required shortening for some frequently used beta-lactams, assuming a CRRT with extracorporeal creatinine clearance of 25 ml/min, normal protein binding and normal non-renal clearance. The altered pharmacokinetics of critically ill patients introduces a considerable degree of uncertainty, but the low toxicity profile of most beta-lactams allows to err in the upper direction.

The carbapenem imipenem has a low protein binding resulting in a high sieving coefficient.

However, it also has a substantial non-renal clearance, that is decreased in patients with chronic renal failure, but preserved in the early phase of ARF [82]. The extracorporeal clearance fraction of imipenem will therefore only be clinically significant during CRRT with a creatinine clearance of more than 25 ml/min [83–85]. Imipenem is administered together with cilastatin in order to minimize renal uptake (toxicity) and degradation by dehydropeptidase. In patients with normal organ function both substances have comparable pharmacokinetics [86]. However, since the non-renal clearance of cilastatin is lower than that of imipenem, dosage adaptation of imipenem will result in the accumulation of cilastatin in patients with reduced renal function [83, 84]. During CRRT the absolute extracorporeal clearance is higher for imipenem than for cilastatin because it has a lower protein binding. However, due to the lower non-renal clearance of cilastatin, its fractional extracorporeal clearance is higher, resulting in a significant elimination and hence decreased accumulation during CRRT [83–85, 87, 88].

Meropenem has a very low protein binding resulting in a sieving coefficient approaching the unity. The order of magnitude of its non-renal clearance is such that the fractional extracorporeal clearance during CRRT mounts to 35–55% of total body clearance. Due to time-dependent killing the anuric dosing interval should therefore be shortened by approximately 40% [89–91] (Table 4).

GLYCOPEPTIDES

Although vancomycin has a predominant renal elimination, it also has a considerable non-renal clearance accounting for approximately 30% of the total body clearance. This non-renal clearance is decreased in chronic renal failure and in the latter phase of ARF, but is preserved during the first 7–10 d of ARF [92]. Studies on patients receiving vancomycin during CRRT report non-renal clearances between 9 and 35 ml/min [69, 93, 94]. Vancomycin has a low protein binding resulting in a sieving coefficient of 0.7 to 0.8 [7, 63, 96], although lower values have also been reported [95]. Based on theoretical predictions, the extracorporeal removal of vancomycin increases to 50% of the total body clearance [6], corresponding with the literature data [69, 92, 93]. Since glycopeptides are time-depending antibiotics [3, 4, 57], dosage adaptation is preferentially performed by decreasing the anuric dosing interval with 50% (Table 4). Vancomycin has a molecular weight of about 1450 daltons, explaining why, despite a comparable creatinine clearance, its extracorporeal removal is higher with hemofiltration than with hemodialysis [97]. The difference between hemofiltration and hemodialysis is more pronounced with higher dialysate flow rates [5]. Together with the toxicity of vancomycin and the altered pharmacokinetics in critically ill patients, this explains why serial monitoring of serum levels remains essential when vancomycin is administered to patients undergoing CRRT.

Teicoplanin has a high protein binding of 90% explaining the low extracorporeal removal demonstrated by Hillaire-Buys *et al.* [98]. However, the non-renal clearance is limited explaining why extracorporeal removal may become important with more efficacious extracorporeal techniques [99] (Table 4).

MACROLIDES AND CLINDAMYCIN

The major route for the elimination of both clindamycin and the macrolides (erythromycin, clarithromycin, azithromycin) is the liver [44, 100, 101]. In addition, clindamycin, erythromycin and clarithromycin have an important protein binding [44, 100] and hence no dosage adapatation is required during CRRT.

ANTIVIRAL AGENTS

Ganciclovir has a low PB and low non-renal clearance resulting in important extracorporeal elimination with CRRT [102, 103] and requiring dosage adaptation (Table 4). However, because of its toxicity and the occurrence of resistant strains, it would be ideal to control plasma levels. Acyclovir, on the other hand, has an important non-renal clearance reducing the contribution of extracorporeal elimination and avoiding the necessity for dosage adaptation.

ANTIFUNGALS

Most antifungals such as amphotericin B, itraconazole and ketaconazole have a high protein binding and/or an important non-renal clearance and do not require dosage adaptation for extracorporeal removal during CRRT [104–106]. Exceptions are flucytosine and fluconazole. Flucytosine has a very low protein binding and non-renal clearance, resulting in a substantial extracorporeal clearance and Fr_{EC}. The dose during CRRT with creatinine clearance of 25 ml/min should therefore be 20 times higher than the anuric dose. The same accounts for fluconazole where, as mentioned before, clearance values during CRRT may reach values observed in healthy volunteers [52–55] (Table 4).

Conclusions

This chapter describes the basic principles governing extracorporeal drug removal with CRRT. Protein binding and non-renal clearance are the major factors determining whether or not extracorporeal drug elimination with CRRT is clinically significant. Knowledge of these pharmacokinetic parameters and a few simples formulas allows calculation of the required dosage adaptation, as shown in Table 4 for some frequently used antimicrobials. These calculations are less inaccurate for hemodialysis than for hemofiltration, due to the molecular weight- and time-dependency of the diffusion process. Table 4 is inevitably incomplete, but application of the described principles will help the clinician in correctly dosing those drugs that have been omitted or new antimicrobials that will come on the market. The calculated doses should take into account eventual treatment interruptions and the residual renal function. Variations of pharmacokinetic parameters, frequently encountered in critically ill patients, constitute a source of error and hence monitoring of plasma levels remains indispensable for drugs with potential toxicity. Apart from dosage adaptation, pharmacologic management of these patients should include a restriction in the use of drugs, giving preference to those with low toxicity and non-renal elimination, limitation of treatment duration and careful clinical monitoring for effect and toxicity.

References

1. Schetz M. Classical and alternative indications for continuous renal replacement therapy. Kidney Int 53(Suppl 66):S96, 1998.
2. Thijs A, Thijs LG. The pathogenesis of renal failure in sepsis. Kidney Int 53(Suppl 66):S34, 1998.
3. Moise PA, Schentag JJ. Pharmacokinetic and pharmacodynamic modelling of antibiotic therapy. Curr Opin Infect Dis 11:673, 1998.
4. Burgess DS. Pharmacodynamic principles of antimicrobial therapy in the prevention of resistance. Chest 115:S19, 1999.
5. Reetze-Bonorden P, Bohler J, Keller E. Drug dosage in patients during continuous renal replacement therapy: pharmacokinetic and therapeutic considerations. Clin Pharmacokinet 24:362, 1993.
6. Schetz M, Ferdinande P, Van den Berghe G, Verwaest C, Lauwers P. Pharmacokinetics of continuous renal replacement therapy. Intensive Care Med 21:612, 1995.
7. Golper TA, Marx MA. Drug dosing adjustments during continuous renal replacement therapies. Kidney Intern 53, Suppl 66:S165, 1998.
8. Böhler J, Donauer J, Keller F. Pharmacokinetic principles during continuous renal replacement therapy: drugs and dosage. Kidney Intern 56(Suppl 72):S24, 1999.
9. Vozeh S, Schmidlin O, Taeschner W. Pharmacokinetic drug data. Clin Pharmacokinet 14:254, 1988.
10. Bodenham A, Shelly MP, Park GR. The altered pharmacokinetics and pharmacodynamics of drugs commonly used in critically ill patients. Clin Pharmacokinet 14:347, 1988.
11. van Dalen R, Vree TB. Pharmacokinetics of antibiotics in critically ill patients. Intensive Care Med 16(Suppl 3):S235, 1990.

12. Park GR. Pharmacokinetics and pharmacodynamics in the critically ill. Xenobiotica 23:1195, 1993.
13. Fry DE. The importance of antibiotic pharmacokinetics in critical illness. Am J Surg 172:S20, 1996.
14. McKindley DS, Hanes S, Boucher BA. Hepatic drug metabolism in critical illness. Pharmacotherapy 18:759, 1998.
15. Power BM, Forbes AM, van Heerden PV, Ilett KF. Pharmacokinetics of drugs used in critically ill adults. Clin Pharmacokinet 34:25, 1998.
16. Benet LZ, Mitchell JR, Sheiner BS. Pharmacokinetics: the dynamics of drug absorption, distribution and elimination. In Goodman Gilman A, Rall TW, Nies AS, Taylor P (eds). The pharmacological basis of therapeutics. Eight edn, Singapore: McGraw-Hill, 1991:3.
17. Rudy AC, Brater DC. Pharmacokinetics. In Chernow B (ed). The Pharmacologic Approach to the Critically Ill Patient. Third edn, Baltimore: Williams & Wilkins, 1994:3.
18. Triginer C, Izquierdo I, Fernandez R, Rello J, Torrent J, Benito S, Net A. Gentamicin volume of distribution in critically ill septic patients. Intensive Care Med 16:303, 1990.
19. Marik PE. Aminoglycoside volume of distribution and illness severity in critically ill septic patients. Anaesth Intensive Care 21:172, 1993.
20. Debord J, Voultoury JC, Lachatre G, Favereau JP, Gay R. Pharmacokinetics and dosage regimens of amikacin in intensive care unit patients. Int J Biomed Comput 36:135, 1994.
21. Fernandez de Gatta MM, Mendez ME, Romano S, Calvo MV, Dominguez Gil A, Lanao JM. Pharmacokinetics of amikacin in intensive care unit patients. J Clin Pharm Ther 21:417, 1996.
22. Hess MM, Boucher BA, Laizure SC, Stevens RC, Sanders PL, Janning SW, Croce MA, Fabian TC. Trimethoprim-sulfamethoxazole pharmacokinetics in trauma patients. Pharmacotherapy 13:602, 1993.
23. McKindley DS, Boucher BA, Hess MM, Croce MA, Fabian TC. Pharmacokinetics of aztreonam and imipenem in critically ill patients with pneumonia. Pharmacotherapy 16:924, 1996.
24. Cornwell EE, Belzberg H, Berne TV, Gill MA, Theodorou D, Kern JW, Yu W, Asensio J, Demetriades D. Pharmacokinetics of aztreonam in critically ill surgical patients. Am J Health Syst Pharm 54:537, 1997.
25. Gous AG, Dance MD, Lipman J, Luyt DK, Mathivha R, Scribante J. Changes in vancomycin pharmacokinetics in critically ill infants. Anaesth Intensive Care 23:678, 1995.
26. Gomez CM, Cordingly JJ, Palazzo MG. Altered pharmacokinetics of ceftazidime in critically ill patients. Antimicrob Agents Chemother 43:1798, 1999.
27. Golper TA, Vincent HH, Gleason JR, Vos MC. Drug removal during high-efficiency and high-flux hemodialysis. In Bosch JP, Stein JH (eds). Hemodialysis. High-efficiency treatments. New York: Churchill Livingstone. Contemporary Issues in Nephrology 27:175, 1993.
28. Rolan PE. Plasma protein binding displacement interactions – why are they still regarded as clinically important? Br J Clin Pharmacol 37:125, 1994.
29. Gibson TP. Renal disease and drug metabolism: an overview. Am J Kidney Dis 8:7, 1986.
30. Elston AC, Bayliss MK, Park GR. Effect of renal failure on drug metabolism by the liver. Br J Anaesth 71:282, 1993.
31. Lee CS, Marbury TC, Benet LZ. Clearance calculations in hemodialysis: application to blood, plasma and dialysate measurements for ethambutol. J Pharmacokinet Biopharmx 8:69, 1993.
32. Rumpf KW, Rieger J, Ansorg R, Doht B, Scheler F. Binding of antibiotics by dialysis membranes and its clinical relevance. Proc Eur Dial Transpl 14:607, 1978.
33. Kraft D, Lode H. Elimination of ampicillin and gentamicin by hemofiltration. Klin Wochenschr 57:195, 1979.
34. Kronfol NO, Lau AH, Barakat MM. Aminoglycoside binding to polyacrylonitrile hemofilter membranes during continuous hemofiltration. ASAIO Trans 33:300, 1987.
35. Cigarran-Guldris S, Brier ME, Golper TA. Tobramycin clearance during simulated continuous arteriovenous hemodialysis. Contrib Nephrol 93:120, 1991.
36. Colton CK, Henderson LW, Ford CA, Lysaght MJ. Kinetics of hemodiafiltration. I. *In vitro* transport characteristics of a hollow-fiber blood ultrafilter. J Lab Clin Invest 85:355, 1975.
37. Colton CK. Analysis of membrane processes for blood purification. Blood Purif 5:202, 1987.
38. Ofsthun NJ, Colton CK, Lysaght MJ. Determinants of fluid and solute removal during hemofiltration. In Henderson LW, Quellhorst EA, Baldamus CA, Lysaght MJ (eds). Hemofiltration. Berlin: Springer-Verlag, 1986:17.
39. Klinkmann H, Vienken J. Membranes for dialysis. Nephrol Dial Transplant 10(Suppl 3):39, 1995.

40. Phillips GJ, Davies JG, Olliff CJ, Kingswood C, Street M. Use of *in vitro* models of haemofiltration and haemodiafiltration to estimate dosage regimens for critically ill patients prescribed cefpirome. J Clin Pharm Therap 23:353, 1998.
41. Schroeder TH, Krueger WA, Hansen M, Hoffmann E, Dieterich HJ, Unertl K. Elimination of meropenem by continuous hemo(dia) filtration: an *in vitro* one-compartment model. Int J Artif Organs 22:307, 1999.
42. Sigler MH, Teehan BO, Van Valckenburgh D. Solute transport in continuous hemodialysis: a new treatment for acute renal failure. Kidney Intern 32:562, 1987.
43. Lam YWF, Banerji S, Hatfield C, Talbert RL. Principles of drug administration in renal insufficiency. Clin Pharmacokinet 32:30, 1997.
44. Benet LZ, Williams RL. Design and optimization of dosage regimens: pharmacokinetic data. In Goodman Gilman A, Rall TW, Nies AS, Taylor P (eds). The pharmacological basis of therapeutics. Eight edn, Singapore: McGraw-Hill, 1991:1650.
45. Bellomo R, Baldwin I, Cole L, Ronco C. Preliminary experience with high-volume hemofiltration in human septic shock. Kidney Int 53(Suppl 66):S182, 1998.
46. Fillastre JP, Singlas E. Pharmacokinetics of newer drugs in patients with renal impairment. Clin Pharmacokinet 20:293, 1991.
47. St Peter WL, Redic-Kill KA, Halstenson CE. Clinical pharmacokinetics of antibiotics in patients with impaired renal function. Clin Pharmacokinet 22:169, 1992.
48. Keller F, Giehl M, Frankewitsch T, Zellner D. Pharmacokinetics and drug dosage adjustment to renal impairment. Nephrol Dial Transplant 10:1516, 1995.
49. Shuler C, Golper TA, Bennett WM. Prescribing drugs in renal disease. In Brenner BM (ed). The Kidney. Fifth edn, Philadephia: Saunders, 1996:2653.
50. Aronoff GR, Berns KS, Brier ME, Golper TA, Morrison G, Singer I, Swan S, Bennett WM. Drug prescribing in renal failure. Dosing guidelines for adults. Fourth edn, American College of Physicians, Philadelphia, 1999.
51. Keller F, Böhler J, Czock D, Zellner D, Mertz AKH. Individualized drug dosage in patients treated with continuous hemofiltration. Kidney Intern 56(Suppl 72):S29, 1999.
52. Nicolau DP, Crowe H, Nightingale CH, Quintiliani RQ. Effect of continuous arteriovenous hemodiafiltration on the pharmcokinetics of fluconazole. Pharmacotherapy 14:502, 1994.
53. Scholz J, Schulz M, Steinfath M, Hover S, Bause H. Fluconazole is removed by continuous venovenous hemofiltration in a liver transplant patient. J Mol Med 73:145, 1995.
54. Valtonen M, Tiula E, Neuvonen PJ. Effect of continuous venovenous haemofiltration and haemodiafiltration on the elimination of fluconazole in patients with acute renal failure. J Antimicrob Chemother 40:695, 1997.
55. Pittrow L, Penk A. Pharmacokinetics and dosage of fluconazole in continuous haemofiltration (CAVH, CVVH) and haemodialysis (CAVHD, CVVHD). Mycoses 41(Suppl 2):86, 1998.
56. Moore RD, Lietman PS, Smith CR. Clinical response to aminoglycoside therapy: importance of the ratio of peak concentration to minimal inhibitory concentration. J Infect Dis 155:93, 1987.
57. Ebert SC, Craig WA. Pharmacodynamic properties of antibiotics: application to drug monitoring and dosage regimen design. Infect Control Hosp Epidemiol 11:319, 1990.
58. Barza M, Ioannidis JP, Cappelleri JC, Lau J. Single or multiple daily doses of aminoglycosides: a meta-analysis. BMJ 312:338, 1996.
59. Ferriols-Lisart R, Alos-Alminana M. Effectiveness and safety of once-daily aminoglycosides: a meta-analysis. Am J Health Syst Pharm 53:1141, 1996.
60. Hatala R, Dinh TT, Cook DJ. Single daily dosing of aminoglycosides in immunocompromised adults: a systematic review. Clin Infect Dis 24:810, 1997.
61. Zarowitz BJ, Anandan JV, Dumler F, Jayashankar J, Levin NL. Continuous arteriovenous hemofiltration of aminoglycosides in critically ill patients. Clin Pharmacol 26:686, 1986.
62. Armendariz E, Chelluri L, Ptachcinski R. Pharmacokinetics of amikacin during continuous veno-venous hemofiltration. Crit Care Med 18:675, 1990.
63. Davies SP, Kox WJ, Brown EA. Clearance studies in patients with acute renal failure treated by continuous arteriovenous haemodialysis. Contrib Nephrol 93:117, 1991.
64. Robert R, Rochard E, Malin F, Bouquet S. Amikacin pharmacokinetics during continuous veno-venous hemofiltration Crit Care Med 19:588, 1991.

65. Ernest D, Cutler DJ. Gentamicin clearance during continuous arteriovenous hemodiafiltration. Crit Care Med 20:586, 1992.
66. Kihara M, Ikeda Y, Takagi N, Fujita H, Shibata K, Masumori S, Shiratori K, Umemura S, Shionoiri H, Ishii M. Pharmacokinetics of single-dose intravenous amikacin in critically ill patients undergoing slow hemodialysis. Intensive Care Med 21:348, 1995.
67. Forrest A, Nix DE, Goss TF, Birmingham MC, Schentag JJ. Pharmacodynamics of intravenous ciprofloxacin in seriously ill patients. Antimicrob Agents Chemother 37:1073, 1993.
68. Journois D, Chamu D, Drevillon C, Dru M, Ballereau M, Safran D. Pefloxacin and metabolites removal in continuous hemofiltration with dialysis. Contrib Nephrol 93:124, 1991.
69. Davies SP, Azadian BS, Kox WJ, Brown EA. Pharmacokinetics of ciprofloxacin and vancomycin in patients with acute renal failure treated by continuous haemodialysis. Nephrol Dial Transplant 7:848, 1992.
70. Fish DN, Bainbridge JL, Peloquin CA. Variable disposition of ciprofloxacin in critically ill patients undergoing continuous arteriovenous hemodiafiltration. Pharmacotherapy 15:236, 1995.
71. Capellier G, Cornette C, Boillot A, Guinchard C, Jacques T, Blasco G, Barale F. Removal of piperacillin in critically ill patients undergoing continuous venovenous hemofiltration. Crit Care Med 26:88, 1998.
72. de Clari F. Ceftriaxone pharmacokinetics during continuous arteriovenous haemofiltration [letter]. J Antimicrob Chemother 27:394, 1991.
73. Keller E, Bohler J, Busse Grawitz A, Reetze Bonorden P, Krumme B, Schollmeyer P. Single dose kinetics of piperacillin during continuous arteriovenous hemodialysis in intensive care patients. Clin Nephrol 43(Suppl 1):S20, 1995.
74. Rohde B, Werner U, Hickstein H, Ehmcke H, Drewelow B. Pharmacokinetics of mezlocillin and sulbactam under continuous veno-venous hemodialysis (CVVHD) in intensive care patients with acute renal failure. Eur J Clin Pharmacol 53:111, 1990.
75. Weiss LG, Cars O, Danielson BG, Grahner A, Wikström B. Pharmacokinetics of intravenous cefuroxime during intermittent and continuous arteriovenous hemofiltration. Clin Nephrol 30:282, 1988.
76. Davies SP, Lacey LF, Kox WJ, Brown EA. Pharmacokinetics of cefuroxime and ceftazidime in patients with acute renal failure treated by continuous arteriovenous haemodialysis. Nephrol Dial Transplant 6:971, 1991.
77. Allaouchiche B, Breilh D, Jaumain H, Gaillard B, Renard S, Saux MC. Pharmacokinetics of cefepime during continuous venovenous hemodiafiltration. Antimicrob Agents Chemother 41:2424, 1997.
78. Lau AH, Pyle K, Kronfol NO, Libertin CR. Removal of cephalosporins by continuous arteriovenous ultrafiltration (CAVU) and hemofiltration (CAVH). Int J Artif Organs 12:379, 1989.
79. Kroh UF, Lennartz H. Evaluation and first validation study on a simplified drug dosage algorithm for multiple organ failure patients. Ren Fail 14:579, 1992.
80. Kroh UF, Lennartz H, Edwards DJ, Stoeckel K. Pharmacokinetics of ceftriaxone in patients undergoing continuous veno-venous hemofiltration. J Clin Pharmacol 36:1114, 1996.
81. van der Werf TS, Mulder PO, Zijlstra JG, Uges DR, Stegeman CA. Pharmacokinetics of piperacillin and tazobactam in critically ill patients with renal failure, treated with continuous veno-venous hemofiltration (CVVH). Intensive Care Med 23:873, 1997.
82. Mueller BA, Scarim SK, Macias WL. Comparison of imipenem pharmacokinetics in patients with acute or chronic renal failure treated with continuous hemofiltration. Am J Kidney Dis 21:172, 1993.
83. Keller E, Fecht H, Böhler J, Schollmeyer P. Single-dose kinetics of imipenem/cilastatin during continuous arteriovenous haemofiltration in intensive care patients. Nephrol Dial Transplant 4:640, 1989.
84. Vos MC, Vincent HH, Yzerman EP. Clearance of imipenem/cilastatin in acute renal failure patients treated by continuous hemodiafiltration (CAVHD). Intensive Care Med 18:282, 1992.
85. Tegeder I, Bremer F, Oelkers R, Schobel H, Schuttler J, Brune K, Geisslinger G. Pharmacokinetics of imipenem-cilastatin in critically ill patients undergoing continuous venovenous hemofiltration. Antimicrob Agents Chemother 41:2640, 1997.
86. Drusano GL, Standiford HC. Pharmacokinetic profile of imipenem/cilastatin in normal volunteers Am J Med 78(Suppl 6a):47, 1985.
87. Przechera M, Bengel D, Risler T. Pharmacokinetics of imipenem/cilastatin during con-

tinuous arteriovenous hemofiltration. Contrib Nephrol 93:131, 1991.

88. Kihara M, Ikeda Y, Shibata K, Masumori S, Ebira H, Shiratori K, Ueda S, Takagi N, Umemura S, Shionoiri H, Ishii M. Pharmacokinetic profiles of intravenous imipenem/cilastatin during slow hemodialysis in critically ill patients. Clin Nephrol 42:193, 1994.
89. Krueger WA, Schroeder TH, Hutchison M, Hoffmann E, Dieterich HJ, Heiniger A, Erley C, Wehrle A, Unertl K. Pharmacokinetics of meropenem in critically ill patients with acute renal failure treated by continuous hemodiafiltration. Antimicrob Agents Chemother 42:2421, 1998.
90. Thalhammer F, Schenk P, Burgmann H, El Menyawi I, Hollenstein UM, Rosenkranz AR, Sunder-Plasmann G, Breyer S, Ratheiser K. Single-dose pharmacokinetics of meropenem during continuous venovenous hemofiltration. Antimicrob Agents Chemother 42:2417, 1998.
91. Tegeder I, Neumann F, Bremer F, Brune K, Lotsch J, Geisslinger G. Pharmacokinetics of meropenem in critically ill patients with acute renal failure undergoing continuous venovenous hemofiltration. Clin Pharmacol Therap 65:50, 1999.
92. Macias WL, Mueller BA, Scarim SK. Vancomycin pharmacokinetics in acute renal failure: preservation of nonrenal clearance. Clin Pharmacol Ther 50:688, 1991.
93. Reetze-Bonorden P, Böhler J, Kohler C, Schollmeyer P, Keller E. Elimination of vancomycin in patients on continuous arteriovenous hemodialysis. Contrib Nephrol 93:135, 1991.
94. Santre C, Leroy O, Simon M, Georges H, Guery B, Beuscart C, Beaucaire G. Pharmacokinetics of vancomycin during continuous hemodiafiltration. Intensive Care Med 19:347, 1993.
95. Bellomo R, Ernest D, Parkin G, Boyce N. Clearance of vancomycin during continuous arteriovenous hemodiafiltration. Crit Care Med 18:181, 1990.
96. Joy MS, Matzke GR, Frye RF, Palevsky PM. Determinants of vancomycin clearance by continuous venovenous hemofiltration and continuous venovenous hemodialysis. Am J Kidney Dis 31:1019, 1998.
97. Jeffrey RF, Khan AA, Prabhu P, Todd N, Goutcher E, Will EJ, Davison AM. A comparison of molecular clearance rates during continuous hemofiltration and hemodialysis with a novel volumetric continuous renal replacement system. Artif Organs 18:425, 1994.
98. Hillaire-Buys D, Peyriere H, Lobjoie E, Bres J, Ossart M, Despaux E. Influence of arteriovenous haemofiltration on teicoplanin elimination. Br J Clin Pharmacol 40:95, 1995.
99. Wolter K, Claus M, Wagner K, Fritschka E. Teicoplanin pharmacokinetics and dosage recommendations in chronic hemodialysis and in patients undergoing continuous veno-venous hemodialysis. Clin Nephrol 42:389, 1994.
100. Davey PG. The pharmacokinetics of clarithromycin and its 14-OH metabolite. J Hosp Infect 19(Suppl A):29, 1991.
101. Hoffler D, Koeppe P, Paeske B. Pharmacokinetics of azithromycin in normal and impaired renal function. Infection 23:356, 1995.
102. Bastein O, Boulieu R, Bleyzac N, Estanove S. Clinical use of ganciclovir during renal failure and continuous hemodialysis. Intensive Care Med 20:47, 1994.
103. Gando S, Kameue T, Nanzaki S, Hayakawa T, Nakanishi Y. Pharmacokinetics and clearance of ganciclovir during continuous hemodiafiltration. Crit Care Med 26:184, 1998.
104. Coronel B, Persat F, Dorez D, Moskovitchenko JF, Peins MA, Mercatello A. Itraconazole concentrations during continuous haemodiafiltration. J Antimicrob Chemother 34:448, 1994.
105. Humphreys H, Oliver DA, Winter R, Warnock DW. Liposomal amphotericin B and continuous venous-venous haemofiltration [letter]. J Antimicrob Chemother 33:1070, 1994.
106. Tomlin M, Priestley GS. Elimination of liposomal amphotericin by hemodiafiltration [letter]. Intensive Care Med 21:699, 1995.
107. Van der Auwera P, Santella PJ. Pharmacokinetics of cefepime: a review. J Antimicrob Chemother 32(Suppl B):103, 1993.

SECTION 3: INFECTION CONTROL/EPIDEMIOLOGY

J. Rello

17. FUNDAMENTALS OF INFECTION CONTROL AND SURVEILLANCE STRATEGIES FOR THE ICU

Charles E. Edmiston, Jr

Introduction

The mission of a hospital infection control program is to ensure continuous improvement in the delivery of patient care. This is done through a structured surveillance, which reviews, analyzes, and reports nosocomial infection rates. It is the overall intent of the program to identify and reduce the risk of acquiring and transmitting infections among patients, staff, physicians, other health care professionals and visitors to the institution. There are in essence three specific goals of a hospital infection control program. The first goal involves the protection of the patient, which is accomplished through ensuring that a low risk exists for the acquisition of a nosocomial infection. This has become a daunting exercise in the presence of a high-risk patient population coupled with an environment that fosters the development of widespread antibiotic resistance. However, there is substantial published data demonstrating that an effective infection control program results in a reduced infection rate, increased case-specific patient survival, fewer complications and a reduction in hospitalized days [1]. Within the ICU environment there are numerous examples of opportunities where infection control interventional practices may occur. For instance, ICU patients are at high risk of acquiring a nosocomial urinary tract infection (NUTI), ventilator-associated pneumonia (VAP), or catheter-related-blood stream infection (CR-BSI). Infection control activities that focus upon reducing the risk of these infections reduce morbidity and improve patient outcomes.

The second goal of an infection control program is to prevent the spread of infection from patients to health care workers and other individuals within the hospital environment. Many of the strategies that are used to accomplish this goal require an expertise that is above and beyond those needed for routine surveillance. By tradition, institutional-based infection control programs have a broad scope of practice that encompass a broad interdisciplinary framework (Table 1).

The infection control practitioner must be able to communicate effectively with a wide range of health care professions. Often this involves documenting the need for patient isolation or identifying the reasons for the use of personal protective equipment. In addition, the infection control department must work in close cooperation with employee health services when infectious exposures become an issue. Finally, employee education from top to bottom is an important function of each infection control team member and knowledge of effective teaching strategies is extremely helpful in carrying out this task.

Finally, in today's manage care environment, infection control teams represent a significant financial investment to the institution. The

TABLE 1. Interdisciplinary responsibilities of the infection control team within the hospital environment

The Scope of Practice of the Infection Control Program
• Data analysis – epidemiology and statistics
• Microbiology – clinical laboratory
• Infectious disease – surveillance
• Occupational health – policies
• Central supply – disinfection, sterilization and processing
• Administration – management and communication
• Patient care – policies and procedures
• Staff development – inservices

financial commitment associated with developing a highly trained and professional group of infection control practitioners is offset by the ability of that team to reduce the risk of nosocomial infections within the health care setting. Approximately two million nosocomial infections occur each year in the United States. These infections are responsible for significant morbidity, mortality and cost. The estimated increased length of stay (LOS) associated with a nosocomial pneumonia is between 6 to 30 days, while the LOS associated with a CR-BSI is from 7 to 21 days. This translates into a significant monetary burden to the institution, since the cost of managing a nosocomial pneumonia is in the range of $4500 to $5000 and treating a CR-BSI may cost as much as $50,000. This does not even begin to address the associated mortality, which is between 23% to 50% for CR-BSI and pneumonia [2, 3]. Therefore, an effectively managed infection control program can have a positive socioeconomic impact within the institution. This is especially true in the critical care environment where the myriad of patient risk factors can contribute to high morbidity with associated adverse clinical outcomes.

Measuring the Impact

Recently, new, innovative technologies have emerged, which claim to reduce the risk of infection within the critical care arena. It goes without saying that most of these technologies are more expensive than standard devices or practices. However, while cost may always be a sentinel factor in the current health care environment, it is important to determine what, if any benefits may be derived by these new technologies and will they have a measurable impact on reducing nosocomial infection rates within selected units or patient populations. An example of this process involves the use of antiseptic or antibiotic bonded catheters for central venous access. As discussed earlier nosocomial bloodstream infections, especially in the critically ill associated with increased length of stay (LOS), higher risk of mortality and increased hospital costs. The attributed mortality associated with central lines has been reported to be 25%, with an additional LOS of 6.5 days in the SICU and an average cost of $28,690 per survivor [4]. A hypothetical comparison is shown in Table 2 investigating the infection control and cost effectiveness of two antiseptic/antibiotic bonded catheters versus a conventional central venous catheter (CVC).

It would appear that catheter B is superior in preventing catheter related-blood stream infections compared to a convention CVC. However, it should be noted that true efficacy is only apparent when sufficient statistical power is present in the study design. It is unlikely that a catheter study with less than 300 devices divided between three arms will provide that level of confidence. However, from a simple cusorary examination, use of catheter A reduced the actual number of CR-BSI by a factor of 2.5, while catheter B reduced the number of actual CR-BSI by a factor of 8.3. If the actual cost of treating a CR-BSI in the SICU is $28,690, then approximately $114, 760 or $172,140 savings could be realized by adopting catheters A or B. It is likely that these types of comparisons will occur with greater frequently as newer innovative technologies impinge upon the critical care environment. The infection control team can and should play a central role in the development of protocols and guidelines for the evaluation of devices

TABLE 2. Comparison of colonization and catheter related-blood stream (CR-BSI) infections between conventional CVC and antiseptic/antibiotic coated catheters (A and B) in the SICU

Device (CVC)	N	Colonization	CR-BSI Rate	Cost ($)
Conventional device[a]	94	32%	8%	25
Coated Catheter A	101	23%	3%	45
Coated Catheter B	90	8%	1%	75

[a] Silastic Hickman catheter.

or technologies that as suggested reduce the nosocomial infection rate. In addition, we should recognize that the maximal benefit derived from the adoption of such innovative technology into our clinical practice is dependent entirely upon which patient populations are studies. In the case of antibiotic/antiseptic coated/bonded catheters, one approach that may be deemed most cost effective is to restrict the use of such devices to patients who are within the highest risk category for CR-BSI, ICU and immunosuppressed patients [5, 6].

Responsibilities of the Infection Control Team Professionals

An effective infection control program represents an interdisciplinary endeavor (Table 1) encompassing the fields of epidemiology, medicine, microbiology, pathology, nursing, and administration [7, 8]. All infection control personnel need to have knowledge and experience in the following areas. The amount of time that the infection control team spends in routine infection surveillance, prevention and control activities relates to:

- Needs of the patient population
- Risk factors of the patient population
- Complexity of the service or unit
- Adherence requirement of federal, state and local laws and regulations governing the infection control program
- Educational needs of the staff

The team is required to collect, review and analyze surveillance data and to identify current trends of nosocomial infections. In addition, the infection control program should be viewed as an agent of change through the active participation of team members on appropriate institutional committees. This participation should result in:

- Development, review and revision of isolation guidelines as per accepted standard practice and to enforce all policies and procedures relating to isolation guidelines
- Active collaboration and consultation with all disciplines and departments to promote infection control principles into effective policies and procedures
- The development of mechanisms for evaluating the impact of new technologies and procedures as they relate to infection control (see pages 245–252)
- The ability to utilize hospital administration as a resource for implementing infection control polices and procedures

The infection control personnel must be knowledgeable of the published literature on the epidemiology and pathogenesis of nosocomial infections, incorporating this informational base into their current practice.

Infection Control Surveillance Criteria

The purpose of infection control surveillance whether global or unit specific is to develop and maintain a database of the institutional nosocomial experience. Pragmatically, surveillance attempts to define the endemic rate of infectious events within the institution. This is a dynamic process, which is in a constant state of flux; in part due to changes in patient care services, which may be impacted by new technology or changes in personnel. Surveillance will also monitors changes that occur above the endemic level. Often these changes are compared to some benchmark such as the nosocomial infection rates developed by the National Nosocomial Infection Surveillance (NNIS) program administered by the Centers for Disease Control and Prevention (CDC) in Atlanta [9]. A significant component of the infection control surveillance program is the feedback or dialogue, which occurs between the infection control staff and the health care provider. This is generally acknowledged as the interventional component, whereas the infection control personnel reviews with the clinical staff, risks factors associated with care of the patient, while suggesting appropriate strategies that attempt to reduce the overall risk of infection. The measure of a successful and effective surveillance program is whether or not implementation of focused prevention and control policies result in decreasing future nosocomial risks.

Surveillance Strategies in the Nosocomial Environment

Numerous surveillance techniques have been proposed for monitoring the rates of infection within a hospital and critical care environments.

- Hospital-wide or global surveillance
- Targeted or focused surveillance
- Periodic or intermittent surveillance
- Prevalence surveillance

Adoption of one or more of these techniques is dependent upon the goals and priorities of the institution. In addition, the type of surveillance performed will also be dependent upon the level of institutional resources including both monetary and personnel. The advantages and disadvantages of the three surveillance strategies are listed below:

A. Hospital-wide surveillance
Advantages
- Provide infection data from all sites within the institution
- Establishes baseline data and identifies outbreaks early
- Clearly identifies patterns

Disadvantages
- Expensive, time consuming and labor intensive
- Generates large amount of data often with little clinical significance
- Reduces staff time for other important activities

B. Targeted surveillance
Advantages
- Highly flexible and mobile
- Can focus on patients with highest risk
- May include all hospital sites if surveillance is rotated
- Less labor intensive than hospital-wide surveillance

Disadvantages
- Less opportunity for defining hospital-wide baseline rates
- May miss initial outbreaks or clusters outside surveillance areas

C. Periodic surveillance
Advantages
- Flexible for staff, increasing opportunities for other activities
- Allows staff to define long-term goals and objectives

Disadvantages
- Possibility that infection clusters may be missed
- Little or no consistent baseline data

D. Prevalence
Advantages
- Documents trends in nosocomial infections
- Used to identify risk factors
- Rapid and with relative low cost
- Data may be used to target future areas of surveillance

Disadvantages
- Unable to compare prevalence rates with incidence rates

- Outbreaks or clusters may be missed
- Provides information for a limited time interval

Few institutions have the available resources to provide complete hospital-wide or global surveillance. Therefore, targeted or focused surveillance has become common-place in our health care institutions. At our institution we use a combination of site-specific and unit-specific surveillance to monitor nosocomial infection rates. Site-specific monitoring focuses on specific sites of infections such as respiratory tract, urinary tract, bloodstream or surgical site infections. In-hospital as well as post-discharge surveillance of surgical site infections is monitored in this manner. Unit-specific surveillance is designated for high-risk patient areas such as the ICUs and other units including the hematology-oncology services or the bone marrow transplant service. Studies have demonstrated that high-risk patient populations have the highest nosocomial infection rates often with significant morbidity and mortality. Therefore, it would be perceived as prudent to focusing surveillance efforts on this high-risk patient population. Periodic surveillance is less time consuming than either hospital-wide or targeted, however failure to miss sentinel clusters is a common fault of this surveillance strategy. Often this surveillance strategy may be combined with targeted so that the opportunity for missing a cluster is greatly reduced. Finally, prevalence surveillance is used to define the number of active infections within a specific time period. In this method of surveillance all new and existing infections are tabulated which results in a rate (prevalence) that is higher than the true incidence rate. However, this strategy may be useful for studying specific risk factors, device-associated infections or the prevalence of selected antibiotic resistant pathogens within a defined patient population [7].

Frequently, several different strategies may be used within a single institution depending upon its particular goals or needs. In the end, however, the limiting factor most often is time and personnel commitments to other endeavors of the infection control program.

Data Collection, Analysis and Reporting

The process of data collection must be epidemiologically sound and driven by definable events such as CR-BSI or other device-related infections. The actual data source documents are numerous and highly variable within a given institution (Table 3).

It is interesting to note that total chart review, Kardex screens and review of cultural results is associated with the highest level of sensitivity for detecting nosocomial infections [10, 11]. With the present widespread (inappropriate) use of antibiotics, it should come as no surprise that review of antibiotic use patterns is associated with documented infection less than 60% of the time. This is also true for fever, which as a single

TABLE 3. Source documents for identifying nosocomial infections during infection control surveillance

	Source Documentation	
Patient	Laboratory	Administration
Physical examination	Microbiology	Admissions
Medical record	Serology	Risk assessment
Nursing Kardex	Pathology	Outpatient clinics
Clinical rounds	Antibiogram data	Employee health
Medication record		
Radiology report		
Operative report		

sentinel indicator of infection is relatively poor. In the case of surgical wound surveillance direct observation of the wound by a trained practitioner is the most accurate means of detecting a surgical site infection. Reliance upon a single source document to detect a nosocomial infection may often lead to underestimating the true incidence of infection. No single surveillance strategy will detect 100% of nosocomial infection, however, in the case of ICU surveillance a focus review of positive blood cultures would likely detect most catheter-related blood stream infections. The development of an effective surveillance program requires experience and knowledgeable infection control practitioners who recognize that in the case of surgical wound infections, direct observation is preferable to reviewing culture reports. Therefore, the most effective strategy for detecting nosocomial infections will usually involve sifting through a combination of sources within the health care institution.

Comparison of Institutional Rates to National Benchmarks

In 1970, the National Nosocomial Infection Surveillance (NNIS) system was established and presently almost 300 hospitals contribute surveillance data for aggregation into a national database [9]. Data is collected using standardized protocols and encompasses Centers of Disease and Prevention (CDC) definitions that include both laboratory and clinical-based criteria. For over 20 years the NNIS program included hospital-wide surveillance but has recently eliminated that component from its program. The future focus will be on high-risk patient populations that include adult and pediatric ICU, high-risk nursery (HRN) and surgical site infections (SSIs). Data is collected from all sites of infection in the ICUs and HRN with an emphasis on device-related infections. A fourth component of the NNIS surveillance program is the reporting of the most common pathogens associated with bloodstream, pneumonia, and urinary tract infection in the ICU. A subset of 41 hospitals from the NNIS system participate in a parallel program, called the Intensive Care Antimicrobial Resistance Epidemiology (ICARE) Project which assesses antimicrobial usage and emerging patterns of resistance within the ICU environment. This program evaluates the use of selected antimicrobial within the ICU setting by ranking usage based upon the defined daily dose [12].

Strategies for the Prevention and Surveillance of Nosocomial Infections in the ICU

CATHETER RELATED-BLOOD STREAM INFECTIONS (BSI)

Table 4 identifies the eight most common microbial pathogens isolated from bloodstream infections in the medical ICU (MICU), surgical ICU (SICU), trauma and burn units [9].

The coagulase-negative staphylococci are the most common pathogens isolated from ICU bloodstream infections. This finding is consistent with previous studies that have found the coagulase-negative staphylococci to be the most common pathogen in device-associated infections. The enterococci have vaulted from an insignificant pathogen less than 20 years ago to the second most common pathogen associated with at-risk ICU patients. *Staphylococcus aureus* is now the third most common bloodstream pathogen reported in the ICU, followed by *Candida albicans*, an organism that less than 15 years ago rarely was associated with infection in the critical care environment. Three members of the Enterobacteriaceae, *Enterobacter* spp., *Klebsiella pneumoniae*, and *E. coli* round out the top eight positions.

Table 5 reports the central line-associated BSI rate for selected ICUs as tabulated by the NNIS system [9]. The rate of catheter-related bloodstream infection ranges from a low of 4.1 per 1000 catheter days in non-academic medical/surgical ICUs to over 12 in burn units.

TABLE 4. Eight most common pathogens isolated from bloodstream infections in medical, surgical, trauma, and burn ICUs, January 1992–May 1999 (NNIS)

	ICU (Percentage)			
Pathogen	Medical	Surgical	Trauma	Burn
CNS[a]	35.7	36.1	31.1	13.9
Staphylococcus aureus	14.0	10.4	12.1	17.6
Enterococus spp	16.5	15.3	11.9	15.5
Candida albicans	6.3	4.5	3.0	4.4
Enterobacter spp	3.1	5.8	10.4	11.2
Ps. aeruginosa	3.6	4.1	4.3	9.5
K. pneumoniae	3.9	4.0	3.4	3.3
E. coli	2.1	2.2	2.9	3.3

[a] CNS, coagulase-negative staphylococci.

TABLE 5. Central line-associated BSI rate for medical, combined medical/surgical, surgical, trauma, and burn ICUs, January 1992–May 1999 (NNIS)

Type of ICU	Number of Units	Central Line-Associated BSI Rate[a]
Medical	124	6.1
Medical/Surgical		
Teaching	72	6.0
Nonteaching	138	4.1
Surgical	146	5.6
Trauma	21	7.3
Burn	17	12.2

[a] [Number of central line-associated BSI/Number of central line days] ×1000.

The variation in these rates is in part a reflection of the intrinsic risk factors that are present in this patient population. However, failure to adhere to basic principles of maximal barrier precautions at the time of line insertion and poor catheter management is also in part responsible for some CR-BSI seen in the ICU. While the pathogenesis of CR-BSI has been characterized as multifactorial, the two major mechanisms responsible for line infection involves migration of microorganisms at the site of insertion into the cutaneous tract resulting in extraluminal colonization and contamination of catheter hub which causes intraluminal colonization [5, 14].

Surveillance and treatment strategies for catheter-related infection is dependent upon the clinical presentation. A localized infection involving a port or tunnel infection requires catheter removal. While infection localized to the exit site can usually be managed with local measures such as warm moist compresses, increasing the frequency of site care and in some cases oral antibiotics. The general treatment strategies for catheter-related infections can be characterized as follows [5]:

Exit Site Infections

Present with symptoms of erythema, tenderness or purulence within 2 cm of site. Treatment is local with warm compresses, daily site care and oral antibiotics.

Tunnel Infections

Characterized by erythema, tenderness or purulence >2 cm from the site. This will require catheter removal.

Pocket (Implantable Port) Infections

Will present with erythema and necrosis over the port reservoir or purulent exudate in subcutaneous pocket. This requires port removal and antibiotic therapy.

CR-BSI
Requires semiquantitative/quantitative culture with 5– to 10–fold difference between central and peripheral cultures, with no other sign of infection elsewhere and associated with defervescence upon catheter removal. CNS – can be managed with *in situ* treatment (antibiotic lock) and systemic antibiotic. Infection due to yeast, *S. aureus* or polymicrobial recurrent infection – requires catheter removal.

Treatment of a CR-BSI is more complex than management of a localized infectious process. The fundamental question with CR-BSI is: does the line have to be removed? In situations where long-term access is required, successful treatment without removal has been reported in the literature. Removal of an infected catheter is warranted when there is a documented fungal infection, persistent bacteremia following antibiotic therapy, polymicrobial infection or infection with a highly virulent pathogen such as *Staphylococcus aureus* [5, 13–16]. Staphylococcal infections involving *Staphylococcus epidermidis* can often be managed with an antibiotic lock, that utilizes a high intraluminal dose of antibiotic, which remains within the lumen of the catheter for period of up to several hours [17, 18].

The cornerstone of preventing CR-BSI is grounded in the basic principles of infection control: judicious handwashing and aseptic technique. Rigorous attention to aseptic principles such as maximal barrier precautions upon insertion and dedicated personnel to provide line care has repeatedly been shown to result in decreased infection. While newer technological developments in the area of wound care and the use of antiseptic/antibiotic impregnated devices has been suggested to reduce the risk of CR-BSI, there is no substitution for meticulous catheter care [5]. Details on specilia techniques of presention will be found elsewhere (pages 587–596).

To minimize the risk of contamination, all line insertions must be performed under rigorous maximal barrier precautions. This includes using sterile drapes (large), gowns, masks and gloves. Several prospective studies have demonstrated that a significant reduction in catheter colonization and bacteremia can be achieved using a rigorous aseptic protocol. While several surface antiseptics have been used to reduce skin contamination at the insertion site, a 3 to 5 minute cleansing with chlorhexidine has been shown to be superior to elemental iodine or an iodophor [5, 13]. Chlorhexidine is presently not available in a commercial preparation for use at the catheter exit site, however, it is likely to be available for this purpose in the near future. The 2% aqueous preparation has been shown to be superior to either alcohol or povidone iodine in preventing catheter-related infections. Two points are worth considering, first chlorhexidine exhibits an excellent residual activity compared to other compounds and this agent is not neutralized by blood, serum or blood proteins.

Historically, routine guideline wire exchanges were proposed as a means to reduce CR-BSI. However, present recommendations do not support this practice since intraluminal colonization of the previous line may serve as a source of contamination for the new line via guidewire insertion [13]. In general, central lines should only be removed when clinical expedient, while peripheral lines may be replaced at a 72 hour interval [5]. Routine skin asepsis and appropriate site care have been shown to be efficacious in limiting microbial growth and colonization of the catheter. At present, either gauze or transparent dressings appear to be equally effective when used appropriately [19]. It has been shown that creating a subcutaneous tract and tunneling the catheter is associated with a significant decrease in catheter-related infections [5, 13]. However, it should be pointed out that use of a dedicated IV team for care and maintenance of lines has been shown to reduce infection rates in intravascular devices [20, 21].

The consensus is now clear that the hub is an important portal for intraluminal colonization of the catheter (see pages 573–586). Catheter hub care mandates the use of aseptic technique during tubing changes and other manipulations. The hub should be cleansed with an antiseptic agent such as 70% isopropyl alcohol or 10% povidine-iodine solution before accessing the system [5]. Mechanical cleansing action alone has been found to be effective in removing most pathogens. Needless systems have been introduced to reduce the risk of sharps injuries to health care workers. Because of a concern of infection with some of needless devices it has been recommended that additional education efforts are required that focuse upon the effective maintenance of these new, innovative and at times complex devices (22, 23).

Identification of the type of catheter-related infection in a standardized manner is one key to improving patient outcomes. An understanding of the etiology and pathogenesis is also important as a basis for developing prevention and treatment guidelines. Over the past 20 years it has become evident that both the exit site and the hub can be implicated in the etiology of CR-BSI. In addition, while many innovative technologies are currently available for the prevention of infection, there is no substitution for aseptic technique and meticulous adherence to catheter care protocols.

Nosocomial Pneumonia

Table 6 identifies the eight most common microbial pathogens isolated from pneumonia in the medical ICU, surgical ICU, trauma and burn units [9]. Pneumonia ranks as the number two most common nosocomial infection accounting for significant morbidity and mortality. Patients receiving mechanically assisted ventilation constitute the population at highest risk for infection (24).

Two organisms, *Staphylococcus aureus* and *Pseudomonas aeruginosa* stand out as the number one and number two most common pathogens associated with pneumonia in the ICU. *Enterobacter* ranks third followed by *K. pneumoniae*, *Candida albicans*, *E. coli* and *H. influenzae* (tied for sixth) and rounding out the group is *Enterococcus*.

TABLE 6. Eight most common pathogens isolated from pneumonia in medical, surgical, trauma and burn ICUs, January 1992–May 1999 (NNIS)

	ICU (Percentage)			
Pathogen	Medical	Surgical	Trauma	Burn
H. influenzae	1.5	4.4	7.4	6.6
Staphylococcus aureus	21.4	17.0	18.1	24.7
Enterococcus spp	1.7	1.8	1.1	1.9
Candida albicans	5.0	3.9	1.5	2.8
Enterobacter spp	8.6	12.8	13.4	8.0
Ps. aeruginosa	21.2	17.2	17.1	21.5
K. pneumoniae	7.7	7.2	7.0	5.3
E. coli	3.5	4.9	4.4	3.4

In addition to these organisms, *Serratia marcescens* and *Proteus* spp. are frequently recovered from respiratory tract cultures in patients clinically diagnosed with nosocomial pneumonia. Diagnosis of nosocomial bacterial pneumonia is problematic especially in the patient on mechanically assisted ventilation. A consensus recommendation proposes standardized criteria for diagnosing pneumonia based on direct rather than clinical evidence and includes the following [25]:

- Bronchoscopically acquired protective specimen brush (PSB) with quantitative culture
- Bronchoalveolar lavage (BAL)
- Protected BAL (pBAL)

The sensitivity of these various procedures is reported to vary from 70% to 100% with a specificity of 60% to 100%. The PSB is widely accepted as a reference method in diagnosing pneumonia in mechanically ventilated patients. However, false positive findings have been reported and may be related to prior antibiotic therapy. Table 7 reports the ventilator-associated pneumonia (VAP) rate for selected ICUs as tabulated by the NNIS system [9]. Patients receiving continuous mechanical ventilation

TABLE 7. Ventilator-associated pneumonia rate for medical, combined medical/surgical, surgical, trauma, and burn ICUs, January 1992–May 1999 (NNIS)

Type of ICU	Number of Units	Ventilator–Associated Pneumonia Rate[a]
Medical	121	8.2
Medical/Surgical		
Teaching	71	12.4
Nonteaching	138	10.3
Surgical	146	14.6
Trauma	21	16.9
Burn	17	19.9

[a] [Number of ventilator-associated pneumonia/number of ventilator days] × 1000.

have a significantly greater risk of developing nosocomial pneumonia than patients not receiving ventilatory support. The pathophysiology of ventilator-associated pneumonia follows a rather predictable course beginning with colonization of the airway and tracheal bronchitis, patients often present with acute respiratory distress or sepsis [26]. The attributed mortality rate hovers somewhere around 25% but a myriad of confounding variables make an accurate assessment difficult. However, mortality rates related to pneumonia have been reported to be significantly greater among patients with MRSA infection [27]. In addition, numerous risk factors have been identified that are independently associated with VAP, these include presence of intracranial pressure monitors, alteration of gastric pH, changing ventilator circuitry every 24 hours, aspiration, reintubation, underlying COPD and use of ventilators for greater than 72 hours. One approach to reducing the incidence of VAP has been directed at reducing the potential microbial contamination originating from the gastrointestinal tract. Two approaches involve the use of selective gut decontamination, which reduces the microbial burden in oropharyngeal and proximal GI tract while the other strategies involve stress ulcer prophylaxis using rimantadine.

It is unlikely that frequent, routine changes of ventilator circuitry will reduce the incidence of VAP. The current policy at our institution is to change the circuitry once a week unless the patient has an excessive production of secretions. One should not underestimate the role that hands play in cross-contamination as a mechanism for transmission of nosocomial pathogens. Cross-contamination has been well documented to occur during tracheal suctioning and manipulation of ventilator circuitry or endotracheal tubes. Therefore, aseptic technique (handwashing) is essential when caring for patients on ventilator support. In addition, it is important to note that devices associated with respiratory therapy or diagnostic examination need to be clean/sterilized/disinfected properly since they may service as a vehicle for dissemination of nosocomial pathogens to at-risk patients. Finally, patient position has been proposed as a simple means for reducing the rate of VAP. A semi-recumbent position (45 degrees) is associated with a lower risk for VAP compared to patients in a surpine position [25]. The use of antimicrobial prophylaxis to prevent nosocomial pneumonia is highly questionable and may lead to emergence of antimicrobial resistance. More detailed information on these issues will be found in chapter 43 (pages 707–718).

Nosocomial Urinary Tract Infections

Table 8 identifies the eight most common microbial pathogens isolated from urinary tract infections in the medical ICU, surgical ICU, trauma and burn units [9]. Nosocomial urinary tract infections (NUTIs) are the most common hospital-acquired infection with the majority occurring following instrumentation. Indwelling urethral catheters that drain into an open system are associated with a higher rate of infection than closed systems.

While acute urinary tract infections may be perceived as benign and often resolves with removal of the catheter, a significant number of these patients receive antibiotic therapy. The

TABLE 8. Eight most common pathogens isolated form urinary tract infections in medical, surgical, trauma and burn ICUs, January 1992–May 1999 (NNIS)

Pathogen	ICU (Percentage)			
	Medical	Surgical	Trauma	Burn
CNS[a]	2.3	1.9	3.5	2.1
Staphylococcus aureus	1.8	1.3	1.7	2.6
Enterococus spp	14.2	14.5	15.5	8.1
Candida albicans	20.8	16.3	10.8	8.4
Enterobacter spp	4.1	6.2	6.5	6.7
Ps. aeruginosa	9.7	13.1	13.5	20.0
K. pneumoniae	6.3	6.1	4.5	4.7
E. coli	13.7	14.6	20.1	13.7

[a] CNS, coagulase-negative staphylococci.

TABLE 9. Urinary catheter-associated UTI rate for medical, combined medical/surgical, surgical, trauma, and burn ICUs, January 1992–May 1999 (NNIS)

Type of ICU	Number of Units	Urinary catheter-associated UTI rate[a]
Medical	124	7.6
Medical/Surgical		
Teaching	71	6.8
Nonteaching	140	4.5
Surgical	146	5.6
Trauma	21	7.7
Burn	17	10.1

[a] [Number of urinary catheter-associated UTI/number of urinary catheter days] × 1000.

widespread use of antibiotics in patients who may be colonized rather than truly infected contributes to antimicrobial pressure within the unit increasing the risk of emergence of antibiotic resistance, potential superinfection or the emergence of yeast (*Candida*) infections. It is interesting to note that *Candida albicans* is the number one uropathogen in both medical and surgical ICUs. At present, there has been a significant increase in the use of antifungal agents within these units. This practice has generated considerable debate, since the criteria for antifungal (*Candida*) therapy is often less than rigorous. Recovery of *Candida* from the urine (in the ICU patient) does not by itself suggest disseminated disease. While it is possible to base antifungal treatment strategies on risk factor stratification, ICU patients almost certainly express multiple risk factors in the absence of clinical disease. In addition, very few institutions perform routine susceptibility testing of candidal isolates and empiric dosing is based upon "expert" opinion rather than institutional MIC data. Therefore, we are left with the premise that often colonization alone, is the sole criteria for treatment and that current dosing guidelines may or may not resolve true clinical infections. There is no doubt that *Candida* has emerged as an important pathogen in the ICU and in selected patients there is an associated high morbidity and mortality. However, appropriate treatment guidelines are lacking and the current practice pattern seems to favor a "high-index of suspicion" whenever the organism is recovered in culture from a non-sterile site.

Table 9 reports the urinary catheter-associated UTI rate for selected ICUs as tabulated by the NNIS system [9]. While infection can occur by a variety of mechanisms, intraluminal migration can be reduced through the use of a closed urinary drainage system. The use of surveillance cultures in catheterized patients is viewed by some practitioners as an effective strategy for the early diagnoses of urinary tract infections, however, this policy has contributed to the widespread abuse of antibiotics in the ICU. As a biomaterial, urinary catheters become rapidly colonized in asymptomatic patients and surveillance cultures should never be used as the sole criteria for therapy. It is not unusual within the ICU to see up to a third of patients whose length of stay is great that 5 days become colonized with yeast (*Candida*). Several new urinary catheters have appeared on the market, which tout antibiotic/antiseptic coatings and suggest that use of these devices will reduce an institution's nosocomial infection rate by making the device resistant to bacterial colonization [28]. Unfortunately, in the clinical evaluation of these devices there is often failure to differentiate between colonized and truly infected patients. It is possible that these devices will have the greatest impact on those patient populations, which require long–term indwelling lines. However, further studies are warranted before these devices completely replace traditional Foley catheters.

Efforts to reduce the risk of NUTIs in the ICU must consider the following recommendations: (a) ongoing educational efforts are required to ensure that personnel are competent in catheter insertion and care, (b) attention focused on appropriate infection control practices that emphasize aseptic technique including hand washing, and (c) ensure an unobstructed urinary flow while maintaining closed sterile drainage.

Isolation Guidelines – Rationale and Practice

Isolation procedures have been developed to prevent the transmission of communicable and infectious diseases to patients, health care workers and visitors. The revised CDC "Isolation Precautions in Hospitals," recognizes a two-tiered system of precautions, Standard Precautions and Transmission-Based Precautions [29]. Standard precautions apply to all patients and represent a standard of care that is in compliance with basic infection control practices. This standard applies to all blood, body fluids, secretions, excretions, non-intact skin surfaces and mucous membranes. Strict adherence to Standard Precautions will effectively reduce the transmission of microorganisms from both recognized and unrecognized sources of infection. In addition to the appropriate use of gloves, masks, eye/face shields, gowns and handling of patient equipment, standard precautions also address management/cleaning of the patient-care environment and sharps injury protection of health care professionals. Transmission-based precautions are implemented when a patient has a documented or is suspected of having being infected or colonized with a "highly transmissible or epidemiologically important pathogen." Transmission-based precautions are always used in addition to standard precautions. The CDC has recommended three specific categories of transmission-based precautions: airborne, droplet and contact. Currently, our institutional Infection Control Committee has implemented a fourth category for vancomycin-resistant enterococci (VRE), Special Isolation Precautions. Table 10 identifies the standard and transmission-based precaution categories.

TABLE 10. Isolation precautions and microbial criteria for isolation

Precaution	Category and Microbiological Criteria
Standard	formerly designated as Universal Precautions
Transmission-based	a. Contact Multidrug-resistant bacteria Methicillin-resistant *S. aureus* (MRSA) *Cl. difficile* Infectious Diarrhea *Herpes* Zoster (immunocompromised)[a] Hemorrhagic viral infection
	b. Airborne[a] (prevent dissimination of particles ≤5 micron) Measles (rubeola) Varicella (disseminated Zoster) Tuberculosis
	c. Droplet (prevent dissemination of particles >5 microns) *H. influenzae* (pneumonia or meninigitis) *N. meningitidis* (pneumonia or meninigitis) Pertussis Influenza Rubella and mumps
	d. Special Isolation vancomycin-resistant enterococci (VRE)

[a] Requires that patient be placed in negative pressure room.

Fundamental Principles of Isolation Precautions

Airborne precautions (for known or suspected TB patient) requires patient placement in a negative pressure room (private) and all doors must be kept closed during the period of isolation. All health care professionals caring for known or a suspected TB patient must wear a N95 respirator mask. If the patient is to be transported within the hospital he (she) must wear a surgical mask when outside of the negative pressure room. A patient may be removed from airborne isolation under the following conditions: (a) receiving effective therapy (TB) for at least two weeks and is improving clinically, (b) has had three consecutive negative sputum smears collected on different days to rule out TB, or (c) a negative BAL. Droplet precautions require that the patient be placed in a private room or in cohort isolation. All health care workers are required to wear a surgical mask when working or coming within three feet of the patient. The patient must wear a surgical mask when being transported within the hospital. Patients must remain in droplet precaution isolation for duration of illness (viral) of following 24 hours of effective antibiotic therapy (bacterial).

Contact precautions dictate that the patient be placed in a private or cohort isolation. All personnel or visitors must wear gloves when entering the room and remove gloves upon leaving the patient's room. Hands must be washed with an antimicrobial soap immediately upon removal of the gloves. Gowns are to be worn if it is anticipated that your clothing will have substantial contact with the patient, environmental surfaces, if the patient is incontinent, has diarrhea, an ileostomy, colostomy or excessive wound drainage. Gowns are removed before leaving the patient's environment. Efforts should be made to ensure that dedicated patient equipment (blood-pressure cuffs, stethoscopes, etc) not be shared with other patients. If not disposable, these items must be thoroughly cleaned and disinfected before use on other patients. Contact precautions cannot be discontinued unless a negative culture is obtained 48 hours after stopping antibiotics. Patients with *Clostridium difficile* diarrhea must be symptom free or have a negative stool toxin assay.

Due to the significant increase in vancomycin-resistant enterococci (VRE) among high-risk patient populations (listed below) our institution has adopted Special Isolation Precautions for VRE patients.

Patient Populations at Increased Risk for Acquiring Vancomycin-resistant Enterococci (VRE)

- Receiving prolonged antimicrobials and/or vancomycin therapy
- Critically ill patients or those with severe underlying disease or immunosuppression
- ICU patients
- Oncology or transplant patients/wards
- Prolonged hospital stay
- Patients having intra-abdominal or cardiothoracic surgical procedures
- Patients with intravascular devices

Special precautions require private or cohort isolation, dedicated patient equipment, all persons must wear gloves and gowns, patients are restricted to their rooms and travel within the hospital only if absolutely necessary. All flat surfaces within the patient's environment must be thoroughly cleaned with a disinfectant cloth at least once per shift. Strict handwashing is required with an antimicrobial agent before and after leaving the patient's room. When the patient is discharged or leaves isolation the entire room is thoroughly cleaned with an effective disinfectant before another patient enters the room. To discontinue isolation three negative stool specimens are required (at least 1 week apart) from stool, rectal or perirectal area and from any other body site that was known to be colonized with VRE. There is a significant potential for widespread environment contamination with VRE and therefore strict enforcement of isolation policies is required to reduce transmission within the institution.

Isolation precautions should be based upon current epidemiologic information that identifies transmission patterns of infectious agents within the hospital environment. The current guidelines from the CDC are intended to recognize the importance of body fluids in the transmission of nosocomial infections, while addressing adequate precautions for traditional routes of transmission (ie. droplet, airborne and contact). Finally, isolation policies should always be viewed as evolutionary in nature, subject to review and update as further data is available on the acquisition and transmission of infectious agents within the hospital environment. For detailed information are refer readers to chapter 18 (pages 331–390).

Antimicrobial Use Policies and the Infection Control Practitioner

Within the critical care environment there has always been an intimate relationship between antimicrobial use policies and infection control practices. The traditional role of the infection control practitioners had been to work closely with physicians, nurses and other health care professionals to facilitate control and prevention of transmission of infectious agents among patients, to staff and visitors within the health care facility. It is also appropriate for the infection control staff to maintain a close, collaborative relationship with the clinical pharmacist when tracking emerging patterns of resistance within the critical are environment. Within our institution, members of the infection control team routinely participate in antimicrobial audits in high-risk patient care areas. In 1999, the infection control team was responsible for documenting a high incidence of vancomycin-resistance enterococci (VRE) among selected immunosuppressed patients on a single unit. The various isolates were collected and genotyped using pulsed-field gel electrophoresis (PFGE) which documented that several of the strains were identical, suggesting a complete breakdown in infection control practices within the unit. In addition, based upon our vancomycin audit, glycopeptide usage in this patient population was the highest (based on total grams and duration) in the institution. An alternative antibiotic use policy was presented to the attending staff physicians that resulted in a dramatic reduction (80%) in vancomycin use among patients on this unit. In addition, the infection control staff met with nursing and environmental services to heighten awareness of the problem and to review current policies and procedures relating to patient care and housekeeping practices. The impact of this comprehensive yet collegial effort has resulted in a sharp reduction in both the emergence of new cases and dissemination of existing clones over the past 12 months.

Antimicrobial resistance is a global problem, unfortunately the magnitude of the problem is not fully realized as evidence by the continuous pattern of antimicrobial use in both the ICU and non-ICU settings. The ICU provides a daunting environment for those practitioners interested in reducing inappropriate antibiotic use. A recent report has documented that within the hospital environment, the ICU is an epicenter for antimicrobial resistance and that selected microbial populations recovered from the ICU express higher levels of resistance than non-ICU strains [12]. This is often a difficult issue to assess and current attitudes regarding appropriate antimicrobial use are steeped in ignorance, apathy or both. In the spring of 1995, the Hospital Infection Control Practice Advisory Committee (HICPAC) published in the Federal Register what amounted to a national action plan for preventing the spread of vancomycin-resistance in the hospital environment. The recommendations from this committee addressed four separate areas: (1) education, (2) role of the hospital microbiology laboratory, (3) prevention and control strategies, and (4) directives for prudent vancomycin use [30]. This was in many ways a unique document that in part reflected upon an agenda for future interdisciplinary strategies aimed at reducing the acquisition and dissemination of resistant pathogens within the health care environment. These recommendations have stimulated other professional societies such as the Infectious Disease Society of American, Society for Healthcare Epidemiology of America, Surgical Infection Society, American Society for Microbiology and the Association for Professionals in Infection Control and Epidemiology to develop policies, procedures and indicators of appropriate antimicrobial use [31]. The original HICPAC recommendations should be viewed as a blue print for leadership in infection control, formulary restraint and microbiological support for preventing the emergence, acquisition and dissemination of all resistant nosocomial pathogens [32]. Therefore, the original (traditional) scope of practice (Table 1) for infection control professionals has been expanded to encompass the documentation of emerging trends of resistance within the hospital environment and the development of interventional strategies aimed at preempting future emerging patterns of resistance.

References

1. Scheckler WE, Brimhall D, Buck AS, Farr BM, *et al.* Requirements for infrastructure and essential activities of infection control and epidemiology in hospitals: a consensus panel report. Infect Control Hosp Epidemiol 19:114, 1998.
2. Jarvis WR. Selected aspects of the socioeconomic impact of nosocomial infections. Infect Control Hosp Epidemiol 17:552, 1996.
3. Gaynes RP. Surveilance of nosocomial infections: a fundamental ingredient for quality. Infect Control Hosp Epidemiol 18:475, 1997.
4. Pittet D, Tarara D, Wenzel R. Nosocomial bloodstream infections in the critically ill patients. J Am Med Assoc 271:1598, 1994.
5. Krzywda EA, Andris DA, Edmiston CE. Catheter Infections: diagnosis, etiology, treatment, and prevention. Nutr Clin Pract 14:178, 1999.
6. Pearson ML, Abrutyn E. Reducing the risk for catheter-related infection; a new strategy. Ann Intern Med 127:294, 1997.
7. Pottinger JM, Herwaldt LA. Basic Surveillance – an overview. Infect Control Hosp Epidemiol 18:513, 1997.
8. Gaynes RP, Solomon S. Improving hospital-acquired infection rates: the CDC experience. Jt Comm J Qual Improv 22:457, 1996.
9. Hospital Infection Program, Centers for Disease Control and Prevention. National nosocomial infection surveillance (NNIS) system report, data summary form January 1990–May 1999, issued June 1999. Am J Infect Control 27:520, 1999.
10. Wenzel RP, Osterman CA, Hunting KJ, Gwaltney JM. Hospital-acquired infection, I surveillance in a university hospital. Am J Epidemiol 103:251, 1976.
11. Glenister H, Taylor L, Barlett C, Cooke M, *et al.* An assessment of selective surveillance methods for detecting hospital acquired infection. Am J Med 91(suppl 3B):121S, 1991.
12. Fridkin SK, Gaynes RP. Antimicrobial resistance in intensive care units. Clin Chest Med 20:303, 1999.
13. Hospital Infection Control Practice Advisory Committee, Centers for Disease Control and Prevention. Guidelines for prevention of intravascular device-related infections. Infect Control Hosp Epidemiol 17:438, 1996.
14. Grosbell IB. Central venous catheter-related sepsis: epidemiology, pathgenesis, diagnosis, treatment and prevention. Intensive Care World 11:55, 1994.
15. Corso F, Wolfe BM. Complications in vascular access devices. Nutr Clin Practice 8:143, 1993.
16. Widmer AF. Intravenous-related infections. In Wenzel RP (ed). Prevention and Control Nosocomial Infections. Williams & Wilkins: Philadelphia, 1997:771.
17. Benoit JL, Carandang G, Sitrin M, *et al.* Intraluminal antibiotic treatment of central venous catheter infections in patients receiving nutrition at home. Clin Infect Dis 21:1286, 1995.
18. Krzywda E, Andris D, Edmiston CE, Quebbeman EJ. Hickman catheter sepsis: efficacy of antibiotic lock therapy. Infect Control Hosp Epidemiol 16:596, 1996.
19. Maki DG, Rinder M. Evaluation of dressing regimens for prevention of infection with peripheral venous catheters. Gauze, a transparent polyurethane dressing, and an iodophor-transparent dressing. J Am Med Assoc 258: 2396, 1987.
20. Faubion WC, Wesley JR, Khaldi N, Silva J. Total parenteral nutrition catheter sepsis: impact of the team approach. J Parenter Enteral Nutr 10:642, 1986.

21. Tomford JW, Hershey CO, McILaren CE, Porter DK, *et al.* Intravenous therapy team and peripheral venous catheter-associated complications. A prospective control study. Arch Intern Med 144:1191, 1984.
22. Danzig LE, Short L, Collins K, *et al.* Bloodstream infections associated with needleless intravenous infusion systems and total parenteral nutrition. J Am Med Assoc 273:1862, 1995.
23. Larson EL, Cheng G, Choo JTE, Merz W. *In-vitro* survival of skin flora in heparin locks and needleless valve infusion devices. Heart Lung 22:459, 1993.
24. Edmiston CE. Nosocomial infections: bacterial pneumonia. In Atlee JL (ed). Complications in Anesthesia. W.B. Saunders: Philadelphia, 1999: 208.
25. Guidelines for prevention of nosocomial pneumonia. MMWR (RR-1):1, 1997.
26. Craven DE, Kunches LM, Kilinsky V, Lichtenberg DA, *et al.* Risk factors for pneumonia and fatality in patients receiving continuous mechanical ventilation. Am Rev Respir Dis 133: 792, 1986.
27. Rello J, Torres A, Ricart M, Valles J, *et al.* Ventilator-associated pneumonia by Staphylococcus aureus. Am J Respir Crit Care Med 150:1545, 1994.
28. Darouiche RO. Anti-infective efficacy of silver-coated medical prostheses. Clin Infect Dis 29:1371, 1999.
29. Hospital Infection Control Practices Advisory Committee, Centers for Disease Control and Prevention. Guideline for isolation precautions in hospitals. Infect Control Hosp Epidemiol 17:53, 1996.
30. Hospital Infection Control Practices Advisory Committee, Centers for Disease Control and Prevention. Recommendations for preventing the spread of vancomycin resistance. Infect Control Hosp Epidemiol 16:105, 1995.
31. Shlaes DM, Gerding DN, John JF, Craig WA, *et al.* Society for Healthcare Epidemiology of America and Infectious Disease Society of American Joint Committee on the Prevetion of Antimicrobial Resistance. Guidelines for the prevention of antimicrobial resistance in hospitals. Infect Control Hosp Epidemiol 18:275, 1997.
32. Edmiston CE. Vancomycin resistance: when failure becomes an opportunity for leadership. Ann Pharmacother 30:680, 1996.

18. ISOLATION AND HANDWASHING

Rosa M. Lopez, and Maite Ricart

Introduction

Infection control measures are developed for decreasing the risk of transmission of micro-organims. These measures, such as handwashing and gloving, respiratory and eye protection, or patient placement make up the fundamentals of isolation precautions. Isolation precautions are based on epidemiological information on transmission of infection in hospitals. The importance of all body fluids, secretions and excretions in the transmission of nosocomial pathogens, and that infections can be transmitted by airborne, droplet and contact routes is well known. Isolation practices are designed to interrupt spread of infections by all routes. Infection control and isolation systems for the care of all patients in hospitals regardless of their infection status and for the care of patients documented to be infected or colonized with highly transmissible or epidemiologically important pathogens are in continuous review and modification for adequate guidelines and improvement of their application.

To adopt and to develop adequate precautions is specially important in the Intensive Care Unit (ICU) because of patient characteristics, the high number of invasive procedures performed and the high prevalence of epidemiologically important pathogens. In this chapter precautions and isolation systems are reviewed in detail.

Scope of the problem

Transfer of pathogens via person-to-person contact is thought to be an important route of dissemination in the hospital setting. Bacterial contamination without apparent soiling can be acquired during routine contact with patients and transferred to other patients. As a result, hand hygiene or hand antisepsis and the use of barrier precautions are cornerstones for the prevention and control of infection.

As ICUs are areas associated with greatly increased risk of nosocomial infections, the improvement of infection control practices is the key of prevention. Although recently doubts have been raised as to the effectiveness of isolation as a measure of prevention in nosocomial infections [1], the vast majority of hospitals all over the world clearly recommend its use [2]. The aim of isolation is to prevent the dissemination of the microorganisms from one patient to another. But it is not the only measure that should be implemented; any step that helps to lessen the resistance of micorganism should be carefully considered, especially those outlined in the Antibiotic Treatment Policies and Basic Techniques for Infection Control [3]. It is well known that insufficient handwashing and the misuse of gloves are among the primary causes of infection in our hospitals.

Handwashing

Handwashing, a tecnique defined as a vigorous, brief rubbing together of all surfaces of lathered hands, followed by rinsing under running water [4], is the most important procedure in reducing the risk of microorganism transmission [5, 6].

The aims of handwashing are: to eliminate pathogens from hands after contact with contaminated surfaces or other sources of contamination, to prevent transmission of microorganisms from patient to patient and from patient to health care workers and to prepare personnel hands before operative procedures.

The microbial flora of the skin consists of resident and transient microorganisms. The resident microorganisms (or colonizing flora) survive and multiply in the skin and are not easily removed by mechanical friction. The transient flora (or contaminatig flora) are microorganisms sporadically isolated from the skin, where they only survive for a limited period of time but can be transmited by hands [7, 8]. Handwashing with plain soap and detergents removes many transient flora effectively [9–11]. Washing hands as promptly and thoroughly as possible between patient contact and after contact with blood, body fluids, secretions, excretions, and equipment or articles contaminated by them is an important component of infection control [12]. The recommended handwashing technique depends on:

- The purpose of the handwashing (the procedure to be performed)
- The intensity of contact with patients or fomites
- The degree of contamination that is likely to occur as a result of this contact
- The susceptibility of patients to infection [13].

The goal of Hygienic handwashing is to eliminate the transient flora. Rubbing lathered hands with plain soap for at least 15 seconds is recommended. Plain soap removes dirt and can physically remove a certain proportion of microbes from skin, but it does not kill bacteria. Antiseptic agents are necessary to kill or inhibit microorganisms.

Hand antisepsis can be performed with handwashing when soaps or detergents that contain antiseptics are used, or by use of alcohol-containing antiseptic handrubs. The primary action of antimicrobial soap includes both mechanical removal and killing or inhibition of both transient and resident flora, but the effect of antiseptic handrubs is only to destroy or inhibit flora, without any effect on soil. The effect on resident flora depends on contact time and antiseptic used [14].

Surgical hand scrub is performed to remove transient flora and reduce resident flora for prolonged surgical procedures, using agents that demonstrate residual activity. The most effective duration for scrubbing is debateable, but it is thought to be about five minutes. This is long enough to remove dirt and should offer the contact time needed to achieve the desired antimicrobial effect as well [15] (Table 1).

Hands should be rinsed to remove residual soap and then completely dried. Drying can remove microorganisms that persist after handwashing [16]; furthermore, wet hands can

TABLE 1. Hand cleaning

Type	Objective	Method
Hygienic handwash	To remove soil and transient microorganisms	Plain soap or detergent for at least 15″
Hand antisepsis	To remove or destroy transient microorganisms	Antimicrobial soap or detergent* or alcohol-based handrub for at least 15″
Surgical hand scrub	To remove or destroy transient flora and reduce resident flora	Antimicrobial soap or detergent for at least 5′ or alcohol-based handrub for at least 30″°

° Previous detergent wash for first scrub of the day or when hands are soiled by organic matter.

* The effect in resident flora will depend on handwash duration and antiseptic used.

transfer bacteria more readily than dry ones [17, 18].

Many antimicrobial agents are available for these procedures, though no single agent is ideal for all uses [19–25]. The choice depends on the characteristics of each agent (mode of action, spectrum of activity, rapidity of action, remaining activity, inactivation by organic matter, safety and toxicity, preparations available) and the efficacy desired in each particular situation. Moreover, guidelines for hand hygiene should be adapted to the particular needs of each hospital in accordance with its epidemiological patterns, and the infection control commitee has to stipulate when particular agents should be used to decontaminate hands. The characteristics of the mot frequently used antimicrobials are summarized in Table 2.

A number of studies report that use of soap and water for frequent daily handwashing may cause skin desquamation, resulting in increased shedding of viable bacteria [26–28]. Moreover, compliance with handwashing policies seldom exceeds 40% [29–32]. The loss of time for patient care may be another reason for poor compliance. Washing hands with an antiseptic soap takes three to four times longer than simply disinfecting with an alcoholic solution [33]. The

TABLE 2. Selection of antiseptics

Antiseptic	Activity	Formulation	Speed	Estability	Toxicity	Persistence
Alcohols	G+, G− bacteria HIV, CMV, enteroviruses M. Tuberculosis Fungi*	60%–90% by weight	15″–2′	Neutralized by organic matter	Minimum cutaneous absortion. Skin drying and dermatitis	No
CHG	G+, G− bacteria Enveloped viruses Fungi*	4% in detergent base or 0.5% in alcohol base preparations	1–2′	Ph-dependent (5.5–7) Reduced in presence of inorganic anions or non-ionic surfactants	Minimal skin absortion. Rarely allergic manifestations. Ototoxicity if instilled into middle ear	Yes >6 h.
Iodine-Iodophors	G+, G− bacteria Enveloped and non-enveloped viruses Fungi M. tuberculosis* spores°	1–2 mg/l of free iodine	1–2′	Reduced in presence of organic matter, or when exposed to the light	Often allergic manifestations detected. Skin irritation. Induction of hypothyroidism in newborns	No
Phenol (Hexachloro phene)	G+, G− bacteria Viruses Fungi M. tuberculosis°	0.5–3%	>2′	Reduced in presence of organic matter. Must to be protected of light	High skin absortion. Neurotoxic	Yes
Phenol (Triclosan)	G+, G− bacteria Viruses* Fungi°	0.3–2%	>2′	Minimally affected by organic matter	Moderate skin absortion. Rarely allergic manifestations.	Yes

* Variable.
° Poor.
From references [19–25].

two major hand antiseptics in use today are alcoholic rubs and medicated soaps or foams containing chlorhexidine (CHG). Alcohols have the most rapid antimicrobial effect and, unlike CHG, are equally effective against gram-positive and gram-negative microorganisms. A disadvantage of pure alcohol is its drying effect on the skin and the absence of a residual activity. Therefore, a combination of the rapid effect of alcohol and the persistence of CHG would seem to offer a desirable antiseptic combination [37]. Recently developed alcohol-based handrubs combine agents with long persistence in skin (chlorhexidine) and skin protectors. Besides, the addition of emollients has the advantage of enhancing the antimicrobial action of antiseptics by slowing evaporation and prolonging their action [38, 39]; as a result, some authors, particularly in Europe, report that alcohol-based handrubs are much more effective in killing bacteria and most viruses [34–36]. Unfortunately, these products cannot be used if hands are dirty because they have no effect on soiling and should not be used as an alternative to handwashing when hands are soiled with organic matter. Nonetheless, they are a good complement to handwashing in the ICU where personnel are in frequent contact with a high number of different patients and have limited time for traditional handwashing.

In addition to handwashing or hand antisepsis, gloves play an important role in reducing the risk of transmission of microorganisms. Gloves reduce the risk of exposure to contaminated matter, reduce the likehood that microorganisms on the hands of personnel will be transmited to patients, and reduce cross-transmission. Gloves must be changed between patient contact and hands should be washed after gloves are removed, because gloves may have non-apparent defects or may be torn during use, and hands can become contaminated during glove removal [40, 41].

Handwashing and wearing gloves are the most basic and effective barrier precautions, and are known to substantially reduced cross-infection between ICU patients [42–44]. But, because of the complexity of the epidemiology and modes of disease transmission, because of the need to curb the spread of infection by all routes, and finally, because of the need to protect both patients and health care workers, other isolation precautions are recommended in hospitals.

Isolation

The various stages and characteristics of nosocomial infection make it necessary to continue modifying isolation guides and recommendations. The first guidelines in the United States were published in 1877 [45], approving the use of separate quarters for contagious patients. In the middle of the 1960s only those assigned to patients with tuberculosis remained in use [46]. At the end of the 1960s it became the norm to isolate patients in individual rooms inside general hospitals. In the 1970s, the first manuals on isolation and precaution differentiated between seven types: Strict Isolation, Respiratory Isolation, Enteric Precautions, Wound and Skin Precautions, Discharge Precautions, Blood Precautions, and Protective Isolation [47, 48].

At the beginning of the 1980s, new problems arose concerning the resistance of several common microorganisms to antibiotic treatment in hospitals, especially in special care units such as the ICU [49]; because of these changes, the first committees for Infection Control were set up inside the centers themselves. In 1985, the Universal Precautions were developed, for use with all patients, on account of the rising number of patients testing positive for HIV or Hepatitis B or C, and in 1987 the Blood and Body Fluid Precautions were introduced [50, 51].

In the 1990s, these two sets of measures merged into one: Standard Precautions, which could be applied to all patients. These precautions have led to a substantial fall in the number of patients requiring measures other than isolation. Another major change has arisen during recent years: the reduction of the aforementioned seven types of isolation [47, 48] into only three categories of Transmission-based Precautions: Airborne Precautions, Droplets Precautions, and Contact Precautions which are used as an additional form of the Standard Precautions in very specific patients [12].

A detail that seems to have escaped us in the midst of all these changes is the use of the word Precaution with regard to the word Isolation. Experience has demonstrated that contagious patients run the risk of becoming phychologically isolated from the rest of the hospital community, including health workers, doctors and family members. Therefore, good epidemiologic knowledge and a good dose of common sense are required, as in an awareness of both the physical and the psychological needs of the patient at all times, especially if one is dealing with children.

In order to apply Isolation Precautions it is necessary to take into account the five universally recognized principal Transmission Routes [12], though it should not be forgotten that a particular microorganism can be transmitted in more than one of these ways:

A. Contact Transmission: The most frequent mode of transmission in hospitals. It may occur via:

Direct-contact: Involves skin-to-skin contact and physical transfer of microorganisms between a susceptible host and an infected or colonized person

Indirect-contact: Involves contact of a susceptible host with a contaminated intermediate object, usually inanimate (instruments, needles, dressings, gloves)

B. Droplet Transmission: This is in fact a form of contact transmission, but the pathogen transfer mechanism to the host is rather different. For this reason it is considered a separate route of transmission. Large droplets (more than five micras in size) are generated from the source person primarily during coughing, sneezing or talking or during the performance of certain procedures such as suctioning and bronchoscopy. Transmission occurs when droplets containing microorganisms are propelled a short distance through the air and deposited on the host. This kind of droplet does not remain suspended in the air; special air handling and ventilation are not required to prevent droplet transmission. So this transmission must not be confused with airborne transmission.

C. Airborne Transmission: This occurs via the dissemination of either airborne droplet nuclei – small particle residue (5 micras or smaller) of evaporated droplets containing microorganisms that remain suspended in the air for long periods of time – or dust particles containing the infectious agent. Microorganisms can be dispersed widely by air currents and may become inhaled by a susceptible host in the same room as, or at a distance from the source patient. Therefore, special air handling and ventilation are required to prevent this kind of transmission.

D. Common Vehicle Transmission: Occurs when microorganisms are transmitted by contaminated items (e.g. food, water, medications, etc).

E. Vectorborne Transmission: Occurs when vectors (mosquitoes, flies, rats, etc) transmit microorganisms. In most regions in the world, this route is of less significance in a hospital setting.

Recommendations

STANDARD PRECAUTIONS

These precautions are designed to reduce the risk of transmission of microorganisms from both recognized and unrecognized sources of infection in hospitals. They should be applied to all patients receiving care in hospitals, regardless of their diagnosis or presumed infection status. Standard Precautions apply to blood, all body fluids, secretions and excretions (except sweat), non-intact skin and mucous membranes [12].

A. Handwashing: The main recommendation for the prevention of infection in hospitals. For this reason we discuss it thoroughly in this chapter.

B. Gloves: Wear clean gloves (they don't need to be sterile), when touching blood, body fluids or contaminated items. Wear sterile gloves just before touching non-intact skin and mucous membranes. Change gloves between tasks on the same patient after contact with materials that contain a high concentration of microorganisms. Remove gloves promptly after use, and wash hands immediately to avoid transfer of microorganisms to other patients or environments.

C. Mask, Eye protection, Face Shield: All these protective items must be used during procedures that are likely to generate splashes or sprays of blood or body fluids.

D. Gown: Wear a clean gown (it does not need to be sterile) to protect skin and clothes during procedures that are likely to generate splashes and sprays of blood or body fluids.

E. Patient-care Equipment: Handle used equipment soiled with blood or body fluids in a manner that prevents skin and mucous membrane exposure, contamination of clothing, and transfer of microorganisms to other patients and environments. Ensure that single-use items are discarded properly.

F. Environmental Control: Ensure that the hospital has adequate procedures for the routine care, cleaning and disinfection of environmental surfaces, beds and other frequently touched surfaces. Ensure that these procedures are being followed.

G. Linen: Handle, transport and process used linen soiled with blood or body fluids in a manner that prevents skin and mucous membrane exposures and contamination of clothing. Avoid transfer of microorganisms to other patients.

H. Occupational Health: 1. Take care to prevent injuries when using needles, scalpels and other sharp instruments or devices. Never recap used needles. Do not remove used needles from disposable syringes by hand. Do not bend, break, or otherwise manipulate used needles by hand. Place used needles, disposable syringes and other sharp items in appropriate puncture-resistant containers.

2. Use mouthpieces and resuscitation bags as alternatives to mouth-to-mouth resuscitation methods.

CONTACT PRECAUTIONS

These precautions are designed to reduce the risk of transmission by direct or indirect contact. Follow these Precautions in addition to Standard Precautions for patients known or suspected to be infected or colonized with important microorganisms that can be transmitted by this transmission route [12]. Examples are: Enteric: *Clostridium difficile*. Skin: *Herpes simplex virus*, Impetigo, Major abscesses, cellulitis or decubiti, *Pediculosis*, *Scabies* and *Zoster*.

A. Patient Placement: Place the patient in a private room (if not possible, those with active infections with the same microorganism may be placed together). If this cohorting is not feasible, consider the epidemiology of the microorganism and the patient population when determining patient placement.

B. Gloves and handwashing: Wear clean gloves (they don't need to be sterile) when entering the room. Change gloves after contact with infective material. Remove gloves before leaving the room. Wash hands immediately with antimicrobial soap or a waterless antiseptic agent if washing hands is impossible [3, 13]. Do not touch anything that has been in contact with the patient after removing gloves and washing hands.

C. Gown: Wear a clean gown (it does not need to be sterile) when entering the room if you anticipate that your clothing will have substantial contact with the patient or with the items in the room. Remove the gown before leaving and ensure that clothing does not come into contact with environmental surfaces.

D. Patient transport: Limit the movement and transport of the patient from the room; essential journeys only. If the patient is transported out of the room, ensure that precautions are maintained. Warn the people who are to receive the patient.

E. Patient-care Equipment: When possible, restrict use of the equipment to a single patient or cohort of patients infected or colonized with the same pathogen. If this is not possible, clean and disinfect the equipment carefully.

DROPLET PRECAUTIONS

These measures are designed to reduce the risk of the transmission of infectious agents via large droplets (larger than five micras). Follow these precautions in addition to Standard Precautions for a patient known or suspected to be infected with microorganisms transmitted by droplets that can be generated by patients during coughing, sneezing or talking [12], or during the performance of procedures such as suctioning. Examples: *Neisseria meningitidis, Haemophilus influenzae*, *Pertussis*, *Mumps*, *Rubella*.

A. Patient Placement: Place the patient in a private room (if not possible, patients who have active infections with the same microorganism may be placed together). If this cohorting is not feasible, maintain a spatial separation of at least three feet between patients and visitors. Special air handling and ventilation are not necessary. The door can remain open.

B. Mask: Wear a mask when working within three feet of the patient (for logistical reasons, some hospitals require wearing a mask on entering the room).

C. Patient transport: Limit the movement of the patient from the room; essential journeys only. If transport is necessary, the patient must wear a mask. Warn the people who are to receive the patient.

AIRBORNE PRECAUTIONS

These measures are designed to reduce the risk of airborne transmission of infectious agents. Use these precautions in addition to Standard Precautions for a patient known or suspected to be infected with microorganisms transmitted by droplets that remain suspended in the air and that can be dispersed widely by air currents within a room or over a long distance [12]. Examples are: Tuberculosis, Measles, Varicella.

A. Patient Placement: Place the patient in a private room. If possible, this room must have:

- Monitored negative air pressure in relation to the surrounding areas
- 6 to 12 air changes per hour
- Appropriate discharge of air outdoors or monitored high-efficiency filtration of room air before the air is circulated to other areas in the hospital [52].

Keep the room door closed. Cohorting can be used if a private room is not available. If cohorting is not desirable, consult with infection control professionals [12].

B. Respiratory Protection: Wear respiratory protection (mask with high filtration capacity, e.g. N95 respirator) when entering the room of a patient with known or suspected infectious pulmonary tuberculosis [12–53]. Susceptible persons should not enter the room of patients known or suspected to have measles or varicella, but if there is no alternative, they should also wear respiratory protection. Visitors should be limited; visitors must wear respiratory protection. Remove the mask after leaving the room [53].

C. Patient Transport: Limit the movement and transport of the patient from the room:

essential journeys only. If transport is necessary, the patient must wear a surgical mask, or a bacterial filter if on mechanical ventilation [12, 53].

IMMUNOCOMPROMISED PATIENTS

Immunocompromised patients vary in their susceptibility to nosocomial infections, depending on the severity of immunosuppression. The use of Standard Precautions for all patients and Transmission-based Precautions for specified patients should reduce the acquisition of microorganisms from other patients and environment. In cases of severe neutropenia, consult with infection control professionals [52].

Conclusions

Standard Precautions are the primary strategies for nosocomial infection control, and are designed for the care of all patients in hospitals regardless of their diagnosis or presumed infection status. Transmission-based Precautions are additional strategies designed to complement the Standard Precautions and are used in patients known or suspected to be infected or colonized with epidemiologically important microorganisms that can be transmitted by airborne or droplet transmission or by contact with dry skin or contaminated surfaces. Given this synthesis, a large number of patients that previously required specific precautions are now cared for without special manipulations. A large number of patients require the same standard precautions and this is easier for staff to apply because it allows the adoption of a routine in the care and contact with patients and because of the limited number of patients that will require additional precautions. Moreover, the three groups of Transmission-based Precautions are very specific in their recommendations and are better known by health care workers than previous guidelines. However, because the epidemiology of some diseases, particularly those with a respiratory component of transmission, is not well known or well defined, low compliance or controversial practices are detected, especially if resources are not adequate or when patients are not diagnosed. Compliance with empiric Transmission-based Precautions is usually inadequate, probably as they involve extra work.

Most research has been guided by the problems concerning effectiveness and compliance with handwashing as well as other isolation precautions. Reports indicating poor compliance are often taken to suggest that personnel fail to wash their hands or wear gloves or manipulate gowns correctly because of lack of time (i.e. heavy workload), a shortage of facilities (e.g. sinks often inconveniently placed), inadequate resources such as nurse ratio or close single room for each patient in the ICU, damage to hands skin (additionally, allergic reactions to gloves), and ignorance of or disagreement with the recommendations (training usually improves compliance, but only temporarily). Probably all these factors contibute. Greater familiarity with the routes of disemination and fuller knowledge of the barrier precautions or control measures will improve them.

Providing better hand care facilities, faster and more effective antiseptics with better skin protection, ready availability of adequate supplies and resources, better design of the area and rooms, and continuous personnel education promoting research into infection control practices, would improve compliance with precaution recommendations.

However, there is no system of isolation that is applicable to all ICUs. Each hospital has to customize the recommendations to their type of patients and to the resources at their disposal.

References

1. Olmsted R. Are isolation precautions necessary to prevent transmission of multidrug-resistant organisms? Infectious Disease News, 1998.
2. Schlaes DM, Gerding DN, John JF, Craig WA, Borstein DL, *et al.* Society for Healthcare Epidemiology of America and Infectious Diseases Society of America Joint Commettee on the prevention of antimicrobial resistance: Guidelines

for the prevention of antimocrobial resistance in hospitals. 25:584, 1997.
3. Goldmann DA, Weinstein RA, Wenzel RP, Tablan OC, Duma RJ, *et al*. Strategies to prevent and control the emergence and spread of antimicrobial-resistant microorganisms in hospitals. JAMA 275:234, 1996.
4. Garner JS, Simmons BS. Guideline for handwashing and hospital environmental control. Infect Control 7:231, 1985.
5. Larson EL. A casual link between handwashing and risk infection? ICHE 9:28, 1988.
6. Rotter ML. Hygienic hand disinfection. Infect Control 5:18, 1984.
7. Salzman TC, Clark JJ, Likemm L. Hand decontamination of personnel as a mechanism of cross-infection in nosocomial infections with antibiotic-resistant *Escherichia coli* and *Klebsiela-Aerobacter*. Antimicrob Agents Chemother 2:97, 1967.
8. Casewell M, Phillips I. Hands as a route of transmission of *Klebsiella* species. BMJ 11:1315, 1977.
9. Lowbury EJL, Lilly HA, Bull JP. Disinfection of hands, removal of transient organisms. Br Med J 2:230, 1964.
10. Sprunt K, Redman W, Leidy G. Antimicrobial effectiveness of routine handwashing. Pediatrics 52:264, 1973.
11. Ojajarvi J. The importance of soap selection. J Hyg 86:275, 1981.
12. Gardner JS and the Hospital Infection Control Practices Advisory Committee. Guidelines for isolation precautions in hospitals. ICHE 17:53, 1996.
13. Larson EL. APIC guideline for handwashing and hand antisepsis in health care settings. AJIC 23:251, 1995.
14. Pereira LJ, Lee GM, Wade KJ. The effect of surgical handwashing routines on the microbial counts of operating room nurses. Am J Infect Control 18:354, 1990.
15. Association of Operating Room Nurses. Recommended practices: surgical hand scrub. AORN J 52:830, 1990.
16. Ansari SA, Springthorpe VS, Sattar SA, Tostowarky W, Wells GA. Comparison of cloth, paper, and warm air drying in eliminating viruses and bacteria from washed hands. AJIC 19:243, 1991.
17. Marples RR, Towers A. A laboratory model for contact transfer of microorganisms. J Hyg 82:237, 1979.
18. Mackintosh C, Hoffman P. An extended model for transfer of microorganisms via hands: differences between organisms and the effect of alcohol disinfection. J Hyg 92:345, 1984.
19. Larson EL, Morton HE. Alcohols. In Block SS (ed). Disinfection, sterilization and preservation, 4th edn, Philadelphia: Lea & Febiger, 1991: 191.
20. Larson EL, Butz AM, Gullette DL, Laughon BA. Alcohol for surgical scrubbing? ICHE 11:139, 1990.
21. Ayliffe GAJ. Surgical scrub and skin disinfection. Infect Control 5:23, 1984.
22. Denton GW. Chlorhexidine. In Block SS (ed). Disinfection, sterilization and preservation. 4th edn, Philadelphia: Lea & Febiger, 1991:274.
23. Gottardi W. Iodine and iodine compounds. In Block SS (ed). Disinfection, sterilization and preservation. 4th edn, Philadelphia: Lea & febiger, 1991:152.
24. Zamora JL. Chemical and microbiologic characteristics and toxicity of povidone-iodine solutions. Am J Surg 151:400, 1986.
25. O'Connor DO, Rubino JR. Phenolic compounds. In Block SS (ed). Disinfection, sterilization and preservation. 4th edn. Philadelphia: Lea & Febiger, 1991:204.
26. Meers PD, Yeo GA. Shedding of bacteria and skin squames after handwashing. J Hyg 81:99, 1978.
27. Larson EL. Handwashing and skin. Physiologic and bacteriologic aspects. Infect Control 6:14, 1985.
28. Ojajarvi J, Makela P, Rastasalo I. Failure of hand disinfection with frequent hand washing: a need for prolonged field studies. J Hyg 79:107, 1997.
29. Meengs MR, Giles BK, Chisholm CD, Cordell WH, Nelson DR. Hand washing frequency in an emergency department. Ann Emerg Med 23:1307, 1994.
30. Graham M. Frequency and duration of handwashing in an intensive care unit. AJIC 18:78, 1990.
31. Donowitz LG. Handwashing technique in a pediatric intensive care unit. Am J Child Dis 141:683, 1987.
32. Albert RK, Condie F. Handwashing patterns in medical intensive care units. N Engl J Med 304:1464, 1981.
33. Widmer AF. Infection control and prevention strategies in the intensive care unit. Intensive Care Med 20 (suppl4):s7, 1994.
34. Pittet D, Mourouga P, Perneger TV. Compliance with handwashing in a teaching hospital. Ann Intern Med 130:126, 1999.

35. Voss A, Widmer AF. No time for handwashing? Handwashing versus alcoholic rub: can we afford 100% compliance? ICHE 18:205, 1997.
36. Pereira LJ, Leegm, Wade KJ. An evaluation of five protocols for surgical handwashing in relation to skin condition and microbial counts. J Hosp Infect 36:49, 1997.
37. Ulrich JA. Clinical study comparing Hibistat (0.5% chlorhexidine gluconate in 70% isopropyl alcohol) and Betadine surgical scrub (7.5% povidone-iodine) for efficacy against experimental contamination of human skin. Curr Ther Res 31:27, 1982.
38. Hobson DW, Woller W, Anderson L, Guthery E. Development and evaluation of a new alcohol-based surgical hand scrub formulation with persistent antimicrobial characteristics and brushless application. AJIC 26:507, 1998.
39. Beck WC. Alcohol foam has a place in the clinical arena. AORN J 50:157, 1989.
40. Goldmann DA. The role of barrier precautions in infection control. J Hosp Infect 18:515, 1991.
41. Doebbeling BN, Pfaller MA, Houston AK, Wenzel RP. Removal of nosocomial pathogens from the contaminated glove: implications for glove reuse and handwashing. Ann Intern Med 109:394, 1988.
42. Conly JM, Hill S, Ross J, Lertzman J, Louie TJ. Handwashing practices in an intensive care unit: the effects of an educational program and its relationship to infection rates. AJIC 17:330, 1989.
43. Klein BS, Perloff WH, Maki DG. Reduction of nosocomial infection during pediatric intensive care by protective isolation. N Engl J Med 320:1714, 1989.
44. Olson B, Weinstein RA, Nathan C, Chamberlin W, Kabis SA. Occult aminoglycoside resistance in *Pseudomonas aeruginosa*: Epidemiology and implications for therapy and control. J Infect Dis 152:769, 1985.
45. Lynch T. Communicable Disease Nursing. St. Louis, MO: Mosby, 1949.
46. Gage ND, London JF, Sider MT. Communicable Disease. Philadelphia, PA: FA Davis, 1959.
47. Palmer MB. Infection control. A Policy and Procedure Manual, 1986.
48. Centers for Disease Control. Isolation Techniques for use in hospitals. 2nd edn, Washington, DC: US Government Printing Office, 1975:80.
49. Schaffner W. Infection control: old myths and new realities. Infect Control 1:330, 1980.
50. Centers for Disease Control. Recommendations for preventing HIV transmission in health-care settings. MMWR 36(2S):1S, 1987.
51. Centers for Disease Control. Update: Universal precautions for prevention of transmission of HIV, HBV and other bloodborne pathogens in health-care settings. MMWR 37:377, 1988.
52. Centers for Disease Control. Draft guidelines for preventing the transmission of tuberculosis in health-care facilities. MMWR 43(RR-13):1, 1994.
53. Department of Health and Human Services. Department of Labor. Respiratory protective devices: final rules and notice. Federal Register 60(110):30336, 1995.

19. STERILIZATION AND DISINFECTION IN THE ICU

Montserrat Sallés and Maite Ricart

Introduction

The mission of asepsia procedures in hospitals is to avoid the transmission of potentially pathogenic microorganisms from patient to patient, from health care personnel to patient, and from patient to personnel. Providing adequate health care with a high level of asepsia and at the same time interrupting the transmission of microorganisms are key steps in the attempts to reduce the incidence of nosocomial infectious diseases. The contamination of medical equipment – due either to inadequate cleaning, disinfecting or sterilizing of medical devices and environmental surfaces, or to inadequate reuse of material – exposes patients to a high risk of nosocomial infection. This risk is particularly high in the Intensive Care Unit (ICU).

Cleaning is the essential first step in disinfection or sterilization. Steam sterilization is the most efficient procedure, because it is non-toxic, fast and low-cost. However, many of the devices and instruments used in the ICU are thermolabile, and so steam sterilization cannot be implemented in this setting. A large proportion of materials are reprocessed using low temperature methods with ethylene oxide (EO) or, more recently, plasma gas (PG), hydrogen peroxide or peracetic acid. Disadvantages such as toxicity, lengthy time of sterilization (in the case of EO) or high cost (in the case of PG) mean that high-level disinfection is often systematically preferred to sterilization for the reprocessing of critical and semicritical devices. Non-critical materials can be disinfected by low-level chemical disinfectants such as sodium hypochlorite (0.1%), ethyl or isopropyl alcohol (70–90%), or an aldehyde (1%). This chapter describes three important procedures for preventing ICU infections.

Sources and Reservoirs

Sources and vehicles of infecting microorganisms in hospitals may be patients, personnel, or inanimate objects such as medical devices, or environmental objects or materials. Before these devices can be used on a patient without risk of infection, the microorganisms present on the surface of the item must be removed.

The main reservoirs of microorganisms are well known. Several studies have also shown the relationship between respiratory tract infections and air or water systems [1–8]. The isolation of some microorganisms suggests the possibility of contamination from sources such as the hands of health care personnel or incorrectly reprocessed equipment and devices. Widespread surface contamination may occur with some pathogens (VRE, VRS, MRSA, *Acinetobacter*); hands may become transiently colonized and cause cross-contamination. So, meticulous cleaning, disinfection or sterilization of medical devices, together with handwashing, will prevent pathogen transmission.

General Principles

Cleaning

Cleaning is defined as the elimination of dirt from an object and the reduction of a significant proportion of the microorganisms present on the surface. Modern technologies have created increasingly sophisticated devices with a wide variety of tools, each of which presents its own particular difficulties for cleaning. Cleaning is the first step in correct disinfection or sterilization. The presence of organic material is one of the main factors that contribute to the failure of equipment disinfection or sterilization, because it blocks the access of chemical agents. However, the mechanical process drags and destroys a high percentage of microorganisms. One study affirms that scrupulous cleaning alone reduces the presence of microbial contamination ions between 99.9% to 99.99% when a flexible fiberbronchoscope was artificially contaminated by *Pseudomonas aeruginosa* and *Mycobacterium tuberculosis*. Another study reported that scrupulous cleaning achieved total HIV elimination on fiberscopes [9, 10]. Cleaning must be done meticulously and as soon as possible, as dirt is more difficult to eliminate when wet than when dry. Not all the equipment needs the same cleaning procedure, so the manufacturer's instructions must be followed in order to avoid damaging the instrument in question. A number of intrinsic factors should be considered when cleaning:

- Water quality: the "harder" the water, the more detergent required to obtain maximum detergent efficiency. Using deionized water avoids equipment corrosion.
- Water temperature: temperatures of between 22°C and 43°C (71°F/109°F) avoid blood coagulation and facilitates the elimination of dirt.
- Mechanical action. Each piece of equipment requires a specific mechanical procedure depending on its physical structure. Because of their fragility, certain instruments cannot be washed with ultrasounds or specific washing machines.

Non-abrasive detergents are recommended for cleaning medical equipment. Detergents are non-ionic, proteolytic products, biodegradable at 80°C, which ensure elimination of organic material and reduce microbial contamination due to the lithium effect. Some studies have proved that enzymatic detergents are more effective than neutral ones on materials of difficult access, because the enzymatic detergent has endopeptidases that hydrolyze the majority of peptide bonds in the protein molecules. As a result, contaminating agents with a proteic base (e.g. pus, or blood) are eliminated. The enzymes present in commercial enzymatic detergents vary: formulas on the market contain proteases, amylases and/or lipases. The enzyme by itself is not a cleanser, but a proteic substance that facilitates cleaning. Once it has performed its role, it can be totally eliminated through the detergent's action. Some products on the market combine enzymes with detergents. Powder detergents should be dissolved in water, otherwise they may block channels of difficult access or may damage equipment due to their high concentration. These detergents contain enzymes which are living products, and so their expiry date must be carefully checked; their active life is shorter than non-enzymatic detergents. Once the equipment has been properly cleaned the next step is either disinfection or sterilization, depending on the classification of the equipment. Cleaning can be manual (Table 1) or mechanical. Mechanical cleaning can be done by different types of washing machines in the Sterilization Unit. There are washers for endoscopes, endoscopy

TABLE 1. Manual cleaning procedure

1. Submerge or soak the tool in a soapy solution.
2. Scrub thoroughly to detach any particles with the help of accessories (scrubs, brushes, etc) to gain full access.
3. Rinse with abundant water to eliminate the rest of emulsified organic matter.
4. Dry properly to avoid possible contamination.

utensils, rubber bands and other utensils. Equipment can also be washed by ultrasound.

Cleaning utensils such as brushes and sponges must be kept under totally hygienic conditions. Therefore, cleaning and disinfection are needed after each use.

Disinfection

Disinfection is the chemical process by which microorganisms are destroyed using chemical products known as disinfectants. The disinfection process may fail if a proper previous cleaning has not been carried out or if the exposure time has not been sufficient for the disinfectant to work. Disinfectants are chemical substances that destroy microorganisms on inanimate equipment, without apparently altering the instruments. Certain germicides such as alcohol can be used as antiseptics and disinfectants.

A number of factors affect the efficiency of disinfectants. Some are intrinsic qualities of microorganisms and disinfectants, and others physical and chemical properties:

1. Number and location of microorganisms; certain locations may be more inaccessible to disinfectants (e.g. channels of endoscopes, etc).
2. Innate resistance to microorganisms from high to low resistance to disinfectants: bacterial spores, non-lipid viruses (e.g. poliovirus, coxsackie), mycobacteria, fungi, lipid viruses (HIV, HBV, herpes virus), vegetative forms of bacteria.
3. Concentration and power of disinfectants.
4. Physicochemical factors (temperature, pH, relative humidity).
5. Organic matter may protect microorganisms from disinfectants, or may diminish the activity of some disinfectants.
6. The correct exposure time to disinfectants must always be respected; otherwise, their activity may be reduced.
7. Microorganisms may produce a thick mass of cells and extracellular materials or biofilms. It has been proved that in the interior of chloride polyvinyl channels some type of microorganism protects itself from the disinfectant action, and becomes a reserve for continued contamination.

Depending on their potential, disinfectants are classified as:

1. High level disinfectants: these inactivate all vegetative forms of microorganisms, including all types of viruses and fungi. They can also destroy some bacterial spores if the exposition time is long enough (7–10 hours).
2. Intermediate level disinfectants: these eliminate all forms of vegetative bacteria: *Mycobacterium tuberculosis* as well as most viruses and fungi, but they do not ensure destruction of bacterial spores.
3. Low level disinfectants: these eliminate most vegetative bacterial forms and some viruses and fungi, but do not guarantee destruction of *Mycobacterium tuberculosis*, non-lipid viruses or bacterial spores.

Depending on their chemical structure, they are classified as:

- Alcohols: ethyl alcohol, isopropyl alcohol
- Aldehydes: formaldehyde, paraformaldehyde, glutaraldehyde
- Biguanides: chlorhexidine
- Chloride derivates: chloramine T, sodium hypochlorite
- Iodine derivates: iodic povidone, iodic alcohol, iodine
- Cationic detergents: quaternary ammonium compounds (benzalkonium chloride, cetrimide)
- Phenol and its derivates
- Gases: ethylene oxide, propiolactone
- Heavy metals: silver and mercury derivates
- Oxidizing agents: peracetic acid, hydrogen peroxide, potassium permanganate.

Disinfectants are selected on the basis of their characteristics, and the requirements for their correct application [11–13]. Bodies such as EPA, FDA and CDC register, regulate and recommend procedures for the choice and application of disinfectants.

We will briefly discuss the characteristics of the most frequently used agents in hospitals to disinfect materials and surfaces.

SODIUM HYPOCHLORITE

A high potential, efficient and economic bactericide of fast but not continuous action. Corrosive, irritates skin and mucous. Becomes inactivated in contact with organic matter. Must be kept in opaque, well-closed containers. The original commercial solution has to be considered when preparing solutions; once prepared, solutions must be thrown away daily because they are unstable. On the market today there are commercial preparations that associate bleach with a compatible detergent. The percentage of concentration to be used is 100 ppm for low level disinfection, and 1000 ppm for high level disinfection.

GLUTARALDEHYDE

A high potential bactericide used for high level disinfection of semicritical clinical utensils and thermosensitive equipment. Used at a 2% alkaline concentration. Does not attack metals, optical lenses, rubber bands or plastics. Recommended exposure time: 20 minutes at environmental temperature. Some authors recommend a 10 minute exposure if the temperature of the solution is 25°C (77°F); others recommend between 20 to 45 minutes in order to destroy mycobacteria. Solutions can be reused the following day, depending on their use, but keeping them for longer than a week is not recommended. Utensils must be totally submerged in the solution. In case of channels or holes with a difficult access a disinfectant solution is injected with a syringe at the moment of submersion; it can thus penetrate all the streams and disinfect the interior and exterior parts of the equipment. There are a variety of glutaraldehyde formulas, but alkaline solutions are preferred to acidic ones due to their anticorrosive properties.

It is a toxic, irritating, allergenic, teratogenic and mutagenic product that may affect DNA. May cause sensitization by contact or inhalation. Its steam may irritate mucouses, pharynx and eyes causing rhinitis, conjunctivitis, cough and bronchospasms to people with a particularly sensitive respiratory tract; may cause occupational asthma. Environmental concentration should not exceed 0.02 ppm. In order to avoid the formation of toxic steams, hot water cannot be used when preparing solutions, and the equipment must be scrupulously rinsed with abundant sterilized water, or soaked in regular water, depending on its use. The product is toxic and all health care workers must take prevention and security measures during manipulation by wearing gloves, facial masks, ocular protection, and whitecoats when anticipating splashing or aerosol.

HYDROGEN PEROXIDE

A powerful bactericide and fast oxidizing agent which facilitates the elimination of organic material. Hydrogen peroxide is considered a high level disinfectant at 6% with phosphoric acid at 0.085%; it is accepted for fiberendoscopies, but not for its accessories. Studies show that hydrogen peroxide at 6% is more effective in high level disinfection of endoscopes than a glutaraldehyde solution at 2%. Hydrogen peroxide is corrosive in concentrations above 8%. Direct contact with the concentrated product irritates eyes, mucous membranes and skin. Steam inhalation may cause inflammation of the respiratory tract.

PHENOL

May be bacteriostatic or bactericidal, depending on its concentration and pH. Phenol is very irritating even after carefully washing the equipment; equipment may retain residues, because phenolics are assimilated by porous materials. Highly absorbable via skin; products are neurotoxic.

QUATERNARY AMMONIUM COMPOUNDS

Low power bacteriostatics which are good cleaning agents. When used as disinfectants nosocomial infections have been reported, due to a contamination of the solutions.

ETHYL ALCOHOL

Intermediate power bactericide, characterized by its fast action. Continued contact on the skin causes irritation and dryness. Alcohol becomes inactive with the presence of organic material. Alcohol evaporates quickly, making a long period of contact difficult. May damage rubber bands and some plastics. Hardens rubber and obscures methacrylate equipment. It is inflammable.

ASSOCIATION OF ALDEHYDE

Usually used at a concentration level of 1%. Gloves must be used for its manipulation and the dissolutions must be prepared with cold water to avoid inhalation of toxic steam. Must not be mixed with other detergents or sodium hypochlorite. May cause dermatitis and sensitization.

Sterilization

Sterilization is the method used to destroy all kind of microorganisms, particularly necessary in equipment that penetrates sterilized cavities. A range of sterilization systems are used in hospitals:

STEAM STERILIZATION

Germicidal action works through denaturalization of proteins. It is the method chosen to reprocess thermostable equipment. The temperature of the process oscillates between 121°C to 132°C (250°F to 270°F) for between 3 to 30 minutes depending on the system (gravity or prevacuum) and whether the equipment is wrapped or not. Advantages: fast, efficient, economic, non-toxic. Disadvantages: unsuitable for thermosensitive equipment.

ETHYLENE OXIDE (EO)

Germicidal action is due to an alkylating process. Used for thermosensitive equipment; requires posterior ventilation. The duration of the ventilation depends on the following variables: composition, configuration, kind of packaging, sterilization and distinctive traits of the ventilation system. Manufacturers should provide thorough information about parameters for ventilating their products. If this information is not available maximum ventilation should be applied, i.e. the period stipulated for the products which are most difficult to ventilate: 12 hours at 50°C (122°F) and 8 hours at 60°C (140°F). Advantages: useful for thermosensitive equipment. Good penetration. Disadvantages: toxic, requires ventilation; cycles are long; expensive. Due to its toxicity all materials must be ventilated, resulting in a long sterilization and ventilation cycle, the shortest lasting 15 hours. Requires specific equipment. The remains of organic material, saline solutions or an excess of humidity in the equipment sterilized with EO may cause the formation of toxic products such as ethylene chlorohydrin or glycol ethylene which are not eliminated even with ventilation.

Currently, new low temperature sterilization methods are offering an alternative to EO because they do not leave toxic residues on the sterilized utensils; subsequent ventilation is not necessary; nor are environmental and personnel security measures. Among these systems are:

PLASMA-GAS

This system uses vaporized hydrogen peroxide at 58%, and high frequency energy through which gas plasma is generated. Its cycles work at a temperature below 50°C (122°F) for 50–65 minutes. Non-corrosive, with fast cycles and a system that generates non-toxic residues (H_2O, O_2), making ventilation and environmental measures unnecessary. But it is not useful for cellulose and clothes, and requires special polypropylene packaging.

VAPOR-PHASE HYDROGEN PEROXIDE

This system uses vaporized hydrogen peroxide at an initial concentration of 30%; sterilizes at a temperature of 39°C (102°F) for 50 minutes. Fast and non-corrosive, but its penetration is lower than ethylene oxide and fluids. Not suitable for cellulose and its derivates.

PERACETIC ACID

A sporicide active at low concentrations (<1%) and at low temperatures. Accepted as a new sterilization method for utensils that can be totally submerged (e.g. endoscopes). Functions at temperatures between 50–56°C (122°F–133°F). Process lasts 20 to 30 minutes, depending on initial temperature, water pressure, and filter status. Non-corrosive, generates non-toxic residues (acetic acid, H_2O, O_2, H_2O_2), and remains active in presence of organic matter, but can only be used for submergible equipment. This system has trays for different types of instruments, allowing their aseptic transport after sterilization.

VAPORIZED FORMALDEHYDE

Another low temperature system (50° to 60°) in a permanent vacuum chamber. Cycles last between 3 and 5 hours. It uses formaldehyde at a concentration of 2%. This system has no toxic impact on the environment. Equipment is ventilated during the same cycle.

Recommendations for Reprocessing Medical Devices

In 1968 Spaulding [11] established a three-category system for the risk of infection of medical devices, based on their degree of contact with the patient: critical, semi-critical and non-critical. Not long afterwards, the CDC adopted the same basic classifying system in their Infection Control Guide [14].

According to this classification critical devices are those that come into contact with sterile tissues or vascular system. The category includes surgical instruments, catheters (vascular, cardiac, urinary), implants, needles, endoscopes that enter sterile tissues (e.g. arthroscopes or laparoscopes) and all endoscope accessories used for diagnostic or therapeutic purposes and which penetrate into mucous membranes (i.e. biopsy forceps, brushes). All respiratory therapy devices, anesthesia equipment and other devices that come into contact with mucous surfaces or broken skin, such as laryngoscopes or bronchoscopes, are defined as semi-critical items. Non-critical devices come into contact with intact skin but not with mucous membranes: for instance, blood pressure cuffs, stethoscopes, infusion pumps, and room furniture. There is generally little risk of transmitting infections to patients by non-critical items, but they may produce a cross-transmission by contaminating hands of health care workers or medical equipment.

Single-use devices should be used whenever possible but reusable devices can be reprocessed depending on their Spaulding category and the level of disinfection required. Semi-critical materials must be sterilized, or at least a high-level disinfection must be performed [11, 14]. High-level disinfection is a procedure defined as the inactivation of vegetative bacteria, viruses, fungi and mycobacteria but not necessarily of bacterial spores. High-level disinfectants are effective against bacterial spores if the exposure time is long enough (up to 10 hours). Intermediate-level disinfectants inactivate *M. tuberculosis*, vegetative bacteria, most viruses and most fungi, but do not necessarily destroy bacterial spores. Disinfection levels are summarized in Table 2.

All materials must be thoroughly cleaned before the sterilization or disinfection stage, because, as mentioned before, the presence of organic matter may impede correct reprocessing. Steam sterilization can achieve an optimal level of decontamination for a range of medical equipment; however, this system cannot be used with thermolabile devices. EO is a good low-heat system for sterilization of thermolabile items, but it is highly toxic. In addition, the system is time consuming since materials must be ventilated in order to eliminate the EO at the end of the process; it may therefore take too long for routine use between patients, or when a large

TABLE 2. Disinfection levels

Disinfection level	Lipid Viruses	Vegetative Bacteria	Fungi	Non-lipid Viruses	Mycobacteria	Bacterial Spores
High	+	+	+	+	+	+*
Intermediate	+	+	+	±	±	−
Low	+	+	±	−	−	−

* Long exposure time.
From references [11–13].

TABLE 3. Low-temperature sterilization methods

Method	Advantages	Disadvantages
Ethylene oxide	Good penetration	Requires material ventilation Long cycles (8–12 hours) Expensive
Paracetic acid liquid	Decomposition products are not harmful Leaves no toxic residue Quick process Remains effective in presence of organic matter	Only for materials that can be immersed Only few instruments can be sterilized in each cycle Does not allow storage
Hydrogen peroxide plasma-gas	Quick process Leaves no toxic residue Non-corrosive	Special packaging are required Cellulose, clothes and liquids cannot be sterilized
Hydrogen peroxide vapor-phase	Quick system Non-corrosive	Lower penetration power Fluids, cellulose and its derivates cannot be sterilized
Formaldehyde vapor	Quick process. No toxic residue Material ventilation in the same cycle	Not accepted in some countries as sterilization system

number of devices are needed. The low temperature sterilization methods currently available are summarized in Table 3. When sterilization is not possible (i.e. because of characteristics of the material, or because there is little material available) a high-level disinfection could be performed if adequate disinfectant concentrations are used. Storage in solutions is avoided, and solutions are discharged daily. According to the Spaulding criteria and HICPAC, high-level disinfection can be achieved using 2% glutaraldehyde for a period of 20′. But because of the complexity of some of these items (such as FFBs) some authors recommend longer exposure times (30′) to guarantee the elimination of microorganisms such as *M. tuberculosis* [9]. After performing a high-level disinfection for semicritical equipment, a final rinse with sterile water is recommended, because microorganisms such as *Legionella* sp. or *Mycobacterium* sp. can contaminate non-sterile water.

High-level disinfection must be used for spirometers, temperature sensors, manual ventilation bag ports, nebulizers and other respiratory devices used on multiple patients [15]. The use of 70% isopropyl alcohol has been reported as adequate to disinfect volume sensors; however, new materials have recently been used in this type of device, and these materials can be sterilized in low temperature systems. It is very important that manufacturers of medical apparatus give specific recommendations regarding cleaning and disinfecting or sterilizing procedures, so as to avoid damage to the instruments [12, 16].

Low-level disinfectants are adequate for non-critical material – devices that only come into contact with intact skin, such as furniture, infusion pumps or external parts of ventilators. This material must be correctly cleaned before disinfection by immersing or soaking the object in soap solution if possible, or using wet gauzes to remove dirty or organic matter. Subsequently, low-level disinfectant should be applied long enough to provide adequate disinfection and then stored to avoid contamination. Low-intermediate disinfection could be achieved by alcohol (ethyl or isopropyl 70–90%), sodium hypochlorite (0.1%), iodophor detergent, phenolic detergent, quaternary ammonium detergent or aldehyde associations (1%).

Sodium hypochlorite is a useful option, but it cannot be used in metals due to its corrosive effect. In addition, it becomes inactivated in contact with organic matter. Iodine derivates also corrode metals, and commercial presentations are usually for performing antisepsia rather than disinfection. Phenolic products are difficult to manipulate because they are easily absorbed by porous materials; the residual disinfectant may irritate tissue even when thoroughly rinsed, and the high rates of skin and mucous absorption may have neurotoxic effects.

Recommendations for Environment

As ICUs are high-risk areas, the use of two aldehydes associated for daily cleaning is recommended. There is no evidence that special disinfectants are required for controlling multidrug-resistant microorganisms. However, it is known that the most common gentamicin-resistant plasmid also codes for resistance to quaternary ammonium disinfectants.

The infection control measures for avoiding water transmission are based on: to keep the internal hospital water system waretight, to maintain residual free chlorine between 0.2 and 0.6 ml/l and to perform periodical cleaning with low-level disinfectants of water containers as well as tapwater in showers and handwashers. Meticulous scrubbing to remove encrusted particles is recommended.

Air transmission is controlled by cleaning and periodically removing the filters, pipes, air collector and air exits, with special attention to cleaning and disinfecting the final pipe sections between the last filter and the air exit to the ICU.

Rules for Storing and Handling Sterile Equipment in the Unit

Equipment should be stored in closed locations to protect it from dust. Before opening the wrapping, make sure it is not wet, dirty or broken; otherwise it cannot be used. The wrapper should be opened aseptically. Ensure that the interior packaging has been chemically controlled. If it is not correct it must be returned and reprocessed in the Central Sterilization Unit.

Conclusions

Rigorous cleaning, followed by a correctly performed disinfection or sterilization process and adequate storage of medical instruments is necessary to reduce the risk of infections. Complete information must be provided and followed in order to guarantee reprocessing of devices and to avoid damage to materials.

The Infection Control Committee at each Health Care Center should set down guidelines for the type of disinfectants to be used, and should also advise on the appropriate concentrations. It should determine the cleaning strategy, bearing in mind the center's epidemiologic pattern, the toxicity of the products and other possible risks to personnel or patients, and should also seek to reduce the environmental impact of chemical residues caused by the process.

References

1. Meenhorst PI, Reingold AL, Groothvis DG. Water-related nosocomial pneumonia caused by *Legionella pneumophila* serogroup 1 and 10. J Infect Dis 152:356, 1985.
2. Armon PM, Chou T, Weil D. Nosocomial Legionnaire's disease caused by aerosolized tap water from respiratory device. J Infect Dis 146: 460, 1982.
3. Irwin RS, Demers RR, Pratter MR. An outbreak of *Acinetobacter* infection associated with the use of a ventilator spirometer. Respir Care 25:232, 1980.
4. Cefai C, Richards J, Gould FK. An outbreak of *Acinetobacter* respiratory tract infection resulting from incomplete disinfection of ventilatory equipment. J Hosp Infect 15:177, 1990.
5. Reeves DS, Brown NM. Mycobacterial contamination of fiberoptic bronchoscopes. J Hosp Infect 30 (suppl):531, 1995.
6. Spach DH, Silverstein FE, Stamm WE. Transmission of infection by gastrointestinal endoscopy and bronchoscopy. Ann Intern Med 118:117, 1993.
7. Weber DJ, Wilson MB, Rutala WA, Thomann CA. Manual ventilation bags as a source of bacterial colonization of intubated patients. Am Rev Respir Dis 142:892, 1990.
8. Gauthier DK, Long M. Colonization of mechanical ventilation bags during use. Am J Infect Control 22:358, 1994.
9. Hanson PJV, Chadwick EP, Gaya H, Collins JV. A study of gluteraldehyde disinfection of fiberoptic bronchoscopes experimentally contaminated with *Mycobacterium tuberculosis*. J Hosp Infect 22: 137, 1992.
10. Hanson PJV, Gor D, Clarke JR. Recovery of the human immunodeficiency virus from fiberoptic bronchoscopes. Thorax 46:410, 1991.
11. Spaulding EH. Chemical disinfection of medical and surgical materials. In Lawrence CA, Block SS (eds). Disinfection, Sterilization and Preservation. Philadelphia: Lea & Febiger, 1968:517.
12. Favero MS, Bond WW. Chemical disinfection of medical and surgical materials. In Block SS (ed). Disinfection, Sterilization and Preservation. 4th edn, Philadelpia: Lea & Febiger, 1991:617.
13. Rutala WA. APIC guideline for selection and use of disinfectants. Am J Infect Control 2:99, 1990.
14. Garner JS, Favero MS. CDC guidelines for hand washing and hospital environment control. Infect Control 7:231, 1986.
15. The Hospital Infection Control Practices Advisory Committee (HICPAC). Guideline for prevention of nosocomial pneumonia. Am J Infect Control 22:247, 1994.
16. Martin MA, Reichelderfer M. APIC guideline for infection prevention and control in flexible endoscopy. Am J Infect Control 22:19, 1994.

20. ANTIBIOTIC RESISTANCE IN THE ICU

H. Lode, R. Erbes, H. Geerdes-Fenge, M. Raffenberg and H. Mauch

Introduction

Patients hospitalized in ICUs are 5–10 times more likely to acquire nosocomial infections than other hospital patients. The frequency of infections at different anatomic sites and the risk of infection vary by the type of ICU, and the frequency of specific pathogens varies by infection site. Contributing to the seriousness of nosocomial infections, especially in ICUs is the increasing incidence of infections caused by antibiotic-resistant pathogens. Antimicrobial resistance has resulted in increased morbidity and mortality as well as higher health care costs. Yearly expenditures arising from drug-resistance in the United States are estimated to approach $4 billion and are rising [1–3].

The emergence of resistance is a result of factors such as increased use and misuse of antimicrobial agents, increased use of invasive devices and procedures, a greater number of susceptible hosts, and lapses in infection control practices leading to increased transmission of resistant organisms. In the hospital, widespread use of antimicrobials in the ICU and for immunocompromised patients has resulted in the selection of multidrug-resistant organisms [1].

Epidemiology

Microorganisms have a remarkable array of mechanisms with which to overcome the effects of antimicrobial agents (Table 1). These include the production of structure-altering or inactivating enzymes (e.g. beta-lactamase- or aminoglycoside-modifying enzymes), alteration of penicillin-binding proteins or other cell-wall target sites, altered DNA topoisomerase targets, permeability mutations, and ribosomal modification [4–7]. Selective pressure resulting from antimicrobial administration can lead to the growth of previously susceptible strains that have acquired resistance or to the overgrowth of strains that are intrinsically resistant. The emergence of *Stenotrophomonas maltophilia* during imipenem therapy is an example of selection of intrinsically antibiotic-resistant strains. In general, resistance is acquired by mutational change or by the acquisition of resistance-encoding genetic material. Increased use of antimicrobial agents in clinical practice as well as the enormous quantities of antibiotics employed in agriculture, fisheries, and animal husbandry provide conditions favorable to the selection of resistance microorganisms [8]. Transferable plasmids may possess genes encoding resistance to a wide range of antimicrobial agents. Thus, for Gram-positive and Gram-negative organisms, a single transfer event can result in the acquisition of several antimicrobial resistance determinants. Virtually all major bacterial pathogens have acquired antimicrobial resistance genes.

The most representative data on nosocomial infection rates have been provided by the National Nosocomial Infection Surveillance (NNIS) System [10]. Surveillance data from ICUs are available from this system for the years 1986 through 1997 [11] and have shown that the relative frequency of different sites of nosocomial infections (ie. ventilator-associated pneumonia, bloodstream infections, urinary tract

TABLE 1. Resistance mechanisms

Antibiotics	Mechanisms	Pathogens	Current Crisis	Future Crisis
β-Lactams Penicillins Cephalosporins Monobactams Carbapenems	Altered penicillin-binding proteins	*S. aureus* *Staphylococcus epidermidis* *S. pneumoniae* *Streptococcus sanguis* *H. influenzae* *N. gonorrhoeae* *N. meningitidis* *E. coli* *P. aeruginosa*	*S. pneumoniae* *S. epidermidis*	*N. meningitidis*
	Reduced permeability	*P. aeruginosa* *E. cloacae* *S. marcescens* *K. pneumoniae* *Klebsiella oxytoca*	*P. aeruginosa* *E. cloacae*	*Serratia marcescens* *K. pneumoniae*
	β-Lactamase	*S. aureus* *S. epidermidis* *Enterococci* *P. aeruginosa* *Enterobacteriaceae* *N. gonorrhoeae* *N. meningitidis* *Moraxella* *Bacteroides* *Acinetobacter*	*Xanthomonas* *Acinetobacter*	*Bacteroides* *N. meningitidis* *Enterobacteriaceae* *Salmonella* *Shigella* *Haemophilus* *Enterococci*
Fluoroquinolones Norfloxacin Ofloxacin Ciprofloxacin	Altered DNA gyrase	*S. aureus* *S. epidermidis* *Enterobacteriaceae* *Pseudomonads*	MRSA	*Pseudomonads* *Enterobacteriaceae* *Haemophilus* *N. gonorrhoeae*
Lomefloxacin	Reduced permeability	*Enterobacteriaceae* *P. aeruginosa*	*Serratia* *P. aeruginosa*	*Enterobacteriaceae*
Macrolides-lincosamides Erythromycin Clindamycin	Methylating enzymes	*Streptococci* *S. pneumoniae* *Enterococci* *Staphylococci*	*Enterococci*	*S. pneumoniae* *Staphylococcus pyogenes* *Staphylococcus agalactiae* *Mycobacterium tuberculosis*
Glycopeptides Vancomycin Teicoplanin	Altered target	*Enterococci* *Leuconostoc* *Lactococcus* *Pediococcus* *Lactobacillus* *Staphylococcus haemolyticus*	*E. faecium*	MRSA Methicillin-resistant *S. epidermidis* Streptococci

From [1].

infections) and the absolute risk of infection (per 1.000 device days) vary by type of ICU; the relative frequency of different nosocomial pathogens varies by site of infection (Table 2); and the site-specific rates of nosocomial infections and similar types of ICUs vary 10- to 20-fold among hospitals [2, 11, 12]. Main concerns in US ICUs are vancomycin resistant *Enterococcus sp* (VRE) [13–15], extended spectrum beta-lactamase-producing Gram-negative bacilli [16], multidrug-resistant *Mycobacteria tuberculosis* [17], fluconazole-resistant *Candida* sp [18] and more recently, strains of *S. aureus* with reduced susceptibility to vancomycin – because such strains have now been isolated in Japan and the United States [19]. This concern has been fueled by multiple reports of outbreaks of infection caused by these pathogens and increasing rates of endemic infection in ICU patients. However, only limited data are available regarding the prevalence of these pathogens in ICUs throughout the United States. Data obtained from the NNIS documents the increasing frequency of VRE in US hospitals [20] (Figure 1). Archibald *et al.* [3] reported the prevalence of drug resistant pathogens isolated from different patient populations of eight hospitals between 1994 and 1995 (Table 3). For five of the antimicrobial pathogen combinations, the percentage of resistant isolates was significantly higher in the ICU than in the two other settings [3].

In the European Prevalence of Infection in Intensive Care (EPIC) study covering 1,417 ICUs with 10,038 patient case reports a total infection rate of 44.8% was observed and 2,604 patients (20.6%) had an ICU-acquired infection: pneumonia (46.9%), lower respiratory tract infection (17.8%), urinary tract infection (17.6%), and blood-stream infection (12%) were the most frequent types of ICU infection reported [21]. Most frequently isolated microorganisms were *Enterobacteriaceae* (34.4%), *Staphylococcus aureus* (30.1%), *Pseudomonas aeruginosa* (28.7%), coagulase-negative staphylococci (19.1%), and fungi (17.1%). Information concerning the patterns of antimicrobial resistance was recorded in the study for *S. aureus*, *P. aeruginosa*, and coagulase-negative staphylococci. Of the 528 ICU-acquired infections associated with *S. aureus*, resistance patterns were reported in 456 (86%). Of these 456 infections, 59.6% were associated with methicillin-resistant *S. aureus* strains (MRSA). In those laboratory-confirmed bacteremias in which *S. aureus* was cultured, 72.4% of strains were MRSAs. The highest prevalences of MRSA were found in Italy (81%) and France (78.4%). Of 504 ICU-acquired infections associated with an appropriate positive

TABLE 2. Major infection sites

Bloodstream		Pneumonia		Surgical Site		Urinary Tract	
Pathogen	%	Pathogen	%	Pathogen	%	Pathogen	%
CoNs	33.5	*Pseudomonas aeruginosa*	17.4	*Enterococcus spp*	15.3	*Escherichia coli*	19.2
S. aureus	13.4	*S. aureus*	17.4	CoNs	12.6	*C. albicans*	14.4
Enterococcus sp	12.8	*Enterobacter sp*	11.4	*S. aureus*	11.2	*Enterococcus sp*	14.1
Candida albicans	5.8	*Klebsiella pneumonia*	6.7	*P. aeruginosa*	10.3	*P. aeruginosa*	11.2
Enterobacter sp	5.2	*Haemophilus influenzae*	4.9	*Enterobacter sp*	9.5	*K. pneumoniae*	
Other	29.3	Other	42.2	Other	41.1	Other	35.3
Total	100.0	Total	100.0	Total	100.0	Total	100.0

From [2].
CoNs = Coagulase-negative staphylococci.

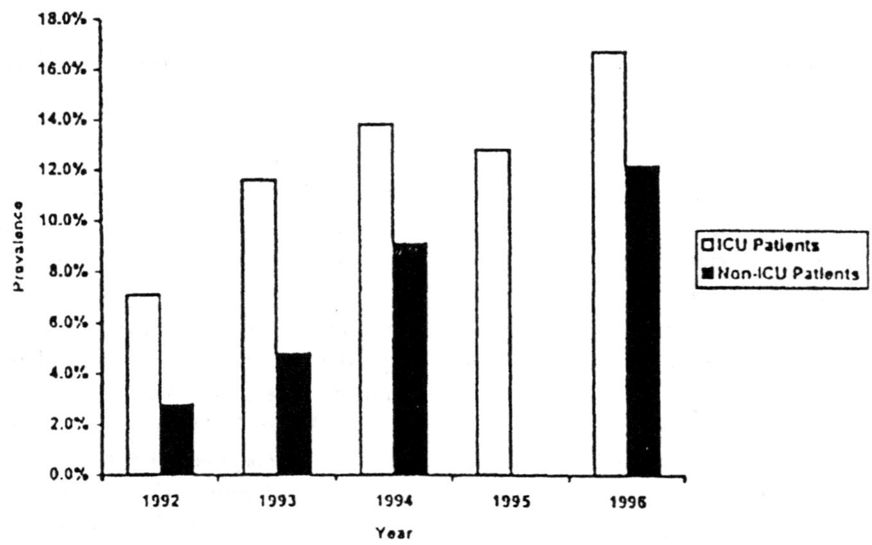

FIGURE 1. Nosocomial Enterococcus in the United States, 1992 through 1996. From Summary of Notifiable Diseases, United States, 1996 *MMWR*.

TABLE 3. Pathogenic combination

	No. of Resistant Isolates/Total No. of Isolates Tested (%)		
Antimicriobial/Pathogen Combination	Inpatients	Outpatients	P Value
Methicillin/coagulase-negative *Staphylococcus*	922/1.881 (49.0)	250/796 (35.9)	<0.01
Methicillin/*S. aureus*	861/2.633 (32.7)	233/1.594 (14.6)	<0.01
Ceftazidime/*Enterobacter cloacae*	145/559 (26.0)	15/126 (11.9)	<0.01
Imipenem/*P aeruginosa*	164/1.368 (12.0)	31/477 (6.5)	<0.01
Ceftazidime/*P aeruginosa*	147/1.889 (7.8)	25/631 (4.0)	<0.01
Vancomycin/*Enterococcus sp*	92/1.459 (6.3)	8/575 (1.4)	<0.01
Ciprofloxacin/*E coli*	16/3.189 (0.5)	28/3.997 (0.7)	NS
Ceftazidime/*E coli*	5/2.348 (0.2)	9/1.887 (0.5)	NS

From [3].

culture of *P. aeruginosa*, patterns of resistance were reported in 410 cases. Of these, 267 isolates (65.1%) were resistant to one or more of the following: gentamicin (46.3% of resistant isolates), imipenem (21.1%), ceftazidime (27.7%), ciprofloxacin (26.3%), or a ureidopenicillin (37.4%). Of the 335 ICU-acquired infections associated with a positive culture of coagulase-negative staphylococci, resistance patterns were reported in 279 cases; 204 isolates (73.1%) were resistant to one or more of the following: methicillin (70.1% of isolates resistant), cefotaxime (68.6%), gentamicin (66.1%), vancomycin (3.5%), and teicoplanin (9.3%) [21].

RISK FACTORS FOR RESISTANCE DEVELOPMENT

Multiple case-control studies have analyzed the risk factors associated with infection or colonization with MRSA or VRE. Both univariate analysis in individual case studies and multivariate analysis have demonstrated that antibiotic exposure and cephalosporin use are risk factors for infection with MRSA [22–24].

Risk factors for ventilator-associated pneumonia caused by potentially drug-resistant bacteria such as MRSA, *P. aeruginosa*, *A. baumannii* and/or *S. maltophilia* were analyzed in 135 consecutive episodes of VAP observed in a single ICU in Paris over a 25 month period. 70–77 episodes were caused by "potentially resistant" bacteria and 58 episodes were caused by "other" organisms. According to logistic regression analysis three variables among potential factors remain significant: duration of mechanical ventilation ≥7 days (OR = 6.0), prior antibiotic use (OR = 13.5), and prior use of broad spectrum drugs (3. generation cephalosporin, fluoroquinolone, and/or imipenem) (OR = 4.1). Although 22 episodes of early-onset VAP in patients receiving no prior antibiotic were caused by antibiotic-susceptible bacteria, 84 episodes of late-onset VAP in patients receiving prior antibiotics were mainly caused by potentially resistant bacteria [25].

Despite high dosages and focused treatment orientated on bacteriologic results it is well-known that specific pathogens like *S. aureus* and *P. aeruginosa* are difficult to eradicate in ventilated patients and these strains will develop resistance in short time during treatment [26].

Multi-drug-resistant *Acinetobacter baumannii* have become a considerable concern in several US and European ICUs. In a national Spanish surveillance system covering 49 Spanish hospitals most VAPs caused by Gram-negative bacilli were due to *P. aeruginosa* (22%) followed by *A. baumannii* (13%); in contrast with *P. aeruginosa*, the pattern of *A. baumannii* distribution was patchy and only 10 of the 49 hospitals had at least three *A. baumannii* episodes [27]. In a case-controlled study from Cleveland 15 cases of *A. baumannii* nosocomial pneumonia were analyzed [28]. Seven of these patients were bacteremic and the mean duration time from admission to the ICU to infection was 12.8 days. Sepsis developed in 35% of the patients and 43% of the case patients died during their hospitalization, with two of those deaths attributed to *Acinetobacter* infection. Univariate analysis showed that prior use of ceftazidime was associated with infection with *Acinetobacter*. However, the epidemiologic pattern of resistant *A. baumannii* strains may vary from hospital to hospital. Individual therapeutic approaches should be customized to each institution [28]. Emerging resistance problems limit the utility of currently available antibacterial agents [29].

Many factors can contribute to the development of bacterial resistance to anti-infective agents, but one of the most important risk factors is repeated exposure to sub-optimal antibiotic concentrations. Pharmacodynamic data, which describe the relationship between drug serum concentration and the pharmacologic effects of the drug, may be useful in designing regimens that minimize the likelihood of exposing pathogens to sub-lethal-drug levels [30, 31]. The pharmacodynamic parameters that correlate with clinical success differ for concentration-dependent drugs whereas those that are relatively concentration independent (Table 4). For fluoroquinolones and aminoglycosides, optimal dosing means maintaining high maximum peak centrum to MIC ratios. Pharmacodynamic data thus predict problems with resistance may arise when fluoroquinolones are used to treat pathogens with high MIC values, such as *Pseudomonas*, because the highest drug levels attained are only approximately four to five times the MIC; the optimal level would be ten times the MIC. For beta-lactam agents, increasing the duration of time above the MIC should help prevent the emergence of resistance. For drugs with relatively short half-lives, levels four to five times the MIC can be maintained over extended intervals by more frequent dosing

TABLE 4. Pharmacodynamic characteristics of antimicrobial agents

Pharmacodynamic Characteristic	Representative Antimicrobial Agents	Goal of Regimen	Parameters Correlating with clinical efficacy
Concentration-dependent killing	Aminoglycosides, fluoroquinolones, metronidazole	Maximize concentrations	Ratio of maximum peak concentration to MIC; ratio of AUC to MIC
Concentration-independent killing	Penicillins, cephalosporins, aztreonam	Maximize exposure time	Time above MIC levels

From [31].

TABLE 5. Infection control

Infection Control Measures
1. Identify reservoir – Colonized and infected patients – Environmental contamination, common sources
2. Halt transmission among patients – Improve hand washing and asepsis – Barrier precautions (gloves, gown) for colonized and infected patients – Eliminate any common source; disinfect environment – Separate susceptible patients – Close unit to new admissions if necessary
3. Halt progression from colonization to infection – Discontinue compromising factors when possible (eg. extubate, remove, nasogastric tube, discontinue bladder catheters, as clinically indicated; rotate IV catheter sites; proper ventilator and pulmonary care)
4. Modify host factors – Treat underlying disease and complications – Control antibiotic use (rotate, restrict, or cease)

From [44].

or by continuous infusion [31]. These pharmacodynamic considerations are only beginning to be tested in clinical setting [32] however, if these pharmacodynamic predictions are confirmed, it will suggest that clinicians need to consider pharmacodynamic properties when choosing antibiotic therapy. Choosing the right dose and dosing interval may also be critical to achieving optimal clinical responses and preventing the emergence of resistant pathogens.

IMPLICATIONS OF RESISTANCE DEVELOPMENT

Infections with resistance microorganisms have serious consequences such as significantly prolonged ICU stays, increased morbidity and health-care costs. However, there is debate about true mortality associated with resistant bacteria, because affected patients frequently suffer from severe or even untreatable underlying conditions [34]. The EPIC study and a group from Brazil showed mortality rates from MRSA three and four times higher than from methicillin susceptible *S. aureus* (MSSA) [35, 36]. whereas others could not confirm these data [37]. In contrast, results for mortality due to vancomycin resistant enterococci (VRE) bacteremia compared with those sensitive to vancomycin (VSE) did not show significant rises in mortality, but significantly longer hospital stays [38]. In comparison with historic controls without VRE bacteremia, however, a risk ratio for mortality of 2.3 for VRE bacteremia was reported [39].

Nosocomial infections with multi-resistant pathogens are usually associated with a high death rate. Physicians in Paris analyzed the relationship between VAP due to *Pseudomonas or Acinetobacter* species and death by comparing the outcomes for patients colonized with these pathogens with those for patients with pneumonia due to these pathogens. Mortality rates were 29% among colonized patients and 73% among patients with VAP [40].

PREVENTION IN CONTROL OF ANTIMICROBIAL RESISTANCE

Concensus statements have been published that delineate strategies to prevent and control the emergence and spread of antimicrobial resistant microorganisms in hospitals [41, 42]. Prevention strategies are based on minimizing the transmission of antibiotic resistant pathogens between patients and developing a program to prevent or reduce antimicrobial resistance (Table 4). The CDC has published general isolation guidelines to minimize the risk of transmission of infection agents from colonized/infected patients to other patients or health-care providers [43]. General and traditional infection control measures in the ICU (and detailed infection control recommendations) have been published to minimize the transmission of MRSA, VRE and *S. aureus* with reduced susceptibility to vancomycin (GISA).

Regarding the use of antibiotics and pharmacological actions that can alter the resistance pattern, the following options exist [47]:

1. To abolish or limit the use of the particular agent(s) and thus try to induce a change in the trend of resistance.
2. To decrease the duration of therapy and thus attempt to change resistance patterns.
3. To manipulate the dose of the antibiotics administered and thus attempt to change the pattern of resistance.
4. To rotate antibiotics and thus to decrease antibiotic pressure.
5. To use antibiotic combinations.

However, all these strategies need to be investigated, developed and validated.

Conclusion

ICUs are generally considered epicenters of antibiotic resistance and the principal sources of outbreaks of multi-resistant bacteria (Chapter 22). Antibiotic resistant bacteria can emerge in three main ways – by acquisition of new genes via transposons or horizontal gene transfer, by selection of resistant variants and by selection of naturally resistant strains. The most important risk factors are deficits in prevention and infection control measures, excessive consumption of antibiotics, the frequent use of invasive devices and the relative density of a susceptible patient population with severe underlying diseases. Infections due to antibiotic-resistant bacteria have a major impact on morbidity and health-care costs. Increased mortality, however, is not uniformly shown for all these organisms: MRSA, *Pseudomonas sp.* and multi-resistant Gram-negative enterobacteria seem to cause higher mortality, in contrast to vancomycin-resistant enterococci (VRE). Programs to prevent and control the development of resistant organisms (Chapter 21) should focus on the implementation of optimal infection control measures (Chapter 18) and some reasonable pharmacological actions to use antibiotics properly.

References

1. File TM. Overview of resistance in the 1990s. Chest 115(Suppl. 3):3, 1999.
2. Weber DJ, Raasch R, Rutala W. The growing importance of antibiotic-resistant pathogens. Chest 115(Suppl. 3):34, 1999.
3. Archibald L, Phillips L, Monnet D, *et al.* Antimicrobial resistance in isolates from inpatients and outpatients in the United States: increasing importance of the intensive care unit. Clin Infect Dis 24:211, 1997.
4. Neu HC. The crisis in antibiotic resistance. Science 257:1064, 1992.
5. Tomasz A. Multiple-antibiotic-resistant pathogenic bacteria: a report on the Rockefeller University Workshop. N Engl J Med 330:1247, 1994.
6. Gold HS, Moellering RC. Antimicrobial-drug resistance. N Engl J Med 335:1445, 1996.
7. Thornsberry C. Trends in antimicrobial resistance among today's bacterial pathogens. Pharmacotherapy 15:3, 1995.
8. Feinman SE. Antibiotics in animal feed – drug resistance revisited. ASM News 64:24, 1998.
9. Shlaes DM, Rice LB. Emerging mechanisms of β-lactam resistance: an update. Infect Dis Clin Prac 15:35, 1995.
10. Emorit G, Culver DH, Horan TC, *et al.* National nosocomial infections surveillance system

(NNIS): description of surveillance methods. AM J Infect Control 19:19, 1991.

11. National Nosocomial Infections Surveillance (NNIS) report. Data summary from October 1986–April 1997, issued May 1997: a report from the NNIS System. Am J Infect Control 25:477, 1997.
12. Mulligan ME, Standiford HC, Kauffman CA. Methicillin-resistant *Staphylococcus aureus:* a consensus review of the microbiology, pathogenesis, and epidemiology with implications for prevention and management. Am J Med 94:313, 1993.
13. Murray BE. Vancomycin-resistant enterococci. Am J Med 102:284, 1997.
14. Eliopoulos GM. Vancomycin-resistant enterococci: mechanism and clinical relevance. Infect Dis Clin North Am 11:851, 1997.
15. Boyce JM. Vancomycin-resistant *enterococcus:* detection, epidemiology, and control measures. Infect Dis Clin North Am 11:367, 1997.
16. Paterson DL, Ko WC, Mohapatra S, *et al.* Klebsiella pneumoniae bacteremia: impact of extended spectrum beta-lactamase (ESBL) production in a global study of 216 patients [abstract]. 37th Interscience Conference on Antimicrobial Agents and Chemotherapy, Sept 28–Oct 1, 1997; Toronto, Ontario, Canada.
17. Flament-Saillour M, Robert J, Jarlier V, Grosset J. Outcome of multi-drug-resistant tuberculosis in France. Am J Respir Crit Care Med 1260:587, 1999.
18. White TC, Marr KA, Bowden RA. Clinical, cellular and molecular factors that contribute to antifungal drug resistance. Clin Microbiol Rev 11:382, 1998.
19. Vedel G, Lervez M, Lemann F, *et al.* Prevalence of *Staphylococcus aureus* and coagulase-negative staphylococci with decreased sensitivity to glycopeptides as assessed by determination of MICs. Eur J Clin Microbiol Infect Dis 9:820, 1990.
20. CDC. Summary of notifiable diseases, United States, 1996. MMWR 45:1, 1997.
21. Vincent J-L, Bihari DJ, Suter PM, Bruining HA, White J, Nicolas-Chanoin M-H, Wolff M, Spencer RC, Hemmer M, for the EPIC International Adisory Committee. JAMA 274:639, 1995.
22. Law MR, Gill ON. Hospital-acquired infection with methicillin-resistant and methicillin-sensitive staphylococci. Epidemiol Infect 101:623, 1988.
23. Hershow RC, Khayr WF, Smith NL. A comparison of clinical virulence of nosocomially acquired methicillin-resistant and methicillin-sensitive *Staphylococcus aureus* bacteriuria in a skilled-care nursing home. Arch Fam Med 3:357, 1994.
24. Washio M, Mizoue T, Kajioka T, *et al.* Risk factors for methicillin-resistant *Staphylococcus aureus* (MRSA) infection in a Japanese geriatric hospital. Public Health 111:187, 1997.
25. Trouillet J-L, Chastre J, Vuagnat A, Jloy-Guillou M-L, Combaux D, Dombret M-C, Gibert C. Ventilator-associated pneumonia caused by potentially drug-resistant bacteria. Am J Resp Crit Care Med 157:531, 1998.
26. Fink MP, Snydman DR, Niederman MS, *et al.*, for the Severe Pneumonia Study Group. Treatment of severe pneumonia in hospitalized patients: results of a multi-center, randomized, double-blind trial comparing intravenous ciprofloxacin with imipenem-cilastatin. Antimicrob Agents Chemother 3:547, 1994.
27. Rello J, Ausina V, Ricart M, Castella J, Prats G. Impact of previous antimicrobial therapy on the etiology and outcome of ventilator-associated pneumonia. Chest 194:1230, 1993.
28. Husni RN, Goldstein LS, Arroliga AC, Hall GS, Fatica C, Stoller JK, Gordon SM. Risk factors for an outbreak of multi-drug-resistant *Acinetobacter* nosocomial pneumonia among intubated patients. Chest 115:1379, 1999.
29. Jones RN. The emergent needs for basic research, education, and surveillance of antimicrobial resistance. Diagn Microbiol Infect Dis 25:1, 1996.
30. Schentag JJ, Birmingham MC, Paladino JA. In nosocomial pneumonia optimizing antibiotics other than aminoglycosides is a more important determinant of successful clinical outcome, and a better means of avoiding resistance. Semin Respir Infect 12:279, 1997.
31. Burgess DS. Pharmacodynamic principles of antimicrobial therapy in the prevention of resistance. Chest 115(Suppl.):19, 1999.
32. Drusano GL. Infection in the intensive care unit: b-lactamase-medicated resistance among Enterobacteriaceae and optimal antimicrobial dosing. Clin Infect Dis 27(Suppl. 1):111, 1998.
33. Thomas JK, Forrest A, Bhavnani SM, *et al.* Pharmacodynamic evaluation of factors associated with the development of bacterial resistance in acutely ill patients during therapy. Antimicrob Agents Chemother 42:521, 1998.
34. Albrich WC, Angstwurm M, Bader L, Gärtner R. Drug resistance in intensive care units. Infection 27(Suppl.):19, 1999.
35. Ibelings MM, Bruining HA. Methicillin-

resistant *Staphylococcus aureus:* acquisition and risk of death in patients in the intensive care unit. Eur J Surg 164:411, 1998.
36. Conterno LO, Wey SB, Castelo A. Risk factors for mortality in *Staphylococcus aureus* bacteremia. Infect Control Hosp Epidemiol 19:32, 1998.
37. Harbarth S, Rutschmann O, Sudre P, Pittet D. Impact of methicillin resistance on the outcome of patients with bacteremia caused by *Staphylococcus aureus*. Arch Intern Med 26:182, 1998.
38. Mainous MR, Lipsett PA, O'Brien M. Enterococcal bacteremia in the surgical intensive care unit. Does vancomycin resistance affect mortality? The John Hopkins SICU Study Group. Arch Surg 132:76, 1997.
39. Edmond MB, Ober JF, Dawson JD, Weinbaum DL, Wenzel RP. Vancomycin-resistant enterococcal bacteremia: natural history and attributable mortality. Clin Infect Dis 23:1234, 1996.
40. Fagon JY, Chastre J, Domart Y, Trouillet JL, Gibert C. Mortality due to ventilator-associated pneumonia or colonization with *Pseudomonas or Acinetobacter species*: Assessment by quantitative culture of samples obtained by a protected specimen brush.
41. Goldmann DA, Weinstein RA, Wenzel RP, *et al.* Strategies to prevent and control the emergence and spread of antimicrobial-resistant microorganisms in hopsitals: a challenge to hospital leadership. JAMA 275:234, 1996.
42. Shlaes DM, Gerding DN, John JF, *et al.* Society of America Joint Committee on the Prevention of Antimicrobial Resistance: guidelines for the prevention of antimicrobial resistance in hospitals. Clin Infec Dis 25:584, 1997.
43. Garner JS. Hospital Infection Control Practices Advisory Committee: guideline for isolation precautions in hospitals. Infect Control Hosp Epidemiol 17:53, 1996.
44. Weinstein RA. Epidemiology and control of nosocomial infections in adult intensive care units. Am J Med 91(Suppl. 3B):17, 1991.
45. Wenzel RP, Reagan DR, Bertino JS, *et al.* Methicillin-resistant *Staphylococcus aureus* outbreak: a consensus panel's definition and management guidelines. Am J Infect Control 26: 102, 1996.
46. CDC. Recommendations for preventing the spread of vancomycin resistance: recommendations of the Hospital Infection Control Practices Advisory Committee (HICPAC) MMWR 44:1, 1994.

21. EPIDEMIC INFECTIONS IN THE ICU: MULTIRESISTANT MICROORGANISMS

Marc J.M. Bonten

Nosocomial problems with antibiotic resistant microorganisms have occurred in several stages over the last 40 years. After the first recognition of antibiotic resistance of *S. aureus* to penicillin in the 1950s, emergence of Gram-negative bacteria resistant to multiple antibiotics became prominent in the 1970s and 1980s. Concerns about (multi-)resistance among nosocomial Gram-positive bacteria re-emerged in the late 1980s. Currently, the most important nosocomial resistance problems on a global scale are caused by methicillin-resistant *S. aureus* (MRSA), vancomycin-resistant enterococci (VRE), *Enterobacteriaceae* with plasmid-encoded extended-spectrum beta-lactamases (ESBL), and *Pseudomonas aeruginosa*.

Intensive Care Units (ICUs) are classically the settings where antibiotics are used most intensively and, as a result, where many problems with antibiotic resistance become evident. Here, I describe the characteristics of nosocomial epidemics of four groups of multi-resistant nosocmial pathogens; VRE, MRSA, ESBL-producing Enterobacteriaceae, and *P. aeruginosa*. Despite the differences in bacterial species, the differences in mechanisms of resistance, the different ecological niches and the different infections caused by these pathogens, there are striking similarities in the variables determining nosocomial spread. The existence of each of these multi-resistant microorganisms and their concurrent spread seem to result from extensive antibiotic use and lapses in compliance with infection control measures. Problems with these bacteria become evident as monoclonal outbreaks, soon followed by establishment of endemicity. Finally, endemicity seems to be established on general hospital wards and in chronic care facilities and nursing homes, creating a continuous influx of colonized patients into special care wards.

Routes of Colonization

Nosocomial infections are usually preceded by colonization. Actually, infections with multiresistant pathogens represent only the tip of the iceberg. When infections emerge, colonization has already occurred in a large proportion of patients. In many ICUs endemicity with multiple resistant pathogens has been established. The proportion of patients being colonized in ICU may be more or less stable, with low or high levels of endemicity, or may fluctuate, with epidemic rises and periods without any patient being colonized. These changes in endemic prevalences of colonization are created by changes in the dynamics of the different routes of colonization. Resistant bacteria may be introduced into the ICU by a single colonized patient or may be introduced on a regular basis, because of a continuous source of colonized patients outside the ICU. In the latter scenario, continuous admission of colonized patients may create an important variable in the dynamics of colonization in ICUs.

Colonization may also be derived from endogenous sources, such as the gut. Pathogens may be part of the normal gut flora, where they reside in low amounts. However, when intestinal ecology is disturbed by illness, or more likely, by antibiotics, resistant bacteria may overgrow and colonize other body sites, such as the respiratory tract. This route of colonization has been demonstrated to be relevant for enteric Gram-negative bacteria and *P. aeruginosa* [1, 2].

Furthermore, microorganisms may be derived from exogenous sources, such as contaminated environment or other colonized patients. Multiple epidemics originating from contaminated surfaces or medical devices have been described. In addition, the concept of cross-colonization is probably known to all physicians working in ICUs. Microorganisms can be transferred from patient to patient via the hands of health care workers and physicians.

Epidemics and the establishment of endemicity of colonization with any pathogen results from the interaction of these four routes of colonization. Although the final result of colonization, e.g. infection, is identical for all pathogens, the relevance of these routes may differ considerably. Different pathogens may have different dynamics of colonization, and for a certain pathogen the dynamics may differ between different wards. For example, the relevance of cross-colonization may differ between wards. Knowledge about the relevance of these different routes is essential when designing infection control strategies.

Vancomycin Resistant Enterococci (VRE)

Enterococci are gram-positive bacteria, which traditionally have been considered to be of low pathogenicity [3]. However, they are among the bacteria most frequently isolated from nosocomial infections. In the National Nosocomial Infections Surveillance System, performed in US hospitals, enterococci accounted for 10% of all clinical isolates reported to the system during the period 1990 until 1993 [4]. Enterococci generally are recovered from urinary tract infections, and in mixed bacterial flora in intra-abdominal infections and wound infections. Occasionally enterococci cause severe infections such as endocarditis, pneumonia and meningitis, and enterococcal bloodstream infections can be associated with a high mortality rate [3, 5, 6]. *E. faecium* and *E. faecalis* account for most clinical enterococcal isolates [3, 7].

Enterococci are intrinsically resistant to many classes of antibiotics (such as semisynthetic penicillinase-resistant penicillins, cephalosporins, trimethoprim-sulfamethoxazole, and clindamycin), and have acquired resistance to even more antibiotics, following the introduction and wide-spread use of these agents [3]. Resistance to vancomycin among enterococci was first reported from Europe in the 1980s [8, 9] and was described to be plasmid-mediated in 1988 [10]. The latter facilitates rapid spread of resistance genes among enterococci and even to staphylococci [11], which, however, has yet only been demonstrated *in vitro*.

There are several phenotypes of vancomycin-resistance. The *vanA* type has high-level resistance to vancomycin and teicoplanin and is usually mediated by self-transferable plasmids that bear transposons (related to Tn1546). The *van*B type remains susceptible to teicoplanin and is transferable by conjugation of large genetic elements from chromosome to chromosome [12].

EPIDEMIOLOGY OF VRE

Percentages of VRE among nosocomial enterococcal isolates in US hospitals increased from 0.4% in 1989 to 13.6% in 1993 in ICUs [13]. A similar increase was noted in non-ICU wards in recent years, especially in large teaching hospitals and initially on the east coast of the US [13]. Initially, outbreaks of VRE-infections were monoclonal and occurred in high-care settings, such as oncology wards, renal units and ICUs [14–20]. However, in many large hospitals, multiple clones of VRE are responsible for high rates of gastrointestinal tract colonization [21–24], and it is estimated that for each patient with a clinical isolate of VRE as many as ten other patients may be colonized. In these settings, intestinal colonization with VRE is now endemic with up to 50% of patients in ICUs colonized [23]. From acute care facilities, dissemination of VRE to long-term care facilities may occur from resident transfer [25].

Epidemiological studies have elucidated, at least in part, why VRE have spread within, and even between, US hospitals so rapidly in recent years. Colonization of the gastrointestinal tract and skin have been demonstrated to be persistent in ill patients, and transient contamination of the inanimate environment (e.g. electronic thermometers, monitoring devices, blood pressure cuffs, stethoscopes, electrocardiographic monitors, bedrails and air cushions [15, 21, 26]) frequently occurs. VRE seem to combine characteristics of three other groups of nosocomial pathogens: persistent colonization of the gastrointestinal tract (similar to multi-resistant Gram-negative bacteria) [27, 28], persistent colonization of the skin (similar to MRSA) [23] and contamination of the inanimate environment (similar to *Clostridium difficile*) [23]. As a result, cross-acquisition via the hands of health-care workers frequently occurs, even when compliance with infection control measures seems reasonable [21, 29]. Moreover, as for MRSA, persistently colonized health care workers [30], and residents of long-term care facilities [31] may serve as sources for multiply resistant enterococci.

The dynamics of VRE-endemicity within an ICU are regulated by the number of colonized patients in the ward (e.g. the colonization pressure), the number of VRE-positive patients that are admitted to the unit, and the use of antibiotics, particularly vancomycin and third-generation cephalosporins, which provide enterococci with a selective growth advantage [29, 32].

INFECTION CONTROL

The Centers for Disease Control and Prevention (CDC) defined measures to limit the spread of VRE, focusing on education of hospital staff, early detection and prompt reporting of VRE, and immediate implementation of appropriate infection-control measures to prevent person-to-person transmission of VRE [33]. For example, VRE-infected or colonized patients should be placed in single rooms or should share a room with another VRE-positive patient; gloves and gowns should be used when contacting these patients or their inanimate environment; gloves and gowns should be removed before leaving the room and hands should be washed immediately with antiseptic soap [33]. The use of gloves and gowns and cohorting of colonized patients had been successful in controlling monoclonal outbreaks of VRE [34, 35], but failed to limit the spread of VRE in an endemic and polyclonal setting, despite enforcement of handwashing resulting in a mean compliance of 50% [21]. In addition to enforcement of infection control measures, use of vancomycin and third-generation cephalosporins, which have been associated with VRE-infections in many studies, should be restricted. A recent study of gastrointestinal tract colonization of mice with VRE suggested that vancomycin and antibiotics with potent antianaerobic activity promoted persistent high-density intestinal VRE colonization, whereas antibiotics lacking potent antianaerobic activity did not [36]. In a hospital in New York state, reduction in the use of vancomycin and third-generation cephalosporins resulted in a decrease of the point prevalence of fecal colonization with VRE from 47% to 15% of the patients [37]. An enhanced infection control program, combining amongst others cohorting of nurses, higher compliance rates with handwashing and restriction of antibiotic use, reduced transmission of VRE in an oncology unit where colonization was endemic. The infection rate of bloodstream infections with VRE decreased from 2.1 to 0.45 infections per 1000 patient-days and colonization decreased from 20.7 to 10.3 patients per 1000 patient-days [38].

Pseudomonas aeruginosa

Pseudomonas aeruginosa is one of the most common and difficult to treat nosocomial pathogens in ICUs. In the EPIC study, a point prevalence study in April 1992 in 1417 ICUs in 17 European countries, *P. aeurginosa* was isolated from 28.7% of cultures associated with ICU-acquired infections [39]. Infections of the lungs occur most frequently, almost always after preceding colonization of the upper respiratory tract [40, 41].

EPIDEMIOLOGY

Respiratory tract colonization with *P. aeruginosa* is endemic in many ICUs worldwide. The intestines are considered the most important endogenous source from where microorganisms reach the respiratory tract via the gastropulmonary route [42, 43], via colonization of the skin, or via transiently colonized hands of health care workers during tending [2, 44–46]. The potential importance of exogenous sources (e.g. contaminated equipment) has been demonstrated repeatedly during outbreaks of infections with *P. aeruginosa* [47–52]. In addition, colonized patients serve as continuous exogenous sources of microorganisms from where other patients can be colonized via cross-acquisition [53].

Acquisition of RTC with *P. aeruginosa* has been associated with the duration of ICU-stay, the necessity and length of mechanical ventilation [41], and by previous antibiotic use, providing *P. aeruginosa* with a selective growth advantage [1, 54]. Furthermore, the risk for cross-acquisition may be associated with the number of other patients in the ward that are already colonized, thereby increasing colonization pressure.

The relative importance of the different routes of colonization in endemic settings has seldom been determined. When combining extensive surveillance with biotyping of multiple isolates, endemicity of *P. aeruginosa* in a Dutch ICU was characterized by polyclonality, with most patients being colonized with unique genotypes [1]. Colonization was frequently present on admission, and when acquired in ICU, the intestinal tract seemed to be more important as a source than was cross-transmission. Although the endemic prevalence was similar to that of VRE in an American medical ICU, the dynamics of colonization appeared to be completely different.

INFECTION CONTROL

Due to the differences in epidemiology between *P. aeruginosa* and other nosocomial pathogens (such as VRE), infection control measures should be tailored to the pathogen of interest. Based on the results of the Dutch study, prevention of colonization in the intestines or the stomach would have little effects on respiratory tract colonization and infection rates with *P. aeruginosa* [1]. Since gastric colonization never preceded respiratory tract colonization, decontamination at this site would not have had any effects on respiratory tract colonization. This confirms the results of studies in which intestinal and gastric decontamination was achieved with topical non-absorbable antibiotics [55, 56]. In fact, analyses of sequences of colonization of bacteria causing ventilator-associated pneumonia have repeatedly shown that the stomach is not an important reservoir for *P. aeruginosa* [57]. A regimen in which colonization of the upper respiratory tract is prevented would be much more effective in preventing pneumonia. Such an approach has been tested twice, and in both studies, oropharyngeal decontamination with non-absorbable antibiotics significantly reduced the incidence of nosocomial pneumonia [58, 59].

Antibiotics have been selected as important risk factors for acquisition of colonization with *P. aeruginosa*. Eradication of the normal human bacteria, including the anaerobic flora, facilitates overgrowth with *P. aeruginosa*. It has been suggested that this anaerobic flora provides colonization resistance to potentially pathogenic bacteria such as *P. aeruginosa* [60]. However, whether a change of first choice therapy from amoxicillin-clavulanic acid to, for example, a second-generation cephalosporin will decrease rates of RTC with *P. aeruginosa* is unknown.

As for all other nosocomial pathogens compliance with infection control measures, such as hand-washing, remain the cornerstone of limiting the spread of *P. aeruginosa*.

Methicillin-Resistant Staphylococcus aureus

Methicillin-resistant *S. aureus* (MRSA) was recognized in the United Kingdom in 1961, rendering glycopetides as the only remaining effective antibiotics for some strains [61]. Resistance to methicillin is based on the mutation of a penicillin-binding protein (PBP2a) and gene (e.g. MecA) [62]. Although MRSA isolates are not considered to be more virulent than MSSA, a delay in appropriate antibiotic therapy, evidently, may influence patient's outcome. Extremely worrisome are the recently reported strains of MRSA with reduced susceptibility to vancomycin, which may be precursors of VRSA [63–66].

EPIDEMIOLOGY OF MRSA

Since the initial description of MRSA, numerous infections and nosocomial outbreaks have been reported from all over the world [67–69]. Infection rates of MRSA, however, have increased especially in recent years. In the National Nosocomial Infections Surveillance System, performed in over 200 US hospitals, the pecentage of nosocomial *S. aureus* isolates resistant to methicillin increased from 2.4% in 1975 to 29% in 1991, and incidence rates were highest in large hospitals [70]. In England and Wales the proportion of MRSA among cases of *S. aureus* bacteremia increased from 1.5% during 1989–91 to 13.2% in 1995 [71].

As most antibiotic-resistant nosocomial pathogens, MRSA is especially prominent in ICUs. The results of the EPIC study, revealed that overall 60% of *S. aureus* infections were caused by MRSA with proportions as high as 81% in Italy and 78% in France [39]. In another study, consecutive isolates of *S. aureus* obtained in 43 laboratories from ten European countries were tested for methicillin-resistance. Overall, 12.8% of the 7333 isolates were resistant to methicillin. Percentages of MRSA were <1% in Denmark and Sweden, <2% in The Netherlands and Switzerland, and >30% in Spain, France and Italy [72].

The anterior nares are the natural niches for *S. aureus*. From here, staphylococci may spread to the skin (especially eczematous lesions), surgical wounds, foreign bodies (e.g. tracheostoma, external fixation devices), burns and the upper respiratory tract [67, 73]. Colonization with MRSA may persist for years, even after discharge from the hospital [74]. The most important mode of transmission of MRSA is via transiently colonized hands of health care workers who acquire the organism after close contact with colonized patients or contaminated equipment [68, 73, 75, 76]. Less frequently, health care workers may act as primary sources of infection when they have acquired nasal colonization with MRSA [45, 67, 68], or patients acquire MRSA via airborne transmission, as demonstrated in burn units [75, 77–79].

INFECTION CONTROL

Several strategies have been implemented to control nosocomial spread of MRSA. Traditional barrier-type precautions (e.g. limited number of patients per room, no room-mates with drainage tubes, hand-washing, and glove use) have been insufficient to limit the spread of MRSA in most parts of the world [73]. However, The Netherlands and Scandinavian countries proved that a policy of extensive surveillance in combination with isolation of infected or colonized patients can successfully prevent MRSA-endemicity [72]. Moreover, a policy of contact isolation in combination with extensive surveillance, enforcement of compliance with infection control measures by staff and active eradication of MRSA-colonization successfully controlled a monoclonal outbreak of MRSA in a neonatal ICU in the US [80]. However, implementation of such a policy will be labor-intensive and costly, and, therefore, require strong support by hospital administrators. Importantly with regard to the financial aspects of nosocomial epidemics, understaffing and overcrowding have been shown to facilitate MRSA-epidemics, probably because more lapses in compliance with infection control measures will occur [81]. French researchers recently calculated the costs and benefits of an MRSA control program in an endemic setting with an admission prevalence of MRSA of 4% [82]. In a case-control study, the mean cost attributable to MRSA infection was US$9275 and a reduction of MRSA infection rate of 14% would make the control program beneficial.

Active eradication of MRSA-colonization from patients and health care workers as a measure to control outbreaks is controversial [73]. Doebbeling *et al.* analyzed the results of six randomized double-blind studies comparing the efficacy of mupirocin ointment in eliminating nasal carriage of *S. aureus* among 339 health care workers with stable nasal colonization. Mupirocin or placebo were applicated for five days, and nasal carriage with *S. aureus* was eliminated in 91% of the volunteers receiving mupirocin, including nine with MRSA, and in 6% of those receiving placebo [83]. However, reports on the emergence of mupirocin resistant strains of MRSA are worrisome [84, 85].

Extended Spectrum Beta-Lactamases in Enterobacteriaceae

As a group, *Enterobacteriaceae* are the most important nosocomial pathogens, frequently causing infections of the urinary tract, the lower respiratory tract, biliary tract and surgical wounds [4]. Enterobacteriaceae have responded to the wide-spread use of β-lactam antibiotics with inactivation of these drugs by β-lactamases (such as TEM-1, TEM-2 and SHV-1 β-lactamases), which are typically plasmid-encoded [62]. These resistances were overcome by the development of second and third generation cephalosporins and combinations of β-lactam antibiotics with β-lactamase-inhibitors. However, in 1982 the first Enterobacteriaceae with resistance to broad-spectrum cephalosporins such as cefuroxime, cefotaxime and ceftazidime were isolated in Europe [86, 87]. These extended-spectrum β-lactamases (ESBLs) arose by point mutations, probably under pressure of widespread use of antibiotics. ESBLs differ in only one or a few amino acids from the original TEM-1, TEM-2 and SHV-1 β-lactamases and are also plasmid-mediated [62]. By now, more than 25 different ESBL have been described [88, 89]. Although the first ESBLs were reported from Europe, they have spread to most continents during the last decade [90]. In the US, resistance rates of *Klebsiella pneumoniae* to ceftazidime in ICUs rose from 3.6% in 1990 to 14.4% in 1993 [91].

EPIDEMIOLOGY

Many nosocomial outbreaks of ESBLs have been reported [92–106]. Most outbreaks occurred in special care wards such as ICUs and oncolgy wards. *Klebsiella pneumoniae* were involved in almost all outbreaks and extensive use of third generation cephalosporins, mostly as monotherapy, frequently was a risk factor [94, 97, 99, 102]. In contrast to outbreaks of VRE and MRSA, some outbreaks of ESBL were caused by the spread of a single ESBL-gene among multiple genotypes of *Enterobacteriaceae* [96, 97, 103], although horizontal spread of bacteria with ESBLs has been described as well [95, 101]. As for MRSA and VRE, environmental contamination may contribute to the epidemiology of *Enterobacteriaceaea* containing ESBL [101, 104]. More recently, situations of endemicity of colonization with ESBL-producing Enterobacteriaceae have been reported [107–110]. For example, in Chicago ceftazidime resistance due to TEM-10 is now endemic among *K. pneumoniae* and *E. coli* and the prevalence of these strains was especially high in nursing home patients [107]. In addition, ESBL-producing Enterobacteriaceae where already endemic in a French ICU in 1990. The risk for patients to acquire these bacteria was 4.2% in the first week and increased to 24% in the fourth weeks, and most cases of colonization were caused by the same strain type [108].

INFECTION CONTROL

With regard to infection control, two aspects are instrumental when attempting to control outbreaks of ESBL-containing Enterobacteriaceae or to prevent nosocomial epidemics. First, as for all other nosocomial pathogens, enforcement of compliance with infection control measures is of keystone importance. Reinforcement of handwashing compliance [92, 111], and glove use [92], barrier precautions [102, 111], and appropriate room disinfection [103] reduced the spread of resistant bacteria.

A limited and rational use of broadspectrum antibiotics such as third generation cephalosporins is the second strategy to prevent and control outbreaks with these bacteria. ESBL-genes can easily be transferred to other bacteria and even other bacterial species, especially in the presence of the antibiotic pressure provided by these agents. In three studies the use of ceftazidime was a risk factor for infection with ESBL-containing microorganisms [97, 99, 102]. Discontinuation of empiric ceftazidime and reduction of cefttzadime use in combination with barrier precautions resulted in a decline of resistant isolates, but they were not completely eradicated [97, 102]. In a smaller outbreak in a pediatric cancer ward, no further cases of infection with resistant strains were detected after a change of empirical therapy from ceftazidime to a combination of amikacin, azlocillin and nafcillin [99]. However, reduction in the use of cephalosporins, as a measure to reduce the incidence of colonization and infection with cephalosporin-resistant *Klebsiella* species, resulted indeed in less colonization and infection at the price of increased imipenem resistance in *P. aeruginosa* [112].

Another approach would be to use intestinal decontamination by non-absorbable antibiotics, as a temporary adjunct to strict hygienic and antimicrobial control measures, to eradicate colonization with multi-resistant bacteria [55].

Theoretical Framework of Colonization in ICU

The dynamics of colonization and bacterial transmission in an ICU can be described using a micro-epidemiological framework based on the transmission dynamics of vector-borne diseases (Figure 1) [113]. Crucial to this concept is that each pathogen has a basic reproductive number, R_0, defined as the average number of secondary cases generated by one primary case in an ICU where no measures of infection control are present. If R_0 is larger than 1, each case will generate more than one new case and the number of patients colonized will increase. The large R_0 the more rapid the rise in new cases, which is typical for epidemic outbreaks. If R_0 is equal to 1 a stable situation will develop (endemicity), and if R_0 is smaller than 1, the pathogen will not spread and stutter to extinction. Implementing infection control measures will change R_0, with the ultimate goal to reduce R_0 to levels lower than 1. Using mathematical modeling as a tool for infection control may have several advantages. It may provide quantitative estimations of the efficacy of different infection control measures and may predict the effects of changes in infection control. Furthermore, it necessitates a very accurate description of the dynamics of colonization in ICUs and identifies our lapses in knowledge. Therefore, modeling can both be hypothesis-testing as well as hypothesis-generating.

As represented in Figure 1, patients in ICU are either colonized or non-colonized. The number of patients in each box is created by the number of patients admitted (without and with colonization on admission) and the length of stay. In addition, patients may switch to the other box when colonization is acquired or lost. When colonization does not vanish, such as is the case for VRE, the admission rate with colo-

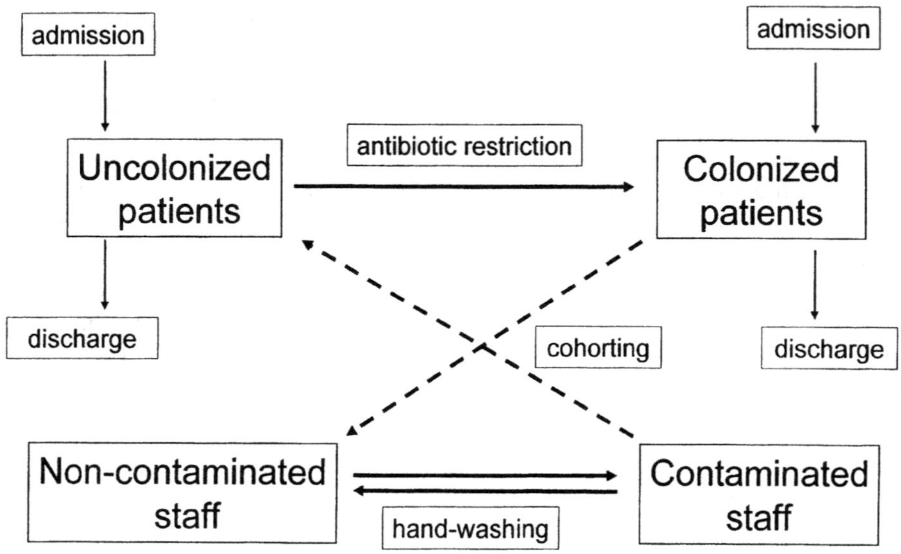

FIGURE 1. The micro-epidemiological framework of pathogen transmission in ICU, based on the transmission dynamics of vector-borne diseases, showing the possible effect of infection control measures. Once patients become colonized they are assumed to remain colonized for the duration of their stay in ICU.

nized patients represents the lower bound of the prevalence of colonization. For example, when there is no cross-transmission ($R_0 = 0$), the number of patients being colonized is equal to the admission rate of colonized patients. However, when there is cross-transmission, the endemic prevalence will increase when R_0 increases (Figure 2).

Cross-transmission occurs after contamination of the hands of health care workers. For this to occur, they must first contact a colonized patient and subsequently a susceptible, non-colonized patient. Infection control measures aim to reduce the possibility of cross-transmission, and these measures can be introduced into the model (Figure 1). For most pathogens, health care workers will only be contaminated shortly. Hand-washing reduces the duration of contamination, and this variable will be influenced by the proportion of occasions that hands are washed and the efficacy of hand-washing in reducing microbial contamination. Theoretically, the endemic prevalence of a pathogen depends on the R_0 value of a pathogen and the compliance with hand-washing (Figure 3). The larger R_0, the higher the compliance rates with hand-washing necessary for infection control. Compliance with hand-washing has been reported repeatedly to be low, with percentages ranging from 28% to 52% for nurses and even lower rates for physicians [114, 115]. Compliance is probably associated with intensity of care [114], suggesting that understaffing may further deteriorate compliance with infection control measures.

Cohorting of health care workers may also be an effective measure of infection control, because it limits the possibilities to contact both colonized and non-colonized patients. The level of cohorting can be expressed as the likelihood that a second patient-contact will be with the same patient. When cohorting is 100%, each patient-contact is with the same patient and cross-transmission can never occur. The cohorting level will be higher for nursing staff (estimated to be 80% in one study [116]) than for physi-

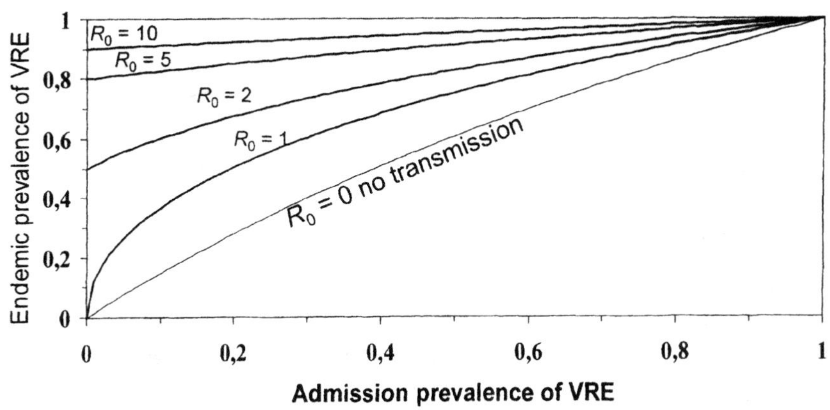

FIGURE 2. The predicted endemic prevalences of colonization with a pathogen according to the admission prevalence and the basic reproductive rate (R_0).

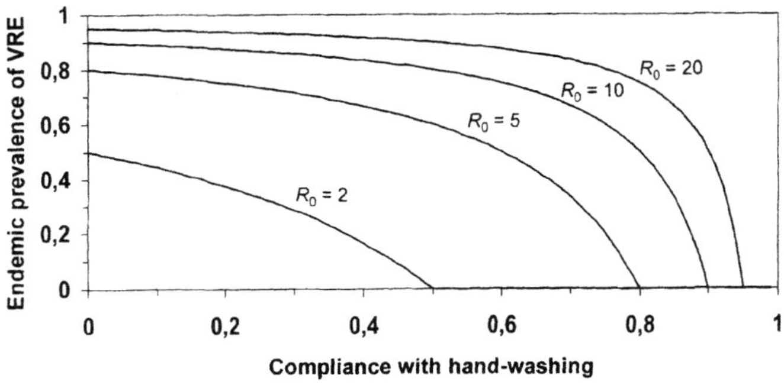

FIGURE 3. The predicted endemic prevalences of colonization with a pathogen according to the compliance rate with hand-washing and the basic reproductive rate (R_0).

cians, since they usually tend all patients in ICU. As for hand-washing, increasing levels of cohorting will be necessary for effective infection control when R_0 increases (Figure 4).

Little is known about the likelihood of acquisition of colonization after contact with either patient or contaminated staff member. However, antibiotic use has frequently been identified as a risk factor for colonization in epidemics of multiple resistant pathogens. Due to the selective growth advantage created by these agents, colonization may be facilitated more easily. In this way, antibiotics may influence the dynamics of colonization in ICU by increasing the occurrence of cross-transmission. In addition, antibiotic use may facilitate colonization from endogenous sources. In these cases there will be no cross-transmission and, as a result, infection control measures such as cohorting and hand-washing will hardly influence endemic prevalence.

Mathematical modeling has only recently been used to describe and investigate epidemiology of pathogens in ICU. The theoretical framework described here was based on epidemiological studies with VRE in a medical ICU

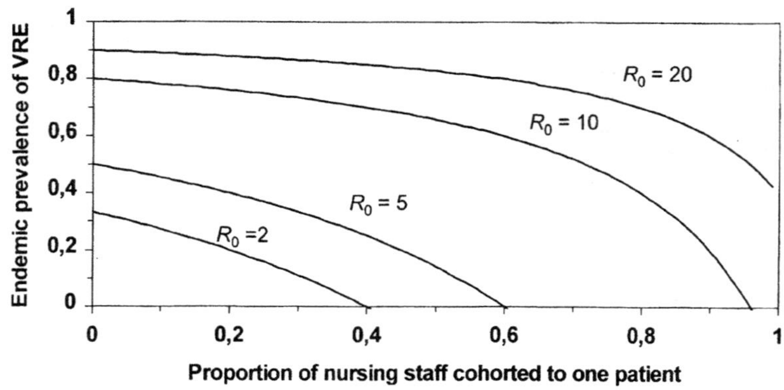

FIGURE 4. The predicted endemic prevalences of colonization with a pathogen according to the level of cohorting of nursing staff and the basic reproductive rate (R_0).

in Chicago where colonization with VRE was endemic [113]. R_0 was calculated to be 3.4 [113]. According to the mathematical model, the endemic prevalence would have been 75% without infection control policies. In fact, with infection control measures, the mean endemic prevalence of VRE-colonization was 36%. Overall, compliance with hand-washing procedures was 50% and cohorting of nurses was estimated to be 80%. The estimated R with infection control measures was 0.7, and it was concluded that the endemic prevalence was stabilized by the constant introduction of colonized patients.

Conclusion

Antibiotic resistant pathogens are an important thread for critically ill patients in ICUs, and this problem is not expected to decrease in the coming years. In contrast, in addition to the well known problem pathogens described in this review, other resistant pathogens will emerge. Anticipated problems for the (near) future include a growing resurgence of multiple resistant Gram-negative bacteria, and increased incidences of infections caused by intrinsically resistant species such as *Stenotrophomonas malthophila* [117] and Acinetobacter species [118, 119]. In addition, a urinary isolate of *Klebsiella pneumoniae* with plasmid-mediated resistance to ciprofloxacin has been described recently [120]. Furthermore, resistance to antimicrobial agents is increasing in anaerobic bacteria [121] and yeasts [122]. Most alarming, however, are MRSA isolates which, after exposure to vancomycin, express various degrees of vancomycin resistance [63–65], and the description of vancomycin tolerance in *Streptococcus pneumoniae* [123].

The results of several studies have suggested that reduction of antibiotic use within in the hospital could decrease nosocomial carriage of these multi-resistant bacteria [37, 97, 99, 102]. Encouraging in this regard is the recent observation that influencing antibiotic use on a national level [e.g. decrease of macrolide use in Finland], could diminish erythromycin resistance in Group A streptococci [124]. In addition, scheduled changes of antibiotic use may reduce levels of antibiotic resistance [125]. Improving compliance with infection control measures may even be harder than decreasing antibiotic use. Several studies have shown that compliance rates with handwashing in ICUs vary from 20% to 40% [115, 126–128], and the lessons of Semmelweis seem to be forgotten [129]. However, exact levels of compliance necessary to prevent cross-transmission are unknown and the effect of the continuous re-introduction of patients colonized with multi-resistant bacteria has not been studied yet. Mathematical modeling of the dynamics of resistant pathogens in ICUs and hospitals may help to a better understanding of this problem, and may help to design effective targeted interventions.

References

1. Bonten MJM, Bergmans DCJJ, Speijer H, Stobberingh EE. Characteristics of polyclonal endemicity of *Pseudomonas aeruginosa* colonization in intensive care units: Implications for infection control. Am J Respir Crit Care Med 160:1212, 1999.
2. Olson B, Weinstein RA, Nathan C, Chamberlin W, Kabins SA. Epidemiology of endemic *Pseudomonas aeruginosa*: why infection control efforts have failed. J Infect Dis 150:808, 1984.
3. Murray BE. The life and times of the Enterococcus. Clin Microbiol Rev 3:46, 1990.
4. Emori TG, Gaynes RP. An overview of nosocomial infections, including the role of the microbiology laboratory. Clin Microbiol Rev 6:428, 1993.
5. Edmond MB, Ober JF, Dawson JD, Weinbaum DL, Wenzel RP. Vancomycin-resistant enterococcal bacteremia: Natural history and attributable mortality. Clin Infect Dis 23:1234, 1996.
6. Maki DG, Agger WA. Enterococcal bacteremia: Clinical features, the risk of endocarditis, and managment. Medicine 67:248, 1988.
7. Moellering RC. Emergence of *Enterococcus* as a significant pathogen. Clin Infect Dis 14:1173, 1992.
8. Uttley AHC, Collins CH, Naidoo J, George RC. Vancomycin-resistant enterococci. Lancet i:57, 1988.
9. Uttley AH, George RC, Naidoo J, *et al.* High-level vancomycin-resistant enterococci causing hospital infections. Epidemiol Infect 103:173, 1989.
10. Leclercq R, Derlot E, Duval J, Courvalin P. Plasmid-mediated resistance to vancomycin and teicoplanin in *Enterococcus faecium*. New Engl J Med 319:157, 1988.
11. Noble WC, Virani A, Cree R. Cotransfer of vancomycin and other resistance genes from *Enterococcus faecalis* NCTC 12201 to Staphylococcus aureus. FEMS Microbiol Lett 93:195, 1992.
12. Leclercq R, Courvalin P. Resistance to glycopeptides in enterococci. Clin Infect Dis 24: 545, 1997.
13. Centers for Disease Control. Nosocomial enterococci resistant to vancomycin – United States, 1989–1993. MMWR 42:597, 1993.
14. Montecalvo MA, Horowitz H, Gedris C, *et al.* Outbreak of vancomycin-, ampicillin-, and aminoglycoside-resistant *Enterococcus faecium* bacteremia in an adult oncology unit. Antimicrob Agents Chemother 38:1363, 1994.
15. Boyce JM, Opal SM, Chow JW, *et al.* Outbreak of multi-drug-resistant *Enterococcus faecium* with transferable vanB class vancomycin resistance. J Clin Microbiol 32:1148, 1994.
16. Edmond MB, Ober JF, Weinbaum DL, *et al.* Vancomycin-resistant *Enterococcus faecium* bacteremia: risk factors for infection. Clin Infect Dis 20:1126, 1995.
17. Jordens JZ, Bates J, Griffiths DT. Faecal carriage and nosocomial spread of vancomycin-resistant *Enterococcus faecium*. J Antimicrob Chemother 34:515, 1994.
18. Moreno F, Grota P, Crisp C, *et al.* Clinical and molecular epidemiology of vancomycin-resistant *enterococcus faecium* during its emergence in a city in southern Texas. Clin Infect Dis 21: 1234, 1995.
19. Biavasco F, Miele A, Vignaroli C, Manso E, Lupidi R, Varaldo PE. Genotypic characterization of a nosocomial outbreak of VanA *Enterococcus faecalis*. Microbial Drug Res 2:231, 1996.
20. Brown AR, Amyes SGB, Paton R, *et al.* Epidemiology and control of vancomycin-resistant enterococci in a renal unit. J Hosp Infection 40: 115, 1998.
21. Slaughter S, Hayden MK, Nathan C, *et al.* A comparison of the effect of universal use of gloves and gowns with that of glove use alone on acquisition of vancomycin-resistant enterococci in a medical intensive care unit. Ann Intern Med 125:448, 1996.
22. Morris JG, Jr, Shay DK, Hebden JN, *et al.* Enterococci resistant to multiple antimicrobial agents, including vancomycin. Establishment of endemicity in a University Medical Center. Ann Intern Med 123:250, 1995.
23. Bonten M, Hayden MK, Nathan C, *et al.* Epidemiology of colonisation of patients and environment with vancomycin-resistant enterococci. Lancet 348:1615, 1996.

24. Manso E, de Sio G, Biavasco F, Varaldo PE, Sambo G, Maffei C. Vancomycin-resistant enterococci. Lancet 342:616, 1993.
25. Trick WE, Kuehnert MJ, Quirk SB, *et al.* Regional dissemination of vancomycin-resistant enterococci resulting from interfacility transfer of colonized patients. J Infectious Diseases 180:391, 1999.
26. Livornese LL, Jr, Dias S, Samel C, *et al.* Hospital-acquired infection with vancomycin-resistant *Enterococcus faecium* transmitted by electronic thermometers. Ann Intern Med 117:112, 1992.
27. Bonten MJM, Hayden MK, Nathan C, Rice TW, Weinstein RA. Stability of vancomycin-resistant enterococcal genotypes isolated from long-term-colonized patients. J Infect Dis 177:378, 1998.
28. Montecalvo MA, de Lencastre H, Carraher M, *et al.* Natural history of colonization with vancomycin-resistant *Enterococcus faecium*. Infect Control Hosp Epidemiol 16:680, 1995.
29. Bonten MJM, Slaughter S, Ambergen AW, *et al.* The role of "colonization pressure" in the spread of vancomycin-resistant enterococci. An important infection control variable. Arch Intern Med 158:1127, 1998.
30. Rhinehart E, Smith NE, Wennerstein C, *et al.* Rapid dissemination of beta-lactamase-producing, aminoglycoside-resistant *Enterococcus faecalis* among patients and staff on an infant-toddler surgical ward. New Engl J Med 323:1814, 1990.
31. Elizaga ML, Beezhold D, Hayden MK, *et al.* The prevalence of colonization with vancomycin-resistant enterococci among hospitalized residents of long-term care facilities. Abstracts of the IDSA 34th annual meeting 101:abstract no 352, 1996.
32. Carmeli Y, Samore MH, Huskins C. The association between antecedent vancomycin treatment and hospital-acquired vancomycin-resistant enterococci. A meta-analysis. Archives Internal Medicine 159:2461, 1999.
33. Centers for Disease Control. Preventing the spread of vancomycin resistance. Report from the Hospital Infection Control Practices Advisory Committee. Federal Register 59:25758, 1994.
34. Torres A, Gatell JP, Aznar E, *et al.* Re-intubation increases the risk of nosocomial pneumonia in patients needing mechanical ventilation. Am J Respir Crit Care Med 152:137, 1995.
35. Handwerger S, Raucher B, Altarac D, *et al.* Nosocomial outbreak due to *Enterococcus faecium* highly resistant to vancomycin, penicillin, and gentamicin. Clin Infect Dis 16:750, 1993.
36. Donskey CJ, Hanrahan JA, Hutton RA, Rice LB. Effect of parenteral antibiotic administration on persistence of vancomycin-resistant *Enterococcus faecium* in the mouse gastrointestinal tract. J Infect Dis 180:384, 1999.
37. Quale J, Landman D, Saurina G, Atwood E, Ditore V, Patel K. Manipulation of a hospital antimicrobial formulary to control an outbreak of vancomycin-resistant enterococci. Clin Infect Dis 23:1020, 1996.
38. Montecalvo MA, Jarvis WR, Uman J, *et al.* Infection-control measures reduce transmission of vancomycin-resistant enterococci in an endemic setting. Ann Intern Med 131:269, 1999.
39. Vincent JL, Bihari DJ, Suter PM, *et al.* The prevalence of nosocomial infection in intensive care units in Europe. Results of the european prevalence of infection in intensive care (EPIC) study. J Am Med Assoc 274:639, 1995.
40. Talon D, Mulin B, Rouget C, Bailly P, Thouverez M, Viel J-F. Risks and routes for ventilator-associated pneumonia with *Pseudomonas aeruginosa*. Am J Respir Crit Care Med 157: 978, 1998.
41. Bonten MJM, Bergmans DCJJ, Ambergen AW, *et al.* Risk factors for pneumonia, and colonization of respiratory tract and stomach in mechanically ventilated ICU patients. Am J Respir Crit Care Med 154:1339, 1996.
42. Heyland D, Mandell LA. Gastric colonization by Gram-negative bacilli and nosocomial pneumonia in the intensive care unit patient: evidence for causation. Chest 101:187, 1992.
43. Inglis TJJ, Sherratt MJ, Sproat LJ, Gibson JS, Hawkey PM. Gastroduodenal dysfunction and bacterial colonization of the ventilated lung. Lancet 341:911, 1993.
44. Widmer AF, Wenzel RP, Trilla A, Bale MJ, Jones RN, Doebbeling BN. Outbreak of *Pseudomonas aeruginosa* infections in a surgical intensive care unit: probable transmission via hands of a health care worker. Clin Infect Dis 16:372, 1993.
45. Boyce JM, Opal SM, Potter-Bynoe G, *et al.* Spread of methicillin-resistant *Staphylococcus aureus* in a hospital after exposure to a health care worker with chronic sinusitis. Clin Infect Dis 17:496, 1993.
46. Noone MR, Pitt TL, Bedder M, Hewlett AM,

Rogers KB. Pseudomonas aeruginosa colonisation in an intensive therapy unit: role of cross infection and host factors. Brit Med J 286:341, 1983.
47. Craven DE, Goularte TA, Make BJ. Contaminated condensate in mechanical ventilator circuits: a risk factor for nosocomial pneumonia? Am Rev Respir Dis 129:625, 1984.
48. Grundmann H, Kropec A, Hartung D, Berner R, Daschner F. Pseudomonas aeruginosa in a neonatal intensive care unit: reservoirs and ecology of the nosocomial pathogen. J Infect Dis 168:943, 1993.
49. File TM, Tan JS, Thomson RB, Stephens C, Thompson P. An outbreak of Pseudomonas aeruginosa ventilator-associated respiratory infections due to contaminated food coloring dye – further evidence of the significance of gastric colonization preceding nosocomial pneumonia. Infect Control Hosp Epidemiol 16:417, 1995.
50. Whitby JL, Rampling A. Pseudomonas aeruginosa contamination in domestic and hospital environment. Lancet i:15, 1972.
51. Favero MS, Carson LA, Bond WW, Petersen NJ. Pseudomonas aeruginosa: growth in distilled water from hospitals. Science 173:836, 1971.
52. Tredget EE, Shankowsky HA, Joffe MA, *et al.* Epidemiology of infections with Pseudomonas aeruginosa in burn patients: The role of hydrotherapy. J Infect Dis 15:941, 1992.
53. Maki DG. Control of colonization and transmission of pathogenic bacteria in the hospital. Ann Intern Med 89:777, 1978.
54. Olson B, Weinstein RA, Nathan C, Chamberlin W, Kabins S. Occult aminoglycoside resistance in Pseudomonas aeruginosa: epidemiology and implications for therapy and control. J Infect Dis 152:769, 1985.
55. Brun-Buisson C, Legrand P, Rauss A, *et al.* Intestinal decontamination for control of nosocomial multiresistant Gram-negative bacilli: study of an outbreak in an intensive care unit. Ann Intern Med 110:873, 1989.
56. Godard J, Guillaume C, Reverdy ME, *et al.* Intestinal decontamination in a polyvalent ICU: a double-blind study. Intens Care Med 16:307, 1990.
57. Bonten MJM, Gaillard CA, de Leeuw PW, Stobberingh EE. Role of colonization of the upper intestinal tract in the pathogenesis of ventilator-associated pneumonia. Clin Infect Dis 24:309, 1997.
58. Pugin J, Auckenthaler R, Lew DP, Suter PM. Oropharyngeal decontamination decreases incidence of ventilator-associated pneumonia: a randomized, placebo-controlled, double-blind clinical trial. J Am Med Assoc 265:2704, 1991.
59. Rodriguez-Roldan JM, Altuna-Cuesta A, Lopez A, *et al.* Prevention of nosocomial lung infection in ventilated patients: use of an antimicrobial pharyngeal nonabsorbable paste. Crit Care Med 18:1239, 1990.
60. Vollaard EJ, Clasener HAL. Colonization resistance. Antimicrob Agents Chemother 38:409, 1994.
61. Barber M. Methicillin-resistant staphylococci. J Clin Pathol 14:385, 1961.
62. Jacoby GA, Archer GL. New mechanisms of bacterial resistance to antimicrobial agents. New Engl J Med 324:601, 1991.
63. Hiramatsu K, Aritaka N, Hanaki H, *et al.* Dissemination in Japanese hospitals of strains of Staphylococcus aureus heterogeneously resistant to vancomycin. Lancet 350:1670, 1997.
64. Smith TL, Pearson ML, Wilcox KR, *et al.* Emergence of vancomycin resistance in Staphylococcus aureus. New Engl J Med 340: 493, 1999.
65. Sieradzki K, Roberts RB, Haber SW, Tomasz A. The development of vancomycin resistance in a patients with methicillin-resistant Staphylococcus aureus infection. New Engl J Med 340:517, 1999.
66. Waldvogel FA. New resistance in Staphylococcus aureus. New Engl J Med 340:556, 1999.
67. Haley RW, Hightower AW, Khabbaz RF, *et al.* The emergence of methicillin-resistant Staphylococcus aureus infections in United States hospitals. Possible role of the house staff-patient transfer circuit. Ann Intern Med 97:297, 1982.
68. Thompson RL, Cabezudo I, Wenzel RP. Epidemiology of nosocomial infections caused by methicillin-resistant Staphylococcus aureus. Ann Intern Med 97:309, 1982.
69. Centers for Disease Control. Methicillin-resistant Staphylococcus aureus. MMWR 30: 140, 1981.
70. Saravolatz LD, Pohlod DJ, Arking LM. Community-acquired methicillin-resistant Staphylococcus aureus infections: a new source for nosocomial outbreaks. Ann Intern Med 97:325, 1982.
71. Speller DCE, Johnson AP, James D, Marples RR, Charlett A, George RC. Resistance to methicillin and other antibiotics in isolates of Staphylococcus aureus from blood and cere-

brospinal fluid, England and Wales, 1989–95. Lancet 350:323, 1997.

72. Voss A, Milatovic D, Wallrauch-Schwarz C, Rosdahl VT, Braveny I. Methicillin-resistant *Staphylococcus aureus* in Europe. Eur J Clin Microbiol Infect Dis 13:50, 1994.
73. Mulligan ME, Murray-Leisure K, Ribner BS, *et al*. Methicillin-resistant *Staphylococcus aureus*: A consensus review of the microbiology, pathogenesis, and epidemiology with implications for prevention and management. Am J Med 94:313, 1993.
74. Frenay HM, Vandenbroucke-Grauls CMJE, Molkenboer MJ, *et al*. Long-term carriage, and transmission of methicillin-resistant *Staphylococcus aureus* after discharge from hospital. Infect Control 22:207, 1992.
75. Crossley K, Landesman B, Zaske D. An outbreak of infections caused by strains of *Staphylococcus aureus* resistant to methicillin and aminoglycosides. II Epidemiologic studies. J Infect Dis 139:280, 1979.
76. Peacock JE, Marsik FJ, Wenzel RP. Methicillin-resistant *Staphylococcus aureus*: introduction and spread within a hospital. Ann Intern Med 93:526, 1980.
77. Boyce JM, White RL, Causey WA, Lockwood WR. Burn units as a source of methicillin resistant *Staphylococcus aureus* infections. J Am Med Assoc 249:2803, 1983.
78. Rutala WA, Katz EBS, Sheretz RJ, Sarubbi FA. Environmental study of a methicillin-resistant *Staphylococcus aureus* epidemic in a burn unit. J Clin Microbiol 18:683, 1983.
79. Farrington M, Ling J, Ling T, French GL. Outbreaks of infection with methicillin-resistant *Staphylococcus aureus* on neonatal and burns units of a new hospital. Epidemiol Infect 105:215, 1990.
80. Jernigan JA, Titus MG, Groschel DHM, Getchell-White SI, Farr BM. Effectiveness of contact isolation during a hospital outbreak of methicillin-resistant *Staphylococcus aureus*. Am J Epidemiol 143:496, 1996.
81. Haley RW, Cushion NB, Tenover FC, *et al*. Eradication of endemic methicillin-resistant *Staphylococcus aureus* infections from a neonatal intensive care unit. J Infect Dis 171:614, 1995.
82. Chaix C, Durand-Zaleski I, Alberti C, Brun-Buisson C. Control of endemic methicillin-resistant *Staphylococcus aureus*. A cost-benefit analysis in an Intensive Care Unit. JAMA 282: 1745, 1999.
83. Doebbeling BN, Breneman DL, Neu HC, *et al*. Elimination of *Staphylococcus aureus* nasal carriage in health care workers: Analysis of six clinical trials with calcium mupirocin ointment. Clin Infect Dis 17:466, 1993.
84. Dawson SJ, Finn LF, McCulloch JE, *et al*. Mupirocin-resistant MRSA. J Hosp Infect 28: 75, 1994.
85. Marples RR, Speller DCE, Cookson. Prevalence of mupirocin resistance in *Staphylococcus aureus*. J Hosp Infect 29:153, 1995.
86. Knothe H, Shah P, Krcmery V, Antal M, Mitsuhashi S. Transferable resistance to cefotaxime, cefoxitin, cefamandole and cefuroxime in clinical isolates of *Klebsiella pneumoniae* and *Serratia marcescens*. Infection 11:315, 1983.
87. Payne DJ, Marriott MS, Amyes SGB. Mutants of the TEM-1 beta-lactamase conferring resistance to ceftazidime. J Antimicrob Chemother 24:103, 1989.
88. Bush K, Jacoby G. Nomenclature of TEM beta-lactamases. J Antimicrob Chemother 39:1, 1997.
89. Medeiros AA. Evolution and dissemination of β-lactamases accelerated by generations of β-lactam antibiotics. Clin Infect Dis 24 (Suppl 1):S19, 1997.
90. Paterson DL, Ko WC, Mohapatra S, *et al*. *Klebsiella pneumoniae* bacteremia: Impact of extended spectrum beta-lactamases production in a global study of 216 patients. Proceedings of the 37th Interscience Conference on Antimicrobial Agents and Chem 328-J-210, 1997.
91. Itokazu GS, Quinn JP, Bell-Dixon C, Kahan FM, Weinstein RA. Antimicrobial resistance rates among aerobic gram-negative bacilli recovered from patients in intensive care units: evaluation of a national postmarketing surveillance program. Clin Infect Dis 23:779, 1996.
92. Brun-Buisson C, Legrand P, Philippon A, Montravers F, Ansquer M, Duval J. Transferable enzymatic resistance to third-generation cephalosporins during nosocomial outbreak of multiresistant *Klebsiella pneumoniae*. Lancet aug 8:302, 1987.
93. Jarlier V, Nicolas MH, Fournier G, Philippon A. Extended broad-spectrum β-lactamases conferring transferable resistance to newer β-lactam agents in Enterobacteriaceae: hospital prevalence and susceptibility patterns. Rev Infect Dis 10:867, 1988.
94. Sirot J, Chanal C, Petit A, Sirot D, Labia R,

Gerbaud G. *Klebsiella pneumoniae* and other Enterobacteriaceae producing novel plasmid-mediated β-lactamases markedly active against third-generation cephalosporins: Epidemiologic studies. Rev Infect Dis 10:850, 1988.

95. Arlet G, Sanson-le Pors MJ, Rouveau M, *et al.* Outbreak of nosocomial infections due to *Klebsiella pneumoniae* producing SHV-4 beta-lactamase. Eur J Clin Microbiol Infect Dis 9: 797, 1990.
96. Papanicolaou GA, Medeiros AA, Jacoby GA. Novel plasmid-mediated beta-lactamase (MIR-1) conferring resistance to oxyimino- and β-methoxy β-lactams in clinical isolates of *Klebsiella pneumoniae*. Antimicrob Agents Chemother 34:2200, 1990.
97. Rice LB, Willey SH, Papanicolaou GA, *et al.* Outbreak of ceftazidime resistance caused by extended-spectrum β-lactamases at a Massachusetts chronic-care facility. Antimicrob Agents Chemother 34:2193, 1990.
98. de Champs C, Rouby D, Guelon D, *et al.* A case-control study of an outbreak of infections caused by *Klebsiella pneumoniae* strains producing CTX-1 (TEM-3) beta-lactamase. J Hosp Infect 18:5, 1991.
99. Naumovski L, Quinn JP, Miyashiro D, *et al.* Outbreak of ceftazidime resistance due to a novel extended-spectrum β-lactamase in isolates from cancer patients. Antimicrob Agents Chemother 36:1991, 1992.
100. Coovadia YM, Johnson AP, Bhana RH, Hutchinson GR, George RC, Hafferjee IE. Multiresitant *Klebsiella pneumoniae* in a neonatal nursery: the importance of maintainance of infection control policies and procedures in the prevention of outbreaks. J Hosp Infect 22:197, 1992.
101. Bauernfeind A, Rosenthal E, Eberlein E, Holley M, Schweighart S. Spread of *Klebsiella pneumoniae* producing SHV-5 beta-lactamase among hospitalized patients. Infection 21:18, 1993.
102. Meyer KS, Urban C, Eagan JA, Berger BJ, Rahal JJ. Nosocomial outbreak of *Klebsiella* infection resistant to late-generation cephalosporins. Ann Intern Med 199:353, 1993.
103. Prodinger WM, Fille M, Bauernfeind A, *et al.* Molecular epidemiology of *Klebsiella pneumoniae* producing SHV-5 β-lactamase: parallel outbreaks due to multiple plasmid transfer. J Clin Microbiol 34:564, 1996.
104. Hobson RP, MacKenzie FM, Gould IM. An outbreak of multiply-resistant *Klebsiella pneumoniae* in the Grampian region of Scotland. J Hosp Infect 33:249, 1996.
105. Pegues DA, Pegues CF, Hibberd PL, Ford DS, Hooper DC. Emergence and dissemination of a highly vancomycin-resistant vanA strain of *Enterococcus faecium* at a large teaching hospital. J Clin Microbiol 35:1565, 1997.
106. Dunne WM, Wang W. Clonal dissemination and colony morphotype variation of vancomycin-resistant *Enterococcus faecium* isolates in metropolitan Detroit, Michigan. J Clin Microbiol 35:388, 1997.
107. Schiappa DA, Hayden MK, Matushek MG, *et al.* Ceftazidime-resistant *Klebsiella pneumoniae* and *Escherichia coli* bloodstream infection: A case-control and molecular epidemiologic investigation. J Infect Dis 174:529, 1996.
108. Lucet J-C, Chevret S, Decré D, *et al.* Outbreak of multiply resistant Enterobacteriaceae in an Intensive Care Unit: Epidemiology and risk factors for acquisition. Clin Infect Dis 22:430, 1996.
109. Coudron PE, Moland ES, Sanders C. Occurrence and detection of extended-spectrum beta-latamases in members of the family Enterobacteriaceae at a veterans medical center: Seek and you may find. J Clin Microbiol 35: 2593, 1997.
110. D'Agata E, Venkataraman L, DeGirolami P, Samore M. Molecular epidemiology of acquisition of ceftazidime-resistant Gram-negative bacilli in a nonoutbreak setting. J Clin Microbiol 35:2602, 1997.
111. French GL, Shannon KP, Simmons N. Hospital outbreak of *Klebsiella pneumoniae* resistant to broad-spectrum cephalosporins and beta-lactam-beta-lactamase inhibitor combinations by hyperproduction of SHV-5 beta-lactamase. J Clin Microbiol 34:358, 1996.
112. Rahal JJ, Urban C, Horn D, *et al.* Class restriction of cephalosporin use to control total cephalosporin resistance in nosocomial Klebsiella. JAMA 280:1233, 1998.
113. Austin DA, Bonten MJM, Slaughter S, Weinstein RA, Anderson RM. Vancomycin-resistant enterococci in Intensive Care hospital settings: Transmission dynamics, persistence and the impact of infection control programs. Proc National Academy of Sciences USA 96:6908, 1999.
114. Pittet D, Mourouga P, Perneger TV. Compliance with handwashing in a teaching hospital. Ann Inter Med 130: 126, 1999.
115. Albert RK, Condie F. Hand-washing patterns

in medical intensive-care units. New Engl J Med 304:1465, 1981.

116. Bonten MJM, Austin DJ, Weinstein RA, Anderson RM. Quantifying changes in infection control programs in intensive care hospital settings: Number of health care workers affects patient outcome. (submitted).
117. Spencer RC. The emergence of epidemic, multiple-antibiotic-resistant *Stenotropho-monas (Xanthomonas) maltophilia* and *Burkholderia (Pseudomonas)* cepacia. J Hosp Infect 30 (Suppl):453, 1995.
118. Bergogne-Bérézin E, Joly-Guillou ML. Hospital infection with *Acinetobacter spp.*: an increasing problem. J Hosp Infect 18:250, 1991.
119. Bergogne-Bérézin E. The increasing significance of outbreaks of *Acinetobacter spp.*: The needs for control and new agents. J Hosp Infect 30 (Suppl):441, 1995.
120. Martinez-Martinez L, Pascual A, Tran J, Jacoby GA. Plasmid-mediated resistance to quinolones. Proc 37th Interscience Conference on Antimicrobial Agents and Chem Addendum: 6-LB-20, 1997.
121. Rasmussen BA, Bush K, Tally FP. Antimicrobial resistance in anaerobes. Clin Infect Dis 24 (Suppl 1):S110, 1997.
122. Sandven P, Bjorneklett A, Maeland A. Susceptibilities of Norwegian *Candida albicans* strains to fluconazole: Emergence of resistance. Antimicrob Agents Chemother 37:2443, 1993.
123. Novak R, Henriques B, Charpentier E, Normark S, Tuomanen E. Emergence of vancomycin tolerance in *Streptococcus pneumoniae*. Nature 399:590, 1999.
124. Seppala H, Klaukka T, Vuopio-Varkila J, *et al.* The effect of changes in the consumption of macrolide antibiotics on erythromycin resistance in group A streptococci in Finland. New Engl J Med 337:441, 1997.
125. Kollef MH, Vlasnik J, Sharpless L, Pasque C, Murphy D, Fraser V. Scheduled change of antibiotic classes. A strategy to decrease the incidence of Ventilator-Associated Pneumonia. Am J Respir Crit Care Med 156:1040, 1997.
126. Gould D. Nurses' hand decontamination practice: results of a local study. J Hosp Infect 28:15, 1994.
127. Doebbeling BN, Stanley GL, Sheetz CT, *et al.* Comparative efficacy of alternative handwashing agents in reducing nosocomial infections in intensive care units. New Engl J Med 327:88, 1992.
128. Simmons B, Bryant J, Neiman K, Spencer L, Arheart K. The role of handwashing in prevention of endemic intensive care unit infections. Infect Control Hosp Epidemiol 11:589, 1990.
129. Jarvis WR. Handwashing – the Semmelweis lesson forgotten? Lancet 344:1311, 1994.

22. CHALLENGES IN OUTBREAK INVESTIGATIONS IN INTENSIVE CARE UNITS

Belinda E. Ostrowky and William R. Jarvis

Abstract

Patients hospitalized in intensive care units (ICUs) are at high risk of developing nosocomial infections. This is a result of severity of the patient's illness and exposure to life-saving invasive devices and procedures. Each year, multiple hospital ICUs experience increases in nosocomial infections that represent an increase in the incidence over expected rates (i.e., nosocomial outbreaks). This chapter will review selected outbreaks affecting ICU populations (organized by pathogen/agent), approaches for investigating and controlling outbreaks in ICU populations, and special issues associated with outbreaks in ICU populations.

Introduction

Epidemic nosocomial infections (or outbreaks) are defined as hospital-acquired infections that represent an increase in incidence over expected rates [1]. Although there is surveillance for nosocomial infections in general, it is unclear what percentage of all nosocomial infections are associated with outbreaks, since few studies have examined the frequency, sites and pathogens involved in hospital outbreaks. Stamm *et al.* estimated in a survey at one US university hospital that patients included in nosocomial outbreaks represented 0.2% of all hospital admissions and 3.7% of all patients who developed a nosocomial infection [2]. Although intensive care unit (ICUs) beds account for a small but increasing fraction (5–10%) of all beds in US hospitals, ICU patients account for a disproportionate percentage of all nosocomial infections [3]. The extent of ICU-related outbreaks also is not well defined, but has been suggested to be high. Wenzel *et al.* performed surveillance for outbreaks at the University of Virginia Hospital and at hospitals participating in the Virginia statewide infection control program for a five year period between 1978 and 1982 [4]. In this study, 10 of 11 outbreaks identified were in ICUs, eight of these outbreaks involved infections of the bloodstream.

The Investigation and Preventions Branch of the Hospital Infections Program (HIP) at the CDC maintains an active training program in the epidemiology of nosocomial infections. As a part of the program, trainees conduct on-site epidemiologic investigations of hospital outbreaks in collaboration with hospital personnel. Requests for assistance are received from hospital, state or local health departments, and ministries of health [5]. Although there are biases in which type and what outbreaks we are invited to assist in, review of on-site epidemic investigations for the decade of the 90s is helpful in defining the scope of ICU-related outbreaks. From January 1990 to December 1999, we investigated 112 outbreaks (8–16 investigations per year), 21 (18.8%) were in ICUs only. Several others included ICU patients along with patients on other hospital wards. Of the 21 ICU outbreaks, 14 were in neonatal ICUs (NICU), 2 in surgical ICUs (SICU), 1 in a pediatric cardiac care unit (CCU), 1 in a post cardiothoracic surgical care unit, 1 in a neurosurgical ICU, 1 in general ICU, and one that involved several ICUs for neonatal-pediatric age patients. The pathogens associated with these 21 outbreaks included bacteria (N = 17) (13 gram negative bacteria, 2 gram-positive, 2 with multiple bacterial), fungi (N = 3), and one outbreak was endotoxin-related septic reactions.

Investigations in the ICU setting can be complicated by intrinsic host factors, such as severity of illness and immunosuppression, treatment regimens, use of multiple medications, and extrinsic factors, such as, invasive procedures and devices. This chapter will review approaches for investigating and controlling outbreaks in ICU populations, selected epidemics affecting ICU populations (organized by pathogen and agents), and special issues associated with epidemics in ICU populations.

Evaluation of Outbreaks in ICUs

DEFINING AND INVESTIGATING AN OUTBREAK

The evaluation of any outbreak begins by confirming whether an outbreak actually exists. Active surveillance for infections in the ICU setting can provide the necessary background/baseline infection rate data and be the source for identifying a potential outbreak. Use of standard definitions of nosocomial infection, such as those used by the CDC's National Nosocomial Infections Surveillance (NNIS) system are essential if inter- or intra-hospital comparisons are to be made [6]. Once a cluster is detected, the medical records of the potential "cases" should be reviewed. From this review, a case definition should be formulated. In addition to a description of the "case" based on signs, symptoms and/or laboratory data, this case definition should include three elements: who is effected (e.g., person), what is the time period over which the "cases" occurred (e.g., time), and what is the place or setting for the "cases" (e.g., place) [1, 7].

Once a case definition is established, case ascertainment should be conducted. Additional cases may be detected by a review of microbiology, pathology, ICU, radiology, pharmacy and infection control records. Next, a line-listing of all potential cases can be produced. The listing should include each patient, date of illness, location of patient and some initial demographic and exposure information, e.g., age, gender, underlying diagnosis, invasive procedures and devices, and service. Plotting the distribution of cases by time, e.g., an epidemic curve, can assist in developing hypotheses about the mode of transmission (Figure 1A and 1B). Before embarking on a major investigation, one should determine whether an outbreak is occurring; rates of infection/events for pre-epidemic and epidemic periods should be calculated and compared.

Since transfer of patients between hospital wards is common, it may be difficult to attribute an outbreak to a particular ward, such as an ICU.

TABLE 1. Approach to recognition and investigation of outbreaks in the ICU

1. Surveillance
   - Detection of clusters
2. Determine existence of an outbreak
   - Exclude pseudo-outbreak
   - Define case
   - Case-ascertainment
   - Compare pre-epidemic and epidemic period rates
3. Epidemiologic studies
   - Line-listing
   - Epidemic curve
   - Comparative studies (risk factor assessment)
     - Case-control study
     - Cohort study
4. Additional studies
   - Observational studies
   - Review practices
   - Culture surveys
   - Isolate typing
5. Interventions
6. Assess interventions

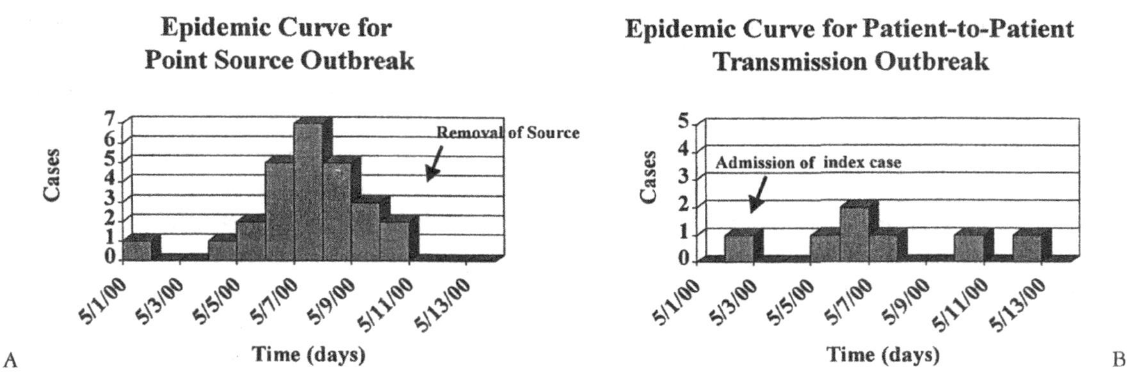

FIGURE 1A and 1B. Illustrate epidemic curves for two types of outbreaks (point source and patient-patient transmission). Figure 1A illustrates a typical point source outbreak in which the number of cases peaks and then disappear when a single source is identified and removed. Figure 1B illustrates an index case and six additional cases developing illness after exposure to the index patient. The epidemic curve is relatively flat, spread over days and has breaks compared to Figure 1A.

Infection rates can be calculated for other areas of the hospital and compared to selected ICUs to aid in identifying the location of the outbreak. In addition, a review of the geographic location of cases using a spot map of the hospital or ICU may suggest the location or pattern of transmission.

Review of the literature and current facility policies should be done to assist in generating hypotheses about the source of the outbreak. In the ICU, patient care may be delivered by many caregivers and patients may require many invasive procedures or devices, e.g., as mechanical ventilation, central venous catheters, or bronchoscopy. Thus, all policies and procedures should be reviewed in detail and with appropriate groups of health care workers (i.e., physicians, nurses, respiratory therapists). All relevant isolates/specimens and suspected sources related to the outbreak should be saved for future testing.

Early Control Measures and Reporting of an Outbreak

There should be two important focuses in an outbreak investigation 1) to find the cause of the outbreak and 2) to control the outbreak while the source/risk factors are being sought [1]. The exact order and extent of investigation and control of an outbreak depends on the associated mortality/morbidity, public health importance, possibility of a common source, characteristics of the pathogen, and resources available. Infection control measures, such as isolation (designated room or area separating case-patients from other patients) or cohorting (sharing of rooms, sections or responsibilities for care based on whether the patient has the condition/infection) of patients and/or healthcare workers (HCWs), may be necessary to control the outbreak and may be just as important as finding the cause. This may require culture surveys to identify all colonized and infected patients and then physically separate the colonized/infected patients from the other patients.

The decision to close an ICU is complicated and should be made on a case by case basis. Although there are no rules, risk from the outbreak versus benefits of continued ICU level of care should be weighed. In general, wards/units should be closed for conditions associated with high mortality or permanent disability, have a clear onset, and that continue despite introduction and compliance with infection control precautions. Investigators should establish criteria for re-opening of the ward/unit before closing the unit. All personnel should comply with local/state/federal laws for reporting outbreaks. In addition, depending on the magnitude, severity, and public health importance (e.g., potentially contaminated product or malfunctioning device) of the outbreak, the outbreak should be reported to local, state or federal health care agencies. These agencies may assist in identifying related infections (i.e., intrinsic product contamination), provide guidance, or provide personnel for onsite assistance in the investigation.

Comparative Studies

After generating hypotheses, additional studies to identify the source of the outbreak may be appropriate. Settings in which these additional efforts should be considered are when resources are available, when the outbreak is associated with high mortality or severe disease, new or unusual pathogens or methods of transmission, and/or outbreaks which continue despite implemented control measures. The choice of type of comparative study will depend on resources, time, and size of the outbreak. If the number of patients in an outbreak is large or the outbreak has persisted over a long period of time and there are many potential associated exposures to review, a case-control may be most appropriate. In this study, case-patients are compared to control-patients who do not have the adverse outcome or infection, but would have had the opportunities for exposure (in the ICU at the same time as case-patients). In ICU outbreaks, since ICU patients are very different from general ward patients, other ICU patients may be the most appropriate control-patients. In some studies, controls may be matched to cases on certain factor(s), such as age, gender, or other factors known to predispose to the outcome. In general, random selection of controls is preferred. Two concerns about matching are that special statistics are needed for matched analyses and that when matching is done, no comparisons can be made between case- and control-patients on the factors on which matching was done.

Review of the medical records of the case-patients should identify several potential sources/risk factors. In the case-control study, the presence or absence of these factors in the case-patients and controls are compared to see if any of these exposures are more likely to be present in cases, suggesting that this may be associated with the outbreak. A pitfall in an ICU outbreak, is that there are so many exposures that can be collected. Only biologically plausible exposures should be evaluated. A rule of thumb is that if an exposure is not present in at least 30%–40% of the cases, even if it is more common in cases than controls, it will not account for enough cases to be the source of the outbreak (attributable risk). Use of standardized data collection forms facilitate the systematic review of exposures of the complicated ICU patients.

In a cohort study, one assesses the entire population (e.g., all ICU patients from June 2000–December 2001) and evaluates what exposures are more common among those who develop disease/infection. If significantly more exposed patients than unexposed patients develop the outcome, than this factor may be not only associated but causally related to the outbreak. This type of study is usually time-consuming, costly, and fewer risk factors can be examined.

ICU patients are complex. They are often severely ill and have underlying illnesses that place them at increased risk for infection. In addition, ICU patients often need life-saving devices and procedures. While these intravenous catheters, ventilators, or surgical procedures are life-saving, they place the patients at increased risk of infection. The use of multiple and prolonged antimicrobial agents can also place these patients at increased risk for infections with antimicrobial-resistant organisms. All of these potential confounding factors (e.g., severity of illness, device and procedure use, antimicrobial exposure, etc.) need to be assessed and controlled for during comparative studies [8].

Observational Studies

Once comparative studies identify a potential source, observational studies may assist in confirming the source or mode of transmission. For instance, if a particular medication is associated with case-patients in comparative studies, intrinsic (e.g., at the time of manufacture) or extrinsic (e.g., after manufacture) contamination of the medication should be evaluated [9]. To confirm intrinsic contamination, cultures of unopened medication should be performed and state health department and federal agencies, such as the Food and Drug Administration (FDA) and CDC should be contacted to see if they have other reports of possible intrinsic contamination. Often inquiries from several hospitals can lead to the identification of intrinsic contamination of a product [10]. If intrinsic contamination is excluded, the pathway of the medication in the hospital and who and how the medication is manipulated in the facility needs to be reviewed in detail to identify potential sources of extrinsic contamination (such as breaches in admixture procedures); observation of healthcare worker preparation and administration of the medication may be helpful.

Laboratory Support and Molecular Tools

Patient laboratory data should be reviewed with microbiology (if an infection) or clinical laboratory personnel. The investigation of an outbreak often is a partnership between epidemiology and laboratory personnel. The first signs of a cluster or outbreak may be identified by an increase in isolation of certain pathogens in the laboratory. In addition, certain laboratory characteristics may aid in identifying cases, for example, an increase in the rate of the isolation of bacterial isolates with unusual microbiologic characteristic, such as non-pigmented *Serratia spp.* isolates or specific antimicrobial susceptibility pattern. Laboratory personnel also may aid in collecting environmental or other cultures, to support data from comparative and observational studies. Often investigation personnel choose to perform extensive cultures of personnel, environmental or other sources before any epidemiologic evaluation. This strategy can be costly. Furthermore, even exhaustive cultures may not identify the cause of the outbreak, without epidemiologic direction. We highly recommend that personnel, product, environment or other culture surveys be based upon the results of epidemiologic studies.

Pseudo-Outbreaks

Pseudoepidemics/pseudo-outbreaks are defined as situations in which hospital personnel perceive an epidemic of true infection is occurring, but with careful investigation, no clinical infection is present [11]. Most pseudoepidemics are caused by errors in processing cultures, such as contamination of specimens during collection, transport or laboratory manipulation. Other pseudo-outbreaks result from surveillance artifact (e.g., changes in infection definitions used, changes in populations cared for in the facility, introduction or changes in laboratory methods used or tests performed) [2]. Two recent pseudo-outbreaks exemplify the types of problems encountered. In the first, a cluster of cultures positive for *Aeromonas hydrophilia* were associated with inadequate disinfection of endoscopes before colonic biopsy [12]. There was a cluster of positive cultures obtained from patients during colonoscopy but a review of the "case-patients" medical records revealed no symptoms consistent with infection. Laboratory and instrument culture data revealed that the patient specimens were being contaminated when they were collected through an *A. hydrophilia* contaminated endoscope. In the second, a pseudo-outbreak of *P. aeruginosa* was traced to extrinsically contaminated lithium heparin bottles resulting in false positive blood cultures [13]. A review of case-patients records revealed that they did not have symptoms consistent with bloodstream infections and cultures of the heparin bottles revealed contamination. Some pseudo-outbreaks involve the healthcare facility as a whole, but may first become apparent in the ICU due to larger numbers of severely ill patients who require more intensive culturing. It also may be more difficult to differentiate a pseudo-outbreak from a real outbreak in the ICU, since these patients may be immunosuppressed making them vulnerable to an array of organisms. In addition, many ICU patients may be colonized with common nosocomial pathogens so that cultures (e.g., sputum, tracheal aspirates) may be positive but true disease attributable to the pathogen isolated is not present.

Review of Epidemic Nosocomial Infections in ICUs

Bacteria are the most common organisms causing nosocomial infections in ICU settings, including epidemics [4, 5]. A wide array of both usual and unusual pathogens have accounted for these ICU outbreaks. The most common gram-negative bacteria are *Pseudomonas*, *Klebsiella*, *Serratia* or *Acinetobacter* species. The most common gram-positive bacteria are the Staphylococcal and Streptococcal species [5]. For both gram-negative and gram-positive organisms, management has become complicated due to antimicrobial resistance among some of the organisms causing nosocomial outbreaks, particularly methicillin-resistant. *S. aureus* (MRSA), vancomycin resistant-*enterococcus* (VRE) and extended spectrum β-lactamase (ESBL) producing *Klebsiella* species [10]. Fungal pathogens, such as *Candida*, *Aspergillus*, or *Malasessezia* species and viruses, such as influenza, or *Respiratory Syncytial Virus* (RSV), have caused outbreaks in the ICU setting [8]. These agents have been associated with a variety of clinical syndromes, including bloodstream infections and sepsis, catheter-associated urinary tract infections, ventilator-associated pneumonias, or meningitis. In addition to infectious agents, ICU outbreaks have been caused by toxins and non-infectious agents.

Gram-Negative Bacteria

Gram-negative bacteria are the most common cause of nosocomial ICU outbreaks [4, 5, 14] (Table 2A). *Pseudomonas aeruginosa* is the third most frequent nosocomial pathogen and is a frequent cause of ICU outbreaks [15]. Contamination of respiratory therapy equipment has frequently been implicated in epidemic transmission of Pseudomonas species [16].

Two recent outbreaks show that Pseudomonas species can be transmitted by a variety of methods. In one outbreak, *P. aeruginosa* was isolated from nine patients in an SICU during November 1990; this rate of isolation was three times higher than that noted previously on this unit [17]. Three patients were infected with the same strain, as defined by identical serotype, pyocin types and molecular methods. The hands of 80 HCWs were cultured and a strain of *P. aeruginosa* identical to that infecting the patients was isolated from the hands of a nurse providing care for all three patients. All environmental, medical device, and ward stock supplies cultured were negative. No clusters of infection with this strain or other strains of *P. aeruginosa* were observed after compliance with handwashing and universal precautions were reemphasized. It could not be determined definitely whether this carriage was the source of the cluster or a consequence of it. The evaluation underscores the importance of routine handwashing by healthcare workers between contacts with different patients [17].

In the second, *P. cepacia* was isolated from 29 patients in two ICUs at one Canadian Hosptial. Twelve infections – five bacteremias, four pneumonias and three urinary tract infections – occurred. The source was presumed to be a contaminated ventilator thermometer. The ventilator thermometers were calibrated in a bath whose water had not been changed for months; cultures of the waterbath were positive for *P. cepacia*.

TABLE 2A. Nosocomial outbreaks in ICUs caused by gram-negative bacteria, 1989–1999

Reference	Pathogen	Type of ICU*	Number of Patient	Site(s) of Infection	Source	Control Measures
[17]	*P. aerginosa*	SICU	9	Multiple sites-wound, pneumonia, urinary tract	Healthcare worker hands	Handwashing, universal precautions
[18]	*P. cepacia*	ICU	29	Multiple sites-bacteremia, pneumonia, urinary	Ventilator thermometer, waterbath	Disinfecting water bath, infection control
[19]	*S. marcescens*	NICU	26	Bacteremias	Hands, invasive procedures	Handwashing, infection control
[20]	*S. marcescens*	NICU	32	Bloodstream, colonization and infection	Contaminated chlorxylenol soap	Removal of 4oz soap bottles
[21]	*Acinetobacter*	NICU/Nursery	8	Bacteremias	Air conditioning	Installation of new air conditioning system
[24]	*Acinetobacter*	5 ICUs	75	Bacteremias/ catheter tip infection	Reusable pressure transducers	High level disinfecting/ sterilization
[25]	*O. Anthropi*	Pediatric Neurosurgical ICU	3	Meningitis	Extrinsic contamination of salt solution, pericardial tissue implants,	Removal of implants; use of sterile solution
[27]	*E. hormaechei*	NICU	10	Colonization/ infections (Bloodstream, Tracheitis)	Environmental contamination, healthcare workers hands	Isolation of patients, environmental cleaning
[28]	Polymicrobial (*Enterobacter cloacae*, *P. aeruginosa*)	NICU	5	Bacteremias	Extrinsic contamination of dextrose multidose vials during manipulation	Review of aseptic technique in use of multidose vials
[29]	Polymicrobial (*E. cloacae*, *P. aeruginosa*, *K. pneumoniae*, *S. marcescens*, *K. oxytoca*)	NICU	9	Bacteremia	Extrinsic contamination of inravenous pressure monitoring equipment	Setting up pressure-monitoring equipment immediately before procedure

TABLE 2A (Continued)

Reference	Pathogen	Type of ICU*	Number of Patient	Site(s) of Infection	Source	Control Measures
[30]	*K. oxytoca*	NICU	10	Bacteremia	Reservoir of colonized patients, suboptimal infection control during injections and transfusions	Cohorting, identifying colonized patients, improving aseptic technique
[31]	*S. Worthington*	NICU	60	Bacteremia and cellulitis	Environment, suboptimal infection control, healthcare worker hands	Handwashing, infection control, aseptic technique for procedures, cohorting
[32]	*S. Infantis*	NICU	27	Bacteremia	Suboptimal infection control, healthcare worker hands	Handwashing, infection control, aseptic technique for procedures, cohorting

*SICU = Surgical intensive care unit.
ICU = General intensive care unit.
NICU = Neonatal intensive care unit.

However, even with elimination of this reservoir, *P. cepacia* was only eradicated from the ICUs after intensive infection control efforts were instituted (e.g., improved handwashing) [18].

Serratia marcescens is a gram-negative bacillus. It is a ubiquitous environmental organism, but is not part of the normal human flora. Several ICU outbreaks have been caused by *S. marcescens*. In the first outbreak, 26 neonates developed gram-negative bacteremia after their admission to the NICU at a 1000 bed general teaching hospital in Guatemala; 23/26 (88%) died. In a cohort study, 81% (13/16) of the patient blood cultures and 57% (4/7) of NICU HCWs handwashing cultures grew *S. marcescens*. Most of the isolates identified were the same two serotypes and had similar antimicrobial resistance profiles. The investigators hypothesized that gram-negative bacteremia occurred after invasive procedures were performed on neonates whose skin became colonized through bathing (non-chlorinated water) or from hands of NICU personnel [19]. In another outbreak, 32 infants in an NICU acquired *S. marcescens* infection or colonization. A case-control study showed that very low birthweight infants with multiple invasive procedures and exposures to certain HCWs were at greatest risk of *S. marcescens* infection or colonization. NICU HCWs carried their own bottles of 1% chlorxylenol soap, which often were left standing inverted in the NICU sink and work areas. Cultures of 16 (31%) of 52 samples of soap and 1 (8%) of 13 sinks yielded. *S. marcescens*. The 16 samples of soap all came from opened 4 oz bottles carried by HCWs, supporting extrinsic contamination. DNA banding patterns of case infant, HCW soap bottle, and sink isolates were identical [20].

Acinetobacter spp. are multi-drug resistant bacteria that grow well in water and cause infections with unexplained, increased summer prevalence [21]. Hospital outbreaks have been related to human reservoirs, where the mode of transmission is controlled by strict adherence to infection control practices or by removal of the environmental reservoir (e.g., respirometer, humidifier) [22]. In one outbreak, eight infants acquired *Acinetobacter spp.* bloodstream infection while in a nursery in the Bahamas; three infants died [23]. A retrospective cohort study showed that patients with peripheral intravenous catheters were more likely to develop *Acinteobacter spp.* bacteremia. Cultures of the nursery air conditioners and settle plates in the nursery grew *Acinetobacter spp.* Review of hospital events found that after the installation of a new air conditioner *Acinetobacter spp.* bacteremias occurred more frequently during months of increased absolute humidity or environment dew points.

Beck-Sague *et al.* reported epidemic bacteremia due to *Acinetobacter baumannii* in five ICUs in one hospital [24]. Logistic regression analysis suggested that the strongest influence on the risk of *A. baumannii* bacteremia was the number of days of intravenous pressure transducer usage. Plasmid analysis showed that patient blood culture and transducer *A. baumannii* isolates were identical. A review of practices showed that transducers were wiped with alcohol in the ICU between patient uses. Since reusable transducers appeared to be the source of this outbreak, recommendations were made for either high level disinfection or sterilization for these types of transducers [24]. Processing and re-use of transducers have been a recurrent cause of nosocomial bloodstream outbreaks [24].

In another outbreak, the infection control service at one hospital detected an increase in the number of *A. calcoaceticus* isolates from ICU patients. The organism was recovered from the respiratory tract in most case-patients. The investigators were able to identify the oxygen and temperature probes of ventilatory circuits as probable sources of the outbreak [22].

New or unusual organisms are often the cause of nosocomial outbreaks. In one such outbreak, three patients contracted *Ochrobactrum anthropi* meningitis at a 232 bed pediatric hospital [25]. *O. anthropi* (formerly CDC group Vd, Achrombacter species) is a motile gram-negative bacillus recently reported to cause nosocomial infections [26]. Neurosurgical patients with pericardial tissue implants were found to be greatest risk of infection. Culture of implants removed from two of the case-patients, an implant at implantation, a non-implanted piece of pericardial tissue, and an unwrapped but unopened bottle of Hank's balanced salt solution grew *O. anthropi*. *O. anthropi* contamination of the tissue occurred due to extrinsic contamination of the Hank's balance salt solution during tissue processing [25].

Enterobacter hormaechei was first identified as a unique species in 1989. In 1996, Wenger *et al.* reported an outbreak of *E. hormaechei* infection/colonization among premature infants in an NICU at a tertiary hospital [27]. The outbreak occurred among vulnerable, low birthweight premature infants. Environmental contamination and lapses in infection control may have facilitated transmission from patient-to-patient by healthcare workers. The outbreak ended after case-patients were isolated from other infants, HCW compliance with infection control practices was increased, cleaning of environmental surfaces was enhanced, and empiric antimicrobial coverage was changed.

Several outbreaks have involved more than one gram-negative pathogen. Archibald *et al.* described a nosocomial outbreak of polmicrobial bloodstream infections caused by *E. cloacae* and *P. aerugenosa* in a NICU in Puerto Rico [28]. The investigation included a retrospective cohort study, assessment of NICU infection control practices, patient HCW exposures to NICU and cultures of the environment and HCWs' hands. Results of these studies led investigators to conclude that a dextrose multidose vial became contaminated during manipulation or needle puncture and that successive use of this contaminated vial for the preparation of infusions for multiple patients may have been responsible for the bloodstream infections.

In another outbreak, nine patients developed gram-negative bacteremia with *E. cloacae*, *P. aerugenosa*, *K. pneumoniae*, *S. marscecens* or *K. oxytoca* following open heart surgery. The investigation suggested that contamination of uncovered pre-assembled pressure equipment by water from a malfunctioning spray hose disinfectant device used to clean the operating room was the most likely the cause. The outbreak was terminated by setting up pressure-monitoring equipment immediately before the procedures and discontinuing use of the hose-disinfectant system [29].

Recent investigations have included four outbreaks related to gram-negative bloodstream infection in ICUs. Three of these four investigations have been in NICUs in international settings, one each in Columbia, Brazil and Indonesia. The outbreak in Cali, Colombia involved *K. pneumonia* bloodstream infections and colonization in a high risk nursery [30]. Approximately 10% of infants in a cohort study had *K. pneumonia* bloodstream infections and 65% of NICU patients were colonized with *K. pneumonia*. Observational studies revealed that HCWs had suboptimal handwashing compliance (76%) and glove use (85%) and failed to use antiseptic techniques during intravenous injection (0%). Cohorting of the *K. pneumonia*-colonized neonates and improving infection control practices terminated the outbreak.

In another outbreak, 60 newborn nursery patients developed genital or peri-anal cellulitis and sepsis at one Indonesian hospital [31]. Predominant bloodstream pathogens were non-typhi Salmonella or Klebsiella species which produced extended-spectrum beta-lactamases. Infection control practices and adherence to aseptic technique were inadequate. A similar outbreak of *Salmonella infantis* multidrug-resistant nosocomial bacteremia in the NICU at two municipal hospitals with high mortality and cost occurred in Brazil. Several breaks in infection control practice and environmental cleaning were observed. Strict adherence to infection control practices and cohorting were effective in terminating nosocomial transmission [32]. In each of these outbreaks, overcrowding, understaffing, inadequate attention to infection control practices, aseptic technique and handwashing facilitated pathogen transmission.

Gram-Positive Bacteria

Gram-positive bacteria are the second most frequently reported cause of epidemic bacterial nosocomial infections. Infections with *streptococcus*, *staphylococcus* and *enterococcus spp.* are the most common [5] (Table 2B). Lannigan *et al.* described a cluster of five episodes of *Steptococcus pyogenes* infection or colonization in adults in an ICU following the admission of a patient with severe cutaneous infection [33]. The situation was controlled by aggressive infection control efforts, including screening of patients and HCWs for *S. pyogenes* by throat culture. HCWs and patients who were culture positive were treated with antimicrobials. Handwashing and environmental cleaning assisted in terminating the cluster. In another outbreak, Nicolle *et al.* describe a cluster of patient with group A Streptococcal bacteremia and pneumonia in an ICU after admission of a patient with group A streptococcal cellulitis and bacteremia [34]. All the streptococcal isolates were the same M- and T-type. The authors speculated that a staff member had been a transient carrier, although none could be confirmed. All patients in the ICU received antimicrobials for group A streptococcus and no further cases were observed. These outbreaks demonstrate how admission of patients with group A streptococcal infection may be a source for additional infections unless appropriate infection control measures are strictly adhered to in the case of such patients.

The traditional challenges in gram-positive infections (especially staphylococci and entero-

TABLE 2B. Nosocomial outbreaks in ICUs caused by gram-positive bacteria

Reference	Pathogen*	Type of ICU**	Number of Patients	Site of Infection	Source	Control Measures
[33]	*S. pyogenes*	ICU	5	Skin	Cross-transmission	Infection control
[34]	Group A Streptococcus	ICU	3	Cellulitis, bacteremia, pulmonary	Possible staff member carrier	Prophylactic antibiotics given to all ICU patients
[35]	MRSA	PICU patients in a SICU	7	Multiple	Cross-transmission	Removal of PICU patients back to own cohorted area
[36]	MRSA	ICU	14	Multiple, including bacteremia/ sepsis	Patient-to-patient	Contact precautions
[39]	MRSA	ICU	6	Colonization/ infection of multiple sites, including skin, catheter tips and line site, tracheostomy sites	Exhaust ducting of adjacent isolation room	Ventilation system repair
[40]	MRSA	NICU	19	16 colonized, three infected (bacteremia, conjunctivitis and dialysis catheter site infection)	Cross-transmission	Contact isolation infection control enhancement
[37]	MRSA	ICU	41	Pneumonia	Intubation, Bronchoscopy	–
[38]	MRSA/Cipro-resistant *S. aureus*	ICU	6	Pneumonia	Selective pressure from antimicrobial use	–
[44]	VRE	Cardio thoracic ICU	6	Infection/ colonization at multiple sites (mediastinal wound, intraortic ballon pump, intravenous catheter tips, urine)	Cross-transmission	Cohorting of patients and staff education, contact precautions
[43]	VRE	MICU	45	VRE colonization	Cross-transmission	Universal glove and gown use

*MRSA = methicillin resistant *Staphylococcus aureus*.
VRE = vancomycin resistant enterococcus.

**ICU = General intensive care unit.
PICU = Pediatric intensive care unit.
SICU = Surgical intensive care unit.
NICU = Neonatal intensive care unit.
MICU = Medical intensive care unit.

cocci spp.) have been complicated by the emergence of antimicrobial resistance in these species. Hospitals participating in the ICU component of the NNIS system, had a 47% and 43% increase, respectively, in the percentage of enterococcal isolates with vancomycin resistance and *S. aureus* isolates with methicillin resistance (MRSA) [15]. Although resistant pathogens may become endemic in ICUs, some of the earliest descriptions of VRE and MRSA in the United States have been outbreaks in ICUs. These pathogens continue to be a problem in the ICU [35–38] (Table 2B). The most important reservoir of MRSA within the hospital setting is the MRSA-infected/colonized patient or HCWs. Person-to-person transmission occurs by transient carriage of MRSA strains on the hands of HCWs. Simple infection control measures, including, identification of colonized patients, proper isolation/cohorting, and handwashing can assist in reducing transmission. For example, Ribner *et al.* reported an outbreak of MRSA in PICU patients after the PICU was consolidated with the SICU [35]. Previously, the pediatric patients had been separate from adult patients. The separation of PICU and SICU patients to their own units halted the acquisition of MRSA in this population. Improvement in the nurse-to-patient ratio and other infection control efforts occurred in both ICUs.

Cotterill *et al.* reported a *S. aureus* outbreak with an unusual source [39]. During a four month period, six patients in an ICU became colonized/infected with MRSA. Four of these patients were nursed sequentially in the same bed on the unit before acquisition of the organism. Investigation led the authors to believe that the exhaust duct of the adjacent isolation room ventilation system (where an MRSA patient was isolated) was faulty and allowed the MRSA to enter the other ICU room. Transmission was terminated once the ventilation system was repaired.

Jernigan *et al.*, describe a NICU MRSA outbreak [40]. Weekly surveillance cultures of the NICU patients for MRSA were performed on all patients; 16 of 331 admissions became MRSA colonized and three developed infection (bacteremia, conjunctivitis or dialysis catheter site infection). All the patient isolates had identical chromosomal patterns and plasmid profiles, which differed from control isolates from patients other floors. Contact isolation and aggressive infection control measures were implemented and the rate of transmission of MRSA from patients on contact isolation was significantly lower than the rate for patients not on contact isolation [40]. This underscores that active surveillance and patient isolation can control these resistant pathogens.

Vancomycin-resistant enterococci (VRE) has caused many outbreaks associated with a wide array of immunosuppressed patient populations, including, oncology, transplant [41, 42] and ICU patients [43, 44]. Severity of illness, underlying disease, duration of hospital stay, exposure to antimicrobials particularly vancomycin and ICU exposure are known risk factors for VRE colonization/infection [42]. Like MRSA, colonized patients play a role in the transmission to other patients. In an outbreak in a cardiothoracic ICU, Karafil *et al.* described six patients with colonization/infection in several body sites, including mediastinal wound and intra-aortic balloon pump [44]. The outbreak was controlled with cohorting of patients and staff, education, and aggressive implementation of contact precautions. In another study, Slaughter *et al.* found that 45 patients acquired VRE colonization in their MICU. The authors found that although universal use of gowns and gloves was no better that use of gloves alone in preventing colonization with VRE, adherence to recommended practices was significantly greater in the former group [43]. These data underscore that infection control is a critical element in controlling VRE outbreaks and endemic VRE in ICUs. The CDC and Hospital Infection Control Practices Advisory Committee (HICPAC) introduced specific recommendations for the prevention of the spread of VRE in 1995 [45]. These recommendations suggest prudent use of vancomycin, VRE educational programs, an active role for the microbiology laboratory in the detection, reporting and control of VRE, and strategies for the prevention and control of nosocomial transmission of VRE. Central to these recommendations is the detection and isolation of patients found to be colonized (identified by screening with peri-anal swab collection and culturing on selective media containing vancomycin) or infected with VRE.

Fungal and Related Pathogens

Because of their severity of illness, use of invasive devices and procedures and widespread exposure to broadspectrum antimicrobials, ICU patients are at increased risk of nosocomial fungal outbreaks. A number of fungal pathogens have been associated with ICU outbreaks. Burnie *et al.* documented an outbreak of systemic candidal infections due to cross transmission with one strain of *Candida albicans* over nine months [46]. The implicated strain was isolated from swabs from the mouth and hands of nurses working in the ICU. Voss *et al.* reported a *C. albicans* outbreak, including four patients with fungemia, occurring in a SICU over a four week period [47]. Genomic DNA typing methods showed that 3/6 patients appeared to be infected with the same *C. albicans* strain. The hands of one HCW were colonized with a strain that was identical to an isolate from a patient before infection of the patient. These and other data show that HCWs hands can become transiently colonized with *Candida spp.* and can transmit those pathogens to other patients in the ICU [48, 49].

Numerous outbreaks of *Apergillus* species have been described, including an outbreak of *A. fumigatus* over five months in an ICU [50]. The source of infection was presumed to be disturbance of accumulated spores in fibrous insulation material above the perforated metal ceiling. An outbreak of *Nocardia asteroides* infections was described in the nephro-urological ICU at a hospital in London [51]. Investigation suggested patient-to-patient transmission, although air and dust samples from ICU were positive for *N. Asteroides*. This ICU was closed and fumigated with fomaldehyde and not re-opened until air samples were negative for *Nocardia*. These outbreaks demonstrate that ICU patients are at risk of invasive fungal infections. Thus, it is important that these high-risk patients be physically separated from construction or other sources (roofs, false ceilings) of environmental fungal pathogens [52].

There have been several ICU outbreaks caused by Malassezia species, a lipophilic fungus commonly found in normal human skin. *M. furfur* has been associated with sporatic episodes of fungemia in patients receiving parenteral lipid emulsions as part of total parenteral nutrition. Richet *et al.* described a cluster of three NICU patients with severe bronchopneumonia associated with respiratory failure, thromobocytopenia, and leukocytosis [53]. A point prevalence survey revealed *Malssezia spp.* colonization in other infants and healthcare personnel and suggested that the organism could be transmitted to or between infants. In 1995, when HCWs at a New Hampshire hospital noticed an increasing number of NICU patients with positive cultures for *M. pachydermitis*, an investigation was initiated [54]. One nurse and 12 pet dogs of HCWs were found to be colonized with the same genotype of *M. pachydermatis* identified in case-patients. *M. pachydermatis* is a fungus that is becoming increasing common in nosocomial infections; it also is a cause of otitis externa in dogs. In this outbreak, it was hypothesized that *M. pachydermitis* was introduced into the NICU by the hands of nurses who had become colonized with *M. pachydermitis* by their pet dogs. As handwashing practices improved, the outbreak was terminated. More recently, three adults in an ICU in Mexico City developed simultaneous folliculitis with *M. pachydermitis* reportedly from fomites [55].

Viral Pathogens

A variety of viral pathogens have caused nosocomial outbreaks in ICU patients. Respiratory

TABLE 2C. Nosocomial outbreaks in ICUs caused by fungal pathogens

Reference	Pathogen	Type of ICU*	Number of Patients	Site of Infection	Source	Control Measures
[46]	*C. albicans*	NICU	13	Bloodstream	Hands/Healthcare workers	Handwashing, Change in hand antisepsis
[47]	*C. albicans*	SICU	6	4 Bloodstream, catheter site, meningitis	Hands/Healthcare worker	–
[50]	Aspergillus	ICU	2	Invasive disease	Ceiling spores	Environmental leaning
[51]	*N. asteroides*	ICU	6	Abdominal abscesses and pulmonary disease	Patient-to-patient Environment Hands/Healthcare worker	ICU closed, Fumigated with formaldehyde
[53]	*M. furfur*	NICU	3	Pneumonia	Patient-to-patient Hands/Healthcare worker	Enhanced infection control
[54]	*M. pachydermatis*	NICU		Bloodstream	Colonized healthcare workers and pet dogs Hands	Handwashing
[55]	*M. pachydermatis*	ICU	3	Skin	Fomites	Enhanced infection control

*NICU = Neonatal intensive care unit.
SICU = Surgical intensive care unit.
ICU = General intensive care unit.

Syncytial Virus (RSV), hepatitis, herpes and enteroviruses are the most common. In an outbreak of hepatitis A in an ICU in a regional hospital in North Queensland, seven people were infected including two patients, two close contacts of the index patient and three ICU nursing staff [56]. The index case was admitted with an overdose an multiple trauma; he was not suspected to be incubating hepatitis A. The outbreak was traced to inadequate precautions by HCWs while handling the index patient's bile. In another outbreak at a London hospital, hepatitis B infections occurred in operating room and ICU staff following the emergency admission of an unconscious bisexual drug addict who was incubating hepatitis B [57].

In another outbreak, a series of acute *herpes simplex* virus (HSV) infections occurred among nurses and patients in a PICU in two separate clusters in a hospital in Kentucky. The investigation suggested that PICU personnel risked acquiring serious herpetic infection from patients and vice versa unless recommended infection control precautions were followed, including identification of HSV infected patients, glove and barrier precaution use by HCWs and identification and exclusion of HCWs with active HSV infections, i.e., on hands and exclusion of these personnel from work [58].

Non-parenteral transmission of *Cytomegalovirus* (CMV) is unusual. However, an outbreak at a New York hospital was traced to an infant with congenital CMV who lived only eight hours [59]. Transmission occurred to four other infants who were in the NICU at the same

TABLE 2D. Nosocomial outbreaks in ICUs caused by viral pathogens

Reference	Pathogen	Type of ICU*	Number of Patients	Site of Infection	Source	Control Measures
[56]	Hepatitis A	ICU	7 (including 2 staff members)	Systemic	Unrecognized patient	Enhanced infection control measures
[57]	Hepatitis B	ICU	5	Systemic	Unrecognized patient	Enhanced infection control measures
[58]	Herpes Simplex Virus	PICU	2 clusters of patients and staff	Localized, skin	Patient and healthcare workers	Enhanced infection control measures, removal of infected healthcare workers
[59]	Cytomegalovirus	NICU	5	Systemic	Direct and indirect patient contact	Enhanced infection control measures
[60]	Echovirus 11	NICU	4	Systemic, respiratory, myocarditis	Introduction by pregnant mother Cross-transmission	Identification of patients, enhanced infection control measures
[62]	Influenza	NICU	5	Systemic	Cross-transmission	Identification of patients, enhanced infection control measures
[67]	Respiratory Syncytial Virus	PICU/ Liver transplant	17	Pulmonary	Cross-transmission	None, surveillance
[68]	Respiratory Syncytial Virus and Echovirus 7	NICU	73 RSV 20 Echovirus 7	Pulmonary and systemic	Cross-transmission	Enhanced infection control measures, active surveillance
[70]	Respiratory Syncytial Virus	MICU	5	Pulmonary	Cross-transmission	Enhanced infection control, active surveillance

* ICU = General intensive care unit.
PICU = Pediatric intensive care unit.
NICU = Neonatal intensive care unit.
MICU = Medical intensive care unit.

time; two infants died. Direct or indirect contact was thought to be the mode of spread.

Numerous nosocomial outbreaks of echovirus infections have been described in NICUs since the 1970s [60, 61]. One of these outbreaks involved four neonates at a special-care baby unit in Cambridge Maternity Hospital. Clinical infection in the babies varied, but included hypotonia, fever, poor feeding, myocarditis, and lower respiratory tract abnormalities. The proposed cause of the outbreak was introduction of the virus to the maternity hospital by a pregnant woman with mild or asymptomatic infection. The laboratory aided in prompt diagnosis of infection, and infection control measures aided in termination of the outbreak. Outbreaks of influenza A have been described in NICUs involving infants with clinical signs and symptoms indistinguishable from those seen in bacterial sepsis [62].

Viruses account for nearly 50% of the nosocomial infections in pediatric patients [63]. Of respiratory virus outbreaks, those caused by RSV are the most common [64]. Nosocomial RSV transmission can result in increased morbidity and mortality for all affected infants, but has particularly serious consequences for premature infants up to age six months, immunosuppressed patients, infants with congenital heart disease and post-surgical patients [64–66]. Pohl *et al.* retrospectively reviewed 17 of 493 children who received liver transplantation between 1985 and 1991 and developed post-transplant RSV infections [67]. Thirteen developed nosocomial infections while convalescing from their transplant; two children died for progressive pulmonary disease. Early onset of infection after transplant and pre-existing lung disease predicted more severe disease. Wilson *et al.* reported concurrent outbreaks of RSV and Echovirus 7 in an NICU, including infants with dual infection [68]. During a six month period, 73 infants were identified with RSV infections. During the same period, Echovirus 7 was cultured from 20 infants, six infants had concurrent RSV and Echovirus 7, and seven had both, but not concurrently. This dual outbreak persisted for months despite initial infection control measures, due to a lack of a rapid diagnostic test for enteroviruses, asymptomatic patients, and the logistics of handling a dual pathogen outbreak in a confined setting.

Several studies have assessed the efficacy of various control measures in preventing nosocomial RSV infection. Handwashing alone should prevent most nosocomial RSV or other viral infections. Since handwashing compliance is often poor, however, other preventative measures may be needed (gloves, gowns, eye-nose goggles, exclusion of HCWs with upper respiratory tract symptoms from working with immunosupressed patients, limiting visitors). The efficacy of many of these measures has not been fully evaluated [52, 64, 69].

Adults who are immunocompromised, aged, institutionalized, and/or have underlying medical disease may also be at increased risk for severe RSV infections. Guidry *et al.* evaluated intubated adults in an MICU who were admitted for pneumonia, asthma or chronic obstructive pulmonary disease for evidence of RSV infection (70). Five of 11 intubated patients had RSV-positive respiratory secretions. In addition, 1/7 MICU employees with acute respiratory symptoms and 4/48 ward patients in the facility had RSV-positive secretions. Their conclusion was that patients may be admitted to facilities with unknown RSV and can be the source of nosocomial spread of RSV within a facility.

Non-Infectious Nosocomial Epidemics in ICUs

In 1984, the HIP, CDC investigated three clusters of an unusual syndrome in premature infants in three NICUs. In each NICU, the illness affected only premature infants. In these infants, ascites and/or hepatomegaly, direct hyperbilirubinemia, renal insufficiency, and/or thrombocytopenia developed.

A cohort study identified the receipt of a newly introduced, intravenous vitamin E preparation, E-Ferol* (distributed by O'Neil, Jones, and Feldman Pharmaceuticals, St. Louis, MO) (used to prevent retroperitoneal fibroplasia), as the major risk factor associated with disease [71]. This investigation resulted in a nationwide recall of intravenous E-Ferol and no further episodes were reported.

Distribution of Infections by Site

In adult and pediatric ICUs, the most common endemic infections are pneumonias, urinary tract and bloodstream infections [15]. In contrast, the distribution of endemic nosocomial infections among newborns differs from adults and older

* Use of a trade name and commercial sources is for identification only and does not imply endorsement by the Public Health Service or the Department of Health and Human Services.

children. Among NICU infants, the most frequent are bloodstream infections, followed by pneumonia and then infections of the ears, eyes and nose [15, 64]. Risk factors for the three main sites of nosocomial infection are summarized in Table 3.

Nosocomial Bloodstream Infections and Intravascular Device-Related Infections

Intravascular catheters have become life-saving devices in ICU patients. They are used to administer intravenous fluids, medications, blood products, and parenteral fluids and to monitor the hemodynamics of critically ill patients. However, the use of intravascular devices frequently can be complicated by a variety of local and systemic infectious complications. An estimated 200,000 nosocomial bloodstream infections occur each year [72]. Most nosocomial bloodstream infections are related to the use of an intravascular device, with bloodstream infection rates being substantially higher among patients with intravascular devices than among those without such devices. The most common pathogens isolated from bloodstream infections in hospital participating in the ICU component of NNIS system were coagulase-negative staphylococcus (37.3%), Enterococcus spp. (13.5%), and *S. aureus* (12.6%) [15]. The incidence of and potential risk factors for intravascular device-related infections vary by the type of device (Table 3) and therapy infused through the device. For example, tunneled central venous catheters (CVCs) and totally implantable intravenous devices are believed to have a lower risk of infection than non-tunneled central venous devices [72].

A number of ICU outbreaks have been associated with intravenous pressure monitoring devices, particularly use of reusable transducer domes and transducers [24]. Nosocomial bacteremias and outbreaks associated with these systems led to the development of disposible domes [73]. Subsequently the risk has been reduced greatly in ICUs through the introduction and use of totally disposible transducer systems [72]. However, despite this measure, outbreaks continue to be reported, including an outbreak of Flavobacterium species sepsis associated with contaminated pressure transducers [74]. The mode of transmission was unclear, but was speculated to be from the contaminated transducers to HCWs and then to patients during invasive procedures, such as collection of blood gas specimens.

Catheter-related bloodstream infections remain one of the most important complications of total parenteral nutrition (TPN) therapy, and reported rates of infection during TPN vary widely. Because TPN solutions commonly contain dextrose, amino acids, and/or lipid emulsions, they are more likely than conventional intravenous fluids to support microbial growth of certain microbial species, if contaminated. Lipid emissions particularly are suited for the growth of specific bacteria and yeasts [75, 76]. Patients receiving lipid solutions (e.g., lipidic Anphotencins or propofol) seem to be at increased risk of coagulase-negative staphylococcal bloodstream infection [75].

Nosocomial Pneumonia/Ventilatory-Associated Pneumonia

ICU patients are also at increased risk of nosocomial pneumonia [16]. Most reported outbreaks of nosocomial pneumonia in ICUs have involved common hospital pathogens, such as gram-negative bacilli or *S. aureus*, spread via contact transmission from HCWs, patients and inanimate environment. Devices used for respiratory therapy can also serve as potential sources for transmission of pathogens. Numerous outbreaks have been traced to contamination of respiratory therapy equipment or solutions used during operating or cleaning of these medical devices, including jet nebulizers, mechanical ventilator circuits, portable room humidifiers, resuscitation bags, or ventilator temperature probes [16, 77, 78]. Most of these outbreaks have resulted from inadequate disinfection or sterilization of the

TABLE 3. Factors associated with nosocomial infections, by site

Infection Site/Source	Factors
Intravenous device-related infections[1]	
Peripheral catheters	Venous catheters
	Inflammation at the catheter site
	Catheter <4 days
	Catheter insertion by cutdown
	Site of catheter insertion (greater risk in femoral area)
Non-tunneled central venous catheters (CVCs)	Number of catheter lumen
	Site of catheter insertion
Central arterial catheters	Duration of catheterization (greater than 3, 5, 7 days)
	Colonization of the skin insertion site
	Introducer left in place >5 days
	Catheter insertion in the operating room with submaximal barrier precautions
	Site of catheter insertion (jugular vs subclavian)
Tunneled CVCs	Number of catheter lumen
	Duration of catheterization
	Number of manipulations
	Neutropenia in cancer patients
Nosocomial bacterial pneumonia[2]	Host/Patient:
	Extremes of age
	Severity of illness-including immunosupression
	Underlying chronic lung disease or coma (enhance colonization with microorganisms)
	Exposures:
	Administration of antimicrobials
	Admission to the ICU
	Conditions favoring aspiration or reflux:
	Impaired airway reflexes
	Endotracheal intubation
	Nasogastric tubes
	Supine position
	Depressed level of consciousness
	Reintubation or self extubation
	Conditions requiring prolonged use of mechanical ventilatory support and exposure to respiratory equipment or colonized healthcare workers hands
	Factors that impede adequate pulmonary toilet:
	Upper abdominal or thoracic surgery
	Immobilization due to trauma or illness
Catheter-associated urinary tract infections[3]	Method and duration of catheterization
	Quality of catheter care
	Host susceptibility
	Advanced age
	Debilitation
	Postpartum state

Adapted from:
[1] [72].
[2] [52].
[3] [85].

medical equipment between patient uses or the improper use of tap water in respiratory care devices. For example, an outbreak of *Burkholderia cepacia* lower respiratory tract colonization and infection occurred in ICU patients in various geographic locations throughout one hospital [77]. Forty-four patients became colonized or infected over an 11 month period, whereas *B cepacia* had been isolated from only 13 patients in the preceding 48 months. After a review of case-patients, environmental cultures revealed the source to be an extrinsically contaminated albuterol nebulization solution. Polymerase chain reaction-ribotyping confirmed the genetic relatedness of the *B. cepacia* patient and contaminated albuterol isolates. In another outbreak, a multistate nosocomial outbreak of *Ralstonia pickettii* colonization was reported associated with an intrinsically contaminated respiratory care solution [78]. From February 1 through April 30, 1998, personnel at four hospitals in three states reported a total of 34 patients colonized with *Ralstonia picketti*. All but one had been exposed during endotracheal suctioning to a 0.9% saline solution manufactured by one company. Following an epidemiologic investigation, culture of previously unopened vials of the saline solution yielded *R. pickettii*. All product and patient isolates were genotypically related by pulsed-field gel electrophoresis analysis. The Federal Drug Administration (FDA) recalled the product. The contaminated saline solution was manufactured at one plant that had been associated with a similar outbreak in 1983.

Bronchoscopic procedures are frequently performed in ICU patients for diagnosis and therapy. Outbreaks of infection and/or pseudoinfection associated with bronchoscopes are well documented and most commonly caused by improper cleaning and disinfection procedures or contamination of endoscopes [16, 79]. For example, a pseudo-outbreak due to non-tuberculous mycobacteria was traced to a contaminated water tank of a machine used to clean and disinfect fiberoptic endoscopes [80]. Forty-six bronchoscopies performed on 41 patients during a six-month period yielded 16 specimens positive for acid-fast bacilli. Four patients in the beginning of the pseudo-outbreak were treated for presumed tuberculosis until negative sputum cultures on these patients were obtained. Several of the patient isolates were identified as *Mycobacterium chelonae* or *M. gordonae*, all in-patients with no clinical signs of mycobacterial disease. Control of the pseudo-outbreak was achieved by disinfection of the implicated water tank in the cleaning machine. In another outbreak, 15 patients had positive cultures for *M. abscessus* without evidence of infection following endoscopy. A CDC investigation revealed that *M. abscessus*-positive cultures were significantly more likely to be obtained during bronchoscopy than gastroendoscopy and during procedures using bronchoscopes disinfected in an automated washer rather than by other methods. *M. abscessus* was recovered from the automated washer, the inlet water feeding the washer, and a flexible bronchoscope. Environmental and case-patient isolates were identical by molecular typing [81]. The New York Department of Health received reports from patients at local health-care facilities of three episodes bronchoscopy specimens culture-positive for *M. tuberculosis*, *M. intercellulare* or *P. aeruginosa* in 1996 and 1998. Between patient uses, bronchoscopes had been cleaned, visually inspected, leak tested, and processed by STERIS System 1 processor (STERIS, Mentor, Ohio). The investigation revealed problems related to using automated reprocessing machines, including inadequate device-specific training and use of the wrong set-up or connector systems [82]. Recently, nosocomial transmission of multi-drug resistant *M. tuberulosis* has been documented in an outbreak among eight patients in South Carolina. Inadequate cleaning and disinfecting of the bronchoscope after the procedure performed on a patient led to subsequent false positive cultures in two patients and transmission of infection to two other patients [79].

In addition, several pathogens that cause nosocomial pneumonia are presumed to be transmitted by droplet spread or airborne droplets from specific environmental reservoirs. Epidemics of *Legionella pneumonia* have been associated with contamination of hospital water supplies and/or cooling towers [83].

Nosocomial Urinary Tract Infection

The urinary tract is the most common site of endemic nosocomial infection [84]. Most of these infections (66–86%) follow instrumentation of the urinary tract, predominately urinary catheterization. An estimated four million patients annually receive urinary catheterization and are thus at risk for catheter-associated infection and its complications [85]. The most common nosocomial pathogens isolated from urinary tract infections in hospital participating in the ICU component of NNIS system were *E. coli* (17.5%), *C. albicans* (15.8%), and *Enterococcus spp.* (13.8%) [15]. Many of these microorganisms are part of the patient's endogenous bowel flora, but they can also be acquired by cross-contamination from other patients, solutions, or nonsterile equipment. One of the most important infection control measures for limiting urinary tract infections, is to limit use of urinary tract catheters and thus limit the size of the population at risk [85]. This may be difficult in ICUs, where patients are severely ill, and require other invasive procedures and devices. It would be difficult to care for patients without urinary catherization due to the need to carefully measure urinary output and due to sedation (possibly iatrogenic) which would interfere with urinary continence. If urinary catherization is essential, education of HCWs about prevention guidelines, monitoring of HCWs compliance, and removing the catheter as soon as possible can reduce the risk of infection.

Special Issues/Complicating Issues

Risk Adjustment

INTRINSIC FACTORS – SEVERITY OF ILLNESS

A patient's predisposition for becoming infected is strongly influenced by certain risk factors, such as personal characteristics (intrinsic) and exposures (extrinsic). Intrinsic risk factors are those that are inherent to the patient, such as underlying disease, severity of illness, and advanced age. Knowledge of intrinsic host factors is useful because separate risk-specific rates can be calculated which allow the comparison of nosocomial infection rates among patients with similar risks. The Acute Physiology and Chronic Health Evaluation (APACHE II) and Diagnosis Related Groups (DRG) are two well-known indices for severity of illness used to predict the risk of death among ICU patients and resource utilization, respectively [14, 86, 87].

ADJUSTMENT FOR EXPOSURES-DEVICES, PROCEDURES, LONGER LENGTH OF STAY, AND ICU TYPE

Although many extrinsic risk factors contribute to nosocomial infection, the factors that have been most frequently implicated and studied are certain high risk medical interventions, such as surgical procedures or use of invasive devices. There are several explanations as to why patients with such exposures may be at increased risk of infection, including that those who require invasive devices have more severe underlying illness and that devices/procedures provide a pathway for micro-organisms from the environment to enter the body, facilitate the transfer of pathogens from one part of the patient's body to another, and act as inanimate foci where pathogens can proliferate [88–90].

Since exposure to devices, procedures and longer length of hospital stay may increase a patient's risk of infection, accounting for these factors may aid when evaluating rates of infections. Calculating nosocomial infection rates in ICU patients, using patient-days (ICU patient-days) as the denominator partially adjusts for average length of stay. To reduce the confounding effects of device exposure (when making interhospital comparisons), infection control personnel can use device-days as denominators for site-specific rates (e.g., ventilatory-days for ventilator-associated pneumonia rates, central-line days for central line-associated bloodstream infection rates, and urinary catheter days for catheter-associated urinary tract infection rates) [88].

The type of ICU has also been consistently important in NNIS analyses. For example, the distribution of PICU and NICU device-associated infection rates are different from one another and both differ from adult ICU rates. Because birthweight is a well-described intrinsic risk factor for infection, rates are calculated for each of three birthweight groups in the high risk nursery component, i.e., <1500 g, 1500–2500 g, and 2500 g [87, 91]. Since nosocomial infection rate distributions vary by type of ICU, care should be taken when making inter- or intra-hospital infection rate comparison.

CENTRAL VENOUS CATHETER (CVC)-ASSOCIATED BLOODSTREAM INFECTION RISK AND STAFFING

Bacterial colonization of the skin at the site of intravascular catheter insertion has been shown to be a major risk factor for CVC-associated infection [92, 93]. Meticulous care of the CVC and the CVC insertion site by a dedicated team decreases the risk of bloodstream infection [72]. Since nurses provide most of the manipulation and care of the patient's CVC, the level of care provided by SICU nursing staff may be critical for prevention of primary bloodstream infections in ICU patients. Several studies have documented a higher risk of bloodstream infection in ICU patients when the nurse-to-patient ratio decreases [94, 95]. Archibald *et al.* investigated a *S. marcescens* outbreak in a pediatric cardiac ICU in 1994 and 1995. The nococomial infection rate was most strongly correlated with patient census but was also strongly associated with the nursing hours : patient day ratio [95]. When 28 patients with bloodstream infections (case-patients) were compared to 99 randomly selected patients (controls) hospitalized ≥ three days in the same SICU, case-patients were significantly more likely than controls to be hospitalized during a five month period when there was lower regular nurse-to-patient ratio and higher pooled-nurse-to-patient ratios than during an eight month reference period [96]. These data suggest that, in addition to other factors, nurse staffing composition (i.e., pooled-nurse-to-patient ratio) may be related to primary bloodstream infection risk. This may be particularly important in an era of cost containment and healthcare reform, when the number of or level of training of ICU nurses may be decreasing.

NEUROSURGICAL MONITORING

Patients in neurosurgical ICUs maybe at risk from infection due to procedures and devices which may provide a direct portal of entry of pathogens into the central nervous system [97]. Guidelines exist to minimize the risk of infection from intravascular devices, however, no guidelines exist regarding the care of neurosurgical devices, such as external ventricular catheters [EVCs]. These devices are placed in a cerebral ventricle to monitor intra-cranial cerebrospinal fluid (CSF) pressure and to regulate intra-cranial pressure therapeutically by draining CSF when the pressure is unacceptably high. EVC usually are tunneled subcutaneously, placed in a lateral ventricle, and attached to tubing connected to a transducer system. Trick *et al.* described a recent investigation of *P. aeruginosa* ventriculitis among eight patients at a community hospital neurosurgical ICU. All had percutaneous EVCs. A cohort study suggested a single HCW contaminated the EVCs insertion sites. Affected patients were unlikely to have an occlusive dressing at the EVC insertion site. The authors suggested that a sterile occlusive dressing and proper infection control may decrease the risk of ventriculitis in patients with EVCs [98].

SURGICAL CARE – ANESTHETICS

Propofol (Diprivan, Stuart Pharmaceuticals, Wilmington, Delaware), an intravenous anesthetic used in ICUs and operating rooms for patient sedation, has been implicated as the cause of outbreaks of post-operative infection or acute febrile illness due to extrinsic contamination of the product by anesthesia personnel [99]. These outbreaks were associated with Propofol without preservative. Propofol presented a risk for infection because it is lipid-based (a good bacterial growth media), contained no preservatives, is stored at room temperatures, and is supplied in vials that may be used for multiple patients. A preservative containing product now exists, nevertheless, infection control personnel should investigate the manner in which products without preservatives are handled in ICUs to avoid potential outbreaks.

ANTIMICROBIAL RESISTANCE AND COLONIZATION VS INFECTION

Antimicrobial resistance is emerging as a serious clinical challenge in healthcare facilities throughout the United States and the world [15, 100]. The increasing rates of antimicrobial resistant nosocomial pathogens have been seen particularly in ICUs, where patients have known risk factors that predispose them to infections with resistance pathogens, including extensive antimicrobial exposure, prolonged hospital/ICU stay, and multiple invasive procedures and devices [45]. In hospitals participating in the NNIS ICU component, data suggest that the proportion of *S. aureus* isolates resistant to methicillin, oxacillin, or nafcillin (MRSA) continues to rise and is more than 50% [15]. In addition, the rate of VRE has not slowed and about one quarter of all enterococcal infections in ICU patients are caused by strains which are resistant to vancomycin [15]. As previously mentioned, some of the earliest descriptions of VRE and MRSA in the United States have been outbreaks in ICUs.

Colonization is the presence of a microorganism in or on a host, with growth and multiplication, but without any overt clinical expression or detected immune reaction in the host at the time the microorganism is isolated [101]. Colonization is a natural process in the development of normal flora. In the neonate, this process occurs within days to weeks of delivery, after which neonate's normal flora is similar to that seen in adults [102, 103]. Whether colonization occurs long before or immediately before infection, it can play a major role in development of nosocomial infection [103]. In many instances, colonization is a necessary precedent to infection. Resistant pathogens, such as MRSA and VRE, are important examples of nosocomial pathogens that are often transmitted by the reservoir of unrecognized colonized patients and in which the organism usually colonize the patient before invading and causing disease [103]. ICU patients are especially vulnerable to colonization, due to their long hospital stays, prolonged exposure to antimicrobials, and frequent exposure to invasive devices and procedures. In addition, these nosocomial pathogens can be transmitted via the hands of HCWs in the ICU where patients require extensive care. In ICU outbreaks, education of HCWs about the sources and transmission of these organisms and the importance of handwashing in preventing transmission is essential. In addition, cost-effective methods to identify colonized patients, such as screening cultures, and infection control measures, such as isolation or cohorting of

TABLE 4. Guidelines for the prevention and control of nosocomial infection* from the Centers for Disease Control and Prevention (CDC), Atlanta, GA and the Hospital Infection Control Practices Advisory Committee (HICPAC)

Guidelines for handwashing and hospital environment, 1985 [104]
Guidelines for infection control in healthcare personnel, 1998 [106]
Guidelines for isolation precautions in hospitals, 1996 [105]
Guidelines for prevention of catheter-associated urinary tract infections, 1982 [85]
Guidelines for prevention of intravascular device-related infections, 1996 [72]
Guidelines for prevention of nosocomial pneumonia, 1994 [52]
Guidelines for prevention of surgical site infections, 1999 [107]

*Can be obtained by calling 1-888-232-3299 or on the Hospital Infections Program, CDC webpage at www.cdc.gov/ncidod/hip/default.htm.

these patients, may aid in controlling outbreaks [103].

Prevention

The most important step to prevention and control of nosocomial ICU outbreaks is continuous application of effective infection control and surveillance for infections and unusual clusters of events. Infection control professionals need standard definitions for identifying infections. Systematic review of the data, including calculation of rates of infection should be done and followed over time. When calculating rates of infection one needs to control for exposures such as, devices (e.g. CVC) and length of hospital stay (e.g. rates with patient days as a denominator). Special issues for particular types of ICUs (NICU vs SICU etc.) and types of patients need to be noted when evaluating or comparing at infection rates and attempting to identify causes of any cluster/outbreaks. A systematic review of the problem is the best strategy. While the cause of a cluster/outbreak is sought, implementation of control measures are essential to prevent further pathogen transmission. Handwashing is the cornerstone of any infection control efforts [104]. Proper implementation of recommended infection control measures, such as isolation policies, barrier precautions, environmental cleaning and disinfection/sterilization of medical equipment, should be reinforced [104, 105, 108] (Table 4).

References

1. Beck-Sague C, Jarvis W, Martone W. Outbreak investigations. Infect Control Hosp Epidemiol 18:138, 1997.
2. Stamm W, Weinstein R, Dixon R. Comparison of endemic and epidemic nosocomial infections. Am J Med 70:393, 1981.
3. Edgeworth J, Treacher D, Eykyn. A 25-year study of nosocomial bacteremia in an adult intensive care unit. Crit Care Med 27:1421, 1999.
4. Wenzel R, Thompson R, Landry S, Russell B, Miller P, *et al.* Hospital-acquired infections in intensive care unit patients: An overview with emphasis on epidemics. Infection Control 4:371, 1983.
5. Jarvis W. Nosocomial outbreaks: The Centers for Disease Control's Hospital Infections Program Experience, 1980–1990. Am J Med 91(suppl 3B):101S, 1991.
6. Centers for Disease Control. CDC definitions for nosocomial infections. Am J Infection Control 16:128, 1988.
7. Tafuro P, Ristuccia P. Recognition and control of outbreaks of nosocomial infections in the intensive care setting. Heart and Lung 13:486, 1984.
8. Martone W, Gaynes R, Horan T, Emori T, Jarvis W, *et al.* Nosocomial infection rates for interhospital comparison: Limitations and possible solutions. Infect Control Hosp Epidemiol 12:609, 1991.
9. Bredenberg H, Manangan L, Jarvis W. Selected hospital infections program outbreak investigations, 1994–1998. Infect Control Today August:26, 1999.
10. Wang S, Tokars J, Blanchine P, Carson L, Arduino M, *et al. Enterobacter cloacae* bloodstream infections traced to contaminated human albumin. Clin Infect Dis 30:35, 2000.
11. Richards C, Jarvis W. Lessons from recent nosocomial epidemics. Current Opin Infect Dis 12:327, 1999.
12. Esteban J, Gadea I, Fernandez-Roblas R, Molleja A, Calvo R, *et al.* Pseudo-outbreak of *Aeromonas hydophila* isolates related to endoscopy. J Hosp Infect 41:313, 1999.
13. Namnyak S, Hussain S, Davalle J, Roker K, Strickland M. Contaminated lithium heparin bottles as a source of pseudobacteraemia due to *Pseudomonas flourescens*. J Hosp Infect 41:23, 1999.
14. Jarvis W, Edwards J, Culver D, Hughes J, Horan T, *et al.* Nosocomial infection rates in adult and pediatric intensive care units in the United States. Am J Med 91(suppl 3B):185S, 1991.
15. Centers for Disease Control. National Nosocomial Infections Surveillance (NNIS) system report, data summary from January 1990–May 1999, Issued June 1999. Am J Infect Control 27:520, 1999.
16. Maloney S, Jarvis W. Epidemic nosocomial pneumonia in the intensive care unit. Clinics Chest Med 16:209, 1995.
17. Widmer A, Wenzel R, Trilla A, Bale M, Jones R, Deobbeling B. Outbreak of *Pseudomonas*

aeruginoas infections in a surgical intensive care unit: Probable transmission via hands of a health care worker. Clin Infect Dis 16:372, 1993.

18. Conly J, Klass L, Larson L, Kennedy J, Low D, Harding G. *Pseudomonas cepacia* colonization and infection in intensive care units. Can Med Assoc J 134:363, 1986.
19. Pegues D, Arathoon E, Samayoa B, Del Valle G, Anderson R, Riddle C, *et al.* Epidemic gram-negative bacteremia in a neonatal intensive care unit in Guatemala, Am J Infect Control 22:163.
20. Archibald L, Corl A, Shah B, Schulte M, Arduino M, Aguero S, *et al. Serratia marcescens* outbreak associated with extrinsic contamination of 1% chlorxylenol soap. Infect Control Hosp Epid 18:704, 1997.
21. McDonald C, Banerjee S, Jarvis W, and the National Nosocomial Surveillance System. Seasonal variation of *Acinetobacter* infections: 1987–1996. Clin Infect Dis 29:1133, 1999.
22. Contant J, Kemeny E, Oxley C, Perry E, Garber G. Investigation of an outbreak of *Acinitobacter calcoaceceticus var. anitratus* infections in an adult intensive care unit. Am J Infect Control 18: 288, 1990.
23. McDonald L, Walker M, Carson L, Arduino M, Aguero S, *et al.* Outbreak of *Acinetobacter* spp. bloodstream infections in a nursery associated with contaminated aerosols and air conditioners. Pediatr Infect Dis J 17:716, 1998.
24. Beck-Sague C, Jarvis W, Brook J, Culver D, Potts A, *et al.* Epidemic bacteremia due to *Acinetobacter baumannii* in five intensive care units. Am J Epid 132:723, 1990.
25. Chang H, Christenson J, Pavia A, Bobrin B, Bland L, *et al. Ochrobactrum anthropi* Meningitis in pediatric pericardial allograft transplant recipients. J Infect Dis 173:656, 1995.
26. Alnor D, Frimodt-Meller N, Espersen F, Frederiksen W. Infections with the unusual human pathogen Agrobacterium species and *Ochrbacterum anthropi*. Clin Infect Dis 18:914, 1994.
27. Wenger P, Tokars J, Brennan P, Samel C, Bland L, *et al.* An outbreak of *Enterobacter hormachei* infection and colonization in an intensive care nursery. Clin Infect Dis 24:1243, 1996.
28. Archibald L, Ramos M, Arduino M, Aguero S, Deseda C, *et al. Enterobacter cloacae* and *Pseudomonas aeruginosa* polymicrobial bloodstream infections traced to extrinsic contamination of a dextrose multidose vial. J Ped 133:640, 1998.
29. Rudnick J, Beck-Sague C, Anderson R, Schable B, Miller J, Jarvis W. Gram-negative bacteremia in open-heart-surgery patients traced to probable tap-water contamination of pressure. Infect Control Hosp Epid 17:281, 1996.
30. Richards C, Alonso-Echanove J, Caicedo Y, Jarvis W. *Klebsiella pneumoniae* bloodstream infections and death in a high risk nursery in Cali, Colombia–1999. Oral presentation 39th Interscience Conference on Antimicrobial Agents and Chemotherapy (ICAAC), Abstract No 2088.
31. Parvez F, Roeshadi D, Irmawati L, Sidharta Y, Rosenthal S, *et al.* Investigation of *Salmonella Serotype Worthington* causing cellulities, sepsis, and death in a neonatal intensive care unit, Indonesia. Oral presentation 4th Decennial International Conference on Nosocomial and Healthcare-Associated Infections, Abstract No S-M4-04 Atlanta, GA.
32. Toscano C, Pessoa da Silva C, Santos A, Falcao M, Campos E, *et al.* Nosocomial outbreak of multidrug-resistant *Salmonella Infantis* bacteremia in neonates. Oral presentation 4th Decennial International Conference on Nosocomial and Healthcare-Associated Infections, Abstract No S-M4-05 Atlanta, GA, 2000.
33. Lannigan R, Hussain Z, Austin T. *Streptococcus pyogenes* as a cause of nosocomial infection in a critical care unit. Diag Microb & Infect Dis 3:337, 1985.
34. Nicolle L, Hume K, Sims H, Rosenal T, Sandham D. An outbreak of group A *streptococcal bacteremia* in an intensive care unit. Infect Control 7:177, 1986.
35. Ribner B, Landry M, Kidd K, Peninger M, Riddick J. Outbreak of multiply restraint *Staphylococcus aureus* in a pediatric intensive care unit after consolidation with a surgical intensive care unit. Am J Infect Control 17:244, 1989.
36. Guiguet M, Rekacewicz C, Leclercq B, Brun Y, Escudier B, Andremont A. Effectiveness of simple measures to control an outbreak of nosocomial methicillin-resistant *Staphylococcus aureus* infections in an intensive care unit. Infect Control Hosp Epid 11:23, 1990.
37. Pijol M, Corbella X, Peña C, Pallarés R, Dorca J, *et al.* Clinical and epidemiological findings in mechanically-ventilated patients with methicillin-resistant *Staphylococcus aureus* pneu-

monia. Europ J Clin Microbiol Infect Dis 17:622, 1998.
38. Manhold C, von Rolbicki U, Brase R, Timm J, von Pritzbuer E, *et al.* Outbreak of *Staphylococcus aureus* infections during treatment of late onset pneumonia with ciprofloxacin in a prospective, randomized study. Intens Care Med 24:1327, 1998.
39. Cotterill S, Evans R, Fraise A. An unusual source for an outbreak of methicillin-resistant *Staphylococcus aureus* on an intensive therapy unit. J Hosp Infect 32:207, 1995.
40. Jernigan J, Titus M, Groeschel D, Getchell-White S, Farr B. Effectiveness of contact isolation during a hospital outbreak of methicillin-resistant *Staphylococcus aureus*. Am J Epidemiol 143:596, 1996.
41. Montecalvo M, Shay D, Patel P, Tacsa L, Maloney S, *et al.* Bloodstream infections with vancomycin-resistant enterococci. Arch Intern Med 156:1458, 1996.
42. Shay D, Maloney S, Montecalvo M, Banerjee S, Wormser G, *et al.* Epidemiology and mortality risk of vancomycin-resistant enterococcal bloodstream infections. JID 172:993, 1995.
43. Slaughter S, Hayden M, Nathan C, Hu T, Rice T, Van Voorhis J, *et al.* A comparison of the effect of universal use of gloves and gowns with that glove use alone on acquisition of vancomycin-resistant enterococci in a medical intensive care unit. Ann Intern Med 125:448, 1996.
44. Karanfil L, Murphy M, Josephson A, *et al.* A cluster of vancomycin-resistant enterococci faecium in an intensive care unit. Infect Control Hosp Epid 13:195, 1992.
45. Centers for Disease Control and Prevention. Recommendations for preventing the spread of vancomycin resistance, recommendations of the Hospital Infection Control Practices Advisory Committee (HICPAC). MMWR 41:1, 1995.
46. Burnie J, Odds F, Lee W, Webster C, Williams J. Outbreak of systemic *Candida albicans* in intensive care unit caused by cross infection. Brit Med J Clin Res Ed 290:746, 1985.
47. Voss A, Pfaller M, Hollis R, Rhine-Chalberg J, Doebbeling B. Investigation of *Candida albicans* transmission in a surgical intensive care unit cluster by using genomic DNA typing methods. J Clin Microbiol 33:576, 1995.
48. Pertowski C, Baron R, Lasker B, Werner S, Jarvis W. Nosocomial outbreak of *Candida albicans* sternal wound infections following cardiac surgery traced to a scrub nurse. J Infect Dis 172:817, 1995.
49. Isenberg H, Tucci V, Cintron F, *et al.* Single source outbreak of *Candida tropicalis* complicating coronary bypass surgery. J Clin Microbiol 27:2426, 1989.
50. Humphreys H, Johnson E, Warnock D, Willatts S, Winter R, Speller D. An outbreak of *aspergillosis* in a general ITU. J Hosp Infect 18:167, 1991.
51. Lovett I, Houang E, Burge S, Turner-Warwick M, Thompson F, Harrison A, *et al.* An outbreak of *Nocardia asteroids* infection in a renal transplant unit. Quarterly J Med 50:123, 1981.
52. Centers for Disease Control and Prevention. Guideline for prevention of nosocomial pneumonia. Resp Care 39:1191, 1994.
53. Richet H, McNeil M, Edwards M, Jarvis W. Cluster of *Malassezia furfur* pulmonary infections in infants in a neonatal intensive care unit. J Clin Microbiol 27:1197, 1989.
54. Chang H, Miller H, Watkins N, Arduino M, Ashford D, *et al.* An epidemic of *Malassezia pachydermatis* in an intensive care nursery associated with colonization of health care workers' pet dogs. New Eng J Med 338:706, 1998.
55. Archer-Dubon C, Icaza-Chivez M, Orozco-Topete R, Reyes E, Baez-Martinez R, Ponce de Leon S. An epidemic outbreak of *Malassezia folliculitis* in three adult patients in an intensive care unit: a previously unrecognized nosocomial infection. Int J Derm 38:453, 1999.
56. Hanna J, Loewenthal M, Negel P, Wenck D. An outbreak of Hepatitis A in an intensive care unit. Anaesth Intens Care 24:440, 1996.
57. Shanson D. Hepatitis B outbreak in operating-theatre and intensive care staff. Lancet 2:596, 1980.
58. Adams G, Stover B, Keenlyside A, Hooton T, Buchman T, Roizman B, *et al.* Nosocomial herpetic infections in a pediatric intensive care unit. Am J Epid 113:126, 1981.
59. Gurevich I, Cunha B. Non-parenteral transmission of *Cytomegalovirus* in a neonatal intensive care unit. Lancet 2:222, 1981.
60. Davies D, Hughes C, MacVicar J, Hawkes P, Mair H. *Echovirus-11* infection in a special-care baby unit. Lancet 1:96, 1979.
61. Nagington J, Wreghitt T, Gandy G, Roberston N, Berry P. Fatal echovirus 11 infections in outbreak in special-care baby unit. Lancet 2:725, 1978.

62. Meibalane R, Sedmak G, Sasidharan P, Garg P, Grausz J. Outbreak of *influenza* in a neonatal intensive care unit. J Ped 91:974, 1977.
63. Welliver RC, McLaughlin S. Unique epidemiology of nosocomial infection in a children's hospital. Am J Dis Children 138:131, 1984.
64. Parvez F, Jarvis W. Nosocomial infections in the nursery. Sem Ped Infect Dis 10:119, 1999.
65. Langley J, LeBlanc J, Wang E, Law B, MacDonald N, Mitchell I. Nosocomial *Respiratory Syncytial Virus* infection in Canadian pediatric hospitals: A pediatric investigators' collaborative network on infections in Canada study. Pediatrics 100:943, 1997.
66. Fixler D. *Respiratory Syncytial Virus* infection in children with congenital heart disease: a review. Pediatric Cardiology 17:163, 1996.
67. Pohl C, Green M, Wald E, Ledesma-Medina J. *Respiratory Syncytial Virus* infections in pediatric liver transplant recipients. J Infect Dis 165:166, 1992.
68. Wilson C, Stevenson D, Arvin A. A concurrent epidemic of *Respiratory Syncytial Virus* and *Echovirus* 7 infections in an intensive care nursery. Ped Infect Dis J 8:24, 1989.
69. Karanfil L, Conlon M, Lykens K, Masters C, Forman M, *et al.* Reducing the rate of nosocomially transmitted *Respiratory Syncytial Virus*. Am J Infect Control 27:91, 1999.
70. Guidry G, Black-Payne C, Payne D, Jamison R, George R, Bocchini J. *Respiratory Syncytial Virus* infection among intubated adults in a university medical intensive care unit. Chest 100:1377, 1991.
71. Marton W, Williams W, Mortensen M, *et al.* Illness with fatalities in premature infants: Association with an intravenous vitamin E preparation, E-Ferol. Pediatrics 78:591, 1986.
72. Centers for Disease Control and Prevention. Guideline for prevention of intravascular device-related infections. Am J Infect Control 17:438, 1996.
73. Weinstein R, Stamm W, Kramer L, Corey L. Pressure monitoring devices: overlooked source of nosocomial infection. J Am Med Assoc 236:936, 1976.
74. Hekker T, van Overhagen W, Schneider A. Pressure transducers: an overlooked source of sepsis in the intensive care unit. Intensive Care Med 16:511, 1990.
75. Goldmann D, Martin W, Worthington J. Growth of bacteria and fungi in total parenteral nutrition solutions. Am J Surg 126:314, 1973.
76. D'Angio R, Riechers K, Gilsford R, Constantino J. Effect of the mode of lipid administration on parenteral nutrition-related infections. Ann Pharmacother 26:14, 1992.
77. Reboli A, Koshinski R, Arias K, Marks-Austin K, Stieritz D, Stull T. An outbreak of *Burkholderia cepacia* lower respiratory tract infection associated with contaminated Albuterol nebulization solution. Infect Control Hosp Epidemiol 17:741, 1996.
78. Labarca J, Trick W, Peterson C, Carson L, Holt S, *et al.* A multistate nosocomial outbreak of *Ralstonia pickettii* colonization associated with an intrinsically contaminated respiratory care solution. Clin Infect Dis 29:1281, 1999.
79. Agerton T, Valway S, Gore B, Pozsik C, Plikaytis B, Woodley C. Transmission of a highly drug resistant strain (Strain W1) of *Mycobacterium tuberculosis*: Community outbreak and nosocomial transmission via a contaminated bronchoscope. J Am Med Assoc 278:1073, 1997.
80. Gubler J, Salinger M, von Graevenitz A. Pseudooutbreak of nontuberulous mycobacteria due to a contaminated bronchoscope cleaning machine. Report of an outbreak and review of the literature. Chest 1245, 1992.
81. Maloney S, Welbel S, Daves B, Adams K, Becker S, *et al. Mycobacterium abscessus* pseudoinfection traced to an automated endoscope washer: utility of epidemiologic and laboratory investigation. J Infect Dis 169:1166, 1994.
82. Centers for Disease Control and Prevention. Bronscopy-related infections and pseudoinfections – New York, 1996 and 1998, 1999, MMWR 48:557, 1999.
83. Marrie T, MacDonald S, Clarke K, Haldane D. Nosocomial Legionnaireses' diease: lessons from a four year prospective sudy. Am J Infect Control 19:79, 1991.
84. Martone W, Jarvis W, Edwards J, Culver D, Haley R. Incidence and nature of endemic and epidemic nosocomial infections. Hospital Infections, Fourth Edition, 461, 1998.
85. Centers for Disease Control and Prevention. Guideline for prevention of catheter-associated urinary tract infections. Am J Infect Control 11:28, 1983.
86. Knaus W, Wagner D, Draper E, *et al.* The APACHE III prognostic system, risk prediction of hospital mortality for critically ill hospitalized adults. Chest 100:1619, 1991.

87. Emori G, Culver D, Horan T, Jarvis W, White J, *et al.* National Nosocomial Infections Surveillance (NNIS) System: Description of surveillance methods. Am J Infect Control 19:19, 1991.
88. CDC. Nosocomial infection rates for interhospital comparison: Limitation and possible solutions. Infect Control Hosp Epid 12:609, 1991.
89. Gaynes R, Culver D, Banerjee S, Edwards J, Henderson T. Meaningful interhospital comparisons of infection rates in intensive care units. Am J Infect Control 21:43, 1993.
90. Wenzel R, Osterman C, Donowitz L, Hoyt J, Sande M, *et al.* Identification of procedure-related nosocomial infections in high-risk patients. Rev Infect Dis 3:701, 1981.
91. Gaynes R, Martone W, Culver D, Emori T, Horan T, *et al.* Comparison of rates of nosocomial infections in neonatal intensive care units in the United States. Am J Med 91(suppl 3B):192S, 1991.
92. Kelsey M, Gosling M. A comparison of the morbidity associated with occlusive and non-occlusive dressings applied to peripheral intravenous devices. J Hosp Infect 5:313, 1984.
93. Snydman D, Pober B, Murray S, Gorbea H, Majika J, Perry L. Predictive value of surveillance skin cultures in total-parenteral nutrition-related infection. Lancet 2:1385, 1982.
94. Fridkin S, Pear S, Williamson T, Galgiani J, Jarvis W. The role of understaffing in central venous catheter-associated bloodstream infections. Infect Control Hosp Epid 17:150, 1996.
95. Archibald L, Manning M, Bell L, Banerjee S, Jarvis W. Patient density, nurse-to-patient ratio and nosocomial infection risk in a pediatric cardiac intensive care unit. Pediatr Infect Dis J 16:1045, 1997.
96. Roberts J, Fridkin S, Blumberg H, Anderson B, White N, *et al.* The influence of the composition of the nursing staff on primary bloodstream infection rates in a surgical intensive care unit. Infect Control Hosp Epid 21, 2000.
97. Mayhall C, Archer N, Lamb V, Spadora A, Baggett J, *et al.* Ventriculostomy-related infections: A prospective epidemiologic study. New Engl J Med 310:553, 1984.
98. Trick W, Kioski C, Howard K, Cage G, Tokars J, Yen B, *et al.* Outbreak of *Pseudomonas aeruginosa* ventriculitis among patients in a neurosurgical intensive care unit. Infect Control Hosp Epid 21:204, 2000.
99. Bennett S, McNeil M, Bland L, Arduino M, Villarino M, *et al.* Postoperative infections traced to contamination of an intravenous anesthetic, Propofol. New Engl J Med 333:147, 1995.
100. Burwen D, Banerjee S, Gaynes R. Ceftazidime resistance among selected nosocomial Gram-negative bacilli in the United States. J Infect Dis 170:1622, 1994.
101. Brachman P. Epidemiology of nosocomial infections, Hospital Infection, 2nd edn. Boston, MA: Little, Brown and Co, 1986.
102. Goldmann D. Bacterial colonization and infection in the neonate. Am J Med 70:417, 1981.
103. Jarvis W. The epidemiology of colonization. Infect Control Hosp Epid 17:47, 1994.
104. Centers for Disease Control and Prevention. Guideline for handwashing and hospital environmental control. Am J Infect Control 14:110, 1986.
105. Centers for Disease Control and Prevention. Guideline for isolation precautions in hospitals. Am J Infect Control 24:24, 1996.
106. Centers for Disease Control and Prevention. Guideline for infection control in healthcare personnel. Am J Infect Control 26:289, 1998.
107. Mangram A, Horan T, Pearson M, Silver L, Jarvis W. Guideline for prevention of surgical site infection. Infect Control and Hospital Epid 20:247, 1999.
108. Fridkin S, Welbel S, Weinstein R. Magnitude and prevention of nosocomial infections in the intensive care unit. Infect Dis Clinics North Am 1:479, 1997.

SECTION 4: INFECTIOUS DISEASES EMERGENCIES

M. Kollef

23. SEPTIC SHOCK

Jonathan Cohen

Introduction

This chapter is concerned with the diagnosis and immediate treatment of patients with septic shock. Most clinicians will have a mental image of this condition and would expect to have little difficulty in recognizing it from the end of the bed, but despite this there is no universally accepted definition. Indeed, when clinical investigators attempt to arrive at a consensus there are wide variations in terms. Thus, a necessary preface to this chapter is a brief discussion of the controversy surrounding the nomenclature of these syndromes.

Sepsis is the systemic response to infection, brought about by activation of the host inflammatory processes. Clinical features of sepsis include fever (or hypothermia), leukocytosis (or leukopenia), tachycardia, and tachypnea. Perhaps surprisingly, there is no "case definition" as such; indeed, there is a wide variation in the clinical manifestations of this response, and no single attribute or group of attributes are obligatory components [1]. In an attempt to address this problem a consensus conference met and identified a constellation of clinical features that they referred to as SIRS (the Systemic Inflammatory Response Syndrome) [2]. Although useful in that it drew attention to a common clinical pattern seen in ICU patients, SIRS has been criticized because it is much too sensitive and because it embraces a wide range of possible causes. Sepsis – i.e. infection – is one cause of SIRS, but many other non-infective processes (blood transfusion, trauma, pancreatitis etc) can cause the same clinical picture.

Severe sepsis/sepsis syndrome. These terms are used to describe sepsis associated with organ dysfunction, hypoperfusion or hypotension. Hypoperfusion abnormalities may include, but are not limited to, lactic acidosis, oliguria, and an acute alteration in mental state. These definitions have provided the basis for the inclusion criteria for most of the clinical trials of adjunctive agents in sepsis that have been carried out during the last 10 years, and as such have been the subject of much discussion. While some have argued that sepsis syndrome is a valid clinical entity [3] others have pointed out that it results in the inclusion of such a diverse population of patients that it is too imprecise and serves no useful purpose [1].

Septic shock. Septic shock is universally recognized as the most severe end of the spectrum of systemic syndromes induced by infection, yet remarkably, there is no agreed definition. Indeed the late Roger Bone, one of the doyens of this field, actually wrote "Septic shock should not be viewed as a single entity . . ." [4]. In the same paper, Bone defined septic shock as ". . . simply [sic] the deranged metabolic state that arises from systemic sepsis in a hypotensive patient unresponsive to fluid management". Others have written that septic shock is ". . . the development of arterial hypotension (systolic arterial pressure below 90 mmHg or mean arterial pressure below 60 mmHg) associated with signs of tissue hypoperfusion (increased blood lactate levels >2 mEq/l, oliguria, altered mentation etc) [1].

It is not my purpose here to resolve these dilemmas, but rather to draw attention to the inadequacy of the current use of these terms. Certainly there is broad agreement that septic shock first, implies the presence of infection, and secondly, describes a severe illness in which there is multiple organ dysfunction and a mortality rate which may be as high as 75%. This chapter will focus on the infectious diseases aspects of septic shock; other elements of the management such as cardiovascular support and monitoring are covered elsewhere (see pages 113–126). I will emphasize the practical approach to the diagnosis and management of patients with septic shock, in particular strategies that are currently available in routine clinical practice.

Epidemiology

Sepsis and septic shock have occurred with increasing frequency during the last 15–20 years, much of this being driven by an excess of hospital-acquired (nosocomial) infections [5, 6]. It has been estimated that there are approximately 500,000 cases of sepsis each year in the United States, and that between 150,000 and 250,000 people die directly from the condition. It must be admitted that these figures are imprecise, in large part because of the problems with the definition that were noted above.

The true incidence of septic *shock* is equally difficult to ascertain for similar reasons. Shock is a subset of the larger population of patients with sepsis. In one study of 600 bacteraemic patients which included both community-acquired and nosocomial infections, shock occurred in 20% and was associated with a mortality of 60%, compared to a mortality of just 14% in the non-shocked group [7]. Part of the difficulty is that there is a complex, and at times confusing, relationship between bacteremia, sepsis, and shock. These terms are not synonymous, but in some cases the distinction has become blurred. In the large epidemiological study of SIRS reported by Rangel-Frausto [6] positive blood cultures were found in 69% of patients with shock but just 25% of patients with sepsis. However, in patients with shock the mortality was the same, irrespective of whether they were bacteraemic. In contrast, a somewhat similar study reported by Brun-Buisson *et al.* [8] found that the higher mortality associated with increasing numbers of organ dysfunctions (Relative Risk 4.4 [95% Confidence Interval 1.2–16]) *was* further increased in patients with documented infections (RR 9.4 [1.3–78]). There are several possible explanations for these findings. First, it is important to distinguish studies on bacteremia alone from studies in which all sites of infection are included. Data on secular trends in bacteremia rates and associated mortality [9, 10] are valuable but should not be confused with sepsis studies. Secondly, local epidemiologic factors need to be considered: for instance, a study in which there were a disproportionate number of neutropenic patients would be likely to include a large number of bacteremias caused by *Staph. epidermidis*, an organism of generally low virulence. In contrast, a unit which cared for liver transplant recipients would have a relatively high number of episodes of candidemia, an infection with a much more grave prognosis [10]. Thirdly, there may be differences in the proportion of community- and hospital-acquired infections between different studies. Significant differences occur in the isolation of pathogens from community and hospital-acquired infections [11] and several investigators have reported that nosocomial infections have a higher mortality, certainly in respect of bacteremias [12].

Recently we [13] had an opportunity to analyze data concerning the clinical presentation, microbiologic findings and outcome of a large cohort of patients who had been enrolled in a study of a p55 TNF receptor fusion protein [14]. A total of 444 septic patients were available to study; a subset of 197 were prospectively allocated to a late septic shock group (based on a systolic blood pressure of <90 mmHg or a reduction of <40 mmHg in the absence of other explanations, that did not respond to a fluid challenge and vasopressors). Overall, 61% of patients had a microbiologically documented

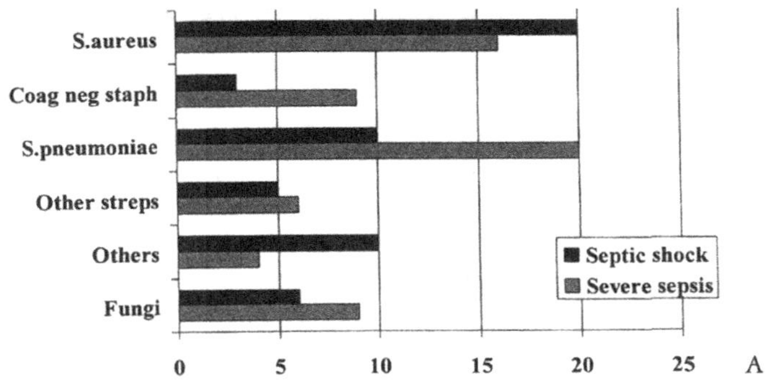

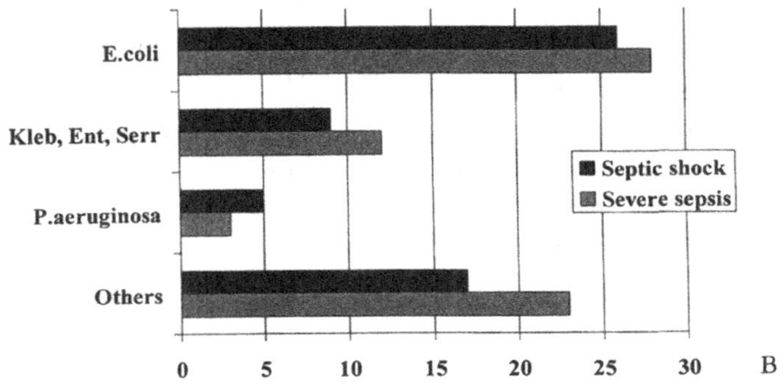

FIGURE 1. A. The distribution of microbial isolates between the severe sepsis and septic shock groups (Gram-positive bacteria and fungi). Reproduced with permission from Cohen J & Abraham E, J Infect Dis 180:116, 1999. B. The distribution of microbial isolates between the severe sepsis and septic shock groups (Gram-negative bacteria). Reproduced with permission from Cohen J & Abraham E, J Infect Dis 180:116, 1999. Kleb = Klebsiella; ENT = Enterobacter, Serr = Servatia.

infection. The proportion of patients with pure Gram-negative (36%), pure Gram-positive (35%) or mixed infections (19%) did not differ between the sepsis and septic shock groups. Furthermore, there were no important differences in the distribution of specific organisms between the two groups (Figure 1). Among Gram-negative bacteria, *E. coli* was the most common isolate, and together with other Enterobacteriaceae was the commonest cause of Gram-negative sepsis. *P. aeruginosa* was notable for the small number of isolates and was not more common in the septic shock group. *Staph. aureus* was the most common Gram-positive isolate; coagulase-negative staphylococci were uncommon. *Strep. pneumoniae* were important causes of sepsis; *Strep. pyogenes* and viridans streptococci were also isolated. Other unusual isolates included anaerobes, *Listeria monocytogenes* and some fungi. Although this large study of nearly 500 patients found no important differences in the pattern of organisms in the sepsis, versus the septic shock group there are some data that suggest that certain bacteria are associated with a higher mortality (summarized in [6]). Candida and enterococcal infections (in particular, vancomycin-resistant *E. faecium*) have high organism-specific mortalities, *Staph. epidermidis* is low. Both *P. aeruginosa* and *Strep. pyogenes* are often associated with a very poor outcome but they occur rather infrequently and it is difficult to obtain statistically significant results. Infec-

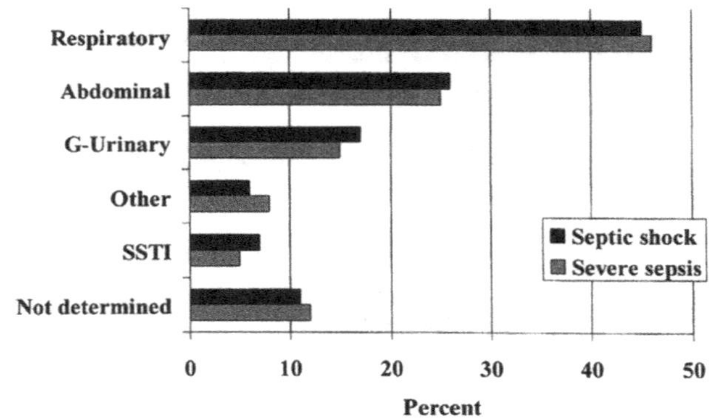

FIGURE 2. Distribution of the primary site of infection between the severe sepsis and septic shock groups. SSTI = skin and soft tissue infections. Reproduced with permission from Cohen J & Abraham E, J Infect Dis 180:116, 1999.

tions with *Stenotrophomonas maltophilia* and *Acinetobacter* are emerging in many units, perhaps in response to antibiotic pressure [15]. At present there are no data to suggest that these bacteria are of particular importance as causes of septic shock.

An analysis of the sites of origin of the infections confirmed data from earlier trials that showed the respiratory tract and intra-abdominal sites to be the most common origins of sepsis. There was no difference in the distribution of the sites between the sepsis and septic shock groups (Figure 2).

Since the test agent showed no significant survival benefit the results of all patients were pooled. As might be anticipated, the overall mortality was higher in the shock group (41.1%) compared to those with sepsis (31.6%). However, it was particularly interesting to look at interactions between the microbiological findings, TNF-α levels and outcome. First, we found that patients with a documented infection had significantly higher TNF-α levels than those from whom no pathogen was isolated (geometric mean [coefficient of variation {CV}] levels were 66 {53%} pg/ml (range, 5–2520) versus 29 {53%} pg/ml (range 5–3310), $p = 0.0001$). Furthermore, in patients with septic shock those with a documented Gram-negative infection had higher TNF-α levels (143 pg/ml) than those with Gram-positive infections (64 pg/ml), $p = 0.004$. These data are of importance for two reasons: first, they show that the difference between "clinically documented" and "microbiologically documented" episodes is not a chance depending on whether a positive culture was obtained in an individual case, but a real and measurable biological difference reflected in different TNF levels. Secondly, it shows that Gram-negative and Gram-positive infections may differ in their biology, and not just represent a "final common pathway" [16].

Diagnosis

The most important reason to make a microbiologic diagnosis in septic patients is to ensure that effective antimicrobial therapy is given. There is good evidence to support the intuitive belief that patients given appropriate therapy are more likely to survive than those given inadequate or inappropriate treatment [17]. Obtaining microbiologic information will also contribute to the local epidemiologic database, without which logical prescribing is difficult, if not impossible. There are substantial differences between intensive care units in the microbial ecology, including for example the prevalence of methicillin-resistant *Staphylococcus aureus* and vancomycin-resistant *Streptococcus faecalis*. Antimicrobial resistance patterns too, vary widely: examples include penicillin resistance in *Streptococcus pneumoniae*, and gentamicin resistance in Enterobacteriaceae. Furthermore, these resistance rates are constantly changing, and an up-to-date awareness of these patterns is obviously essential when considering empiric therapy. Finally, knowledge of the microbial etiology of sepsis may be important in the choice of adjunctive therapies. This is not yet clinical reality, but will clearly be important if, for instance, anti-endotoxin agents ever enter the clinical arena.

There are three key difficulties associated with the diagnosis of infection in patients who appear to be septic.

Establishing infection as the primary cause. The controversies surrounding the definition of sepsis have been discussed above. Establishing that the patient has infection rather than a non-infective cause of SIRS can be extremely difficult. Knowledge of other pathologies that may mimic sepsis and how they may apply to the specific patient can make up for a relative paucity of clinical information. The differential diagnosis of shock due to causes other than infection includes acute myocardial infarction, massive pulmonary embolism, acute blood loss and anaphylaxis. Less common diagnoses are acute hypoadrenalism, diabetic ketoacidosis and some cases of self-poisoning. The diagnosis and management of non-infective shock is beyond the scope of this chapter.

Localizing the site of infection. This may be confounded by the fact there are multiple pathologic processes occurring concurrently or by the frequent use of antibiotics which undermine microbiologic diagnosis. Occasionally the site of infection is occult, for instance when there is sinusitis or deep intra-abdominal infection.

Interpreting the microbiologic findings. Conventional microbiology has many limitations in the ICU patient who may be septic. Principal amongst these is the fact that many organisms isolated from non-sterile sites may represent either colonization of infection – microbiology alone cannot answer this question. Conversely, the microbiology laboratory may report negative findings in samples from sites that are in fact infected, for example because antibiotics have sterilized the specimen.

A CLINICAL APPROACH

Fever is a common sign on the ICU and will often be the first indication of sepsis, although there are many other causes [18]. Practice guidelines for the evaluation of fever on the ICU have recently been published [19].

Focused clinical examination, guided by any risk factors relevant to the individual patient will often reveal potential sources of sepsis and guide subsequent investigation (see pages 19–46). Surgical and traumatic wounds should be exposed and examined for signs of infection. Particular attention should be paid to vascular access sites for signs of phlebitis or cellulitis and to pressure areas or injection sites for evidence of soft tissue infection. Evidence of sinusitis should be sought, and fundoscopy is invaluable in detecting candidal endophthalmitis, a pathognomonic feature of systemic fungal sepsis. Urine in the catheter may be frankly purulent, and the presence of diarrhea may indicate *Clostridium difficile* associated colitis. The importance of repeated, complete physical examination to detect the emergence of new signs cannot be overstated.

DIAGNOSTIC MICROBIOLOGY

Microbiological aspects of infection at specific sites are dealt with in the chapters dealing with those infections (see pages 3–18 and Sections 4–7). Blood cultures are considered below; a more detailed account of the microbiological investigation of sepsis is available [20].

Blood should be obtained for culture whenever there is reason to suspect a clinically significant bacteremia. There are no good data that relate timing of blood cultures with respect to timing of fever. Nevertheless, bacteria are rapidly cleared from blood, and development of fever usually follows an episode of bacteremia by 30–90 minutes, so blood cultures should be taken as soon as possible following a spike of fever.

When a decision has been made to take blood for culture, adherence to a protocol for obtaining the specimen results in lower contamination rates and will also affect yield. Skin should be sterilized prior to venopuncture by swabbing twice with either 70% isopropyl or ethyl alcohol or with an iodine containing solution [20]. Blood should be obtained by venopuncture or if necessary arterial stab. Sites associated with skin contamination (e.g. femoral site) or loss of skin integrity (e.g. dermatological disease) should be avoided. Contamination rates are not significantly higher for blood obtained through a peripheral cannula at the time of insertion and this is acceptable as a means of minimizing the number of venopunctures.

An adequate volume of blood must be obtained. The concentration of bacteremia in adult patients is frequently below one viable organism per ml and may be less than 0.1 organisms per ml, so it is not surprising that the volume of blood obtained for culture is an important variable determining culture yield. In adults, a minimum sample size of 10 ml will optimize yield while increasing the volume above 30 ml is not associated with significantly improved culture rates.

In bacteremia associated with sources other than endocarditis, sensitivity exceeding 99% is reached with either two or three cultures. The taking of only one culture is rarely permissible. Since the rate of contamination of an individual set of blood cultures is finite, ranging from 1% to 4.5%, interpretation of a single isolate of a potentially contaminating organism may be exceedingly difficult. When clinically significant bacteremia is suspected, two or three sets of cultures should be obtained by individual venopunctures. There is no advantage in waiting between them.

NON-SPECIFIC MARKERS OF INFECTION

Traditional markers of infection such as neutrophilia are too non-specific in the ICU setting to be of value in distinguishing sepsis, although marked neutrophilia or failure to mount a neutrophil response may be of prognostic value. Levels of procalcitonin (PCT) and C-reactive protein (CRP) are straightforward to assay. The evidence that these acute phase markers have specificity in differentiating infection from other causes of an inflammatory response has recently been reviewed [21]. In a prospective study of ICU patients, a CRP of 50 mg/l or more had a sensitivity of 98.5% and specificity of 75% in identifying probable or definite sepsis [22]. De Werra *et al.*, also in an ICU population, found PCT levels of 1.5 ng/ml or more had a sensitivity of 100% and specificity of 72% [23]. Two more recent papers illustrate well the difficulty in interpreting the data. Oberhoffer *et al.* [24] reported that PCT was better correlated with TNF-α and IL-6 than was CRP or other clinical parameters such as leukocyte count or fever. Of course, that does not make it better at diagnosing infection. That question was addressed directly in another study of 190 ICU patients, of whom 111 had infection [25]. In this case, CRP was more sensitive and more specific than PCT in identifying infection, although PCT was higher in bacteraemic compared to non-bacteraemic patients, and was particularly elevated in patients with septic shock. In my opinion, such markers can not alone differentiate sepsis from other causes of SIRS, and they should certainly never be used as the sole basis of a decision to use, or not to use antibiotics in a patient who may be septic. Rather, they are a part of a systematic evaluation that includes clinical examination and directed diagnostic techniques. Measurement of PCT or CRP is often most valuable when done sequentially in an individual patient as an aid to following the response to treatment, or as an indicator that a focus of infection remains inadequately treated.

Endotoxemia is present in the blood of about

30% of patients with bacteremia, but endotoxemia does not predict either Gram-negative bacteremia or Gram-negative infection, nor does it predict survival from sepsis. There is some correlation with severity of sepsis, but the level of precision is poor. In the study by Danner *et al.* [26] 43% of 100 septic patients were endotoxin-positive at some point during their ICU stay; however, only 20 patients were positive at study entry. Similar results were obtained by Guidet *et al.* [27] (47% of 93 patients positive) and more recently, by Bates *et al.* [28] (33% of 356 episodes). There are some exceptions: Casey *et al.* [29] observed that 89% of 97 patients had endotoxemia. The mean value was 2.6 EU/ml, equivalent to a value of >200 pg/ml, rather high by most standards. Similarly, an older study by Fink and Grunert [30] of 41 patients found that 38 were endotoxin positive. They were using a turbidometric assay with a sensitivity of 100 pg/ml, so these results are difficult to understand. It is important to note that in most of the clinical studies the cut-off for regarding tests as positive is at a level of approximately 0.1 EU (5–10 pg/ml). This creates ample opportunity for error, either as a result of contamination or by misinterpretation of borderline results [31].

Hurley reviewed a total of 45 studies and used the technique of meta-analysis to calculate the concordance between endotoxemia and Gram-negative bacteremia [32]. His results graphically illustrated the problem. In a hypothetical population of 100 patients with suspected sepsis, of whom 20 have Gram-negative bacteremia, the gelation LAL assay would "correctly" identify 10 of these, but would produce "false" positive results in 10 patients without Gram-negative bacteremia. The newer, chromogenic LAL assay format would be slightly more sensitive, identifying 12 of the 20 with Gram-negative bacteremia, but generating discordant positive results in 24 patients.

The most clear-cut example of the relationship between endotoxemia and outcome is meningococcal disease. Patients with meningococcal meningitis have absent or low levels of endotoxin in the blood, and the mortality is low. In meningococcemia endotoxemia is much more common, and there is a good quantitative relationship between the level of endotoxin in the blood at presentation and the outcome [33]. This relationship is much more difficult to demonstrate in a heterogeneous ICU population. In none of the three recent studies [26–28], did endotoxemia *per se* predict survival. However, in some cases, endotoxemia (but not the precise amount) did correlate with severity of the disease. For instance, in Danner's study the presence of endotoxemia was significantly correlated with a higher plasma lactate, a lower SVR and LVEF, and a greater need for vasopressors. Thus, endotoxemia alone seems not to be helpful in predicting outcome, but a meta-analysis of 11 studies concluded that the combination of Gram-negative bacteremia and endotoxemia did identify a subpopulation of patients at substantially greater risk of dying [32]. The odds ratio (OR) for the risk of dying was 2.3 (95% confidence interval [CI] 1.3–4.0) for endotoxemia without Gram-negative bacteremia, and was 2.0 (95% CI 1.0–3.8) for the converse setting, but increased substantially when both factors were present (OR 6.3, 95% CI 4.0–10.0).

It will be apparent from the foregoing that at the present time, there is no place for routine endotoxin testing in clinical practice. In particular, the positive predictive value of the test is insufficiently high to be of clinical use. It may be that the LAL assay, or one of the newer developments, may be more useful in excluding Gram-negative infection, but that remains to be shown.

Management

GENERAL PRINCIPLES

The immediate priority is to address the three potentially life-threatening issues: airway, breathing and circulation (the so-called ABC of resuscitation). Improvements in supportive care have made an important contribution to the outcome of septic shock. All patients need to have adequate oxygenation and appropriate fluid management, and most will require inotropic and vasopressor therapy. More detailed consideration of these general principles of management can be found in several excellent recent reviews [34–36] and also in pages 113–126.

ANTIMICROBIAL THERAPY

It is perhaps worth re-stating the long-held and probably intuitive view that patients given the correct antibiotics are less likely to die than those treated inappropriately. The evidence for this comes from a series of studies dating back over 30 years and exemplified by a paper from Kreger *et al.* [17]. They analyzed a cohort of 612 patients with Gram-negative bacteremia collected over a 10 year period. Irrespective of the severity of the underlying disease, proper empirical therapy reduced by half the frequency with which shock developed, and the fatality rate was significantly less in the appropriately treated groups compared to those given inappropriate antibiotics (rapidly fatal: 29% vs 77%, ultimately fatal 26% vs 38%, nonfatal 11% vs 29%). It might be argued that such differences would be unlikely to be apparent if the study were to be repeated today, in part because the epidemiology has changed but also because modern antibiotics – and the way they are used – provide such broad spectrum cover that completely inappropriate therapy is very uncommon. However, a recent study from France provides powerful evidence that choosing the correct antibiotic regimen does still have an impact on outcome, and moreover, that infectious diseases expents are more likely to choose the correct regimen than are non-expents. The study was a prospective analysis of 428 episodes of bacteremia seen over one year in a university hospital [37]. "Appropriateness" was defined as therapy that was active *in vitro* against the infecting organism, that was of clinically proven efficacy, and that was given by the intravenous route at appropriate doses. Shock at presentation, a SAPS score of >15 and inappropriateness of the empiric antibiotic regimen were all independently correlated with increased mortality. Initial antibiotic treatment was appropriate in 63% of cases; the figure was 78% for infectious diseases expents compared to 54% for others ($p < 0.001$).

These data show clearly that having a single, "standard antibiotic regimen" for all cases of septic shock is no more logical than it would be to use a single drug for all arrhythmias. The difficulty with sepsis however is that while an electrocardiogram will quickly identify the nature of the rhythm, microbiological diagnosis will usually be delayed 12–18 hours. Immediate antibiotic therapy is essential, but empiric therapy need not mean "blind" therapy, as it is has sometimes been called. The focus of the infection will be a critical piece of information informing the antibiotic choice. Where a patient is presumed to be septic secondary to nosocomial pneumonia, intra-abdominal sepsis or urosepsis for instance, antibiotic choice will be dictated by the local flora related to those sites. Detailed recommendations for the choice of antibiotics will be found in the Section 2 of this book. Here we will restrict the discussion to the initial empiric antibiotic choice in patients with septic shock who are presumed to be bacteremic and/or in whom the focus of infection is not certain.

Consideration of four simple questions will provide much valuable guidance:

1) What is the history and clinical setting? What is the patient's occupation? (Sewer worker, garbage disposal etc.) Is this a post-operative infection, and if so, was it a thoracic, intra-abdominal or pelvic procedure? Was the bowel breached? is there a history of trauma? Are there any other clues to the likely focus?
2) Is this a nosocomial or community-acquired infection? Where was this infection probably acquired? Is there a history of travel? In certain areas of the world, primary resistance

rates in common pathogens are so high that first line antibiotics cannot be trusted.
3) What is the underlying disease, if any? Is the patient neutropenic, or on dialysis?
4) What is the recent microbiologic and antibiotic history? Although one cannot be certain that recent isolates are necessarily the cause of the current episode of sepsis, it is obviously important to be aware if the patient is colonized with *Pseudomonas aeruginosa* or methicillin-resistant *Staphylococcus aureus* (MRSA), for instance. It is also helpful to know the recent antibiotic history, in part because one must assume that whatever is causing the current infection is presumably resistant to those drugs, but also because it may raise the possibility of fungal infection.

This basic information can be assembled quickly and will allow the choice of a suitable regimen. Sometimes the clinical picture is so unambiguous that specific therapy can be given immediately: benzylpenicillin for meningococcaemia, for instance. In general though, a broad spectrum regimen must be chosen.

Adequate cover against Gram-negative bacteria is essential, and can be achieved with a third or fourth generation cephalosporin, penems, quinolones or extended spectrum penicillins such as piperacillin/tazobactam. A key question is whether these agents can be used alone or should be combined with an aminoglycoside. Perhaps surprisingly, there are few good randomized trials that address this question. Many are old, and although some studies have been done in "septicemic" patients none deal specifically with septic shock (a detailed evidence-based review of this topic has recently been published elsewhere [38]). The data, such as they are, indicate that third or fourth generation cephalosporins (such as cefotaxime or ceftazidime) and penems (e.g. imipenem, meropenem) are equally effective and less toxic than aminoglycoside-containing regimens. This is not true for extended spectrum beta-lactamase stable penicillins such as piperacillin/tazobactam, or for quinolones, which need to be given together with an aminoglycoside. Other agents such as aztreonam are highly active but in most units are held in reserve, and in any case will always need to be given with antibiotics providing Gram-positive cover. The need for anti-pseudomonal cover will vary in different circumstances, but where it is judged to be important drugs with specific activity will need to be used (e.g. ceftazidime or a quinolone such as ciprofloxacin).

Considerable discussion has surrounded the suggestion that the rapid lysis of Gram-negative bacteria brought about by certain antibiotics might lead to the release of endotoxin and hence a harmful effect on the patient. There is no doubt that this phenomenon can be demonstrated experimentally [39] and that certain antibiotic classes are more likely to cause this problems than are others [40]. The key question though, is whether this has any clinical relevance in patients with septic shock [41]. Several pieces of evidence suggest that it does not. Patients with meningococcaemia are among those with the highest recorded levels of endotoxin, but there is no evidence that penicillin causes clinically-significant increases in endotoxemia [33, 42], and similar results were obtained in patients with sepsis and septic shock [43, 44]. For the time being, there are no data to support the view that antibiotic choice should be influenced by any consideration of antibiotic-induced endotoxin release.

Gram-positive bacteria can be more problematic. If *Staphylococcus aureus* is strongly suspected then it is wise to include specific agents such as nafcillin (or flucloxacillin in Europe). Combined with an aminoglycoside these still provide good broad empiric cover. If MRSA is a concern then there is little option at present but to use a glycopeptide such as vancomycin. Newer agents such as the oxazolinodones (e.g. linezolid) are likely to be poteutial alternatives. Coagulase-negative staphylococci are not common causes of septic shock but may need consideration in neutropenic patients. Vancomycin must be used.

Streptococcus pneumoniae is no longer uniformly sensitive to benzylpenicillin, and the choice of agent will depend on the local epidemiology where the infection was acquired. However, high-level resistance is still relatively uncommon and most strains with intermediate penicillin resistance will be susceptible to extended spectrum cephalosporins such as cefotaxime. Enterococci (*Streptococcus faecalis* and *S. faecium*) are common co-pathogens in infections arising from the bowel or biliary tract. In general, drugs such as piperacillin/tazobactam will provide adequate cover and at the same time treat the more important enteric Gram-negative rods. Ampicillin-resistant enterococci are usually treated with vancomycin, but vancomycin resistant strains (VRE) are now widespread on many ICUs. Fortunately, it is very uncommon for enterococci (whatever their resistance pattern) to be *solely* responsible for septic shock, so vancomycin should not be used empirically for septic shock just because of the possibility of infection with a VRE, even if the colonization rates on the unit are high.

Anaerobic bacteria usually occur as part of a mixed infection and rarely cause shock alone. Nevertheless, antibiotics active against anaerobes are usually included in regimens in which anaerobic bacteria might be implicated. As a general rule, metronidazole should be used for infections arising below the diaphragm and clindamycin or penicillin for anaerobic chest infections.

Fungi are assuming ever greater importance on the ICU, and *Candida spp* in particular are occasionally isolated from the blood of patients with septic shock. It would be unwise to use an anti-fungal agent as the only empiric agent in a patient with septic shock, but in selected cases (for instance, neutropenic patients who had received extended courses of antibacterials and who were known to be colonized with *Candida*) the addition of an anti-fungal would be reasonable. Fluconazole is an attractive choice because of its lack of toxicity and ease of use; the disadvantage is that some non-albicans species of Candida have diminished sensitivity. A reasonable compromise is to use a high initial dose: 800 mg/day is usually recommended.

In summary then, there are no prospective, randomized controlled clinical trials that compare different empiric treatment strategies specifically in patients with septic shock, and recommendations must be therefore be based on data drawn from other settings. Although single agents such as penems do seem to be effective in bacteremic patients, as discussed above, the considerable mortality associated with septic shock leaves the clinician little room for maneuver. Choice of the correct initial antibiotic regimen is associated with a better outcome, and under these circumstance it will rarely be possible to treat a patient with septic shock with a single drug. A summary of some suitable regimens is provided in Table 1.

OTHER ASPECTS OF TREATMENT

Once the patient has been stabilized it is essential to seek, and where appropriate drain, any focal collections of pus. This process, referred to as source control, is discussed in more detail in Sections 7 and 8.

Coagulation abnormalities are common in sepsis [45] but only require specific therapy if there is uncontrolled bleeding or if a surgical procedure is planned. Antithrombin [46] and activated protein C [47] are two among several anticoagulant agents that have been evaluated as adjunctive agents in sepsis. Their effect probably owes much to anti-inflammatory properties unrelated to coagulation. Antithrombin was ineffective, but a large landomized controlled trial of activated protein C demonstrated a highly significant reduction in 28 day moitality, and this agent is likely to enter clinical practive soon [48].

High-dose steroids (typically, methylprednisolone 30 mg/kg by bolus injection followed by a nine hour infusion) have been evaluated several times as potentially valuable adjunctive agents for patients with septic shock [49–50]. Despite an impressive array of supporting experimental and pre-clinical data, the evidence

TABLE 1. First-line empiric antibiotic regimens suitable for patients with presumed septic shock in whom the primary site of infection is not apparent

Piperacillin/tazobactam *plus* gentamicin[1] (in units with high levels of MRSA it may be necessary to add a glycopeptide initially)
Cephalosporin[2] *plus* gentamicin[1] (metronidazole can be added for suspected intra-abdominal infections)
Nafcillin (cloxacillin) *or* vancomycin[3] *plus* gentamicin[1]. For high suspicion of staphylococcal infection
Vancomycin[3] *plus* fluoroquinolone[4,5] (metronidazole can be added for suspected intra-abdominal infections). Suitable for patients with hypersensitivity to β-lactams

Notes:
General comments: Several other drugs and alternative regimens exist which are equally appropriate. The lack of good quality RCT data means that these are only recommendations. Nevertheless, it is probably helpful to become familiar with just a small number of selected drugs and regimens, rather than try and memorize many equally effective alternatives. These regimens are not intended for circumstances in which the clinical findings point clearly to a specific infection, e.g. meningococcal sepsis or necrotizing fasciitis. Recommendations for these infections will be found in the relevant chapters of the book. Specialist infectious diseases/microbiological advice should be sought at an early stage, and particularly if unusual or opportunistic infection is a possibility.

[1] Gentamicin is the cheapest aminoglycoside; others can be substituted if local resistance patterns show high levels of gentamicin resistance.

[2] Second generation cephalosoporins such as cefazolin are widely used, but in a seriously ill patient, and in particular one who has recently received antibiotics, an extended spectrum agent such as cefotaxime is preferred. If anti-Pseudomonas cover is needed then use ceftazidime.

[3] Vancomycin (or teicoplanin) should only be used empirically if MRSA is suspected on clinical or epidemiologic grounds, or when there is clear evidence of hypersensitivity to β-lactams.

[4] Most experience has been gained with ciprofloxacin, which also has the best anti-Pseudomonal activity.

[5] Carbapenems (imipenem, meropenem) are equally applicable here but are often kept as reserve agents.

from these trials is that steroids given in this way are not beneficial, and indeed may have some harmful effects, such as an increased rate of bacterial superinfection [51]. Very recently there has been a renewed interest in steroid therapy, but used at a significantly lower dose. Bollaert *et al.* have described a series of 41 patients with septic shock requiring catecholamine support and who were treated with hydrocortisone 100 mg intravenously three times daily for five days, or placebo [52]. Although there was no difference in the 28 day survival figures for the two groups, shock reversal was significantly better in the steroid group. A larger trial capable of detecting significant differences in survival has recently been completed and appears to confirm the benefit of this approach (53).

Steroids are just one out of a very long list of experimental agents that have been evaluated as potential therapeutic agents in septic shock [54]. None have proved successful in large, phase III placebo controlled trials, and at the time of writing, none are licensed for clinical use for this indication. Nevertheless, there is intense interest in this therapeutic area from both basic and clinical scientists and from the pharmaceutical industry, and it seems very probable that one or more of these agents will come into routine use in the near futive.

References

1. Vincent J-L. Sepsis and septic shock: update on definitions. In Reinhart K, Eyrich K, Sprung C (Eds). Sepsis. Current perspectives in pathophysiology and therapy. Berlin: Springer-Verlag, 1994:3.
2. Bone RC, Balk RA, Cerra FB, *et al.* Definitions for sepsis and organ failure and guidelines for the use of innovative therapies in sepsis. The ACCP/SCCM Consensus Conference Committee. American College of Chest Physicians/Society of Critical Care Medicine. Chest 101:1644, 1992.
3. Bone RC, Fisher CJ Jr, Clemmer TP, *et al.* Sepsis syndrome: a valid clinical entity. Crit Care Med 17:389, 1989.
4. Bone RC. Definitions and therapy of sepsis. In Reinhart K, Eyrich K, Sprung C (Eds). Sepsis. Current perspectives in pathophysiology and therapy. Berlin: Springer-Verlag, 1994: 228.
5. Forgacs IC, Eykyn SJ, Bradley RD. Serious infection in the intensive therapy unit: a 15 year study of bacteremia. Quarterly J Med 60:773, 1986.
6. Rangel-Frausto M. The epidemiology of bacterial sepsis. Infect Dis Clinics N Am 13:299, 1999.

7. Ispahani P, Pearson NJ, Greenwood D. An analysis of community and hospital-acquired bacteremia in a large teaching hospital in the United Kingdom. Quarterly J Med 63:427, 1987.
8. Brun BC, Doyon F, Carlet J, *et al.* Incidence, risk factors and outcome of severe sepsis and septic shock in adults: a multicenter prospective study in intensive care units. J Am Med Assoc 274:968, 1995.
9. Pittet D, Wenzl RP. Nosocomial bloodstream infections. Secular trends in rates, mortality, and contribution to total hospital deaths. Arch Intern Med 155:1177, 1995.
10. Crowe M, Ispahani P, Humphreys H, *et al.* Bacteremia in the adult intensive care unit of a teaching hospital in Nottinhgam, UK, 1985–1996. Eur J Clin Microbiol Infect Dis 17:377, 1998.
11. Wolff M, Brun-Buisson C, Lode H, *et al.* The changing epidemiology of severe infections in the ICU. Clin Microbiol Infect 3 (Suppl 1):S36, 1997.
12. Roberts FJ, Geere IW, Coldman A. A three-year study of positive blood cultures, with emphasis on prognosis. Rev Infect Dis 13:34, 1991.
13. Cohen J, Abraham E. Microbiologic findings and correlations with serum Tumor Necrosis Factor-α in patients with severe sepsis and septic shock. J Infect Dis 180:116, 1999.
14. Abraham E, Glauser M-P, Butler T, *et al.* p55 Tumor Necrosis Factor Receptor Fusion Protein in the Treatment of Patients with Severe Sepsis and Septic Shock. A randomized controlled multicenter trial. J Am Med Assoc 277:1531, 1997.
15. Hanberger H, Garcia RJ, Gobernado M, *et al.* Antibiotic susceptibility among aerobic Gram-negative bacilli in intensive care units in 5 European countries. J Am Med Assoc 281:67, 1999.
16. Opal SM, Cohen J. Are there fundamental differences of clincal relevance between Gram positive and Gram negative bacterial sepsis? Crit Care Med 27:1608, 1999.
17. Kreger BE, Craven DE, McCabe WR. Gram-negative bacteremia IV. Re-evaluation of clinical features and treatment in 612 patients. Am J Med 68:344, 1980.
18. Circiumaru B, Baldock G, Cohen J. A prospective study of fever in the intensive care unit. Intensive Care Med 25:668, 1999.
19. O'Grady NP, Barie PS, Bartlett JG. *et al.* Practice guidelines for evaluating new fever in critically ill adult patients. Critical Care Med 26:1041, 1998.
20. Llewelyn M, Cohen J. Diagnosis of infection in sepsis. Intensive Care Med 27 (suppl 1): S10, 2001.
21. Carlet J. Rapid diagnostic methods in the detection of sepsis. Infect Dis Clinics N Am 13:483, 1999.
22. Povoa P, Almeida E, Moreira P, *et al.* C-reactive protein as an indicator of sepsis. Intensive Care Med 24:1052, 1998.
23. de Werra I, Jaccard C, Corradin SB, *et al.* Cytokines, nitrite/nitrate, soluble tumor necrosis factor receptors, and procalcitonin concentrations: comparisons in patients with septic shock, cardiogenic shock, and bacterial pneumonia. Critical Care Med 25:607, 1997.
24. Oberhoffer M, Karzai W, Meier-Hellmann A, *et al.* Sensitivity and specificity of various markers of inflammation for the prediction of tumor necrosis factor-α and interleulin-6 in patients with sepsis. Critical Care Med 27:1814, 1999.
25. Ugarte H, Silva E, Mercan D, *et al.* Procalcitonin used as a marker of infection in the intensive care unit. Critical Care Med 27:498, 1999.
26. Danner RL, Elin RJ, Hosseini JM, *et al.* Endotoxemia in human septic shock. Chest 99:169, 1991.
27. Guidet B, Barakett V, Vassal T, *et al.* Endotoxemia and bacteremia in patients with sepsis syndrome in the intensive care unit. Chest 106:1194, 1994.
28. Bates DW, Parsonnet J, Ketchum PA, *et al.* Limulus Amebocyte Lysate assay for detection of endotoxin in patients with sepsis syndrome. Clin Infect Dis 27:582, 1998.
29. Casey LC, Balk RA, Bone RC. Plasma cytokine and endotoxin levels correlate with survival in patients with the sepsis syndrome. Ann Intern Med 119:771, 1993.
30. Fink PC, Grunert JH. Endotoxemia in intensive care patients: a longitudinal study with the limulus amebocyte lysate test. Klinische Wochenschrift 62:986, 1984.
31. Cohen J. The detection and interpretation of endotoxemia. Intensive Care Med 26 (suppl 1):S51, 2000.
32. Hurley JC. Reappraisal with meta-analysis of bacteremia, endotoxemia, and mortality in Gram-negative sepsis. J Clin Microbiol 33:1278, 1995.
33. Brandtzaeg P, Kerrulf P, Gaustad P, *et al.* Plasma endotoxin as a predictor of multiple organ failure

and death in systemic meningococcal disease. J Infect Dis 159:195, 1989.
34. Edwards JD. Management of septic shock. Br Med J 306:1661, 1993.
35. Dellinger RP. Current therapy for sepsis. Infect Dis Clinics N Am 13:495, 1999.
36. Wheeler AP, Bernard GR. Treating patients with severe sepsis. New Engl J Med 340:207, 1999.
37. Byl B, Clevenbergh P, Jacobs F, *et al.* Impact of infectious disaeases specialists and microbiologic data on the appropriateness of antimicrobial therapy for bacteremia. Clin Infect Dis 29:60, 1999.
38. Bochud P-Y, Glauser M-P, Calandra T. Antibiotics in sepsis Intensive Care Med 27 (suppl 1):S33, 2001.
39. Dofferhoff AS, Potthoff H, Bom VJ, *et al.* The release of endotoxin, TNF and IL-6 during the antibiotic treatment of experimental Gram-negative sepsis. J Endotoxin Res 2:37, 1995.
40. Jackson JJ, Kropp H. β-lactam antibiotic-induced release of free endotoxin: *in vitro* comparison of penicillin-binding protein (PBP) 2-specific imipenem and PBP 3-specific ceftazidime. J Infect Dis 165:1033, 1992.
41. Prins JM, van Deventer SJ, Kuijper EJ, *et al.* Clinical relevance of antibiotic-induced endotoxin release. Antimicrob Agents Chemo 38: 1211, 1994.
42. Lehner PJ, Davies KA, Walport MJ, *et al.* Meningococcal septicaemia in a C6-deficient patient and effects of plasma transfusion on lipopolysaccharide release. Lancet 340:1379, 1992.
43. Prins JM, van Agtmael M, Kuijper EJ, *et al.* Antibiotic-induced endotoxin release in patients with Gram-negative urosepsis: a double-blind study comparing imipenem and ceftazidime. J Infect Dis 172:886, 1995.
44. Maury E, Barakett V, Blanchard H, *et al.* Circulating endotoxin during initial antibiotic treatment of severe Gram-negative bacteremic infections. J Infect Dis 178:270, 1998.
45. Levi M, ten Cate H. Disseminated intravascular coagulation. New Engl J Med 341:586, 1999.
46. Eisele B, Lamy M, Thijs LG, *et al.* Antithrombin III in patients with severe sepsis. A randomized, placebo-controlled, double-blind multicenter trial plus a meta-analysis on all randomized, placebo-controlled, double-blind trials with antithrombin III in severe sepsis. Intensive Care Med 24:663, 1998.
47. Roback MG, Stack AM, Thompson C, *et al.* Activated protein C concentrate for the treatment of meningococcal endotoxin shock in rabbits. Shock 9:138, 1998.
48. Bernard GR, Vincent JL, Laterre G-F, *et al.* Efficacy safety of recombinant human activated protein C for severe sepsis. N Engl J Med 344:699, 2001.
49. Hinshaw LB, Peduzzi P, Young E, *et al.* Effect of high-dose glucocorticoid therapy on mortality in patients with clinical signs of systemic sepsis. New Engl J Med 317:659, 1987.
50. Bone RC, Fisher CJ Jr, Clemmer TP, *et al.* A controlled clinical trial of high-dose methylprednisolone in the treatment of severe sepsis and septic shock. New Engl J Med 317:653, 1987.
51. Cronin L, Cook DJ, Carlet J, *et al.* Corticosteroid treatment for sepsis: a critical appraisal and meta-analysis of the literature. Crit Care Med 23:1430, 1995.
52. Bollaert P-E, Charpentier C, Levy B, *et al.* Reversal of late septic shock with supraphysiologic doses of hydrocortisone. Crit Care Med 26:645, 1998.
53. Annane D. Effects of the combination of hydrocortisone and fludrocortisone on mortality in septic shock. Crit Care Med 26:A46, 2001.
54. Cohen J. Adjunctive therapy in sepsis: a critical analysis of the clinical trial programme. Brit Med Bull 55:212, 1999.

24. ACUTE BACTERIAL MENINGITIS

P. Fernández Viladrich

Introduction

Bacterial meningitis is defined as the inflammation of both leptomeninges and the cerebrospinal fluid (CSF) that they contain, when caused by bacterial organisms. As a rule, the infectious process also affects the ependymus and ventricular CSF [1]. The most frequent bacterial meningitis are those due to pyogenic organisms that usually cause the typical clinical picture of acute meningitis with purulent CSF. The purulent aspect of the CSF is due to both bacterial growth and an intense polymorphonuclear response. Other bacterial agents, such as *Brucella melitensis*, *Mycobacterium tuberculosis*, *Treponema pallidum*, *Leptospira* sp and *Borrelia burgdorferi*, can also cause meningitis that often runs a subacute or chronic course and presents with clear CSF showing a predominantly lymphocytic pleocytosis. These agents will not be considered in this chapter.

Epidemiology and Etiology

Acute bacterial meningitis is a frequent disease world-wide [1]. It mainly occurs in the community setting, although it has been progressively frequent in the nosocomial setting [2]. Its incidence varies widely, depending on factors such as age, geographic region, socioeconomic level and, especially, the existence of a hyperendemic or epidemic situation of meningococcal disease, since only meningococcal meningitis may occur in an epidemic form. A recent estimate of the incidence of bacterial meningitis in the USA has been between two and three per 100,000 people per year [3].

Until recently, its incidence had been highest in childhood, especially in children aged from six months to two years [4]. Presently, its epidemiological spectrum has changed in industrialized countries due to the systematic vaccination of infants with the *Haemophilus influenzae* conjugated vaccine. So the incidence of meningitis caused by this organism, which was the most frequent cause of bacterial meningitis in the pediatric population of industrialized countries, has greatly declined [5, 6]. Consequently, bacterial meningitis has become an illness which, in developed countries, prevails in adults [3].

Currently, the most common pathogens causing community-acquired bacterial meningitis at all ages (except in neonates) are *Streptococcus pneumoniae* and *Neisseria meningitidis*, followed by *Listeria monocytogenes* which usually affects both the elderly and those patients with immunosuppressive illnesses or therapies. *H. influenzae*, Group B streptococcus, *Enterococcus* sp., *Staphylococcus aureus*, and Gram-negative bacilli also occasionally infect this immunosuppressed population [1–3]. In the hospital setting, bacterial meningitis mainly constitutes a complication of neurosurgical procedures. The most common causal pathogens are Gram-negative bacilli, both the enterobacteriaceae and the non-fermenting Gram-negative bacilli such as *Pseudomonas aeruginosa* and *Acinetobacter baumannii* that often infect craniotomies and external ventricular drainages and frequently show antibiotic multi-resistance [7–10]. Neurosurgical infection caused by *S. aureus* and coagulase-negative staphylococci occurs with lesser frequency than that caused by Gram-negative bacilli. Streptococci of the *viridans* group, enterococci, and various Gram-positive bacilli, including *Clostridium perfringens*, occasionally infect these patients. In the particular case of CSF shunt infection, the most characteristic causative organisms are *Staphylococcus epidermidis* and *Propionibacterium acnes*, although any other organism can occasionally cause a shunt infection [11, 12].

Pathogenesis

Organisms can reach the central nervous system (CNS) through several pathways [1]. Frequently, they arrive there by hematogenous route from a distant focus of infection. This mechanism is though to occur in the majority of cases of meningococcal and listerial meningitis as well as in many cases of pneumococcal meningitis and meningitis due to *H. influenzae*. In fact, any bacteria can occasionally cause meningitis by that mechanism. Organisms can also reach the CNS from an infectious focus in the vicinity such as otitis media, sinusitis, or when a CSF cranial fistula permits the direct entrance of bacteria into CSF. In up to 30 per cent of brain abscesses and in certain spinal subdural empyemas, purulent meningitis occurs as a consequence of its perforation into ventricular or subarachnoid spaces [13]. In the case of neurosurgical procedures, organisms can be directly seeded during the procedure's performance – for instance, craniotomy or spinal anesthesia – but more frequently they enter CSF during the postoperative period through infection of the surgical wound or through a catheter for ventricular drainage. CSF shunts are usually infected during the surgical procedure, but sometimes the infection occurs later from an infected surgical wound or from gut lesions. Table 1 shows the relationships between the various foci of infection and the etiologic agents.

TABLE 1. Relationship between foci of infection and etiologic agents of bacterial meningitis in adults

Foci of infection	Most frequent etiologic agents
Acute pharyngitis (with or without purpuric lesions)	*Neisseria meningitidis*
Acute otitis media	*Streptococcus pneumoniae*
Cholesteatomatous otitis media*	*Proteus* sp., Streptococcus sp., *Bacteroides* sp.
Chronic sinusitis*	Anaerobic bacteria, Streptococcus sp.
Postraumatic pericranial fistula	*Streptococcus pneumoniae*
Bacterial pneumonia	*Streptococcus pneumoniae*
Dental infection*	*Streptococcus milleri*
Chronic bronquial or lung infection*	Anaerobic bacteria, Streptococcus sp.
Abdominal or urinary infection	*Escherichia coli*, *Klebsiella pneumoniae*
Acute endocarditis	*Staphylococcus aureus*, *S. pneumoniae*
Subacute endocarditis*	*Enterococcus faecalis*, *Streptococcus viridans*
Neurosurgical wound infection	Gram-negative bacilli, *Staphylococcus aureus*
Lumbar puncture or spinal anesthesia	Streptococci of the *viridans* group
Cerebrospinal fluid shunt infection	*Staph. epidermidis, Propionibacterium acnes*
No apparent focus in teenagers	*Neisseria meningitidis*
No apparent focus in the elderly or immunosupressed patients	*Listeria monocytogenes*, *Streptococcus pneumoniae*, *Streptococcus agalactiae*
Any focus in patients with neutropenia or cancer	*Pseudomonas aeruginosa*, Enterobacteriaceae, *Listeria monocytogenes*, Gram-positive cocci

* A focal intracranial suppuration should be ruled out.

Once organisms have reached the CSF, they quickly multiply, and consequently several cytokines are released and create an inflammatory process that increases blood-brain barrier permeability and produces cytotoxic and vasogenic brain edema, intracranial hypertension, ischemic phenomena and neuronal damage. This inflammatory process and its negative consequences may be greatly increased when cell wall fragments are massively released after bacteriolitic antibiotics are administrated. On the other hand, bacterial growth in the meningeal spaces frequently goes on to a secondary bacteremia that may contribute to morbidity. Particularly, hemodynamic instability or shock, if not properly treated, will make worse the neurological process by lowering the cerebral perfusion pressure and increasing brain ischemia [14–16].

Clinical Manifestations

Clinical manifestations are due to the meningeal inflammation and its neurological consequences, the original source of infection, and possible concurrent primary or secondary septicemia.

The characteristic elements of the meningeal syndrome are fever, headache, nausea or vomiting, meningismus, and impairment of consciousness level. Frequently this picture presents incompletely because one of these elements is missing. High fever is the most frequent sign, and it is usually preceded by chills of variable intensity. However, fever may be absent in the elderly and in immunosuppressed patients as well as in those who are in shock or have been given antipyretic drugs. Likewise, meningismus may also be absent during the first few hours of the meningeal process, in deep comatose patients, and also in the elderly or immunosuppressed. Clinical symptoms and signs of meningitis are even more difficult to ascertain in patients who are hospitalized in ICUs after suffering from head trauma or certain neurosurgical procedures. Thus fever may be due to another concurrent infectious process or to intracranial hemorrhage, and meningismus may be absent because of coma or pharmacological relaxation. Contrarily, meningismus may be difficult to evaluate in neurosurgical patients because it may be related to the surgical wound, especially in occipital craniotomies, or to hemorrhage in the subarachnoid space. Moreover, there are several circumstances in which the clinician must be alerted as to the possibility of concurrent bacterial meningitis: the confused or agitated patient with pneumonia, alcoholism or liver cirrhosis in whom abnormal mental or behavioral sings could be attributed to hypoxemia, alcoholic deprivation, or hepatic encephalopathy, or those patients who present with fever and either seizures or an ischemic brain event.

Seizures are a frequent complication of bacterial meningitis. They have repeatedly been associated with higher mortality and neurological sequelae [2, 17–19]. In adults, they occur much more frequently in pneumococcal meningitis than in meningitis caused by other pathogens. Thus about 30% of adults with pneumococcal meningitis convulse [2, 20]. Moreover, the majority of these seizures occur precociously. In my experience, about 10 per cent of adults with pneumococcal meningitis have already convulsed when first visited, and other 20 per cent convulse after antibiotic treatment has been initiated, usually during the first 24 or 48 hours of treatment. Some patients go on to status epilepticus. Additional impairment of the consciousness level and signs of brain herniation also often occur after the initiation of antibiotic treatment. Other neurological complications such as brain infarcts due to cortical thrombophlebitis or arteritis occur in about 15 per cent of adults with bacterial meningitis [21]. In fact, early death related to one of these complications occurring when CSF has already been sterilized by appropriate antibiotic therapy has been a common experience when treating patients with pneumococcal meningitis (and occasionally other types of bacterial meningitis), and may be explained in part by the CSF inflammatory burst mentioned above. That is why, with the intention of preventing these neurological complications, for more than a decade now, we have been administering very early adjunctive therapy (see below) to both all adult patients with suspected pneumococcal meningitis and those with bacterial meningitis of any other etiology showing signs of intracranial hypertension [22].

Of paramount importance are symptoms and signs due to a primary focus of infection, because they are of value both to point to the etiologic agent and to orient the most appropriate approach to the patient. Thus, when bacterial meningitis is preceded by respiratory symptoms a classical meningeal pathogen such as meningococcus, pneumococcus or *H. influenzae* is probably the cause [23]. Meningitis due to *L. monocytogenes* will not usually be preceded by respiratory symptoms. The existence of previous or concurrent sore throat occurs in about 40 per cent of cases of teenagers and adults with meningococcal disease [17]. Pharyngitis, occasionally with a purulent exudate, is frequently found in these cases and may be mistaken for a more banal pharyngeal process. In many cases, it is probably an authentic meningococcal pharyngitis [24, 25].

Acute bacterial meningitis is the most frequent intracranial complication of *acute otitis media* at all ages. In adults, this process is almost exclusively due to *S. pneumoniae* and, conversely, about 35 per cent of adult pneumococcal meningitis are a complication of an attack of acute otitis media [20, 26]. On the other hand, a brain abscess is the most frequent intracranial complication of *cholesteatomatous chronic otitis media*, in which the classical meningeal pathogens are usually not implicated [27]. Thus, in patients with both meningeal signs and otitis, ascertaining the type of otitis has diagnostic and therapeutic consequences. A lumbar puncture should be performed without delay if the otitis media is acute, whereas a computed brain scan should first be performed if it is chronic, in order to rule out a supurative intracranial collection that may have presented as bacterial meningitis. A *pericranial fistula* is likely to be present if the patient has suffered, even many years before, from a cranial or facial trauma, an operation involving either the ethmoid or sphenoid sinuses or the otic cavities, or if they have had CSF rhinorrhea or recurrent episodes of bacterial meningitis. *S. pneumoniae* is also the most frequent cause of bacterial meningitis in this setting, although other respiratory pathogens such as *H. influenzae*, *N. meningitidis* or streptococci of the *viridans* group may also be the cause [26].

Symptoms and clinical signs of meningitis following cranial or spinal surgery are similar to that of community-acquired bacterial meningitis. Inflammatory symptoms and signs at surgical site may be the first alarming sign, and leakage of CSF through the surgical wound often occurs when meningitis develops. CSF leaks may be both a risk factor for developing meningitis during the postoperative period and a consequence of the meningitis itself owing to the accompanying CSF hypertension. Clinical manifestations of catheter-related ventriculitis may be less clear and a high level of suspicion must be maintained in order to reach a precocious diagnosis. Fever is the most constant sign. Any impairment of the previous level of conciousness may also be indicative of CSF infection. In patients who are on ventilatory assistance because of severe head trauma, the appearance of high fever that has no apparent origin should alert to the existence of meningitis. Symptoms of ventriculo-peritoneal shunt infections are usually insidious and mainly consist of subacute and frequently intermittent abdominal pain with moderate fever or without fever at all. Infection of ventriculo-venous shunts manifest more often by subacute or chronic intermittent high fever. Diagnosis of shunt infections is often delayed until significant shunt malfunction occurs, which may cause acute hydrocephalus and rapid worsening of the ventricular infection.

As has been said, septicemia may be both the cause and the consequence of the meningeal infection, and may cause distant infection, such as arthritis or endocarditis, or shock. A maculo-petechial or purpuric skin rash is characteristic of meningococcemia, although it may also be due to other microorganisms.

Diagnosis

When a diagnosis of community-acquired bacterial meningitis is suspected, a lumbar puncture should be performed immediately and the CSF opening pressure must be recorded and its aspect observed. In cases with a non-acute clinical course, especially if a focal neurological deficit or papilledema is found, and in patients who present with a primary focus of infection that characteristically is complicated by a brain abscess, such as chronic cholesteatomatous otitis media, chronic sinusitis, and dental or anaerobic lung infection, a CT brain scan should be performed previously to the lumbar puncture. As stated above, seizures are quite frequent in bacterial meningitis, so in themselves do not constitute an indication for brain scanning prior to practicing lumbar puncture if the illness runs an acute course. Ventricular CSF can be obtained directly through ventricular catheters in patients with catheter-related ventriculitis, or by puncturing the reservoir or valvular system of internal shunts in those suspected of having shunt infection.

CSF may appear either clear or only slightly cloudy during the first few hours of the illness, in some cases of severe meningococcal sepsis with meningitis, in meningitis due to *L. monocytogenes*, and in shunt infections. In these cases, there may be either no CSF cells or only slight pleocytosis. However, white blood cell counts between 1000 and 5000 per microliter are common in fully established bacterial meningitis, with a percentage of polymorphonuclear cells between 90 and 100 per cent. As an exception, a significant percentage of lymphocytic cells are frequently found in meningitis caused by *L. monocytogenes* [28]. Evaluation of CSF pleocytosis may be impossible when hemorrhage into ventricular or meningeal spaces has occurred. CSF protein is usually elevated in bacterial meningitis, the more frequent range being from 1–5 g per liter. Hypoglucorraquia occurs in about 50% of bacterial meningitis cases and CSF glucose is often almost undetectable. However, normal CSF glucose does not rule out a diagnosis of bacterial meningitis.

An urgent CSF Gram stain is especially advised in order to optimize empirical antibiotic therapy. Results are positive in less than 25% of cases of listerial meningitis, in about 50 to 60% of meningococcal, staphylococcal and Gram-negative bacillar meningitis, and in more than 80% of pneumococcal meningitis. CSF cultures are positive in about 70% of meningococcal meningitis and in 85 to 90% of the other etiologies. CSF cultures are often sterile in patients who have received prior effective antibiotic therapy. If the patient has not been treated with antibiotics, sterile CSF cultures may occur in some cases of meningococcal meningitis or in cases of meningitis that are secondary to a brain abscess. This is why in all cases of bacterial meningitis not suggestive of meningococcal disease in which cultures have ultimately been sterile a CT brain scan is then recommended in order to rule out such an abscess even if the illness has apparently been an acute onset. Other diagnostic microbiological techniques such as latex agglutination, co-agglutionation, or contra-immunophoresis have not shown much yield, especially in adults, and therefore have not entered clinical practice. Recent techniques of polymerase chain reaction in CSF could be very useful in selected cases in which etiologic diagnosis has epidemiological implications, as may occur in meningococcal disease [29].

Blood cultures should always be performed in acute bacterial meningitis because if they are positive they will establish the etiologic diagnosis [30]. On occasion, they are the only means of supporting the diagnosis, as sometimes occurs in patients who have suffered from severe cranial trauma and in whom it is not possible to obtain CSF. For instance, in the absence of a respiratory infection, positive blood cultures for *S. pneumoniae* or *H. influenzae* makes the diagnosis of postraumatic bacterial meningitis probable in such circumstances and constitutes an indication for urgent therapy. Frequency of positive blood cultures in bacterial meningitis ranges from 40% in meningococcal meningitis to more than 85% in pneumococcal meningitis. Culture of a pharyngeal secretions swab in Tayer-Martin media is also recommended in suspected meningococcal disease. If positive, it supports that diagnosis if CSF and blood cultures are negative and it indicates appropriate prophylaxis be given to intimate contacts. Gram stain and cultures of specimens from any possibly infected portal of entry, e.g. otorrhea or surgical wound, should also be performed.

Polymorphonuclear leucocytosis is usually found in bacterial meningitis. However, the white cell blood count may be normal or even low. Leucopenia constitutes a bad prognostic sign that indicates severe sepsis, as does thrombocytopenia and impairment of the coagulation factors, as frequently occurs in meningococcal disease. A certain degree of hypopotasemia may also relate to septicemia, and hyponatremia may be due to inappropriate secretion of antidiuretic hormone, more often in children than in adults. A chest radiographic examination should always be performed. Other radiological tests such as CT of paranasal sinuses, CT of the base of the skull, or magnetic resonance imaging of brain will be performed if necessary.

Differential Diagnosis

Several conditions, both infectious and non-infectious, may occasionally be confused with bacterial meningitis [1]. Among the more frequent are acute viral meningitis or meningoencephalitis and acute disseminated encephalomyelitis that may initially present with a predominance of polymorphonuclear cells in CSF. Some cases of tuberculous meningitis of very acute onset may also show this CSF polymorphonuclear predominance. Chemical meningitis, such as that which may be produced when radiological contrasts or certain anesthetics or material from a dermoid or parasite cyst are introduced in the subarachnoid space, can also produce both a clinical syndrome and CSF cytochemical alterations similar to that seen in acute bacterial meningitis. Occasionally, a spontaneous or post-surgical subarachnoid hemorrhage with fever may suggest bacterial meningitis.

Therapy

Bacterial meningitis constitutes a medical emergency that must be rapidly treated in order to minimize both mortality and neurological sequelae. Mortality is high and has not changed significantly over the antibiotic era in spite of the very effective antibiotics we have and the therapeutic developments that are provided in ICUs [2, 31]. Of note is the fact that in developed countries, the overall mortality of pneumococcal meningitis in adults is 30% [2, 20, 21]. This mortality is mainly caused by the above mentioned early neurological complications. All of those neurological complications may also occur in bacterial meningitis of other etiologies, although with lesser frequency than in pneumococcal meningitis. For instance, these complications cause death in a low percentage of patients with meningococcal meningitis (about two per cent overall), the majority of deaths in meningococcal disease being due to fulminant meningococcemia [17]. When these complications, especially brain herniation, do occur, brain damage is frequently irreversible, and measures to lower inflammation and cranial hypertension are usually late. Although a general rule for the treatment of bacterial meningitis is not to delay antibiotic treatment since significant delays will certainly increase mortality and neurological sequelae, precocious antibiotic treatment may not only be insufficient to avoid neurological complications, especially those associated with pneumococcal meningitis, but may even favor their occurrence through their bacteriolitic effect. Therefore, since in these cases the administration of appropriate adjunctive therapy may be even more urgent than that of the antibiotic itself, I will begin with that aspect of therapy. I will consider therapy for community-acquired and nosocomial bacterial meningitis separately.

Therapy for Community-Acquired Meningitis

EARLY ADJUNCTIVE THERAPY

An initial perfusion of mannitol may occasionally be lifesaving by rapidly lowering cranial hypertension [32, 33]. In deeply comatose patients, consciousness level frequently improves rapidly after mannitol has been given. That improvement may be manifested by passing from coma to an agitated state. Moreover, improvement of the bradicardia and respiratory rhythm irregularities that these patients sometimes present may also be observed.

With regard to the anti-inflammatory treatment, there is general agreement about the convenience of administering dexamethasone to children with bacterial meningitis [34]. Dexamethasone has been shown to reduce neurological and audiologic sequelae in children with meningitis due to *H. influenzae* type b [35]. It may be the same for pneumococcal meningitis provided it be given before or at the same time as antibiotic therapy, and even in children with meningococcal meningitis a slight tendency toward a beneficial effect has been observed [36]. In any case, the administration of dexamethasone during the first 48 hours of therapy has not been associated with significant adverse events [36]. On the other hand, early dexamethasone therapy has also been associated with reduced mortality of adult patients with pneumococcal meningitis, but since the experience published so far has been limited [37] and controlled studies are lacking, its indication for purulent meningitis continues to be controversial. However, there is a progressive tendency to recommend the use of dexamethasone in at least some cases of bacterial meningitis in adults. Thus, some authorities consider that its use might be useful in patients with bacterial meningitis who show clinical symptoms and signs of intracranial hypertension as well as in those cases with a positive CSF Gram stain [38]. Indeed, only by following this later recommendation, more than 80% of cases of pneumococcal meningitis and about 60% of those with meningococcal meningitis should receive dexamethasone, since this is the percentage of those with positive CSF Gram stain. In our experience [22], and that of others [39], early adjunctive treatment consisting of a single bolus dose of mannitol (1 g/kg), dexamethasone during the first two to four days (after an initial loading lose of 8 to 12 mg) and sodium phenytoin (18 mg/kg for the first 24 h and then 2 mg/kg every 8 h for 10 days) to prevent seizures has significantly lowered the mortality of pneumococcal meningitis in adults to less than 15%. We therefore recommend such treatment in all cases of suspected pneumococcal meningitis as well as in meningitis of other etiologies when the opening pressure of lumbar CSF is higher than 30 cm of water. Our group has already administered such treatment to many adult patients with bacterial meningitis without significant adverse events. If this therapy is appropriately conducted, many patients with severe neurological disease will improve rapidly and the need for more aggressive measures may be avoided. However, hospitalization in an ICU is obligatory for those patients who convulse in spite of adjunctive therapy in order to better control seizures, in those with other severe neurological complications that require ventilatory support, airways protection or monitoring of cranial hypertension, and, obviously, for those patients who have severe sepsis or shock [40].

ANTIBIOTIC TREATMENT

In those patients with cutaneous lesions suggestive of meningococcal sepsis, antibiotic therapy must be instituted immediately. If not, antibiotic therapy may be delayed as much as 30 minutes in order to perform a CSF Gram stain and institute pre-antibiotic adjunctive therapy when indicated. Initial antibiotic treatment must be based on both the epidemiological and clinical data and the CSF Gram stain result (Table 2). If CSF Gram stain could not be performed, empirical antibiotic therapy will have to based on epidemiological and clinical data alone. For instance, in the absence of purpuric lesions suggesting meningococcal disease, pneumococcal meningitis must be considered, especially if a characteristic pericranial or pneumonic focus is present. Moreover, listeriosis must also be considered in the elderly and/or in immunosupressed patients, as well as in those patients in whom initial CSF shows significant lymphocytic pleocytosis. In diabetic or cirrhotic patients with sepsis and those with neutropenia, cancer or hematological diseases, meningitis due to enterobacteriaceae or *P. aeruginosa* could also occur. Empirical antibiotic treatment can later be modified if the results of cultures yield the etiologic agent.

Meningococcal meningitis must be treated with a broad spectrum cephalosporin such as ceftriaxone, 50 mg/kg every 24 hours, or cefotaxime 50 mg/kg every six or eight hours. This treatment is more convenient than penicillin if the susceptibility of the causal strain to penicillin is not known, since a variable percentage (about 20 per cent in Spain) of meningococci are moderately resistant to this antibiotic (minimal inhibitory concentrations between 0.1 and 1 mg/l) [41]. In penicillin-allergic patients the elective alternative is chloramphenicol, 25 mg/kg q6 h, with a maximum of 4 g a day. However, of great concern is the recent emergence, albeit anecdotal, of high-level chloramphenicol resistance in *N. meningitidis* isolates [42].

Aztreonam, 30 mg/kg every six hours, may also be appropriate for these patients, but it shows reduced activity on penicillin-resistant meningococci [43]. The most recommended duration of treatment for meningococcal meningitis is seven days, although shorter courses such as four days have been shown to be equally safe and efficient [44, 45].

Appropriate antibiotic treatment of pneumococcal meningitis requires knowledge of the causal strain's susceptibility to penicillin and to broad spectrum cephalosporines. By performing an E-test directly on initial culture plates it is possible to have preliminary information about the susceptibility of the causal strain in less than 24 hours [46]. Until that susceptibility is known, the most recommended antibiotic therapy is the combination of a third-generation

TABLE 2. Empiric antibiotic therapy of community-acquired bacterial meningitis in adults based on foci of infection and cerebrospinal fluid Gram stain

Probably etiologic agent	Elective therapy	Alternative therapies
Neisseria *meningitidis*	Ceftriaxone, cefotaxime	Chloramphenicol, aztreonam meropenem*
Streptococcus pneumoniae	High-dose cefotaxime** plus vancomycin	Vancomycin plus rifampin***
Haemophilus influenzae	Ceftriaxone, cefotaxime	Aztreonam
Listeria monocytogenes	Ampicillin plus gentamycin	Cotrimoxazole, meropenem
Enterobacteriaceae	Ceftriaxone, cefotaxime	Aztreonam
Pseudomonas aeruginosa	Ceftazidime plus tobramycin	Aztreonam
Staphylococcus aureus	Cloxacillin or Vancomycin	Vancomycin
Unknown	Ceftriaxone or high-dose cefotaxime** (plus ampicillin)****	Vancomycin plus aztreonam (plus cotrimoxazole)***

* Meropenem might also be a useful alternative therapy for the majority of etiologic agents.
** >300 mg/kg per day.
*** (See [60]).
**** Ampicillin or cotrimoxazole are added if *Listeria monocytogenes* is considered.

cephalosporin with vancomycin [38]. If dexamethasone is concurrently administered, vancomycin at the recommended dosage for adult patients (30 mg/kg per day) does not reach reliable CSF levels [47], and CSF cefotaxime levels may also be insufficient for some cephalosporin-resistant pneumococcal strains [48]. Moreover, it is not certain whether both antibiotics are synergistic against all pneumococcal strains. That is why I recommend that high dose cefotaxime (300–400 mg/kg per day, with a maximum dose of 24 g per day) always be initially administered to adults with pneumococcal meningitis [49]. This is not necessary in children for whom the dosage of vancomycin is higher (60 mg/kg per day) and usually sufficient to cure the infection even if dexamethasone is given concurrently [50]. After results of susceptibility tests are known, antibiotic therapy may be modified (Table 3).

If the causal strain shows penicillin and cephalosporin resistance, a second lumbar puncture must be performed at 36–48 hours of treatment, in order to assess the evolution of CSF cultures and to test CSF antibiotic levels and/or bactericidal titers. The usual length of therapy for pneumococcal meningitis is 10 days. If the patient has a CSF pericranial fistula, he must be promptly operated on in order to avoid new episodes of bacterial meningitis. In such a circumstance, pneumococcal vaccination has been shown to be inefficient in preventing recurrent episodes of pneumococcal meningitis even when caused by pneumococcal strains of the serotypes included in the vaccine [51].

Meningitis due to *L. monocytogenes* is best treated with the combination of ampicillin (250 mg/kg per day) with gentamycin (5–6 mg/kg per day) [52]. If gentamycin is administered on a once-a-day schedule, higher CSF levels will be reached and higher bactericidal activity will possibly be achieved. For penicillin-allergic patients, the elective antibiotic consists of a high dose of cotrimoxazole that may be administered orally if necessary. The length of therapy for listerial meningitis ranges from three to six weeks, depending on both the immunological status of the patient and the presence of listerial cerebritis. In order to rule out this process, that a magnetic resonance of the brain should be performed on all patients with this disease.

H. influenzae meningitis must be treated with a third-generation cephalosporin. Ten days of therapy are usually sufficient. Community-acquired meningitis caused by enterobacteriaceae (more often *E. coli* or *Klesiella pneumoniae*) are rare, and may occur as a complication of bacteremia from urinary, intestinal or Klebsiella pulmonary origin, usually in patients with diabetes

TABLE 3. Antibiotic therapy for adult meningitis caused by *Streptococcus pneumoniae*

Organism susceptibility	Elective therapy	Alternative therapies
Penicillin-sensitive*	Penicillin G	Chloramphenicol**, Vancomycin plus rifampin
Penicillin-resistant and:		
Cefotaxime-sensitive^	Cefotaxime, Ceftriaxone	Vancomycin plus rifampin
Cefotaxime-resistant^^	High-dose cefotaxime plus vancomycin	Vancomycin plus rifampin

* MIC of penicillin <0.12 mg/l.
** If the causal strain is chloramphenicol-sensitive.
^ MIC of cefotaxime <1 mg/l.
^^ MIC of cefotaxime ≥1 mg/l.

mellitus or chronic alcoholism. A third-generation cephalosporin also constitutes the elective treatment, which must be extended to three or four weeks. Community-acquired *S. aureus* meningitis usually occurs in the setting of endocarditis, septicemia or spinal abscess. High intravenous dose of mafcillin or cloxacillin for 2 to 4 weeks is usually necessary. In the case of concurrent brain abscesses, rifampin may be added. Streptococcal (non-pneumococcal) meningitis is, at present, rare. Processes such as infective endocarditis, brain abscess, pericranial fistula or colonic neoplasm should be ruled out [53]. Depending on the underlying process, a minimum of two weeks of therapy is usually necessary. As a significant percentage of streptococci of the *viridans* group (especially *S. mitis*) are nowadays partially or highly penicillin-resistant [54], antibiotic therapy of streptococcal meningitis will depend on the susceptibility of the causal strain to penicillin. Enterococcal meningitis must be treated with the combination of ampicillin with gentamycin.

Therapy of Hospital Acquired-Meningitis

ADJUNCTIVE THERAPY

The administration of mannitol and/or dexamethasone is not usually necessary in neurosurgical patients when their infected CSF flows through an infected cranial or spinal surgical wound or through an external ventricular drainage since intracranial hypertension is, in part, relieved by this mechanism. Moreover, many patients operated on for craniotomy are already receiving corticosteroid therapy when meningitis occurs during the postoperative period. When meningitis has occurred as a complication of a cranial or spinal surgical wound infection and local suppuration exists, debridement of the infected wound must be undertaken as soon as possible after beginning antibiotic therapy. In the case of catheter-associated ventriculitis, change of the catheter is usually necessary and must be performed after the infection of the ventricular CSF has been controlled, or immediately if at 24 or 48 hours of antibiotic therapy the clinical status of the patient has not improved. In patients with CSF shunt infection and signs of shunt malfunction it is often necessary either to externalize the distal catheter or to withdraw the shunt and insert a ventricular catheter to relieve the hydrocephalus. This maneuver also relieves the ventriculitis itself.

ANTIBIOTIC TREATMENT

For meningitis-ventriculitis complicating neurosurgical procedures, if CSF Gram stain does not show organisms or it is not possible to perform this procedure, empirical antibiotic therapy must cover Gram-positive cocci, including MRSA and enterococci, and Gram-negative bacilli, including *P. aeruginosa*. In this setting, a frequently recommended treatment is the combination of ceftazidime (50 mg/kg every eight hours) with vancomycin. However, if multi-resistant Gram-negative bacilli such as some strains of *A. baumannii* or *P. aeruginosa*, or broad spectrum beta-lactamase producing enterobacteriaceae, are prevalent in a particular hospital setting, other antibiotics such as meropenem (2 g every eight hours for adults) alone or combined with tobramycin or amikacin may be more appropriate than ceftazidime for empirical treatment [55]. Occasionally, the intraventricular administration of aminoglycosides or colistin are necessary to cure those infections [56]. A few cases of central nervous system infection caused by multidrug-resistant *Pseudomonas aeruginosa* and *Acinetobacter baumannii* have been cured with intravenous colistin therapy [57].

The length of therapy for meningitis occurring in a neurosurgical setting ranges from two to four weeks. Meningitis caused by Gram-negative bacilli usually requires at least three weeks of therapy if relapse is to be avoided. In cases in which the intraventricular administration of antibiotics is necessary, two weeks of therapy might perhaps be sufficient. The initial treatment for CSF internal shunt infections will usually consist of empirical antibiotic therapy and externalization of the distal catheter as indicated above, especially if signs of shunt malfunction are present. This approach will usually control the infection at the ventricular and meningeal spaces but will not eradicate the organisms from catheter surfaces. Therefore, after several days of the most appropriate antibiotic therapy based on knowledge of the etiologic agent and its antibiotic susceptibility, the infected shunt must be entirely removed and another shunt placed on the opposite side if the patient is shunt-dependent. In cases of shunt infection with severe ventriculitis in which CSF infection is not controlled after shunt externalization, the shunt must be urgently removed and a ventricular catheter must be simultaneously placed in the ventricular system of the other side if continuous CSF drainage is necessary.

Future Perspectives

Bacterial meningitis will continue to be a serious disease. The best efforts must be directed to prevention. Thus, more effective meningococcal and pneumococcal vaccines are urgently needed [58]. Neurosurgical techniques must be optimized to the maximum, and special care should be paid to surgical wounds over the postoperative period [59]. Also, more developments in adjunctive therapies, and also perhaps newer bactericidal non-bacteriolitic antibiotics are needed.

References

1. Tunkel AR, Scheld WM. Acute meningitis. In Mandell GL, Bennett JE, Dolin R (eds). Principles and practice of infectious diseases, 4th edn, New York: Churchill Livingstone, 1994:831.
2. Durand ML, Calderwood SB, Weber DJ, *et al.* Acute bacterial meningitis in adults. A review of 493 episodes. N Engl J Med 328:21, 1993.
3. Schuchat A, Robinson K, Wenger JD, *et al.* Bacterial meningitis in the United States in 1995. N Engl J Med 337:970, 1995.
4. Wenger JD, Hightower AW, Facklam RR, Gaventa S, Broome CV. Bacterial meningitis in the United States, 1986: report of a multistate surveillance study. J Infect Dis 162:1316, 1986.
5. Adams WG, Deaver KE, Cochi SL, *et al.* Decline of childhood *Haemophilus influenzae* type b (Hib) disease in Hib vaccine era. JAMA 269:221, 1993.
6. Liptak GS, McConnochie KM, Roghmann KJ, Panzer JA. Decline of pediatric admissions with *Haemophilus influenzae* type b in New York State, 1982 through 1993: relation to immunizations. J Pediatr 130:923, 1997.
7. Kaufman BA, Tunkel AR, Pryor JC, Dacey RG Jr. Meningitis in the neurosurgical patient. Infect Dis Clin North Am 4:677, 1990.
8. Ostabal MI, Suarez Pinilla MA, Sanz Sebastian C, Millastre A. Epidemiological study of nosocomial meningitis. Rev Neurol 24:265, 1996.
9. Pottecher T, Balabaud-Pichon V. Meningites nosocomiales de l'adulte. Ann Franc Anesth Rean 18:558, 1999.
10. Núñez ML, Martinez-Toldos MC, Bru M, Simarro E, Segovia M, Ruiz J. Appearance of resistance to meropenem during the treatment of a patient with meningitis by *Acinetobacter*. Scand J Infect Dis 30:421, 1998.
11. Schoenbaum SC, Gardner P, Shillito J. Infections of cerebrospinal fluid shunts: epidemiology, clinical manifestations, and therapy. J Infect Dis 131:543, 1975.
12. Kaufman BA, McLone DG. Infections of cerebrospinal fluid shunts. In Scheld WM, Whitley RJ, Durack DT (eds). Infections of the central nervous system. New York: Raven Press, 1991:561.
13. Ferré C, Ariza J, Viladrich PF, *et al.* Brain abscess rupturing into the ventricles or subarachnoid space. Am J Med 106:254, 1999.
14. Saez-Llorens X, *et al.* Molecular pathophysiology of bacterial meningitis: Current concepts and therapeutic implications. J Pediatr 116:671, 1990.
15. Quagliarello V, Scheld WM. Bacterial meningitis: Pathogenesis, pathophysiology, and progress. N Engl J Med 327:864, 1992.
16. Pfister HW, Fontana A, Täuber MG, Tomasz A, Sheld WM. Mechanisms of brain injury in bacterial meningitis: workshop summary. Clin Infect Dis 19:463, 1994.

17. Viladrich PF. Enfermedad meningocócica en adolescentes y adultos (Hospital de Bellvitge, 1977–1990). Doctoral Thesis. Universidad de Barcelona, 1993.
18. Casado Flores J, García Teresa MA, Cambra F, *et al.* Estudio prospectivo multicéntrico de la meningitis bacteriana grave pediátrica. Ann Esp Pediatr 47:466, 1997.
19. Lacroix J, Deal C, Gauthier M, Rousseau E, Farrell FA. Admissions to a pediatric intensive care unit for status epilepticus: a 10-year experience. Crit Care Med 22:827, 1994.
20. Viladrich PF, Buenaventura I, Gudiol F, *et al.* Meningitis neumocócica del adulto. Estudio de 141 episodios. Med Clin (Barc) 87:569, 1986.
21. Pfister HW, Feiden W, Einhäupl KM. Spectrum of complications during bacterial meningitis in adults. Arch Neurol 50:575, 1993.
22. Viladrich PF, Gudiol F. Avances en las infecciones del sistema nervioso central producidas por bacterias grampositivas. Rev Clin Esp 194:847, 1994.
23. Carpenter RR, Petersdorf RG. The clinical spectrum of bacterial meningitis. Am J Med 33:262, 1962.
24. Banks HS. Meningococcosis: a protean disease. Lancet ii:635 and 677, 1948.
25. Brandtzaeg P. Pathogenesis of meningococcal infections. In Cartwright K (ed). Meningococcal disease. Chichester: John Wiley, 1995:71.
26. Viladrich PF, Gudiol F, Rufi G, *et al.* Meningitis bacteriana. Etiología y focos de origen de 482 episodios. Med Clin (Barc) 86:615, 1986.
27. Ariza J, Casanova A, Viladrich PF, *et al.* Etiological agent and primary source of infection in 42 cases of focal intracranial suppuration. J Clin Microbiol 24:899, 1986.
28. Sánchez C, Garau J, Viladrich PF, Nogueras A, Liñares J. La listeriosis del adulto: epidemiología, clínica, pronóstico y tratamiento. Med Clin (Barc) 84:533, 1985.
29. Fredricks DN, Relman DA. Application of polymerase chain reaction to the diagnosis of infectious diseases. Clin Infect Dis 29:475, 1999.
30. Coant PN, Kornberg AE, Duffy C, Dryja DM, Hassan SM. Blood culture results as determinants in the organism identification of bacterial meningitis. Pediatr Emerg Care 8:200, 1992.
31. Milhaud D, Bernardin G, Rastello M, Mattei M, Blard JM. Meningites bacteriennes de l'adulte en reanimation medicale. Analyse clinique et etude des facteurs pronostiques. Press Med 25:353, 1996.
32. Horwitz SJ, Boxerbaum B, O'Bell J. Cerebral herniation in bacterial meningitis in childhood. Ann Neurol 7:524, 1980.
33. McDonald JT, Uden DL. Intravenous glycerol and mannitol therapy in children with intracranial hypertension. Neurology 32:437, 1982.
34. Coyle PK. Glucocorticoids in central nervous system bacterial infection. Arch Neurol 56:796, 1999.
35. Odio CM, Faingezicht I, Paris M, *et al.* The beneficial effects of early dexamethasone administration in infants and children with bacterial meningitis. N Engl J Med 324:1525, 1991.
36. McIntyre PB, Berkey CS, King SM, *et al.* Dexamethasone as adjunctive therapy in bacterial meningitis. A meta-analysis of randomized clinical trials since 1988. JAMA 278:925, 1997.
37. Girgis NI, Farid Z, Mikhail IA, *et al.* Dexamethasone treatment for bacterial meningitis in children and adults. Pediatr Infect Dis J 8:848, 1989.
38. Quagliarello VJ, Scheld WM. Treatment of bacterial meningitis. N Engl J Med 336:708, 1997.
39. Almirante B, Cortés E, Pigrau C, *et al.* Terapeútica y evolución de la meningitis neumocócica del adulto. Estudio de una serie reciente de 70 episodios. Med Clin (Barc) 105:681, 1995.
40. Alvarez-Lerma F, Cisneros JM, Viladrich PF, *et al.* Indications for admission to the intensive care service of adult patients with severe infections. Enf Infecc Microbiol Clin 16:423, 1998.
41. Sáez-Nieto JA, Vázquez JA, Marcos C. Meningococci moderately resistant to penicillin. Lancet 336:54, 1990.
42. Galimand M, Gerbaud G, Guibourdenche M, Riou JY, Courvalin P. High-level chloramphenicol resistance in *Neisseria meningitidis*. Lancet 339:868, 1998.
43. Pérez Trallero E, García Arenzana JM, Ayestarán Y, Muñoz Baroja I. Comparative activity *in vitro* of 16 antimicrobial agents against penicillin-susceptible meningococci and meningococci with diminished susceptibility to penicillin. Antimicrob Agents Chemother 33:1622, 1989.
44. Viladrich PF, Pallarés R, Ariza J, Rufi G, Gudiol F. Four days of penicillin therapy for meningococcal meningitis. Arch Intern Med 146:2380, 1988.
45. Viladrich PF. Las meningitis meningocócicas. Neurología 12:181, 1997.
46. Viladrich PF. Tratamiento y evolución de la meningitis causada por neumococos resistentes a

la penicilina. Rev Clin Esp 196, monográfico 2:9, 1996.

47. Viladrich PF, Gudiol F, Liñares J, *et al.* Evaluation of vancomycin for therapy of adult pneumococcal meningitis. Antimicrob Agents Chemother 35:2467, 1991.
48. Friedland IR, Klugman KP. Cerebrospinal fluid bactericidal activity against cephalosporin-resistant *Streptococcus pneumoniae* in children with meningitis treated with high-dosage cefotaxime. Antimicrob Agents Chemother 41: 1888, 1997.
49. Viladrich PF, Cabellos C, Pallarés R, *et al.* High doses of cefotaxime in treatment of adult meningitis due to *Streptococcus pneumoniae* with decreased susceptibilities to broad-spectrum cephalosporins. Antimicrob Agents Chemother 40:218, 1996.
50. Klugman KP, Friedland IR, Bradley JS. Bactericidal activity against cephalosporin-resistant *Streptococcus pneumoniae* in cerebrospinal fluid of children with acute bacterial meningitis. Antimicrob Agents Chemother 39:1989, 1995.
51. Viladrich PF, Cabellos C, Martos A, Martinez Lacasa JT, Gudiol F. Lack of efficacy of pneumococcal vaccine in preventing pneumococcal meningitis due to cerebrospinal fluid leaks. 32nd Interscience Conference on Antimicrobial Agents and Chemotherapy (ICAAC), October 1992, Anaheim, California, USA. (Abstract no. 1282).
52. Cherubin CE, Appleman MD, Heseltine PNR, *et al.* Epidemiologic spectrum and current treatment of listeriosis. Rev Infect Dis 13:1108, 1991.
53. Cabellos C, Viladrich PF, Corredoira J, Verdaguer R, Ariza J, Gudiol F. Streptococcal meningitis in adult patients: current epidemiology and clinical spectrum. Clin Infect Dis 28:1104, 1999.
54. Alcaide F, Liñares J, Pallarés R, *et al. In vitro* activities of 22 beta-lactam antibiotics against penicillin-resistant and penicillin-susceptible viridans group streptococci isolated from blood. Antimicrob Agents Chemother 39:2243, 1995.
55. Fernández Viladrich P. Papel de meropenem en la meningitis bacteriana. Enf Infecc Microbiol Clin 15 (Suppl):5761, 1997.
56. Viladrich PF, Corbella X, Corral L, Tubau F, Mateu A. Successful treatment of ventriculitis due to carbapenen-resistant *Acinetobacter baumannii* with intraventricular colistin sulfomethate sodium. Clin Infect Dis 28:916, 1999.
57. Levin AS, Barone AA, Penço J, *et al.* Intravenous colistin as therapy for nosocomial infections caused by multidrug-resistant *Pseudomonas aeruginosa* and *Acinetobacter baumannii.* Clin Infect Dis 28:1008, 1999.
58. Frasch CE. Meningococal vaccines: Past, present and future. In Cartwright K (ed). Meningococcal disease. Chichester: John Wiley, 1995:245.
59. Korinek AM. Risk factors for neurosurgical site infections after craniotomy: a prospective multicenter study of 2944 patients. Neurosurgery 41:1073, 1997.
60. Viladrich PF, Tubau F, Cabellos C, *et al.* Vancomycin plus rifampin for therapy of adult pneumococcal meningitis. Clin Microbiol Infect 5 (suppl 3):250: (abstract no. P616), 1999.

25. ACUTE INFECTIVE ENDOCARDITIS

Jason L. Sanchez and Russell Little

Introduction

According to classical definitions from the pre-antibiotic era, infective endocarditis (IE) was divided by the acuity of presenting symptoms and the rapidity of clinical evolution toward the anticipated lethal outcome. Patients with "acute" endocarditis had an abrupt onset and progression to death in less than six weeks. Patients with slowly developing symptoms were subdivided into categories of "subacute" or "chronic" endocarditis associated with a slowly progressing but also uniformly fatal illness lasting from several months to over two years [1]. The clinical features of acute endocarditis often included a hectic, rapidly deteriorating clinical course and dramatically invasive infection with destruction of heart valves and embolic complications early in the disease [2]. Before the introduction of echocardiography, about half of all IE cases were diagnosed only at autopsy [3]. Currently IE represents the fourth leading cause of life-threatening infectious disease syndromes (after urosepsis, pneumonia and intra-abdominal sepsis) [4]. The microorganisms most often associated with acute IE are *Staphylococcus aureus*, *Streptococcus pneumoniae*, β-hemolytic streptococci (groups A, B, C and G), *Neisseria gonorrhea* and *Neisseria meningitidis*. Enterococcal, as well as nosocomial and prosthetic-valve endocarditis are not as easily classified by their acuity but they often require support and management in intensive care units (ICU), so they are included here. We will review some basic concepts of the IE disease process and diagnosis as well as the clinical features and treatment of patients with this group of life-threatening infections.

Diagnosis

PATHOPHYSIOLOGY OF IE

Intracardiac pressure gradients that induce turbulent blood flow are detected clinically as heart murmurs, some of which are recognized risk factors for the development of endocarditis (Table 1). In the usual sequence of events, turbulent blood flow results in endothelial damage followed by platelet and fibrin deposition at the site of damage forming a focus of nonbacterial thrombotic endocarditis. Transient bacteremia (or fungemia) with organisms that display tissue adhesion structures leads to microbial attachment and inclusion in the platelet/fibrin thrombus to form a vegetation. These vegetations may enlarge through the formation of successive layers of clot and microorganisms. Colonies of bacteria or fungi within a vegetation are relatively resistant to host defenses (e.g. phagocytosis) and to antibiotic penetration. This unique microbial environment within the vegetation determines the need for prolonged therapy with high doses of microbicidal agents to achieve a microbiological cure in patients with IE.

PRESENTING SIGNS AND SYMPTOMS

Patients with IE usually have evidence of turbulent blood flow from congenital or acquired cardiovascular lesions. Table 1 shows a hierarchy of cardiac anatomical risk factors for the development of IE. In the US, mitral valve prolapse (MVP) remains the most common cardiac abnormality predisposing to IE [5]. However, new echocardiographic criteria have reduced the estimated prevalence of MVP in the general

TABLE 1. Cardiac risk factors for infective endocarditis [5]

High risk
Prosthetic heart valve
Previous episode of infectious endocarditis
Cyanotic congenital heart disease
Ventricular septal defect
Patent ductus arteriosis
Coarctation of the aorta
Aortic regurgitation or stenosis (including bicuspid aortic valve)
Mitral regurgitation
Intermediate risk
Mitral valve prolapse with regurgitation
Mitral stenosis
Tricuspid regurgitation or stenosis
Pulmonary stenosis
Hypertrophic obstructive cardiomyopathy
Aortic atherosclerosis or bicuspid valve with minimal stenosis or regurgitation
Low risk
Mitral valve prolapse without regurgitation
Trivial valvular regurgitation with structurally normal heart
Atrial septal defect
Cardiac pacemaker

population of ambulatory subjects from about 15% using the old criteria to 2.4% with the new criteria [6].

The clinical evolution of acute IE usually accompanies the development of systemic signs of infection such as fever, malaise, anorexia, weight loss, etc. In dental cases symptoms typically occur within two weeks of dental manipulation but the time to diagnosis may be quite long (median time of five weeks) [5]. There may be focal signs of embolization, such as nailbed splinter hemorrhages, and skin, mucous membrane or conjunctival petechiae. In most cases there will be evidence of an immunological reaction to infection (elevated blood levels of acute phase reactants, such as C-reactive protein (CRP) and ferritin) and a high erythrocyte sedimentation rate (ESR). Anemia may be lacking in patients who present acutely and embolic inflammatory skin lesions such as Osler's nodes and Janeway lesions are seen in a minority of patients.

CULTURES

The hallmark of IE is *continuous* bacteremia or fungemia. Consequently blood cultures are a crucial part of the diagnostic workup. Two goals should be satisfied, identification of the etiologic agent and demonstration of its continuous presence in the blood. The latter can be confirmed by obtaining positive blood cultures at two or three different times and different vascular access sites. Confounding factors may result in either false-positive or false-negative blood cultures. False-positive cultures are usually the result of contamination of blood samples obtained after inadequate skin site disinfection [7] or from a colonized central venous catheter [8, 9]. Patients with IE may have negative blood cultures that persist for several days or even a week, induced by the prior administration of antibiotics. Isolation of the etiologic microorganism is so important in diagnosis and therapy that it may justify additional blood culture sampling while withholding empirical antimicrobials temporarily in a patient who continues to have fever. However, delay in the initiation of antimicrobial therapy may be contraindicated in patients with a deteriorating clinical course especially if there is aortic valve involvement or if they develop signs of congestive heart failure which carries a high risk of poor outcomes including death [10].

ECHOCARDIOGRAPHY

The widespread use of echocardiography, especially transesophageal echocardiography (TEE), has had a major impact on the approach to the diagnosis of IE. TEE has particularly improved the diagnosis of PVE because shadowing artefacts are often produced by mechanical valves when viewed by transthoracic echocardiography (TTE). Increasing use of TEE can also be attributed to the prominent role of echocardiography in the Duke criteria for the diagnosis of IE (discussed below) and to the proposed cost-effectiveness of TEE in determining the duration of antibiotic therapy in patients with central venous catheter-associated *S. aureus* bacteremia [11].

DIAGNOSTIC CRITERIA, SENSITIVITY AND SPECIFICITY

The diagnosis of IE is associated with a wide variety of often subtle and sometimes nonspecific clinical findings. Competing diagnostic criteria have been proposed by different groups of investigators whose purpose was to define guidelines for clinical studies of IE. However, attempts to apply these criteria to a particular patient can lead to confusion about the necessary components of the work-up and exaggerated doubts about the clinical diagnosis of IE. For example, the criteria proposed by von Reyn *et al.* (also called the Beth Israel criteria) [12] dictate that a "definite" diagnosis of IE should be based on the histopathology of tissues from surgery or autopsy or results from culture of an embolized vegetation. In practice, these diagnostic criteria are seldom satisfied. Even the diagnosis of "probable" IE by the Beth Israel criteria requires detection of a new regurgitant murmur in addition to other findings. The more recently proposed Duke criteria for the diagnosis of IE are more sensitive and clinically useful, but they too were explicitly formulated to serve as entry criteria for patients in epidemiological studies and clinical trials of IE [13]. Accordingly the Duke guidelines permit a diagnosis of IE based on a variety of combinations of stipulated clinical criteria. For example, a "definite" diagnosis of IE can be established by blood cultures yielding a typical organism (e.g. *S. aureus*, viridans streptococci etc.) and an echocardiogram showing an oscillating intracardiac mass (in the absence of an alternative anatomical explanation). The validity of the Duke criteria have been independently confirmed by several groups [14–17]. Other publications have noted the high negative predictive value (at least 92%) of the Duke criteria [18] and a greater sensitivity than the Beth Israel criteria in the diagnosis of native valve IE [17] and PVE [19].

Etiologic Agents of Acute IE

STAPHYLOCOCCUS AUREUS

S. aureus is the most common cause of bacteremia in US adults [20] and of IE in tertiary-care hospitals. This form of endocarditis is characterized by community-acquisition, absence of an apparent primary focus and the presence of metastatic foci of infection. In nonaddicts, 95% of cases involve the mitral and/or the aortic valve [21]. Congestive heart failure complicates *S. aureus* left-sided endocarditis in 35–60% of patients and this may warrant valve replacement surgery [21]. The metastatic complications of *S. aureus* endocarditis include septic arthritis, osteomyelitis, pericarditis, renal and/or splenic or brain abscesses. In addition arterial emboli may occur early in the course of infection resulting in cerebral infarcts or subarachnoid hemorrhage from rupture of a mycotic aneurysm.

In injection drug users methicillin-susceptible *S. aureus* causes approximately 60% of native valve endocarditis. However, methicillin-resistant *S. aureus* (MRSA) strains have become more common in some urban addict populations with community-acquired bacteremia and IE [22]. Among addicts with staphylococcal IE, 50–90% are seen first in the Emergency Department often with a history of 5–10 days of fever, arthralgias, myalgias and a murmur of tricuspid valve insufficiency. A consequence of tricuspid valve *S. aureus* IE is the occurrence of septic pulmonary emboli, sometimes with cavitation or sometimes only multifocal pulmonary infiltrates. Although radiographic findings related to septic pulmonary emboli from the tricuspid valve may be prominent, positive physical findings on chest examination are relatively uncommon and pathologic murmurs may be absent initially [23]. The prognosis for *S. aureus* tricuspid valve IE in injection drug users is very favorable and the mortality rate (with treatment) is generally less than 5%. Two week courses of parenteral antibiotic therapy are usually sufficient and valve replacement is rarely required [4, 23, 24].

Therapy of *S. aureus* IE should usually be with a penicillinase-resistant penicillin (e.g. oxacillin, nafcillin, cefazolin) and an aminoglycoside or vancomycin alone if there is confirmed β-lactam allergy (Table 2). Because patient histories of penicillin-allergy are often uncertain or inaccurate, allergy skin testing and desensitization to a β-lactam antibiotic by an experienced medical specialist should be considered. Synergy between β-lactams and aminoglycosides can be demonstrated with most *S. aureus* strains and combination therapy usually result in a shorter time to the clearing of bacteremia [25]. Target peak and trough levels of either gentamicin or tobramycin should be 3 ug/ml and <1 ug/ml, respectively and 2–3 aminoglycoside doses per day (1 mg/kg/dose for tobramycin and gentamicin) should be used in patients with normal renal function in preference to single daily dosing [26]. Aminoglycoside therapy can generally be discontinued after surveillance blood cultures (on synergistic therapy) become negative and

TABLE 2. Summary of acute native valve IE pathogens and recommended antimicrobial therapy

Pathogen	Frequency	Recommended Rx	Dosage and Route	Duration of Rx
S. aureus	Common	[§]TV: oxacillin or nafcillin	2 g every 4 h IV	2–4 weeks
		plus optional gentamicin	1 mg/kg every 8 h IV	3–5 days
		*cefazolin or other 1st generation cephalosporin	2 g IV every 8 h IV	2–4 weeks
		plus optional gentamicin	1 mg/kg every 8 h IV	3–5 days
		or vancomycin alone	15 mg/kg twice each day IV	4–6 weeks
S. aureus	Common	[§]MV, AV: oxacillin or nafcillin plus optional gentamicin *cefazolin or other 1st generation cephalosporin plus optional gentamicin or vancomycin alone	[§]Same as for TV	4–6 weeks
Enterococcus sp.	10–15%	aqueous penicillin G	18–30 million U/24 h IV	4–6 weeks
		or ampicillin	12 g/24 h IV	
		plus gentamicin	1 mg/kg every 8 h IV	
Enterococcus sp.	10–15%	*vancomycin	15 mg/kg twice each day IV	4–6 weeks
		plus gentamicin	1 mg/kg every 8 h IV	
		or plus streptomycin	7.5 mg/kg every 12 h IM	
Enterococcus sp.	Variable	[¶]ampicillin	18–24 g continuous IV infusion	8–12 weeks
S. pneumoniae	1–3%	aqueous penicillin G or	12–24 million U daily IV	4 weeks
		ceftriaxone	1–2 g every 12–24 h IV	
N. meningitidis	≪1%	ceftriaxone or aqueous	1–2 g every 12 h IV	2–4 weeks
		penicillin G	12–24 million U daily IV	
N. gonorrhea	<1%	ceftriaxone	1–2 g every 12 h IV	4 weeks
GAS	<1%	aqueous penicillin G	12–24 million U daily IV	4 weeks
GBS	<1%	aqueous penicillin G	12–24 million U daily IV	4–6 weeks

[§] Abbreviations in the table as follows: TV = Tricuspid valve, AV = Aortic valve, MV = Mitral valve, GAS = group A streptococci, GBS = group B streptococci.

* In patients with β-lactam allergy.

[¶] In presence of HLAGR.

a beneficial clinical response has occurred. However, this applies only to native valve infection and to organisms that are susceptible to both aminoglycoside and a β-lactam. Although tricuspid valve IE can usually be treated effectively with shorter courses of intravenous (IV) antibiotics (< two weeks), patients with aortic or mitral valve infection should receive at least four weeks of parenteral antibiotic therapy [26]. However, if the organism displays high-level aminoglycoside resistance (HLAGR), then synergistic therapy is not possible and the treatment interval should be extended to 4–6 weeks of either vancomycin or a penicillinase-resistant β-lactam (oxacillin, nafcillin or cefazolin) alone (Table 2) [26].

ENTEROCOCCUS SP.

Enterococci are members of the normal bowel and biliary flora and under most conditions they are considered to be minimally invasive. However, they are responsible for 10–15% of all cases of IE, some of which conform to the definition of "acute or subacute" endocarditis [27]. In recent years the incidence of enterococcal blood stream infections and the consequent risk of endocarditis has increased and it is expected to continue increasing. This trend is thought to result from improvements in sustaining critically ill patients and the increasing use of medical devices that breach the normal anatomical barriers to infection (e.g. skin and the gastrointestinal mucosa). The increased prevalence of enterococcal isolates that are resistant to β-lactams, aminoglycosides and vancomycin has greatly complicated the treatment of these infections.

Enterococci display inherent resistance to antibiotics, in particular they are resistant to cephalosporins, aminoglycosides and penicillinase-resistant β-lactams. Because no single agent is bactericidal for enterococci, standard therapy for enterococcal IE has traditionally relied on combining an aminoglycoside (e.g. gentamicin or tobramycin) and a cell-wall active agent such as ampicillin or vancomycin for 4–6 weeks of IV therapy (Table 2) [26]. Using synergistic antibiotic combinations, microbiological cures have been achieved in 72–79% of cases of enterococcal IE compared with cure rates in the range of 40% with the use of cell-wall agents alone (ampicillin, penicillin or vancomycin) [29]. The emergence of enterococci with HLAGR (e.g. MIC >2000 ug/ml for gentamicin) has denied access to microbicidal therapy and greatly reduced the probability of cure [29]. Enterococci with HLAGR now comprise >50% of isolates in some institutions. A survey of hospitals in the US revealed that HLAGR was found to vary from 27 to 70% of enterococcal isolates in different centers [30]. In addition, the increasing resistance to β-lactam and glycopeptide (e.g. vancomycin) antibiotics has rendered some enterococcal infections untreatable and has spurred the search for new therapies.

Enterococcal IE is typically community-acquired, resulting from an endogenous source of bacteremia (e.g. cholecystitis or urinary tract infection). Nosocomial bacteremia is less likely to result in enterococcal IE. The mean age of patients with enterococcal IE tends to be older (60–70 years) and predisposing cardiac valvular disease is common. The mean duration of symptoms prior to diagnosis of enterococcal IE was 24 days with 44% presenting within 10 days and 24% presenting with signs of heart failure. Enterococcal IE of the aortic valve tends to be more aggressive in its course and has a higher associated mortality, frequently requiring early surgical intervention [31].

The treatment of enterococcal IE depends on the antibiotic susceptibility of the particular isolate. Penicillin (or ampicillin) and gentamicin is generally accepted as the drug combination of choice (Table 2) [26]. A preference by some experienced clinicians for ampicillin over penicillin rests on its typical two-fold superior potency *in vitro* but it has not been shown that this minor difference is clinically significant. Ampicillin or penicillin are preferred over vancomycin (plus an aminoglycoside). Ampicillin (12–18 g/24 h) is administered either by daily continuous infusion or divided into six IV doses and gentamicin, which is also administered in divided dosing (1 mg/kg q8h IV for patients with normal renal function) rather than single daily dosing (Table 2) [26]. Optimal gentamicin peak and trough blood levels are 3 ug/ml and <1 ug/ml, respectively. If a particular enterococcal isolate is high level gentamicin resistant (MIC >2000 ug/ml), streptomycin susceptibility should always be determined since this agent may be effective in 30–50% of gentamicin-resistant strains. Streptomycin dosing in patients with normal renal function is 7.5 mg/kg q12h. If HLAGR is documented, the preferred treatment is high dose ampicillin, possibly even by continuous infusion [26] (18–24 g/day IV) for 8–12 weeks. Vancomycin administration at 30 mg/kg/day divided into two doses should be substituted in the treatment of HLAGR strains (Table 2) in patients with confirmed β-lactam allergy or if the enterococcal isolate displays ampicillin resistance that (rarely) cannot be overcome by the use of ampicillin/sulbactam (to inhibit β-lactamase). High dose ampicillin has resulted in a cure rate of approximately 50% and those failing therapy should be considered for surgical treatment [26]. The optimal regimen for enterococcal IE caused by organisms resistant to both β-lactams and glycopeptides (e.g. vancomycin-resistant enterococci, VRE) is unknown. Multiple antibiotic combinations have been used in animal models with none showing consistent efficacy. Newer agents such as quinupristin/dalfopristin have anecdotal successes and failures in the treatment of VRE strains. Consideration should be given to early surgical intervention in selected patients with resistant organisms, especially if the aortic valve or a prosthetic valve is involved or if cardiac decompensation is present [26, 31].

STREPTOCOCCUS PNEUMONIAE

Pneumococci rarely cause IE. Only 1–3% of all IE cases reported in the antibiotic era are attributable to this agent [32]. However, pneumococcal IE is almost always an acute, aggressive infection that tends to affect the aortic and/or mitral valves. It often results in heart failure or shock and frequently requires prompt or even emergent valve replacement. Osler's classic triad included pneumococcal pneumonia, meningitis and endocarditis in an alcoholic individual. The mortality rate from pneumococcal IE remains very high [32–34] and in a recently published review of 182 evaluable cases, the overall mortality rate was 63% despite the availability of highly effective antimicrobial agents [32]. The aortic valve was involved in 74% of cases and in 13%, two or more valves were affected. Valve perforation and parivalvular abscess occurred in approximately 1/3 of cases. Identified risk factors for invasive pneumococcal disease include tobacco use, recent respiratory infection, chronic pulmonary diseases as well as conditions of impaired systemic host defenses such as extremes of age, malnutrition or glucocorticoid therapy. Chronic disorders that are risk factors for invasive *S. pneumoniae* infection include cirrhosis, renal insufficiency, diabetes mellitus, alcoholism, human immunodeficiency virus (HIV) infection, sickle-cell disease and other congenital or acquired immunodeficiencies [32]. It is unknown whether pneumococcal polysaccharide vaccine protects against pneumococcal IE. No formal recommendations for optimal empirical therapy can be made but in accordance with current recommendations for the treatment of pneumococcal meningitis it is prudent to initiate therapy with ceftriaxone and vancomycin until the results of susceptibility testing can be obtained [32, 35]. For β-lactam susceptible pneumococcal strains, four weeks of IV therapy with high dose penicillin (20M units each day in divided doses [34]) or ceftriaxone (1 g. IV bid) have been successful (Table 2) [32].

NEISSERIA SP.

In a recent review it was found that only 31 cases of *N. meningitidis* IE were reported in the literature during the past 50 years suggesting that meningococci very rarely cause IE [36]. The cited review also suggests that meningococcal IE has become even less common since the advent of antibiotics despite the fact that several thousand cases of meningococcemia occur in the US each year. Most patients with meningococcal IE are normal hosts with normal heart valves and without distincitive risk factors for endocarditis or for *Neisseria* sp. infection. However, a report from the Netherlands found that 31 (46%) of 67 patients older than five years of age with invasive meningococcal infections (not just IE) were reported to have complement deficiency [37].

Most cases of meningococcal IE involve mitral or aortic valves and the frequency of systemic embolic complications is high. Patients with meningococcal IE often present with purpuric skin lesions, arthralgias and signs of acute sepsis and fever [38]. In 26 cases reported by Firestone, cures were achieved in only five patients but there were questions about the validity of diagnosis and length of follow-up in two of these cases [38]. Optimal antibiotic therapy has not been established. Both penicillin and ceftriaxone have been successful and courses of four to six weeks of IV therapy were suggested by the authors of reported cases (Table 2) [36].

Endocarditis due to infection with *N. gonorrhea* is less rare than that due to *N. meningitidis* accounting for <1% of cases of IE. It usually occurs in young adults as a complication of disseminated gonococcemia and infection of an anatomically normal aortic, mitral or tricuspid valve [39]. It is often an aggressive infection with a high rate of perivalvular abscess formation, precipitous deterioration despite appropriate therapy, heart failure and death (19% mortality rate) [40]. The propensity for complicated cardiac infections increases the urgency and value of TEE early in the diagnostic workup [41]. Pre-existing disseminated gonococcal infection is sometimes suggested by petechial skin rashes and/or tenosynovitis. Bacterial hepatitis, meningitis and myocarditis may occur coincidently with this form of acute IE. Disseminated gonorrhea is more common in women than men and cases of gonococcal IE have been reported during pregnancy, and in women with SLE. Unusual features that have been described include involvement of all four valves simultaneously, prosthetic-valve infection and association with terminal complement component deficiencies [40]. Because of the high frequency of penicillin-resistant strains of *N. gonorrhea*, ceftriaxone has become the initial therapy of choice (Table 2) [42].

β-HEMOLYTIC STREPTOCOCCI (GROUPS A, B, C AND G)

In reviews [43–45], *Streptococcus pyogenes* (group A streptococci, GAS) comprised less than 1% of all cases of IE although there have been reports of locally higher frequencies related to clusters of patients who use injection drugs [43, 44]. In both addict and nonaddict patients GAS endocarditis tends to present as an acute, aggressive, short-term febrile illness. IE cased by GAS tends to occur in patients without previous valvular abnormality. It has often been reported as "probable" endocarditis in patients with sustained GAS bacteremia but without a definite vegetation by echocardiography. A recent review of cases of IE due to GAS claimed that only 69 cases have been reported since the introduction of penicillin into clinical medicine [45]. In injection drug-users IE is almost always on the tricuspid valve and the mortality rate is low, 5–10% [43, 44]. In non-addicts as well as a small percentage of addicts it may occur on the mitral or aortic valves. Left-heart IE caused by GAS often has a rapidly progressive course with embolic complications and a high mortality-rate (>20%) even with appropriate therapy. GAS continue to be uniformly susceptible to penicillin and high-dose penicillin G is the regimen of choice (Table 2). A patient history of β-lactam allergy should probably be confirmed by skin testing and if confirmed, penicillin desensitization in consultation with an experienced specialist, should be considered. Most surviving patients received 4–6 weeks of IV antibiotic therapy (Table 2).

β-Hemolytic streptococci other than GAS have also been reported to cause IE [46]. Group B streptococci (*Streptococcus agalactiae*) occur most commonly and they outnumber the reported cases of IE due to GAS. Sixty-two well described cases were reviewed in one publication [47]. These patients were characterized by: high frequency of underlying heart disease (about 55%), diabetes mellitus, gastrointestinal neoplasms, frequent occurrence of large arterial thrombi and a high mortality rate (about 40%). Over one-half of the patients presented with acute endocarditis. All β-hemolytic streptococci, including the GAS, have maintained their susceptibility to penicillin and this antibiotic remains the drug of choice, although some have recommended penicillin plus an aminoglycoside for use in selected cases of group B streptococcal etiology [2]. Early surgery may also be indicated.

Nosocomial IE

Although staphylococci mainly cause community-acquired infections, they are also the major cause of nosocomial IE, accounting for 50–70% of cases, while coagulase-negative staphylococci, enterococci, Gram-negative organisms and *Candida* sp. also occur commonly [48, 49]. The most common sources of nosocomial blood stream infection leading to IE are colonized or contaminated intravascular devices. Other important sources include wound infections and instrumentation of an infected GU tract [48, 49]. Some cases occur following nosocomial blood stream infection in patients with prosthetic heart valves. One prospective study of IE due to *S. aureus* found that 46% of bacteremia cases were nosocomial in origin and that 12.4% of the *S. aureus* bacteremias led to documented IE [50]. Compared with community-acquired staphylococcal IE, nosocomial IE tends to occur in older, more critically ill patients. Fever is the most consistent symptom and vascular embolic phenomena are less common. Dialysis patients represent a special risk group for nosocomial bacteremia because of the frequent need to access their blood stream. Persistent *S. aureus* bacteremia, for more than two to three days on appropriate antibiotic therapy, should prompt an endocarditis evaluation. Attempts to reduce the incidence of nosocomial blood stream infection are critical.

The mortality of nosocomial IE is high, approximately 50% [48–51]. Prompt removal of intravascular devices (e.g. central venous catheters) is important for prevention of nosocomial IE, and for the termination of line-associated bacteremia/fungemia. Vascular catheter removal is especially important when the etiologic agent is *S. aureus* or *Candida* sp. or when another implantable device is present (e.g. prosthetic heart valve, pacemaker, orthopedic hardware).

Prosthetic Valve Endocarditis

The overall lifetime risk of developing prosthetic-valve endocarditis (PVE) is approximately 3–6%. The risk is similar for mechanical and bioprosthetic-valves and is not associated with valve position (aortic vs mitral) [52]. Coagulase-negative staphylococci (predominantly *S. epidermidis*) are the major causes of valve infection during the first year after surgery and most of these isolates are resistant to methicillin and oxacillin [53]. *S. aureus* is also an important cause of PVE accounting for approximately 10–20% of cases [53]. IE that develops within two months of cardiac surgery is often associated with an identifiable source of postoperative infection such as an intravascular catheter, chest-tube or sternal-wound infection. PVE cases presenting later than two months after valve replacement can be community-acquired and, if so, are less likely to have an obvious portal of entry for the infecting organism. The early onset cases begin at the valve sewing ring-annulus interface and as a result are often complicated by invasive perivalvular infection, necrosis of the valve-annulus, dehiscence and dysfunction of the prosthetic valve [53]. These complications often lead to an acute clinical presentation and a high mortality [52–56].

The clinical features of PVE are usually similar to those associated with native-valve IE.

Fever remains the most common presenting symptom [54]. Its presence alone, even if apparently explained by another source, should prompt an evaluation for IE. Signs and symptoms of hemodynamic compromise frequently accompany the presentation of PVE resulting commonly in admission to the ICU. TEE is an especially important, often urgent, diagnostic modality in PVE because of its superior visualization of posterior cardiac structures, its avoidance of acoustic shadowing and its higher resolution. It often permits the detection of perivalvular or myocardial abscess, mycotic aneurysm and valve dehiscence with regurgitation. However, TTE may still provide better visualization of the anterior aspect of a prosthetic aortic valve as well as additional functional information.

Management of PVE depends on the causative organism, the presence or absence of prosthetic valve malfunction (e.g. dehiscence, regurgitation) and the hemodynamic status of the patient. Prompt surgical evaluation should be obtained. Delay of surgery in an attempt to sterilize the valve or reduce the microorganism burden with antibiotics is associated with increased mortality [55, 56]. Surgery is also indicated for fungal PVE and for persistent fungemia despite optimal antimicrobial therapy. Some authorities advocate an expanded role for early surgical intervention in all cases of PVE [57, 58].

The recommended antibiotic regimen for methicillin-resistant staphylococcal PVE is vancomycin, rifampin and gentamicin, and for methicillin-sensitive staphylococcal PVE, nafcillin or oxacillin, rifampin and gentamicin are recommended [26]. Antibiotic therapy should be started, even if it reflects empirical choices, as soon as possible and surveillance blood cultures obtained daily to assure that clearing of bacteremia occurs promptly. Persistent bacteremia (or fungemia) may constitute an indication for removal of the infected prosthesis. The treatment of Gram-negative bacilli and other less common etiologic agents for PVE should comply with the need, in all cases, for prolonged administration of microbicidal agents and should be dictated by the *in vitro* susceptibility pattern of the etiologic agent [26, 54, 57].

References

1. Osler W. Malignant endocarditis. Lancet 1:415, 459, 505, 1885.
2. Bayer AS, Scheld WM. Endocarditis and intravascular infections. In Mandell, Bennett and Dolan (eds). Principles and Practice of Infectious Diseases, 5th edn, Churchill Livingstone, New York, 2000: 857.
3. Watanakunakorn C. Editorial response: Increasing importance of intravascular device-associated *Staphylococcus aureus* endocarditis. Clin Infect Dis 28:115, 1999.
4. Bayer AS, Bolger AF, Taubert KA, Wilson W, Steckelberg J, Karchmer AW, Levison M, Chambers HF, Dajani AS, Gewitz MH, Newburger JW, Gerber MA, Shulman ST, Pallasch TJ, Gage TW, Perrieri R. Diagnosis and management of infective endocarditis and its complications. Circulation 98:2936, 1998.
5. Durack DT, Kaplan EL, Bisno AL. Apparent failures of endocarditis prophylaxis. Analysis of 52 cases submitted to a national registry. JAMA 250:2318, 1983.
6. Freed LA, Levy D, Levine RA, Larson MG, Evans JC, Fuller DL, Lehman B, Benjamin EJ. Prevalence and clinical outcome of mitral-valve prolapse. N Eng J Med 341:1, 1999.
7. Little JR, Murray PR, Traynor PS, Spitznagel E. A randomized trial of povidone-iodine compared with iodine tincture for venipuncture site disinfection: Effects on rates of blood culture contamination. Am J Med 107:119, 1999.
8. Bryant JK, Strand CL. Reliability of blood cultures collected from intravascular catheter versus venipuncture. Am J Clin Path 88:113, 1987.
9. DesJardin JA, Falagas ME, Ruthazer R, Griffith J, Wawrose D, Schenkein D, Miller K, Snydman DR. Clinical utility of blood cultures drawn from indwelling central venous catheters in hospitalized patients with cancer. Ann Intern Med 131: 641, 1999.
10. Douglas JL, Dismukes WE. Surgical therapy of infective endocarditis on natural valves. In Kaye D (ed). Infective Endocarditis. Second edn, New York: Raven Press, 1992: 397.
11. Rosen AB, Fowler VG, Corey GR, Downs SM, Biddle AK, Li J, Jollis JG. Cost-effectiveness of transesophageal echocardiography to determine

the duration of therapy for intravascular catheter-associated *Staphylococcus aureus* bacteremia. Ann Intern Med 130:810, 1999.

12. Von Reyn CF, Levy BS, Arbeit RD, Friedland G, Crumpacker CS. Infective endocarditis: An analysis based on strict case definitions. Ann Intern Med 94(part 1):505, 1981.
13. Durack DT, Lukes AS, Bright DK, the Duke Endocarditis Service. New criteria for diagnosis of infective endocarditis: Utilization of specific echocardiographic findings. Am J Med 96:200, 1994.
14. Bayer AS, Ward JI, Glinzton LE, Shapiro SM. Evaluation of new clinical criteria for the diagnosis of infective endocarditis. Am J Med 96: 211, 1994.
15. Hoen B, Selton-Suty C, Danchin N, Weber M, Villemot J-P, Mathieu P, Floquet J, Canton P. Evaluation of the Duke criteria versus the Beth Israel criteria for the diagnosis of infective endocarditis. Clin Infect Dis 21:905, 1995.
16. Hoen B, Beguinot I, Raboud C, Jaussaud R, Selton-Suty C, May T, Canton P. The Duke criteria for diagnosing infective endocarditis are specific: analysis of 100 patients with acute fever or fever of unknown origin. Clin Infect Dis 23:298, 1996.
17. Heiro M, Nikoskelainen J, Hartiala JJ, Saraste JK, Kotilainen PM. Diagnosis of infective endocarditis: Sensitivity of the Duke vs von Reyn criteria. Arch Intern Med 158:18, 1998.
18. Dodds GA, Sexton DJ, Durack DT, Bashore TM, Corey GR, Kisslo J, the Duke Endocarditis Service. Negative predictive value of the Duke criteria for infective endocarditis. Am J Cardiol 77:403, 1996.
19. Nettles RE, McCarty DE, Corey GR, Li J, Sexton DJ. An evaluation of the Duke Criteria in 25 pathologically confirmed cases of prosthetic valve endocarditis. Clin Infect Dis 25:1401, 1997.
20. Weinstein MP, Towns ML, Quartey SM, Mirrett S, Reimer LG, Parmigiani G, Reller LB. The clinical significance of positive blood cultures in the 1990s: A prospective comprehensive evaluation of the microbiology, epidemiology and outcome of bacteremia and fungemia in adults. Clin Infect Dis 24:584, 1997.
21. Karchmer AW. Staphylococcal endocarditis. In Kaye D (ed). Infective Endocarditis. Second Edn, Raven Press, 1992: 225.
22. Levine DP, Crane LR, Zervos MJ. Bacteremia in narcotic addicts at the Detroit Medical Center. II infectious endocarditis: a prospective comparative study. Rev Infect Dis 8:374, 1986.
23. DiNubile MJ. Short-course antibiotic therapy for right-sided endocarditis caused by *Staphylococcus aureus* in injection drug users. Ann Intern Med 121:873, 1994.
24. Robbins MJ, Soeiro R, Frishman WH, Strom JA. Right-sided valvular endocarditis: etiology, diagnosis and an approach to therapy. Am Heart J 111:128, 1986.
25. Korzeniowski O, Sande MA, the National Collaborative Endocarditis Study Group. Combination antimicrobial therapy for *Staphylococcus aureus* endocarditis in patients addicted to parenteral drugs and in nonaddicts. Ann Intern Med 97:496, 1982.
26. Wilson WR, Karchmer AW, Dajani AS, Taubert KA, Bayer A, Kaye D, Bisno AL, Ferrieri P, Shulman ST, Durack DT. Antibiotic treatment of adults with infective endocarditis due to streptococci, enterococci, staphylococci and HACEK microorganisms. JAMA 274:1706, 1995.
27. Scheld WM, Mandell GL. Enigmatic enterococcal endocarditis. Ann Int Med 100:904, 1984.
28. Hricak V, Kovacik J, Marx P, Fischer V, Krcmery V. Endocarditis due to *Enterococcus faecalis*: Risk factors and outcome in twenty-one cases from a five year national survey. Scand J Infect Dis 30:540, 1998.
29. Arthur M, Courvalin P. Genetics and mechanism of glycopeptide resistance in enterococci. Anti-microb Agents Chemotherap 37:1563, 1993.
30. Pfaller MA, Jones RN, Doern GV, Sader HS, Kugler KC, Beach ML. Survey of blood stream infections attributable to gram-positive cocci: frequency of occurrence and antimicrobial susceptibility of isolates collected in 1997 in the United States, Canada, and Latin America for the SENTRY Antimicrobial Surveillance Program. Diagn Microbiol Infect Dis 33:283, 1999.
31. Rice LB, Calderwood SB, Eliopoulos GM, Farber BF, Karchmer AW. Enterococcal endocarditis: A comparison of prosthetic and native valve disease. Rev Infect Dis 13:1, 1991.
32. Aronin SI, Mukherjee SK, West JC, Cooney EL. Review of pneumococcal endocarditis in adults in the penicillin era. Clin Infect Dis 26:165, 1998.
33. Ugolini V, Pacifico A, Smitherman TC, Mackowiak PA. Pneumococcal endocarditis update: analysis of 10 cases diagnosed between 1974 and 1984. Am Heart J 112:813, 1986.
34. Powderly WG, Stanley SL Jr, Medoff G. Pneumococcal endocarditis: report of a series and

review of the literature. Rev Infect Dis 8:786, 1986.
35. Paris MM, Ramilo O, McCracken GH. Management of meningitis by penicillin-resistant *Streptococcus pneumoniae*. Antimicrob Agents Chemother 39:2171, 1995.
36. Abusbeih G, Nickle HH. Meningococcal endocarditis due to dental caries in a previously healthy adult. Infect Dis Clin Practice 7:353, 1998.
37. Fijen CA, *et al.* Complement deficiencies in meningococcal infection. Clin Infect Dis 28:98, 1999.
38. Firestone GM. Meningococcus endocarditis. Am J Med Sci 211:556, 1946.
39. Wall TC, Peyton RB, Corey GR. Gonococcal endocarditis: A new look at an old disease. Medicine 68:375, 1989.
40. Jackman JD, Glamann DB. Gonococcal endocarditis: twenty five-year experience. Am J Med Sci 301:221, 1991.
41. Sobel JL, Maisel AS, Tarazi R, Blanchard DG. Gonococcal endocarditis: assessment by transesophageal echocardiography. J Am Soc Echocardiog 10:367, 1997.
42. Black JR, Brint JM, Reichart CA. Successful treatment of gonococcal endocarditis with ceftriaxone. J Infect Dis 157:1281, 1988.
43. Savage D, Brown J. Endocarditis due to group A streptococcus. Am J Med Sci 282:98, 1981.
44. Barg NL, Kish MA, Kauffman CA, Supena RB. Group A streptococcal bacteremia in intravenous drug abusers. Am J Med 78:569, 1985.
45. Burkert T, Watanakunakorn C. Group A streptococcus endocarditis: report of five cases and review of the literature. J Infect 23:307, 1991.
46. Baddour LM and the Infectious Diseases Society of America's Emerging Infections Network. Infective endocarditis caused by β-hemolytic streptococci. Clin Infect Dis 26:66, 1997.
47. Gallagher PG, Watanakunakorn C. Group B streptococcal endocarditis: Report of seven cases and review of the literature, 1962–1985. Rev Infect Dis 8:175, 1986.
48. Fernandez-Guerrero ML, Verdejo JA, de Gorgolas M. Hospital-acquired infectious endocarditis not associated with cardiac surgery: an emerging problem. Clin Infect Dis 20:16, 1995.
49. Chen S, Dwyer DE, Sorrell TC. A comparison of hospital and community-acquired infective endocarditis. Am J Cardiol 70:1449, 1992.
50. Fowler VG, Li J, Corey GR, Boley J, Marr KA, Gopal AK, Kong K, Gottlieb G, Donovan CL, Sexton DJ, Ryan T. Role of echocardiography in evaluation of patients with *Staphylococcus aureus* bacteremia: Experience with 103 patients. J Am Coll Cardiol 30:1072, 1997.
51. Lamas CC, Eykyn S. Suggested modifications to the Duke criteria for the clinical diagnosis of native valve and prosthetic valve endocarditis: Analysis of 118 pathologically proven cases. Clin Inf Dis 25:713, 1997.
52. Calderwood SB, Swinski LA, Waternaux CM, Karchmer AW, Buckley MJ. Risk factors for the development of prosthetic valve endocarditis. Circulation 72:31, 1985.
53. Karchmer AW. In Korzeniowski OM (ed). Atlas of Infectious Diseases. Vol 10, Cardiovascular Infections, Philadelphia, PA: Current Medicine, 1998: 5.2.
54. Fisher EA, Fisher LL, Fuster V, Goldman ME. Infective endocarditis: New perspectives on an old disease. Infect Dis Clin Practice 7:12, 1998.
55. Chastre J, Trouillet JL. Early infective endocarditis on prosthetic valves. Eur Heart J 16: (suppl B):32, 1995.
56. Wolf M, Witchitz S, Chastang C, Regnier B, Vaschon F. Prosthetic valve endocarditis in the ICU; prognostic factors of overall survival in a series of 122 cases and consequences for treatment decision. Chest 108:688, 1995.
57. Yu VL, Fang GD, Keys TF, Harris AA, Gentry LO, Fuchs PC, Wagener MM, Wong ES. Prosthetic valve endocarditis: Superiority of surgical valve replacement versus medical therapy only. Ann Thorac Surg 58:1073. Vongpatanasin W, Hillis L, Lange RA. Prosthetic heart valves. N Eng J Med 335:407, 1996.
58. Vlessis AA, Hovaguimian H, Jagges J, Ahmad A, Starr A. Infective endocarditis: Ten year review of medical and surgical therapy. Ann Thorac Surg 61:1217, 1996.

26. FALCIPARUM MALARIA

Charles Feldman and Guy A. Richards

Abstract

Malaria is one of the most common infectious diseases in the world today and *Plasmodium falciparum* is responsible for most of its mortality. Infection with *P. falciparum* has a wide variety of potential clinical consequences which depend on the age of the patient, their degree of immunity and the duration of infection. More recently it has been noted that polymorphism in both host and parasite impacts on disease pathogenesis and presentation. While highly active anti-malarial agents are available for the treatment of infection, control through parasite and insect vector prevention measures has become largely ineffective due to mosquito and parasite mutation with subsequent development of resistance. The potentially substantial socio-economic and clinical benefits of effective vaccine development underlines the need for future emphasis to be placed on immunoprophylaxis.

Introduction

Malaria is one of the most common infectious diseases in the world and *Plasmodium falciparum* is the organism responsible for most of the mortality. It has been estimated that malaria causes approximately 1–2 million deaths per annum, most of these occurring in children [1–3]. *Plasmodium falciparum*, *Mycobacterium tuberculosis* and measles compete for the title of the single most important pathogen causing human morbidity and mortality in the world today [1, 2]. Infection with *Plasmodium falciparum* has a wide variety of potential clinical consequences [3–5].

Factors that may influence presentation include the age of the patient, their degree of immunity and the duration of infection [5]. In holo- or hyper-endemic areas, most adults and older children are partially immune and the disease burden is mainly in children in the first few years of life [5, 6]. The greatest mortality is between the ages of 1–3 years [5]. Parasitization may be almost universal in this age group and effects range from an asymptomatic infection, to a febrile illness, or even life-threatening disease [6]. In areas of low endemicity, severe malaria occurs in both adults and children and non-immune travelers and migrant workers are also vulnerable [5]. In adults infected with falciparum malaria for the first time, the range of clinical syndromes is wide and may include specific and multi-organ failure [6].

The Organism

Malaria is a protozoal disease caused by several species of *Plasmodium* which are spread by mosquitoes of the genus *Anopheles* [3]. *Plasmodium falciparum* is one of the four species of *Plasmodium* causing human infection. The period from inoculation to the apperance of parasitemia (prepatent period) is usually 9–13 days for *P. falciparum*, but may be longer, particularly in those who have been on ineffective prophylaxis [3]. During feeding the female mosquito injects saliva, within which malaria sporozoites are carried, into the skin. Within minutes the sporozoites penetrate into hepatocytes and produce tissue schizonts (also known as meronts). After

5–7 days, each tissue schizont has produced 30,000 daughter merozoites that enter the circulation, invade erythrocytes and form ring trophozoites [3]. Using hemoglobin as energy, development occurs after 48 hours into late trophozoites (larger and lacier in appearance), early blood schizonts (division begins) and then mature schizonts [3]. The erythrocytes then lyse and merozoites are released into the circulation to invade other red blood cells [3]. In non-immune individuals, the process is amplified 20-fold with each cycle. When parasitemia reaches 10–50 trophozoites per microliter, it is detectable on thick blood films, ending the prepatent period [3]. After several cycles, some trophozoites differentiate into sex cells or gametocytes, which are infectious to the mosquito. The gametocyte of *P. falciparum* is characteristically banana-shaped. If male and female gametocytes are taken up by the mosquito, they mate, migrate through the midgut wall and form an oocyst which eventually leads to the release of about 1000 sporozoites after 5–8 days [3]. These invade the salivary glands of the mosquito to complete the cycle at the next blood meal [3].

The time from first inoculation to first symptoms is the incubation period [3]. Its length depends on the patient's immune status and is usually 1–2 days longer than the prepatent period. In non-immune patients, symptoms may occur even before parasitemia is present. The other extreme is premunition where partial immunity is associated with asymptomatic parasitemia [3].

Epidemiology

Malaria persists in those parts of the world where the population of Anopheline mosquitoes as well as the infected human population remain above the critical density required for sustained transmission. Approximately 40% of the world's population are at risk of acquiring malaria, resulting in 300–500 million cases annually [3]. In Africa alone approximately 200 million cases occur every year, with a mortality of approximately one million. In rural Africa one in 20 children die from malaria before the age of five years [3]. Compounding the problem of malaria control in the developing world is the presence of drug resistance, and resistance of mosquitoes to insecticides [3].

Malaria also afflicts individuals in South East Asia, Latin America and South America. In 1992 approximately 75% of malarial infections were acquired in Africa, 17% in Asia, 4% in Central America and the Carribean and 1% each in South America, North America, and Oceania [3]. In developed countries such as the United States, malaria largely occurs as a result of importation from other countries in the blood of immigrants, visitors, military personnel and occasionally also from importation of infected mosquitoes [3].

Recently there has been renewed interest in epidemiological aspects of falciparum malaria [7]. It is recognized that there are clear-cut distinctions between severe and non-severe disease and between the different forms of severe disease [8]. An important question is why *Plasmodium falciparum* causes severe infection in some, but not all patients. This relates partly to age, prior exposure to the parasite and aspects of the immune response [5–9]. Most interestingly, it is now recognized that many of the differences in response may relate to diversity or polymorphism in both host and parasite [6–8, 10–14] which may impact on disease pathogenesis. Genetic characteristics of the host and parasite are thought to be the major determinant of the outcome of a malaria infection. For example, in the host, possession of hemoglobin AS genotype influences the risk of both cerebral malaria and severe anemia [7], whereas possession of certain HLA genotypes (eg HLA-B53) may be linked to resistance to these two complications [10, 11]. Susceptibility to both these complications is linked to polymorphism in the promoter sequence for the tumor necrosis factor (TNF) gene [13, 14], whereas susceptibility to each of these complications individually is influenced by mutations at other sites [7]. Also, different strains of *P. falciparum* have been shown to vary in their ability to induce production of host TNF, and this may determine the clinical severity of the infection [12]. In addition, clonal phenotypic variation with antigenic switching is linked to, and may alter, adhesive properties of the parasite and this may be an important mechanism of immune evasion [6]. Finally, specific adhesive and linked antigenic types may be associated with severe infection [6].

Severe Malaria

The manifestations of severe *P. falciparum* infection are shown in Table 1. There has been much debate in the literature with regard to the definition of severe malaria. The need for such a definition is to alert health care workers to the presence of life-threatening disease, and also to ensure uniformity of definition for epidemiological and research purposes [5]. In this regard it is recognized that no single definition would satisfy all clinical situations and that age and immune status affect the significance of certain features such as height of pyrexia and level of parasitemia. However, the World Health Organization (WHO) has defined very precisely the clinical and laboratory features which should raise the suspicion of severe falciparum malaria [5]. These include:

TABLE 1. Manifestations of severe *Plasmodium falciparum* infection

- Cerebral malaria
- Convulsions
- Severe anemia
- Blackwater fever
- Renal failure
- Pulmonary edema
- Metabolic acidosis
- Hyperthermia
- Coagulation disturbances
- Hyperparasitemia
- Hypoglycemia
- Septicemia/Bacteremia
- Gastrointestinal bleeding
- Aspiration pneumonia

1) Cerebral malaria – unrousable coma not attributable to any other cause in a patient with falciparum malaria.
2) Severe anemia – normocytic anemia with hematocrit <15% or haemoglobin <5 g/dl in the presence of parasitemia of >10,000 µl.
3) Renal failure – urine output of <400 ml in 24 hours in adults or 12 ml/kg/24 hours in children failing to improve after rehydration and a serum creatinine of >265 µmol/l (>3.0 mg/dl).
4) Pulmonary edema or adult respiratory distress syndrome.
5) Hypoglycemia – whole blood glucose <2.2 mmol/l (<40 mg/dl).
6) Circulatory collapse or shock – systolic blood pressure <50 mmHg in children and <70 mmHg in adults with cold, clammy skin or core-skin temperature difference >10°C.
7) Spontaneous bleeding – from gums, nose, gastrointestinal tract and other sites and/or substantial laboratory evidence of disseminated intravascular coagulation.
8) Repeated generalized convulsions – more than two observed within 24 hours despite cooling.
9) Acidemia – arterial pH < 7.25 or acidosis defined as plasma bicarbonate concentration <15 mmol/l.
10) Macroscopic hemoglobinuria – if definitely associated with malaria and not due to oxidant antimalarial drugs in patients with erythrocyte enzyme defects such as glucose-6-phosphate dehydrogenase (G6PD) deficiency.
11) Postmortem confirmation of the diagnosis by histological examination of a needle necropsy of the brain.

One or more of these features in the presence of asexual parasitemia suggests severe falciparum malaria [5].

Pathogenesis of Severe Disease and Cerebral Malaria

The adhesive properties that the parasite confers on the host's erythrocytes appear to play a central role in malaria pathogenicity [15–17]. As the parasite grows in the red blood cells it induces the expression of surface ligands that mediate adhesion to the endothelium of post-capillary venules and this results in sequestration of the parasite within the peripheral circulation [15, 16]. In addition, some isolates cause receptors to be expressed on non-infected red cells, leading to rosette formation, and still others induce expression of adhesion molecules on other parasitized cells causing auto-agglutination [15]. These phenomena can lead to obstruction to local blood flow and/or cause local metabolic disturbances, such as the production of lactic acid, which may manifest as organ-specific dysfunction [15–17]. The endothelial receptors recognized thus far include; platelet glycoprotein CD36, intracellular adhesion molecule 1 (ICAM-1), thrombospondin (TSP), endothelial leukocyte adhesion molecule 1 (ELAM-1 or e-selectin) and vascular cell adhesion molecule 1 (VCAM-1) [15, 16]. ICAM-1 and e-selectin are of particular importance in cerebral malaria. The receptor on infected erythrocytes that mediates adhesion to the endothelial cell is a very large malarial protein called pfEMP1 [15].

A number of theories have been forwarded to explain the mechanisms of cerebral malaria [2, 15–25]. Initially it was assumed that it was simply a mechanical effect related to sludging of parasitized red blood cells within the vasculature, causing decreased cerebral perfusion, and resulting in hypoxia and coma [16]. Other theories have included altered microvascular permeability, secondary to malarial "toxins" or mediators such as kinins causing cerebral edema and coma but this has largely been discounted [20]. Immunological mechanisms were considered following the detection of immune complexes and complement in affected brains [5, 19] and still others have investigated the possibility that disseminated intravascular coagulation (DIC) [19] or endotoxemia [21] may be involved. More recently Clarke and co-workers have proposed the cytokine theory of human cerebral malaria [23–25]. They recognized that cytokines such as TNF and interleukin (IL)-1 when overproduced could themselves cause clinical syndromes such a seen in human malaria [23–25]. Many of these may simply be manifestations of a severe systemic inflammatory response syndrome. Products of schizogony have been shown to trigger release of TNF and IL-1 and serum levels of these cytokines correlate with the severity of malaria infection, including the presence of cerebral symptoms [23–25]. The cytokine theory is also consistent with the concept of sequestration of parasites in the cerebral circulation in that schizogony could cause higher local levels of cytokines and their products [25]. Sequestration, however, may not be essential to the development of cerebral malaria according to the cytokine theory [25]. Cytokines themselves may alter cerebral function through the local generation of nitric oxide (NO), which may act as a vasodilator to increase intracranial pressure and which may also function as a false neurotransmitter [24, 25]. It is also important to consider that septic encephalopathy may be a feature of any severe critical illness and may be indistinguishable clinically from cerebral malaria [26].

Laboratory Diagnosis of Malaria

For the laboratory diagnosis of malaria, thick and thin blood smears should be made as per standard procedures [3, 27]. Thick smears are 20–40 times more sensitive and should be used for screening. Thin smears fixed with methanol, to preserve erythrocyte morphology, and Giemsa stained allow speciation as well as determination of the level of parasitemia [3, 27]. Various clues to distinguish falciparum malaria on thin smear include the finding of small tight rings, applique forms and banana-shaped gametocytes.

Parasitemia should be quantified and counted on thin smears as parasites per 1000 red blood cells corrected to percentage [3, 27]. After initiation of treatment, parasitemia should be followed regularly until resolution to confirm therapeutic efficacy. The time from initiation of treatment until thick smears are repeatedly negative is called the parasite clearance time (PCT). A number of newer techniques have been developed for the diagnosis of malaria including quantitative buffy coat methods, antigen capture, enzyme linked immunosorbent assay, polymerase chain reaction and indirect flourescent antibody tests [3, 27].

Treatment of Severe and Complicated Malaria

If possible, patients with severe or cerebral malaria should be treated in an intensive care unit (ICU) [4]. Treatment should be initiated as rapidly as possible, and should not necessarily await parasitological confirmation of the diagnosis if this is likely to be delayed [4]. Patients should be weighed in order to determine drug dosages accurately [4]. Careful fluid management is essential and may be aided by the placement of a central venous catheter and a urinary catheter. A flow-directed balloon catheter would be ideal in the critically ill patient in the ICU setting. Hyperpyrexia >38.5°C should be treated with tepid sponging, fanning and a cooling blanket [4].

The drug treatment of severe or complicated malaria is shown in Table 2 [3–5, 28, 29]. Parenteral antimalarial drugs are recommended initially at least until there is clear evidence of clinical improvement and oral medication is tol-

TABLE 2. The parenteral treatment of severe and complicated falciparum malaria

Drug	Regimen
Chloroquine*	Chloroquine 10 mg base/kg by constant infusion over 8 hours followed by 15 mg base/kg over 24 hours
Quinine (intravenous)	Quinine dihydrochloride salt 20 mg/kg intravenously in 200 ml 5% dextrose and/or saline over 4 hours (loading dose) followed by quinine dihydrochloride salt 10 mg/kg infusion over 4 hours every 8 hours (maintenance dose) beginning 8 hours after start of the loading dose, until patient can take oral medication.
	ALTERNATIVE** Quinine dihydrochloride salt 7 mg/kg intravenously over 30 minutes (loading dose) followed immediately by 10 mg/kg infusion over 4 hours repeated 8 hourly (maintenance dose) until patient can take oral medication.
Quinidine (intravenous)	Quinidine base 15 mg/kg intravenously over 4 hours (loading dose) followed by quinidine base 7.5 mg/kg over 4 hours (maintenance dose) every 8 hours beginning 8 hours after start of loading dose, until patient can take oral medication.
	ALTERNATIVE** Quinidine base 10 mg/kg intravenously over 1–2 hours (loading dose) followed immediately by 0.02 mg/kg/min by infusion (maintenance dose) for 72 hours or until patient can take oral medication.***
Artemesinin derivatives	
Artesunate	2.4 mg/kg IVI or IM bolus initially followed by 1.2 mg/kg at 12 hours and 24 hours then 1.2 mg/kg daily for 5–7 days. **OR**
Artemether	3.2 mg/kg IM initially followed by 1.6 mg/kg IM daily for 5–7 days.

* For the parenteral treatment of severe malaria in cases of drug-sensitive infections; if any doubt treat as for resistant infections.
** Alternative regimens suggested particularly in the ICU setting.
*** The same dosing regimen has also been reported for the quinidine salt (reference 5).

erated. Quinine is the drug of choice in most of the tropical world. In some countries, such as in the United States, quinidine may be the drug of choice. An intravenous loading dose of either agent is recommended to achieve therapeutic levels rapidly since most deaths occur within the first 48 hours of therapy [3–5, 28, 29]. A total of seven days medication is required which may be completed with oral quinine or quinidine. Artemesinin and its derivatives, although not yet licenced in many areas, appear to be exciting new agents for the treatment of severe and multidrug-resistant malaria [30–35]. Many studies have confirmed their efficacy in malaria treatment [32–35] and recently there have been suggestions that combination treatment of malaria with these agents, together with standard therapy, may be associated not only with more rapid cure of severe infections but limitation of the development of drug resistance [30].

Chloroquine may be used in areas where the infection is known to be sensitive to this agent [3–5, 29]. Other drugs that are sometimes recommended as additional therapy include doxycycline which should be added in areas of relative quinine resistance, and parenteral sulfadoxine-pyrimethamine [28]. Tetracyclines are contraindicated in pregnancy and childhood. Where initial response to therapy is poor, halofantrine or mefloquine have been recommended [4, 5]. Other agents that have been used in treatment but which are now no longer recommended include dexamethasone, mannitol, heparin and dextran [2, 4, 36, 37].

Cerebral Malaria

In many parts of the world cerebral malaria is said to be the most common clinical presentation of severe malaria in man, with a mortality in the region of 20%, or greater, and accounting for 80% of deaths [4, 5]. However, in some parts of Africa, anemia is a more common severe manifestation particularly in children. Cerebral malaria has been defined as the presence of unrousable coma classified according to the Glasgow coma scale (GCS) with exclusion of other encephalopathies such as bacterial meningitis and viral encephalitides and confirmation of infection with *P. falciparum* [2, 4]. Patients falling within this definition manifest with features of a diffuse symmetrical encephalopathy.

In adults cerebral malaria tends to develop after several days of fever and other non-specific symptoms [2, 5]. In children it tends to be more acute in onset, usually after less than two days [2, 5]. It may start dramatically with a generalized convulsion followed by persistent unconsciousness. Post-ictal coma should resolve within 30 minutes, but coma due to cerebral malaria usually persists for 24–72 hours. The most common neurological picture of cerebral malaria is that of a bilateral symmetrical upper motor neuron lesion with increased muscle tone and reflexes [5].

Various forms of posturing may be observed, including decerebrate and decorticate rigidity [4, 5]. These may occur in hypoglycemic and normoglycemic patients. While neck rigidity and photophobia do not tend to occur, mild neck stiffness is not uncommon [2, 4, 5]. Neck retraction and opisthotonus may, however, occur in both adults and children [5]. Corneal and eyelash reflexes and pupillary responses are usually normal in adults, but disorders of conjugate gaze are common [4, 5]. The gag reflex is usually maintained but abdominal reflexes are invariably absent. This latter may be a valuable clinical sign [4, 5]. Papilloedema is not a feature of cerebral malaria, probably reflecting the fact that raised intracranial pressure is not found in the majority of patients early in the course of the illness [4, 5, 38]. Forcible jaw closure and bruxism are common [4, 5].

Studies in children recovering from cerebral malaria have shown neurological sequelae in approximately 10% or more of cases and these occur especially with infections that were complicated by hypoglycemia [2, 5]. Hemiplegia, cortical blindness, behavior disturbances, cranial nerve lesions, extrapyramidal tremor, polyneuropathy, mononeuritis multiplex, Guillain-Barre syndrome, and prolonged coma have all been described as neurological sequelae of patients with cerebral malaria [2, 5].

The APACHE II severity of illness scoring index has been used to predict the mortality of patients with cerebral malaria. Using a cut-off score of 24, the index stratified patient mortality with an accuracy of >95%. In that study high APACHE II score, deep unconsciousness, acute renal failure and acidemia were identified as poor prognostic factors [39].

Convulsions

Convulsions may occur in as many as 50% of cases of cerebral malaria and are more common in children [4]. In children it may be difficult to differentiate febrile convulsions from those due to cerebral malaria and the possibility that they may be related to hypoglycemia should also always be considered [4]. Convulsions are usually generalized, but other types, including focal seizures, may occur [4]. Generalized convulsions appear to impact negatively on the outcome.

The role of prophylactic anticonvulsants in patients with cerebral malaria is under investigation. A single dose of phenobarbitone (200 mg in adults and 3.5 mg/kg in children by intramuscular injection on admission) appears effective [4]. Once seizures occur they should be managed in the usual way. Treatment may initially be with intravenous diazepam (10 mg in adults and 0.15 mg/kg in children), together with maintenance of the airway and cooling of the patient [4]. Recent studies of generalized convulsive status epilepticus have suggested that 0.1 mg/kg lorazepam, or 15 mg/kg phenobarbitol, or diazepam 0.15 mg/kg followed by 18 mg/kg phenytoin, are all acceptable initial treatment regimens [40].

Severe Anemia

The occurrence of anemia is invariable in patients with severe falciparum malaria [4, 5]. It is due to hemolysis of parasitized red blood cells, shortened survival of unparasitized cells and bone marrow dysfunction [4]. Certain red cell enzyme defects, such as G6PD deficiency, may increase susceptibility to antimalarial oxidant-induced hemolysis, and Coombs positive hemolytic anemia and microangiopathic hemolytic anemia also occur [4]. It is recommended that patients should be transfused if the hematocrit falls below 20% [4]. The choice of either whole blood or packed cells would depend on the fluid requirements of the individual patient. Since there is often a requirement for additional clotting factors and platelets in patients with severe malaria, fresh blood rather than stored bank-blood is preferable [4]. In patients who are actively bleeding, platelet or cryoprecipitate transfusions may also be necessary. Transfusion should be carefully monitored to prevent fluid overload with its associated complications and in some patients with normal renal function low dose loop diuretics (e.g. furosemide 20 mg) may be administered during the transfusion to prevent its occurrence [4].

Blackwater Fever

This was previously described as the occurrence of unusually severe intravascular hemolysis with hemoglobinuria in patients with other severe manifestations of falciparum malaria, including renal failure, hypotension and coma, despite relatively low levels of parasitemia [4, 5]. The condition was attributed to some form of immunological response to quinine or one of the other anti-malarial agents, but it is also possible that it may have represented unrecognized G6PD deficiency [4, 5]. No special treatment of hemoglobinuria is currently recommended, although alkalinization of the urine may be desirable [4].

Renal Failure

Some degree of renal dysfunction, as manifested by a raised serum creatinine, is common in patients with severe falciparum malaria [41, 42]. This may be related to hypovolemia and blackwater fever, but more commonly occurs in association with a high parasite count in which the mechanism is said to be a reduction in renal capillary blood flow [4]. A variety of glomerular lesions have been described, however the clinical course of all three forms of renal failure is usually that of acute tubular necrosis [4, 5, 41, 42]. The management is similar to that of renal failure in other critical care settings. Attention should be given to fluid status, electrolytes and acid-base balance. If there is anuria or oliguria after fluid replacement, increasing intravenous doses of furosemide should be given in an attempt to increase urine output [4]. The indications for dialysis are also similar to those of other situations and include severe hyperkalemia, fluid overload, metabolic acidosis and uremia [4, 41, 42].

It has been recommended that the doses of antimalarials should be reduced in patients with renal failure [4]. This was based on the observation of high plasma concentrations of quinine in patients with renal failure. However, this was probably due to impaired hepatic clearance as a consequence of severe infection, rather than impaired renal clearance which has not been documented to occur even in patients with moderately elevated serum creatinine levels [4]. A suggested dosing regimen is: initial dose 20 mg/kg of intravenous quinine dihydrochloride (salt) over four hours followed by 10 mg/kg every eight hours [4]. The infusion volume may be reduced to 50–100 ml of 5% dextrose. After the second day the dose should be reduced to 5 mg/kg eight hourly [4]. Hemodialysis removes quinine and in this situation the dose should remain 10 mg/kg every eight hours [4]. There does not appear to be a need to alter the dose of chloroquine in patients in renal failure, even in those on hemodialysis [4].

Pulmonary Edema

This is a particularly serious consequence of severe falciparum malaria and is often fatal [4, 5]. It is similar in most respects to the acute respiratory distress syndrome (ARDS) and hyperparasitemia (>10%) and pregnancy are important predisposing factors [4]. The pathogenesis is not entirely clear, but as it is associated with a normal/low pulmonary capillary wedge pressure it is most likely due to an increase in pulmonary capillary permeability, as occurs with ARDS [4, 5]. The first indication of the onset of this condition is an increase in the respiratory rate, which precedes the development of any of the other chest signs [4, 5]. Careful fluid management is the cornerstone of the prevention and management [4]. Hemodynamic monitoring by means of a central venous catheter and in particular the Swan Ganz flow directed balloon catheter, which allows accurate measurement of pulmonary artery and pulmonary capillary wedge pressures, may aid in management of fluid status.

Metabolic Acidosis

Metabolic acidosis is common in patients with pulmonary edema, although it may also occur in its absence [4]. The mechanism is not entirely certain and it may occur even in the absence of significant hypoxia or hypoperfusion [4]. It appears to be due to tissue hypoxia as a consequence of stagnant flow of parasitized red blood cells through capillary beds [4]. Other factors may include impaired hepatic blood flow (a site of lactate disposal) and high cytokine levels (TNF leads to lactate production) [4]. In addition, the malaria parasite itself produces large amounts of lactate as a by-product of glycolysis. Therapy should include correction of hypotension and hypoxemia, if present [4]. Acidosis should only be corrected if the pH falls below 7.15 since sodium bicarbonate infusion may worsen pulmonary oedema due to the large sodium load [4]. The prognosis of patients with severe lactic acidosis is poor [4].

Hyperthermia

Progressively increasing body temperature may be associated with convulsions, delirium and coma [4]. High fever increases metabolic demand which may further compromise tissues damaged by stagnant capillary blood flow [4]. Heat stroke may be associated with permanent neurological sequelae [4]. Patients with cerebral malaria often improve with a decrease in the temperature which may be achieved by tepid sponging, fanning and cooling blankets [4].

Coagulation Disturbances

While thrombocytopenia is very common in severe falciparum malaria, in most cases it does not appear to be an indicator of disseminated intravascular coagulation as it usually occurs in the setting of normal coagulation and without evidence of bleeding [4, 5]. It appears that the previous concerns of an important pathogenic role for DIC in severe falciparum malaria were exaggerated and that full blown DIC with bleeding probably only occurs in 5% or less of patients with severe malaria [4, 5].

Hyperparasitaemia

Patients with a blood parasitemia of >10% are at increased risk for the complications of severe malaria [4]. This risk is proportional to the degree of parasitemia [4]. It has been suggested that such patients should have an exchange blood transfusion [4, 43]. This recommendation is not based on large prospective randomized studies, but follows the recommendations of individual case reports and is confounded in some cases by patients with malaria with higher levels of parasitemia who recover without transfusion and in others by the fact that total parasite burden may not be reflected in the peripheral smear [3, 4, 43]. It has also been noted that facilities for full exchange transfusions (6–8 units of blood) may not be widely available but in these situations partial exchange transfusion (e.g. four units) could possibly be undertaken [2, 4].

Hepatic Dysfunction

While abnormalities in "liver function tests" are quite common in patients with severe malaria, true hepatic dysfunction is uncommon and if present is mild [4]. Raised bilirubin levels are often noted and are mostly due to hemolysis [4]. Raised serum levels of aspartate aminotransaminase may also be associated with haemolysis. Occasional patients with severe falciparum malaria do, however, have marked jaundice with raised serum levels of both aspartate and alanine aminotransferases in addition to prolonged prothrombin time [4]. These patients may have true hepatic dysfunction contributed to by hemolysis and DIC [4].

Hypoglycemia

Hypoglycemia is a commonly reported complication in severe malaria [4, 5]. It occurs in particular in two situations [4, 5, 44]. Firstly it may occur in pregnant women, where in addition to neurological sequelae it may also cause foetal distress [4, 5]. Unless it has been prolonged and very severe it is associated with a good prognosis and responds well to glucose administration. Secondly, hypoglycemia may occur in severely ill patients and be associated with severe anemia, jaundice, hyperparasitemia, lactic acidosis and coma [4, 5]. Quinine-induced stimulation of insulin release may be an important mechanism of hypoglycemia, but other factors, including glucose consumption by the parasite may be contributory factors [4, 5, 44]. Other mechanisms that have been considered as possible cause of hypoglycemia include depleted hepatic glycogen stores and inhibition of hepatic gluconeogenesis [5]. Many of the usual clinical features of hypoglycemia are absent, or are masked by or interpreted as the symptoms of malaria, but whenever levels of consciousness deteriorate in patients with malaria, hypoglycemia should be suspected [4, 5, 44]. Treatment with intravenous 50% glucose often results in improvement of the level of consciousness but glucose requirements may be high and infusions of 10–20% glucose, preferably through a central venous catheter may be required to maintain adequate blood levels [4].

Bacteremia/Septicemia

Gram-negative microorganisms are frequently cultured from the blood of patients with severe malaria [4, 5]. While there is often no apparent source for these organisms it is possible that they may arise via translocation through ischemic bowel. In addition these patients often have central venous and urinary catheters in place [4, 5]. The manifestation of bacteremia vary from asymptomatic to severe septic shock [4]. A recent study has shown a high incidence of bacterial infection in patients with falciparum malaria presenting in shock [45]. The previously described "algid malaria" is very reminiscent of Gram-negative sepsis and it has been suggested that they may represent one and the same condition [4, 5]. Many authorities recommend both conventional antibiotics and antimalarial agents in the initial therapy of patients with severe malaria [4].

Gastrointestinal Bleeding

This complication has been noted particularly in patients who have been given high-dose corticosteroids, and is thought to be due to gastric erosion [2, 4, 36]. It should be treated in the usual way together with the infusion of fresh blood [4].

Aspiration Pneumonia

This complication may occur in any patient with a decreased level of consciousness and is particularly common in severe malaria since these patients often vomit [4]. The latter may be associated with convulsions or be due to antimalarial agents and these patients should be nursed on their side. Antiemetics may be given but their efficacy has not been consistently demonstrated [4]. If aspiration does occur, the upper airway should be cleared and parenteral antibiotics initiated [4]. A chest radiograph may help differentiate this condition from pulmonary edema/ARDS.

Special Considerations in Pregnancy

Falciparum malaria is a particularly dangerous disease in pregnancy, especially during the second and third trimester [4]. The mortality of cerebral malaria is approximately 40% in pregnant women and both mother and foetus may die despite aggressive treatment [3, 4]. Pregnant women are at particular risk of hypoglycemia and pulmonary edema [3, 4]. The exact mechanism by which pregnancy enhances the susceptibility to and the risk of complicated disease is not certain but red cells containing mature forms of the asexual parasites are found in the placenta and may significantly compromise placental function [4]. Treatment should start immediately and the potential teratogenic or abortifacient properties of quinine and chloroquine in this severe situation should be ignored and in any case are considered by many authorities to have been largely exaggerated [3–5]. Blood glucose levels should be measured frequently and where possible fetal monitoring should be undertaken [4]. Some clinicians favor cesarian section or induction of labor if the foetus is viable [4].

Special Considerations in Children

Children tend to have a shorter disease course and progress much more rapidly than adults to severe malaria [3]. Hypoglycemia, seizures, severe anemia and sudden death are more common, whereas renal failure, pulmonary edema and jaundice are less likely than in adults [3, 4, 5]. Although respiratory distress does not appear in the original WHO definition of severe malaria it is recognized by clinicians treating children with malaria as an important sign which is not usually due to pulmonary edema or ARDS [46–48]. It has also been termed the malaria hyperpneic syndrome [46]. Possible causes include cardiac failure, co-existent pneumonia, direct sequestration of parasites in the lungs, or as a sign of cerebral malaria [48]. It is important to remember that the clinical features of pneumonia and malaria, both common causes of childhood morbidity and mortality in the developing world, overlap considerably and many children fulfilling the WHO criteria for pneumonia may actually have malaria [7, 49]. The majority of cases of respiratory distress in children are associated with lactic acidosis and this is well documented as a poor prognostic factor [48, 50]. After cerebral malaria, 9–26% of children may have neurologic sequelae of which half will resolve completely [2, 3, 51]. Hypoglycemic children are at greater risk of neurologic sequelae and/or death [3]. It is important to remember in the treatment of children with malaria, that drug dosages need to be modified [3].

Conclusions

The enormous cost in lives as well as the cost of treatment, makes malaria a considerable socioeconomic burden. Control of the disease through parasite and insect vector control measures have become largely ineffective due to mosquito and parasite mutation with subsequent development of resistance, together with a change in the social behavior of the host [52]. The need for effective control measures has never been greater [52, 53]. Measures to achieve this should include prevention, such as insecticide-impregnated bednets and mosquito repellants as well as targeted chemoprophylaxis, and provision of easy access to early treatment once infection occurs [52–54].

Measures for the future include the possibility of a vaccine which could be anti-parasite or even anti-disease [55–58]. With regard to anti-parasite vaccines, appropriate targets would be the protein molecules used by the parasite to evade host immunity [57]. This has been the basis for adopting an "antigenic cocktail" approach towards obtaining a synthetic or recombinant subunit vaccine [57]. Stage-specific malaria vaccines targeting the pre-erythrocytic stage or the erythrocytic stage have been considered [57]. Other considerations have included transmission-blocking vaccines [58]. One vaccine that has been field-tested in South America is the peptide vaccine, SPf66, which gave substantial protection against *P. falciparum* infection [59]. Two other vaccines undergoing field-tests include a blood stage vaccine and a recombinant circumsporozoite protein vaccine [52, 60]. The possible substantial socioeconomic savings with vaccine use underlines the need for emphasis on immunoprophylaxis.

References

1. Murray CJL, Lopez AD. Mortality by cause for eight regions of the world: global burden of disease study. Lancet 349:1269, 1997.
2. Warrell DA. Cerebral malaria: clinical features, pathophysiology and treatment. Ann Trop Med Parasitol 91:875, 1997.
3. Murphy GS, Oldfield III EC. Falciparum malaria. Infect Dis Clin North Am 10:747, 1996.
4. White NJ, Warrel DA. The management of severe malaria. In Wernsdorfer WH, McGregor I (eds). Principles and practice of malariology. Edinburgh: Churchill Livingstone, 1988:865.
5. World Health Organization. Severe and complicated malaria. Trans R Soc Trop Med Hyg 84:1, 1990.
6. Roberts DJ, Biggs B-A, Brown G, Newbold CI. Protection, pathogenesis and phenotypic plasticity in *Plasmodium faciparum* malaria. Parasitol Today 9:281, 1993.
7. Greenwood BM. The epidemiology of malaria. Ann Trop Med Parasitol 91:763, 1997.
8. Molineaux L. *Plasmodium falciparum* malaria: some epidemiological implications of parasite and host diversity. Ann Trop Med Parasitol 90:379, 1996.
9. Urquhart AD. Putative pathophysiological interactions of cytokines and phagocytic cells in severe human falciparum malaria. Clin Infect Dis 19:117, 1994.
10. Hill AVS, Allsopp CEM, Kwiatkowski D, Anstey NM, Twumasi P, *et al.* Common West African HLA antigens are associated with protection from severe malaria. Nature 352:595, 1991.
11. Hill AVS, Elvin J, Willis AC, Aidoo M, Allsopp CEM, *et al.* Molecular analysis of the association

of HLA B53 and resistance to severe malaria. Nature 360:434, 1992.

12. Allan RJ, Rowe A, Kwiatkowski D. *Plasmodium falciparum* varies in its ability to induce tumor necrosis factor. Infect Immun 61:4772, 1993.
13. McGuire W, Knight JC, Hill AVS, Allsopp CEM, Greenwood BM, *et al.* Severe malarial anemia and cerebral malaria are associated with different tumor necrosis factor promoter alleles. J Infect Dis 179:287, 1999.
14. McGuire W, Hill AVS, Allsopp CEM, Greenwood BM, Kwiatkowski D. Variation in the TNF-α promoter region associated with susceptibility to cerebral malaria. Nature 371:508, 1994.
15. Pasloske BL, Howard RJ. Malaria, the red cell, and the endothelium. Annu Rev Med 45:283, 1994.
16. Berendt AR, Turner GDH, Newbold CI. Cerebral malaria: the sequestration hypothesis. Parasitol Today 10:412, 1994.
17. MacPherson GG, Warrell MJ, White NJ, Looareesuwan S, Warrell DA. Human cerebral malaria. A quantitative ultrastructural analysis of parasitized erythrocyte sequestration. Am J Pathol 119:385, 1985.
18. Miller LH, Good MF, Milon G. Malaria pathogenesis. Science 264:1878, 1994.
19. Philips RE, Warrell DA. The pathophysiology of severe falciparum malaria. Parasitol Today 2:271, 1986.
20. Warrell DA, Looareesuwan S, Phillips RE, White NJ, Warrell MJ, *et al.* Function of the blood-cerebrospinal fluid barrier in human cerebral malaria: rejection of the permeability hypothesis. Am J Trop Med Hyg 35:882, 1986.
21. Usawattanakul W, Tharavanij S, Warrell DA, Looareesuwan S, White NJ, *et al.* Factors contributing to the development of cerebral malaria II. Endotoxin. Clin Exp Immunol 61:562, 1985.
22. Grau GE, de Kossodo S. Cerebral malaria: mediators, mechanical obstruction or more? Parasitol Today 10:408, 1994.
23. Clark IA, Chaudhri G, Cowden WB. Roles of tumour necrosis factor in the illness and pathology of malaria. Trans R Soc Trop Med Hyg 83:436, 1989.
24. Clark IA, Rockett KA, Cowden WB. Proposed link between cytokines, nitric oxide and human cerebral malaria. Parasitol Today 7:205, 1991.
25. Clark IA, Rockett KA. The cytokine theory of human cerebral malaria. Parasitol Today 10:410, 1994.
26. Vespa P. Neurological complications of critical medical illnesses and transplantation. Curr Opin Crit Care 4:69, 1998.
27. Bain BJ, Chiodini PL, England JM, Bailey JW. The laboratory diagnosis of malaria. Clin Lab Haem 19:165, 1997.
28. Molyneux M, Fox R. Diagnosis and treatment of malaria in Britain. Br Med J 306:1175, 1993.
29. White NJ. Current Concepts: the treatment of malaria. N Engl J Med 335:800, 1996.
30. White NJ, Nosten F, Looareesuwan S, Watkins WM, Marsh K, *et al.* Averting a malaria disaster. Lancet 353:1965, 1999.
31. Hoffman SL. Artemether in severe malaria – still too many deaths. N Engl J Med 335:124, 1996.
32. Hien TT, Day NPJ, Phu NH, Mai NTH, Chau TTH, *et al.* A controlled trial of artemether or quinine in Vietnamese adults with severe falciparum malaria. N Engl J Med 335:76, 1996.
33. Mohanty S, Mishara SK, Satpathy SK, Dash S, Patnaik J. α, β-Arteether for the treatment of complicated falciparum malaria. Trans R Soc Trop Med Hyg 91:328, 1997.
34. van Hensbroek MB, Onyiorah E, Jaffar S, Schneider G, Palmer A, *et al.* A trial of artemether or quinine in children with cerebral malaria. N Engl J Med 335:69, 1996.
35. van Vugt M, Brockman A, Gemperli B, Luxemburger C, Gathmann I, *et al.* Randomized comparison of artemether-benflumetol and artesunate-mefloquine in treatment of multidrug-resistant falciparum malaria. Antimicrob Agents Chemother 42:135, 1998.
36. Warrell DA, Looareesuwan S, Warrell M, Kasemsarn P, Intaraprasert R, *et al.* Dexamethasone proves deleterious in cerebral malaria. A double-blind trial in 100 comatose patients. N Engl J Med 306:313, 1982.
37. Hoffman SL, Rustama D, Punjabi NH, Surampaet B, Sanjaya B, *et al.* High-dose dexamethasone in quinine-treated patients with cerebral malaria: A double-blind, placebo-controlled trial. J Infect Dis 158:325, 1988.
38. Looareesuwan S, Warrell DA, White NJ, Sutharasamai P, Chanthavanich *et al.* Do patients with cerebral malaria have cerebral oedema? A computed tomography study. Lancet i:434, 1983.
39. Wilairatana P, Looareesuwan S. APACHE II scoring for predicting outcome in cerebral malaria. J Trop Med Hyg 98:256, 1995.
40. Kapur J. Status epilepticus and seizures. Curr Opin Crit Care 4:83, 1998.

41. Trang TTM, Phu NH, Vinh H, Hien TT, Cuong BM, *et al.* Acute renal failure in patients with severe falciparum malaria. Clin Infect Dis 15:874, 1992.
42. Wilairatana P, Westerlund EK, Aursudkij B, Vannaphan S, Krudsood S, *et al.* Treatment of malarial acute renal failure by hemodialysis. Am J Trop Med Hyg 60:233, 1999.
43. Panosian CB. Editorial response: Exchange blood transfusion in severe falciparum malaria – the debate goes on. Clin Infect Dis 26:853, 1998.
44. White NJ, Warrell DA, Chanthavanigh P, Looareesuwan S, Warrell MJ, *et al.* Severe hypoglycemia and hyperinsulinemia in falciparum malaria. N Engl J Med 309:61, 1983.
45. Bruneel F, Gachot B, Timsit JF, Wolff M, Bedos JP, *et al.* Shock complicating severe falciparum malaria in European adults. Intensive Care Med 23:698, 1997.
46. Newton CRJC, Taylor TE, Whitten RO. Pathophysiology of fatal falciparum malaria in African children. Am J Trop Med Hyg 58:673, 1998.
47. Marsh K, Forster D, Waruiru C, Mwangi I, Winstanley M, *et al.* Indicators of life-threatening malaria in African children. N Engl J Med 332:1399, 1995.
48. Marsh K, English M, Crawley J. The pathogenesis of severe malaria in African children. Ann Trop Med Parasitol 90:395, 1996.
49. O'Dempsey TJD, McArdle TF, Laurence BE, Lamont AC, Todd JE, *et al.* Overlap in the clinical features of pneumonia and malaria in African children. Trans R Soc Trop Med Hyg 87:662, 1993.
50. Allen SJ, O'Donnell A, Alexander NDE, Clegg JB. Severe malaria in children in Papua New Guinea. Q J Med 89:779, 1996.
51. Brewster DR, Kwiatkowski D, White NJ. Neurological sequelae of cerebral malaria in children. Lancet 336:1039, 1990.
52. Greenwood BM. What's new in malaria control? Ann Trop Med Parasitol 91:523, 1997.
53. WHO Malaria Unit. Global malaria control. Bull World Health Organ 71:281, 1993.
54. Brown GV. Chemoprophylaxis of malaria. Med J Aust 159:187, 1993.
55. Playfair JHL, Taverne J, Bate CAW, de Souza JB. The malaria vaccine: anti-parasite or anti-disease? Immunol Today 11:25, 1990.
56. Clark IA, Rockett KA. Immunizing against toxic malarial antigens. Parasitol Today 10:6, 1994.
57. Amador R, Patarroyo M. Malaria vaccines. J Clin Immunol 16:183, 1996.
58. Kwiatkowski D, Marsh K. Development of a malaria vaccine. Lancet 350:1696, 1997.
59. Urdaneta M, Prata A, Struchiner CJ, Tosta CE, Tauil P, *et al.* Evaluation of SPf66 malaria vaccine efficacy in Brazil. Am J Trop Med Hyg 58:378, 1998.
60. Stoute JA, Slaoui M, Heppner DG, Momin P, Kester KE, *et al.*, for the RTS, S Malaria Vaccine Evaluation Group. A preliminary evaluation of a recombinant circumsporozoite protein vaccine against *Plasmodium falciparum* malaria. N Engl J Med 336:86, 1997.

27. TOXIC SHOCK SYNDROMES

Kevin B. Laupland and H. Dele Davies

Introduction

The first description of staphylococcal toxic shock syndrome (TSS) was by Todd *et al.* (1978) in children aged 8 to 17 [1]. Shortly afterwards other reports were published and it became well known as an illness of menstruating women who used tampons [2, 3]. The syndrome is characterized by rapid onset of fever, hypotension and multisystem failure with desquamating rash occurring in convalescence [4]. The majority of early cases reported were menstrually associated (MTSS) but this pattern has been changing with an increasing proportion of cases non-menstrually associated (NMTSS) [5].

In the late 1980s, cases of severe invasive group streptococcal (GAS) infections associated with a similar clinical presentation to staphylococcal TSS began to appear in the literature [6–8]. This streptococcal toxic shock-like or streptococcal toxic shock syndrome (STSS) shares in common features of fever, shock and multisystem organ failure with staphylococcal TSS [4, 9]. In contrast, STSS has no menstrual association, is more common at extremes of age and is a much more lethal condition compared to TSS with case fatality rates of approximately 50% as compared to 5% respectively [5, 10–15]. STSS is occasionally associated with the severe soft tissue infection necrotizing fascitis which has been popularly called "flesh eating disease" by the media [12].

Epidemiology

STAPHYLOCOCCAL TOXIC SHOCK SYNDROME

There have been significant changes in the rates of TSS since its first description two decades ago. In the early 1980s the incidence peaked and there was much public awareness [15]. Case-control studies identified white race, young women (under 20 years), barrier contraceptives, and use of tampons, particularly the superabsorbent variety Rely brand, as risk factors for acquiring TSS [2, 16–18]. The Rely brand tampon was withdrawn from the market in 1980 and there was a temporally associated decrease in TSS incidence from rates of approximately 10 per 100,000 young women in 1980 to 1 per 100,000 in 1986 [2, 15, 19–21].

Following the initial identification of MTSS cases, there were increasing numbers of NMTSS cases reported. The majority of NMTSS cases are nosocomially acquired and the sources of infection may be either genital, such as with postpartum or contraceptive diaphragm associated illness, or non-genital such as with postoperative wound infection, burns, cellulitis, and rarely necrotizing fasciitis [5, 22, 23]. Since the mid 1980s rates of NMTSS have been similar to those for MTSS. The overall incidence of TSS has been less well documented since the late 1980s but rates have probably not increased. The case fatality rate for TSS is variable according to age, gender and whether it is menstrually or non-menstrually associated. In one passive surveillance study conducted between 1980–1986, the case fatality rate for TSS was lowest for vaginally associated disease in young females under 15 years old (2%) and was highest in non-vaginally associated cases in women (13%) and men (17%) over 45 years old [24].

STREPTOCOCCAL TOXIC SHOCK SYNDROME

Group A streptococcal infections have re-emerged in the past 15 years as significant causes of severe infections. Acute rheumatic fever and scarlet fever caused by GAS were common until the middle of the twentieth century but then decreased in incidence for reasons that are not well known. Invasive GAS infections, defined as the isolation of *Streptococcus pyogenes* from normally sterile body sites such as blood or cerebrospinal, pleural, or deep tissue aspirate fluid, are increasingly reported as significant causes of severe morbidity and mortality. Population-based studies have shown that invasive GAS disease in Europe and North America now occurs at an incidence of 2–5 per 100,000 [10–13, 25]. Among cases of invasive GAS infection, STSS occurs in approximately 15% (incidence of 0.2–0.7 per 100,000 population) and necrotizing fasciitis in 3–6% [10, 13].

Although early studies suggested that STSS was more common among healthy young individuals, prospective population-based studies have demonstrated that this is not the case [8, 10, 11, 13]. In the largest prospective population-based study of invasive GAS disease reported, STSS was observed in 5% of children under 15 years old compared to 29% in adults over 75 years old [10]. Furthermore, among patients with invasive GAS disease, those with STSS are more likely to have a chronic underlying illness [10, 13]. The most important chronic co-morbid conditions in invasive GAS infection and STSS include HIV infection, malignancy, heart disease, diabetes, lung disease, and alcohol abuse [10, 13]. Skin trauma or breakdown is observed as a preceding event to invasive GAS disease in approximately one third of cases but the relative risk associated with this is unknown. In children, varicella is the most important documented risk factor for acquisition of invasive GAS disease and necrotizing fasciitis with a relative risk of up to 58 [10, 13, 14].

Approximately one half of patients with necrotizing fasciitis have concomitant STSS, although only one quarter of cases of STSS have necrotizing fasciitis [10, 12, 13]. The most common foci of infection associated with STSS include soft tissue infection, pneumonia, bacteremia with no clinical focus, and septic arthritis [10, 13]. The case fatality rate of invasive GAS infection is markedly increased when associated with STSS with rates of 47–81% identified in population-based studies [10, 13, 25]. Necrotizing fasciitis in the absence of criteria for STSS does not increase the case fatality rate above that for invasive GAS infections alone.

Etiology and Pathogenesis

STAPHYLOCOCCAL TOXIC SHOCK SYNDROME

TSS is caused by toxigenic strains of *Staphylococcus aureus*. The evidence supporting a toxic pathogenesis in TSS includes the clinical findings of multisystem involvement in the absence of systemic infection (positive blood cultures in less than 10% of cases) and the ability to reproduce a TSS-like illness in rabbits using purified *S. aureus* toxins [26, 27]. There is strong evidence implicating toxic shock syndrome toxin-1 (TSST-1) and the staphylococcal enterotoxins as the etiologic agents of TSS [28, 29]. TSST-1 was identified independently by Bergdoll *et al.* [30] and Schlievert *et al.* [31] in 1981 and its role in TSS is widely accepted. This protein is produced by over 90% of MTSS isolates and the majority of NMTSS isolates [28, 31]. The staphylococcal enterotoxins are commonly co-produced with TSST-1 and are likely responsible for the syndrome in non-TSST-1 producing isolates from TSS cases [28, 29]. Staphylococcal enterotoxin B is produced by the majority of NMTSS isolates in which TSST-1 is not produced and is likely the cause of the disease in these cases [5, 29, 32, 33]. TSST-1 negative TSS has a higher case-fatality rate which may reflect the higher rate of co-morbid medical conditions typical of NMTSS patients or the different toxins mediating the illness [28].

It is not clear why TSS emerged as a "new" complication of *S. aureus* infections in the late 1970s. Retrospective have identified that *S. aureus* has had the ability to produce TSST-1 since at least the 1950s [34]. The onset of MTSS in 1980 appears to be closely related to the use of superabsorbent tampons, as these products probably increase the risk of MTSS by altering the vaginal milieu to encourage *S. aureus* colonization and promote toxin production. *In vitro* studies of TSST-1 expression by *S. aureus* have identified that production is highly variable according to the environment and that an aerobic, pH neutral, low magnesium environment optimizes toxin production [35]. Tampons may increase the risk of TSS by promoting these conditions. It is less clear which factors have been involved in the development of NMTSS. It is possible that this condition has been present at a low baseline rate for many years but not widely identified until surveillance for MTSS brought it to attention. MTSS and NMTSS appear to be distinct microbiologically as one clone appears to be responsible for the majority of cases of MTSS whereas isolates from NMTSS are heterogeneous [36, 37].

TSST-1 and the staphylococcal enterotoxins are superantigens which induce widespread immune activation and subsequent shock [38]. In the usual cell mediated immune response, T cells recognize antigen presented by the major histocompatibility complex II positive antigen presenting cells with high specificity. The population of T cells that respond are selected based on the specificity of their T cell receptor which is determined by the combination of the variable gene segments Vα, Vβ, Jα, Jβ and Dβ [38]. However, superantigens bypass the usual antigen presenting process and activate T cells based on Vβ specificity alone [38]. This leads to a relatively non-specific activation of large populations of T cells. For instance, TSST-1 is Vβ2 restricted and may stimulate up to 50% of all T cells [38, 39]. The result of this activation is the release of potent mediators of inflammation including interleukins 1 and 6 and tumor necrosis factor which ultimately lead to the clinical manifestations of TSS.

STREPTOCOCCAL TOXIC SHOCK SYNDROME

The pathogenesis of STSS is less well defined than TSS and it appears to be related to both the invasiveness of the organism as well as to the systemic toxins it produces. Identification of virulence determinants is further complicated by the fact that the same strains that cause severe invasive disease are commonly non-disease associated, and that there is considerable heterogeneity among isolates from different cases of STSS [40]. There also appears to be host genetic susceptibility factors involved with the development of STSS. In one small study, HLA DRB1*02, DQA1*0103 alleles and the DRB1*02-DQA1*0102 haplotype were associated with protection from STSS [41]. Some investigators have hypothesized that non-steroidal anti-inflammatory agents may enhance the progression of invasive GAS infections to STSS by attenuating the early inflammatory response [42]. One small case-control study has found an association between ibuprofen use and development of necrotizing fasciitis and STSS in children following varicella infection [43]. However, most of these children received the ibuprofen attar there was evidence for infection, and this drug use may have been a marker of severity of disease rather than causal.

Unlike in TSS where systemic effects are observed in association with a localized infection, STSS is characterized by severe bacteremic infection. No single factor has been identified that enables *S. pyogenes* to aggressively invade tissue but potential virulence determinants include M proteins and enzymes such as streptokinase, hyaluronidase, deoxyribonucleases and proteinases. Although there is a broad range of M protein types observed with severe GAS disease, M1 and M3 have been observed to occur at higher rates with invasive infection [44–46]. However, the association of specific M-types with severe disease is modest and these proteins may be markers for other yet unidentified invasive factors.

There are a number of exotoxins that may potentially mediate STSS although a single one has not been identified as the cause. The streptococcal pyrogenic exotoxins (SPE) function as superantigens and are structurally related to the staphylococcal enterotoxins [38]. Strains of GAS producing SPE A in North America and SPE C in Europe have been associated with STSS [47, 48]. Mitogenic factor and streptococcal superantigen have been identified from STSS isolates but their role is unclear [49, 50]. Watanabe-Ohnishi *et al.* showed that characteristic Vβ restricted T cell population changes occurred in cases of STSS that were not related to SPE and suggested that an unidentified superantigen may be involved [51].

Diagnosis

The diagnosis of TSS or STSS is based on identifying a syndrome of shock, fever, and multisystem failure with the fulfillment of criteria for one of these conditions. The Centers for Disease Control and Prevention case definition for TSS is shown in Table 1 and the criteria for STSS as defined by the Working Group on Severe Streptococcal Infections are shown in Table 2 [4, 9]. The diagnosis of TSS requires a high index of suspicion because it is a clinical diagnosis having no single diagnostic test and the infection source is often mild or clinically not apparent. The diagnosis of TSS does not require isolation of *S. aureus* from a normally sterile site, although most cases will have evidence of this infection from a non-sterile site. STSS is usually easier to diagnose than TSS because of the often fulminant illness and high rate of blood culture positivity (>90%) in this condition [10]. However, the early presentation of patients who later develop STSS is often non-specific and delays in diagnosis and treatment are not uncommon. Unlike in TSS, definite diagnosis of STSS requires the culturing of GAS from a normally sterile site [4, 9].

TABLE 1. Staphylococcal toxic shock syndrome, case definition*

All of:

1) Fever: Temperature ≥38.9°C
2) Rash: Diffuse macular erythroderma
3) Desquamation: 1–2 weeks after onset of illness, particularly of palms, soles, fingers, and toes
4) Hypotension: Systolic blood pressure <90 mm Hg for adults or <5th percentile by age for children or orthostatic syncope

And

Involvement of three or more of the following organ systems:

A. Gastrointestinal: vomiting or diarrhea at onset of illness
B. Muscular: severe myalgia or creatinine phosphokinase level greater than twice the upper limit of normal
C. Mucous membranes: vaginal, oropharyngeal, or conjunctival hyperemia
D. Renal: BUN or serum creatinine greater than twice the upper limit of normal; or ≥5 white blood cells per high power field in the absence of a urinary tract infection
E. Hepatic: total bilirubin, or transaminase greater than twice the upper limit of normal
F. Hematology: platelets <100,000/mm^3
G. Central nervous system: disorientation or alterations in consciousness without focal neurologic signs when fever and hypotension are absent

And

Negative results on the following tests if obtained:

A. Blood, throat or cerebrospinal fluid cultures; blood cultures may be positive for *S. aureus*
B. Serologic tests for Rocky Mountain spotted fever, leptospirosis, or measles

* Reproduced from [4].

TSS and STSS share many clinical features in common, which may be the result of the shock-state or more specifically related to individual toxin effects. In both of these syndromes, shock

TABLE 2. Streptococcal toxic shock, case definition*

I. Isolation of group A streptococcus (*S. pyogenes*)
  A. From a normally sterile site (e.g. blood, CSF, pleural or peritoneal fluid, tissue biopsy, surgical wound, etc.)
  B. From a non-sterile site (e.g. throat, sputum, vagina, superficial skin lesion, etc.)

II. Clinical signs of severity
  A. Hypotension: systolic blood pressure ≤90 mm Hg in adults or <5 percentile for age in children

and

  B. ≥2 of the following:
  1. Renal impairment (Creatinine >177 μmol/l for adults or twice upper limit of normal for age or baseline level in chronic renal insufficiency)
  2. Coagulopathy (platelets ≤100,000 or disseminated intravascular coagulation)
  3. Liver involvement (transaminases or bilirubin ≥ twice upper limit normal or baseline in preexisting liver impairment)
  4. Adult respiratory distress syndrome (pulmonary infiltrates and hypoxemia without heart failure) or evidence of diffuse capillary leak (generalized edema or pleural or peritoneal effusions with hypoalbuminemia)
  5. Generalized erythematous macular rash that may desquamate
  6. Soft tissue necrosis (necrotizing fasciitis, myositis, or gangrene)

Illness with IA and II (A and B) – definite case
IB and II (A and B) – probable case, if no other etiology defined for illness

* Reproduced from [9].

is multifactorial and may be due to vasodilation, non-hydrostatic protein leakage with subsequent intravascular volume depletion, hypovolemia from diarrhea, vomiting, and fever, and myocardial depression [52–55]. The myocardial dysfunction when it occurs demonstrates the picture of a reversible toxic cardiomyopathy or myocarditis [52–55]. The shock-state commonly leads to renal impairment from pre-renal failure or acute tubular necrosis [56, 57]. Electrolyte abnormalities are non-specific and may include low serum calcium, magnesium, sodium, potassium and phosphate [56, 57]. The elevated transaminase and bilirubin levels commonly observed are most likely related to shock liver [53, 54, 57]. Adult respiratory distress syndrome (ARDS) is more common in STSS but may also occur in TSS [53, 54, 57]. Pleural effusions are more common in STSS than in TSS and may be complicated by empyema [9, 58].

Toxin manifestations that may be independent of the shock-state occur commonly especially in TSS. In TSS the rash is typically a diffuse macular erythroderma with desquamation most pronounced on the hands and soles at approximately 1–3 weeks after illness onset. The rash in STSS is similar but is less common and desquamation occurs less commonly. TSS may be associated with mental status changes ranging from headache to encephalopathy which may lead to persistent cognitive impairment [59]. Vomiting and inflammatory diarrhea are common in TSS, as is sterile pyuria. These may be a result of severe illness or secondary to toxin(s).

Necrotizing fasciitis is a rapidly progressive infection that is often difficult to diagnose clinically. It occurs commonly in association with STSS and is definitely diagnosed if histopathological examination reveals necrosis of fascia with edema and polymorphonuclear infiltrate [12]. This diagnosis may be made clinically if tissue necrosis is or at surgical exploration. In the early stages there may be necrosis of the underlying fascia despite normal overlying skin. Clues to the diagnosis include pain out of proportion to physical findings, edema, and/or erythema in the setting of symptoms and signs of infection including fever, arthralgias and myalgias [60]. Rapid changes in clinical findings are particularly worrisome for this diagnosis. Creatine kinase levels are often elevated but this test is both insensitive and non-specific and therefore inadequate to rule out necrotizing fasciitis. Soft tissue radiograms rarely show air in tissue in

TABLE 3. Comparison of epidemiological and clinical features of TSS and STSS

Feature	TSS	STSS
Risk groups	young women using superabsorbent tampons	extremes of age, chronic underlying disease, alcohol abuse, chickenpox
Case fatality rate	2–17%	47–81%
Bacteremia	<10%	>90%
Etiology	TSST-1, staphylococcal enterotoxins	Poorly defined
Rash	all	minority
Necrotizing fasciitis	rare	common (25%)
Antibiotic treatment	oxacillin or clindamycin	clindamycin and penicillin
IVIG	possible benefit	standard of care

necrotizing fasciitis due to GAS and are unhelpful to exclude this diagnosis. Magnetic resonance imaging has been reported as a possible test to rule out necrotizing fasciitis but performance of this test should not delay definitive diagnosis by surgical exploration and biopsy which is the standard of care [60, 61], Since no symptom, sign or non-invasive investigation reliably rules out a diagnosis of necrotizing fasciitis, surgical exploration should be performed in all cases for which the diagnosis is entertained. The procedure has minimal morbidity but a missed or delayed diagnosis of necrotizing fasciitis has very serious and often lethal consequences.

In both TSS and STSS the differential diagnosis includes a broad range of inflammatory conditions. Rocky Mountain spotted fever caused by *Rickettsia rickettsii*, typhus, meningococcemia, Lyme disease and leptospirosis are all infections associated with rash that may mimic TSS. Toxic epidermal necrolysis, erythema multiforme and Stevens-Johnson syndrome all present with rash and fever. Sepsis from endocarditis or Gram-negative organisms may also be difficult to differentiate from toxic shock. Kawasaki disease is an acute illness of children characterized by fever, rash, lymphadenopathy, oral involvement and peripheral extremity changes that must be differentiated from TSS because this condition is complicated by coronary artery aneurysms in approximately 25% of untreated cases [62, 63].

Treatment

The general principles of treatment of TSS and STSS are similar and may involve supportive care, antibiotics, surgery and intravenous immunoglobulin (IVIG). There have been no randomized trials in the treatment of TSS or STSS and management is based primarily on expert opinion and from experience in related conditions. The spectrum of TSS ranges from relatively mild to severe disease whereas STSS is virtually always severe. In one prospective study, 80% of cases of STSS required ICU care, 60% needed mechanical ventilation and 52% vasopressor support [13]. In all cases of STSS and TSS, if ICU care is not initially undertaken, close monitoring on the hospital ward is required with a low threshold to transfer to ICU care in the event of clinical deterioration.

Supportive care in TSS and STSS is similar to that used for septic shock caused by infection with other organisms, particularly Gram-negatives, as discussed elsewhere in this book. Cardio-respiratory support includes intravenous fluids, inotropes/vasopressors, and mechanical ventilation. Intravenous fluids should promptly be administered to replete intravascular volume. Both colloid (albumin or pentastarch) and crystalloid (normal saline or lactated Ringer's) solutions are useful in restoring cardiac output but larger volumes of crystalloid must be given for equal effect [64]. In patients with TSS or STSS who require several liters of fluid or in those with evidence of diffuse capillary leak, use of colloid may help to reduce tissue edema. When hypotension and poor tissue perfusion persist despite adequate fluid resuscitation, inotropic and/or vasopressor agents are indicated. Placement of a pulmonary artery catheter at this stage is prudent to guide therapy. Fluid infusion should continue to reach an initial goal pulmonary wedge pressure of 10–15 mm Hg [65]. Higher filling pressures may be required depending on individual patient response.

There is no single best inotrope or vasopressor in the toxic shock syndromes and an individualized approach is necessary depending on the clinical response including changes in mentation, tissue perfusion, blood pressure and urine output as well as improvements in serum lactate, cardiac index and systemic oxygen delivery [66, 67]. Dopamine (5–20 µg/kg/min) is recommended as the initial agent of choice but other drugs may need to be introduced. Dobutamine (5–20 µg/kg/min) is useful in the setting of the poor cardiac output state occasionally associated with toxic shock [52]. Norepinephrine (0.01–0.5 µg/kg/min) and epinephrine (0.04–1 µg/kg/min) have both inotropic and vasoconstrictor properties. Phenylephrine acts primarily as a vasopressor with minimal inotropic effect. In addition to fluid and inotrope/vasopressor treatment, cardiorespiratory support includes the use of oxygen to correct hypoxia and mechanical ventilation with paralysis is indicated in severe cases to reduce metabolic demand and ensure adequate ventilation. Close attention should also be paid to nutritional supplementation, and correction of metabolic, hemostatic and renal function abnormalities.

Antibiotic therapy is essential in the treatment of TSS and STSS. For TSS, antibiotics are most important for preventing relapse in MTSS but are usually also needed to treat the local infection in NMTSS [68]. Prompt use of antibiotics in STSS is critical because this is nearly always a systemic infection. *S. aureus* is virtually always resistant to penicillin and in some regions it is commonly methicillin resistant (MRSA). *S. pyogenes* is universally sensitive to penicillin. However, despite *in vitro* susceptibility, in STSS beta-lactam antibiotics may be limited in treatment because of "inoculum effect" [69]. This occurs when the bacteria are present in high concentrations and are in stationary phase with the subsequent reduced production of penicillin binding proteins, the target of beta-lactam antibiotics [69]. Clindamycin is a protein synthesis inhibitor antibiotic that has *in vitro* activity against both *S. aureus* and *S. pyogenes*. It is not affected by the inoculum effect and may also treat toxic shock by inhibiting toxin production. Clindamycin has been shown to be more effective than penicillin in mouse models of GAS myositis and in case-control studies in humans with STSS [70, 71].

We recommend that TSS be treated initially with high dose intravenous oxacillin (2 g q4h) or clindamycin (40 mg/kg/day, up to 900 mg q8h maximum) in beta-lactam allergic patients. In regions with high rates of MRSA, vancomycin (20 mg/kg/day, maximum, 1 g IV q12h) should be included until susceptibility-testing results are available. STSS should be treated with high does intravenous penicillin (100,000–200,000 U/kg/day divided q4h up to 24 million units/day) and clindamycin (40 mg/kg/day up to 900 mg q8h) unless susceptibility testing demonstrates resistance. Generally, 7 to 10 days of intravenous therapy are needed for STSS, while step-down to oral therapy is instituted based on clinical response for TSS. In both TSS and STSS a minimum two-week total treatment regimen is recommended. In some cases it may be difficult to differentiate among TSS, STSS and Gram-negative septic shock in the initial presentation. Our recommendation in this situation is that clindamycin (40 mg/kg/day, maximum, 900 mg IV q8h) should be used with a broad spectrum, β-lactamase resistant agent until microbiologic diagnosis is achieved.

Surgical intervention is commonly required in TSS and STSS. Any localized infection source requires intervention such as removal of tampons or wound packing, or surgical drainage of infected wounds, abscesses or empyema. Necrotizing fasciitis must be treated surgically without delay because this condition is typically fulminant. Adequate drainage and excision of all necrotic tissue is mandatory and often-repeated surgical procedures or daily exploration are needed in the treatment of this condition [10, 13]. Wounds should generally be packed open until the infection has been cured.

IVIG has been suggested as an important treatment in TSS and STSS. Intravenous immunoglobulin contains neutralizing antibodies to staphylococcal and streptococcal superantigens and has anti-cytokine activity [72–75]. One observational study comparing 21 STSS patients treated with IVIG with 32 STSS historical controls showed an increased survival rate for those treated with IVIG at 30 days of 67% vs 34% respectively [72]. Randomized trials of this therapy are unlikely to be performed in the future because of the high mortality rate associated with STSS and the apparent efficacy of IVIG. Therefore, a single dose of IVIG (2 g/kg) is recommended as standard treatment for this condition. Occasionally, repeated doses may be beneficial.

Antibodies to the staphylococcal enterotoxins and TSST-1 are protective for TSS and theoretically IVIG would also be valuable in the treatment of this condition [76, 77]. However, TSS has a much lower rate of morbidity and mortality and IVIG use is a clinical decision alone. In children with TSS or STSS it is important to exclude Kawasaki disease as this condition shares many features with toxic shock and may be diagnosed simultaneously [78, 79]. If there is clinical criteria for Kawasaki disease or evidence of coronary involvement then IVIG is clearly indicated based on its proven efficacy in reducing the risk of developing coronary aneurysms from approximately 23% to 2% [80]. Echocardiography is the screening procedure of choice to detect coronary aneurysms and it is our recommendation that this test be performed routinely on all children with TSS or STSS [62, 81].

Preventive measures may play a role in the management of TSS and STSS. In patients with an initial episode of tampon-associated MTSS, it is prudent to recommend against the further use of tampons. If these products are used then the absorbency and amount of time they are left in place may best be minimized. Careful wound care and prompt treatment of infection in surgical cases may reduce risks for NMTSS. Recurrence occurs in up to one quarter of cases of TSS and there is a potential role for eliminating *S. aureus* asymptomatic carriage in the nares using topical mupirocin [2, 82]. Invasive GAS disease has an estimated household contact transmission risk of 3 per 1000 which is comparable to rates observed for sporadic meningococcal disease [10]. Antibiotic prophylaxis for close contacts of patients with STSS may be beneficial but data is lacking and there is no consensus agreement on whether this prophylaxis should be routinely offered [83]. As a result, individual cases should be reviewed and prophylaxis offered based on risk factor assessment. Consultation with an infectious disease or public health specialist is recommended. If prophylactic treatment is warranted then we recommend clindamycin (20–30 mg/kg/day, up to 300 mg po q8h) orally for 10 days to clear pharyngeal carriage. In children, 16% of all cases of invasive GAS disease are complications of varicella infection and it has been estimated that at least 10% of all invasive GAS in children could be prevented by routine vaccination for varicella at one year of age [14].

References

1. Todd J, Fishaut M, Kapral F, Welch T. Toxic-shock syndrome associated with phage-group-I staphylococci. Lancet 2:1116, 1978.
2. Davis JP, Chesney PJ, Wand PJ, *et al.* Toxic-shock syndrome. Epidemiological features, recurrence, risk factors, and prevention. N Engl J Med 303:1429, 1980.
3. Shands KN, Schmid GP, Dan BB, *et al.* Toxic-shock syndrome in menstruating women. Association with tampon use and staphylococcus aureus and clinical features in 52 cases. N Engl J Med 303:1436, 1980.

4. Centers for Disease Control and Prevention. Case definitions for public health surveillance. MMWR 39(RR–13):33, 1990.
5. Kain KC, Schulzer M, Chow AW. Clinical spectrum of nonmenstrual toxic shock syndrome (TSS): Comparison with menstrual TSS by multivariate discriminant analyses. Clin Infect Dis 16:100, 1993.
6. Cone LA, Woodard DR, Schlievert PM, Tomory GS. Clinical and bacteriologic observations of a toxic shock-like syndrome due to streptococcus pyogenes. N Engl J Med 17:146, 1987.
7. Bartter A, Dascal A, Carrol K, Curley FJ. "Toxic strep syndrome" a manifestation of group A streptococcal infection. Arch Intern Med 148:1421, 1988.
8. Stevens DL, Tanner MH, Winship J, *et al.* Severe group A streptococcal infections associated with a toxic shock-like syndrome and scarlet fever toxin A. N Engl J Med 321:1, 1989.
9. The Working Group on Severe Streptococcal Infections. Defining the group A streptococcal toxic shock syndrome. Rationale and consensus definition. JAMA 269:390, 1993.
10. Davies HD, McGeer A, Schwartz B, *et al.* Invasive group A streptococcal infections in Ontario Canada. N Engl J Med 335:547, 1996.
11. Hoge CW, Schwartz B, Talkington DF, *et al.* The changing epidemiology of invasive group A streptococcal infections and the emergence of streptococcal toxic shock-like syndrome. A retrospective population-based study. JAMA 269: 384, 1993.
12. Kaul R, McGeer A, Low DE, *et al.* Population-based surveillance for group A streptococcal necrotizing fasciitis: Clinical features, prognostic indicators, and microbiologic analysis of seventy-seven cases. Am J Med 103:18, 1997.
13. Zurawski CA, Bardsley MS, Beall B, *et al.* Invasive group A streptococcal disease in metropolitan Atlanta: a population-based assessment. Clin Infect Dis 27:150, 1998.
14. Laupland KB, Davies HD, Low DE, Schwartz B, Green K, The Ontario Group A Streptococcal Study, McGeer A. Does varicella-zoster virus (VZV) infection predispose to invasive or severe invasive group A streptococcal (GAS) infection? Evidence from population-based surveillance in Ontario. 38th Interscience Conference on Antimicrobial Agents and Chemotherapy, San Diego, 1998:Abstract L–95.
15. Schuchat A, Broome CV. Toxic shock syndrome and tampons. Epidemiologic Rev 13:99, 1991.
16. Schlech WF, Shands KN, Reingold AL, *et al.* Risk factors for development of toxic shock syndrome: association with tampon brand. JAMA 248:835, 1982.
17. Osterholm MT, Davis JP, Gibson RW, *et al.* Tristate toxic-shock syndrome study. I. Epidemiologic findings. J Infect Dis 145:431, 1982.
18. Schwartz B, Gaventa S, Broome CV, *et al.* Nonmenstrual toxic shock syndrome associated with barrier contraceptives: report of a case-control study. Rev Infect Dis 2 (suppl 1):S43, 1989.
19. Osterholm MT, Forfang JC. Toxic-shock syndrome in Minnesota: results of an active-passive surveillance system. J Infect Dis 145:458, 1982.
20. Gaventa S, Reingold AL, Hightower AW, *et al.* Active surveillance for toxic shock syndrome in the United States, 1986. Rev Infect Dis 2 (suppl 1):S28, 1989.
21. Latham RH, Kehrberg MW, Jacobson JA. Toxic shock syndrome in Utah: a case-control and surveillance study. Ann Intern Med 96:906, 1982.
22. Chesney PJ, Davis JP, Purdy WK, Wand PJ, Chesney RW. Clinical manifestations of toxic shock syndrome. JAMA 246:741, 1981.
23. Davis JP, Osterholm MT, Helms CM, *et al.* Tristate toxic-shock syndrome study. II. Clinical and laboratory findings. J Infect Dis 145:441, 1982.
24. Broome CV. Epidemiology of toxic shock syndrome in the United States: overview. Rev Infect Dis 2 (suppl 1):S14, 1989.
25. Eriksson BKG, Andersson J, Holm SE, Norgren M. Epidemiological and clinical aspects of invasive group A streptococcal infections and the streptococcal toxic shock syndrome. Clin Infect Dis 27:1428, 1998.
26. Kum WWS, Laupland KB, See RH, Chow AW. Improved purification and biologic activities of staphylococcal toxic shock syndrome toxin-1. J Clin Microbiol 31:2654, 1993.
27. Parsonnet J, Gilllis ZA, Richter AG, *et al.* A rabbit model of toxic shock syndrome that uses a constant, subcutaneous infusion of toxic shock syndrome toxin 1. Infect Immun 55:1070, 1987.
28. Garbe PL, Arko RJ, Reingold AL, *et al.* Staphylococcus aureus isolates from patients with nonmenstrual toxic shock syndrome: evidence for additional toxins. JAMA 253:2538, 1985.
29. Crass BA, Bergdoll MS. Involvement of staphylococcal enterotoxins in nonmenstrual toxic shock syndrome. J Clin Microbiol 23:1138, 1986.

30. Bergdoll MS, Crass BA, Reiser RF, *et al.* A new staphylococcal enterotoxin, enterotoxin F, associated with toxic-shock-syndrome *Staphylococcus aureus* isolates. Lancet i:1017, 1981.
31. Schlievert PM, Shands KN, Dan BB, *et al.* Identification and characterization of an exotoxin from *Staphylococcus aureus* associated with toxic-shock syndrome. J Infect Dis 143:509, 1981.
32. Lee TP, Chang AH, Chow AW. Detection of staphylococcal enterotoxin B among toxic shock syndrome (TSS)- and Non-TSS-associated *Staphylococcus aureus* isolates. J Infect Dis 166:911, 1992.
33. Schlievert PM. Staphylococcal enterotoxin B and toxic-shock syndrome toxin-1 are significantly associated with non-menstrual TSS. Lancet 1149, 1986.
34. Hayes PS, Graves OLM, Feeley JC, *et al.* Production of toxic-shock-associated protein(s) in *Staphylococcus aureus* strains isolated from 1956 through 1982. J Clin Microbiol 20:43, 1984.
35. Schlievert PM, Blomster DA. Production of staphylococcal pyrogenic toxin type C: influence of physical and chemical factors. J Infect Dis 147:236, 1983.
36. Musser JM, Schlievert PM, Chow AW, *et al.* A single clone of *Staphylococcus aureus* causes the majority of cases of toxic shock syndrome. Proc Natl Acad Sci USA 87:225, 1990.
37. See RH, Chow AW. Microbiology of toxic shock syndrome: overview. Rev Infect Dis 2:S55, 1989.
38. Marrack P, Kappler J. The staphylococcal enterotoxins and their relatives. Science 248:705, 1990.
39. Choi Y, Lafferty JA, Clements JR, *et al.* Selective expansion of T cells expressing Vβ2 in toxic shock syndrome. J Exp Med 172:981, 1990.
40. Cockerill FR, MacDonald KL, Thompson RL, *et al.* An outbreak of invasive group A streptococcal disease associated with high carriage rates of the invasive clone among school-aged children. JAMA 277:38, 1997.
41. Guedez Y, Norrby-Teglund A, Low DE, McGeer A, Kotb M. HLA class II alleles associated with outcome of invasive group A streptococcal infections. 37th Interscience Conference on Antimicrobial Agents and Chemotherapy, Toronto, 1997:Abstract G–50.
42. Stevens DL. Could nonsteroidal antiinflammatory drugs (NSAIDs) enhance the progression of bacterial infections to toxic shock syndrome? Clin Infect Dis 21:977, 1995.
43. Zerr DM, Alexander ER, Duchin JS, Koutsky LA, Rubens CE. A case-control study of necrotizing fasciitis during primary varicella. Pediatrics 103:783, 1999.
44. Colman G, Tanna A, Efstratiou A, Gaworzewska ET. The serotypes of *Streptococcus pyogenes* in Britain during 1980–1990 and their association with disease. J Med Microbiol 39:165, 1993.
45. Talkington DF, Schwartz B, Black CM, *et al.* Association of phenotypic and genotypic characteristics of invasive *Streptococcus pyogenes* isolated with clinical components of streptococcal toxic shock syndrome. Infect Immun 61:3369, 1993.
46. Schwartz B, Facklam RR, Breiman RF. Changing epidemiology of group A streptococcal infection in the USA. Lancet 336:1167, 1990.
47. Hauser AR, Stevens DL, Kaplan EL, Schlievert PM. Molecular analysis of pyrogenic exotoxins from *Streptococcus pyogenes* isolates associated with toxic shock-like syndrome. J Clin Microbiol 29:1562, 1991.
48. Musser JM, Hauser AR, Kim MH, *et al.* *Streptococcus pyogenes* causing toxic shock-like syndrome and other invasive disease: clonal diversity and pyrogenic exotoxin expression. Proc Natl Acad Sci USA 88:2668, 1991.
49. Yutsudo T, Murai H, Gonzalez, *et al.* A new type of mitogenic factor produced by *Streptococcus pyogenes*. FEBS Lett 308:30, 1992.
50. Mollick J, Miller G, Musser JM, *et al.* A novel superantigen isolated from pathogenic strains of *Streptococcus pyogenes* with aminoterminal homology to staphylococcal enterotoxins B and C. J Clin Invest 92:710, 1993.
51. Watanabe-Ohnishi R, Low DE, McGeer A, *et al.* Selective depletion of Vβ-bearing T cells in patients with severe invasive group A streptococcal infections and streptococcal toxic shock syndrome. J Infect Dis 171:74, 1995.
52. Fisher CJ, Horowitz BZ, Albertson TE. Cardiorespiratory failure in toxic shock syndrome: effect of dobutamine. Crit Care Med 13:160, 1985.
53. Paris AL, Herwaldt LA, Blum D, *et al.* Pathologic finding in twelve fatal cases of toxic shock syndrome. Ann Intern Med 96:852, 1982.
54. Larkin SM, Williams DN, Osterholm MT, *et al.* Toxic shock syndrome: clinical laboratory, and pathological findings in nine fatal cases. 96:858, 1982.
55. Forni AL, Kaplan EL, Schlievert PM, Roberts RB. Clinical and microbiological characteristics of severe group A streptococcus infections and

streptococcal toxic shock syndrome. Clin Infect Dis 21:333, 1995.
56. Chesney RW, Chesney PJ, Davis JP, *et al.* Renal manifestations of the staphylococcal toxic shock syndrome. Am J Med 71:583, 1981.
57. Demers B, Simor AE, Vellend H, *et al.* Severe invasive group A streptococcal infections in Ontario, Canada: 1987–1991. Clin Infect Dis 16:792, 1993.
58. Demeter SL, Fuenning C, Kline JJ. Pleural effusion in toxic shock syndrome. Ann Intern Med 96:148, 1982.
59. Rosene KA, Kopas MK, Kastner LS, *et al.* Persistent neuropsychological sequelae of toxic shock syndrome. Ann Intern Med 96:865, 1982.
60. Stamenkovic I, Lew DL. Early recognition of potentially fatal necrotizing fasciitis. The use of frozen-section biopsy. N Engl J Med 310:1689, 1984.
61. Zittergruen M, Grose C. Magnetic resonance imaging for early diagnosis of necrotizing fasciitis. Pediatric Emergency Care 9:26, 1993.
62. Laupland KB, Davies HD. Epidemiology, etiology, and management of Kawasaki disease: State of the art. Pediatr Cardiol 20:177, 1999.
63. Committee on Rheumatic Fever, Endocarditis, and Kawasaki Disease of the American Heart Association's Council on Cardiovascular Disease in the Young. Diagnostic guidelines for Kawasaki disease. AJDC 144:1218, 1990.
64. Rackow EC, Falk JL, Fein A, *et al.* Fluid resuscitation in circulatory shock: a comparison of the cardiorespiratory effects of albumin, hetastarch, and saline solutions in patients with hypovolemic and septic shock. Crit Care Med 11:839, 1983.
65. Packman MI, Rackow EC. Optimum left heart filling pressure during fluid resuscitation of patients with hypovolemic and septic shock. Crit Care Med 165, 1983.
66. Bakker J, Coffernils M, Leon M, *et al.* Blood lactate levels are superior to oxygen-derived variables in predicting outcome in human septic shock. Chest 99:956, 1991.
67. Rudis MI, Basha MA, Zarowitz BJ. Is it time to reposition vasopressors and inotropes in sepsis? Crit Care Med 24:525, 1996.
68. Chesney PJ, Crass BA, Polyak MB, *et al.* Toxic shock syndrome: management and long term sequelae. Ann Int Med 96:847, 1982.
69. Eagle H. Experimental approach to the problem of treatment with penicillin. I. Group A streptococcal infection in mice. Am J Med 13:389, 1952.
70. Stevens D. Eagle effect revisited. J Infect Dis 158:23, 1988.
71. Marfin A, Stefonik K, Cieskal P, Hedberg K. Clindamycin, an emerging antibiotic for the treatment of severe invasive group A streptococcal infections. International Conference on Emerging Infectious Diseases. Atlanta, GA, 1998.
72. Kaul R, McGeer A, Norrby-Teglund A, *et al.* Intravenous immunoglobulin therapy for streptococcal toxic shock syndrome – a comparative study. Clin Infect Dis 28:800, 1999.
73. Barry W, Hudgins L, Donta ST, Pesanti EL. Intravenous immunoglobulin therapy for toxic shock syndrome. JAMA 267:3315, 1992.
74. Skansen-Saphir U, Andersson J, Bjork L, Andersson U. Lymphokine production induced by streptococcal pyrogenic exotoxin-A is selectively down-regulated by pooled human IgG. Eur J Immunol 24:916, 1994.
75. Takei S, Arora Y, Walker S. Intravenous immunoglobulin contains specific antibodies inhibitory to activation of T cells by staphylococcal toxin superantigens. J Clin Invest 91:602, 1993.
76. Helgerson SD, Mallery BL, Foster LR. Toxic shock syndrome in Oregon. Risk of recurrence. JAMA 252:3402, 1984.
77. Rosten PM, Bartlett KH, Chow AW. Serologic responses to toxic shock syndrome (TSS) toxin-1 in menstrual and nonmenstrual TSS. Clin Invest Med 11:187, 1988.
78. Davies HD, Kirk V, Jadavji T, Kotzin BL. Simultaneous presentation of Kawasaki disease and toxic shock syndrome in an adolescent male. Pediatr Infect Dis J 15:1136, 1996.
79. Abinum M, Cant AJ. Toxic shock syndrome toxin-secreting *Staphylococcus aureus* in Kawasaki syndrome. Lancet 343:300, 1994.
80. Durongpisitkul K, Gururaj VJ, Park JM, Martin CF. The prevention of coronary artery aneurysm in Kawasaki disease: a meta-analysis on the efficacy of aspirin and immunoglobulin treatment. Pediatrics 96:1057, 1995.
81. Capannari TE, Daniels SR, Meyer RA, Schwartz DC, Kaplan S. The sensitivity, specificity and predictive value of two-dimensional echocardiography in detecting coronary aneurysms in patients with Kawasaki disease. J Am Coll Cardiol 7:355, 1986.
82. Casewell MW, Hill RLR. Mupirocin "pseudomonic acid" – a promising new topical antimicrobial agent. J Antimicrob Chemother 19:1, 1987.

28. MENINGOCOCCEMIA

Pere Domingo and Nicolau Barquet

"No microbe can kill more quickly"
Harry A. Feldman, 1979

Definition

Meningococcemia literally means the presence and isolation of *Neisseria meningitidis* in the blood of a patient. Although it is an invariable phenomenon in the pathogenesis of meningococcal disease, it may in itself dominate the clinical picture. The clinical spectrum of meningococcemia ranges from a clinically inapparent, mostly oligo-symptomatic bacteremia as in benign or inapparent meningococcemia to overwhelming cases with early multiple-organ failure as in fulminant meninococcemia. There are few diseases which cause as much social alarm as meningococcal disease on being detected in a community. Fear of infection is justified by its sudden onset, the speed with which it spreads in the community, the fulminating evolution of some patients and its mortality. *N. meningitidis* can cause death within a few hours of the first symptoms, in a way unlike any other mico-organism [1].

The Meningococcus

N. meningitidis is a Gram-negative diplococcus which typically appears with the adjacent sites flattened to produce a biscuit shape. It is an exclusively human pathogen. This bacterium is considered fastidious in its growth conditions, and tends to readily undergo autolysis. Optimal growth conditions include moist environment at 35–37°C with an atmosphere of 5–10% carbon dioxide. The organism grows well on a number of medium bases including blood agar base, trypticase soy agar, supplemented chocolate agar and Mueller-Hinton agar [2].

An outer membrane composed of lipids, lipo-oligosaccharides and outer membrane proteins surrounds the meningococcus. A polysaccharide capsule produced by the bacteria and attached to this outer membrane envelops pathogenic meningococci. At least 13 meningococcal serogroups have been defined on the basis of polysaccharide capsule antigens: A, B, C, D, H, I, K, L, X, Y, Z, Z′ (29E), and W-135, meningococcal disease usually being caused by serogroups A, B, C, L, X, Y, and W-135 [1]. Based on outer membrane protein composition, at least 20 meningococcal serotypes and 10 subtypes have been identified [3]. Endemic meningococcal disease is caused by a broad number of serotypes in contrast with epidemic disease that is caused by a single serotype [4]. There are other classification systems, based on differential antigenic characteristics of lipo-oligosaccharide with at least 13 immunotypes [5–8]. It is possible to use the antigenic properties of immunoglobulin A1 proteases and pili for additional typing [9].

Serogrouping and serotyping are used to characterize the *N. meningitidis* strains and are very important in the development of vaccines, but cannot be used to determine the origin of epidemic and resistant clones [10]. Multilocus enzyme electrophoresis, DNA fingerprinting and protein chain reaction provide a better insight into the epidemiology and clonal expansion of *N. meningitidis* strains [11–14].

Epidemiology

Meningococcemia obviously shares epidemiological characteristics with other forms of meningococcal disease, especially meningococcal meningitis. It may occur world-wide as sporadic, endemic or epidemic disease [15]. Meningococcal disease causes sporadic or endemic disease in developed countries, such as the United States and Western Europe, with annual incidence rates ranging from 1–3 cases per 100,000 inhabitants, and occasional epidemic periods. Most infections in industrialized countries are caused by strains of serogroups B and C [16].

The annual incidence rate in epidemic period is about 10 times higher (10–25/100,000/year) in developing countries, such as sub-Saharan Africa, and meningococcal disease is usually epidemic with incidence rates above 1000/100,000/year. In these countries, serogroup A meningococcal disease is prevalent [17]. Sub-Saharan Africa extends from Ethiopia in the East, to Senegal in the West, mainly within the range of 300 mm to 1000 mm annual rainfall [18]. Meningococcal disease caused by serogroup A occurs in seasonal annual cycles in this area, with the attack rate rising at the end of the dry season and declining after the beginning of the rainy season, and with large-scale epidemics occurring at wider intervals with irregular patterns [19]. The differences in incidence rates between developed and developing countries reflect the different pathogenic properties of *N. meningitidis* strains and socioeconomic, environmental and climatological differences [20].

Epidemics of meningococcal disease can be caused by clonal *N. meningitidis* strains migrating across continents [21]. The clonal serogroup A meningococcus originated in China and spread to Nepal and India between 1983 and 1987 [10, 22], reached Saudi Arabia in 1987, causing an epidemic among pilgrims during the Hajji in Mecca. The organism was then transported with the Hajjis, leading to epidemics in 1988 in Central Africa and in later years in Eastern Africa [23]. The epidemic spread to South Africa in 1996 [24]. The transfer of strains of the same clonal complex by Hajjis to the United States and Europe did not give rise to epidemics there [25]. It is not known why potential pathogenic strains cause major epidemics in some areas while others are not affected [17]. The occurrence of meningococcal disease would not appear to be determined solely by the introduction of a new virulent *N. meningitidis* strain but also by other factors that enhance transmission and by the susceptibility of the local population [26].

In Spain, the annual notified incidence rates of meningococcal disease over recent years have been around 4–5 cases per 100,000 inhabitants, this rate appearing to have risen following a decade of low endemicity (Figure 1). This suggests that notified cases were well over 2000 in 1997, whereas meningococcal disease caused nearly 3000 deaths from 1980 to 1994. The case-fatality rate of meningococcal disease has been falling steadily for several years, but was still 10% in 1997. Since 1988, incidence of meningococcal disease in Spain caused by serogroup B meningococci has declined, and incidence due to serogroup C meningococci has increased. This change of pattern led to the carrying out of a mass vaccination campaign against serogroup C in Spain during 1996–97. The incidence rates and case-fatality rates in other Western European countries were similar in recent years, with a trend to increase in the late 1990s [27].

However, it is widely known that notified cases clearly underestimate the true incidence of notifiable diseases, and in a recent report from the urban area of Barcelona which covered the years 1987–1992, and in which an active epidemiological search system was used, the rate of undernotification was estimated to be more than 30% of cases [28]. Meningococcal disease has the highest incidence rate in children, especially among those aged one year or less in whom the incidence rate approaches 100 cases per 100,000 inhabitants per annum. This is true for meningococcemia as well as for other clinical forms of

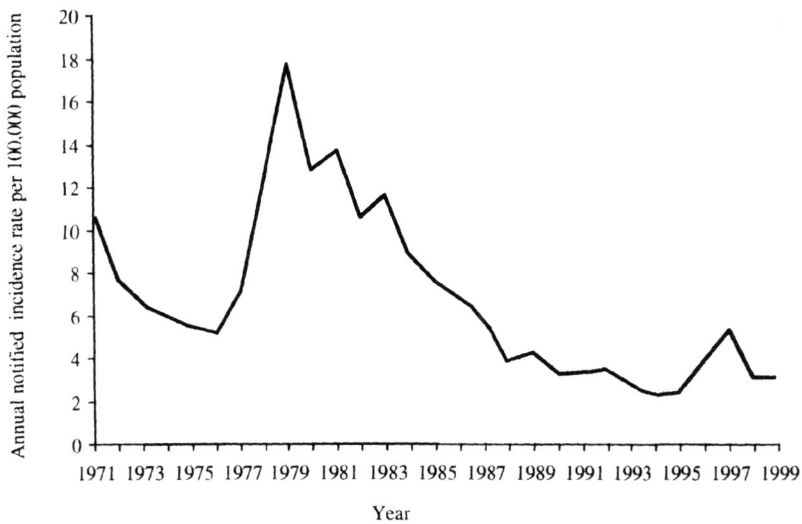

FIGURE 1. Meningococcal disease in Spain (1980–1999): Annual notified incidence rates (Cases reported to the Public Health Service).

meningococcal disease. The risk of contracting meningococcal disease is inversely related to age. After childhood, the incidence rate shows a sharp decline with a second incidence peak during adolescence (age group 15–19 years) (Figure 2) [28]. Meningococcal disease is more frequently seen in patients living in the inner city, where other risk factors for infectious diseases, such as overcrowded homes, poor nutrition and hygiene, low levels of education and low family income, are also prevalent [29].

Several risk factors, which we have grouped in Table 1, have classically been identified for acquiring meningococcal disease, the most serious being exposure to a pathogenic strain of *N. meningitidis* contained in nasopharyngeal secretions of a healthy carrier or patient. Most meningococcal cases acquire the invading strain from a healthy carrier, and secondary cases, i.e. those who acquire the bacterium from another case, constitute no more than 5% of the total number of cases [28]. Unexpectedly, as Osler pointed out as early as 1915, physicians, nurses and other healthcare workers rarely acquire *N. meningitidis* from a patient [30].

Other risk factors for acquiring meningococcal disease include the immune status of the patient, preceding or concomitant *Mycoplasma pneumoniae* or viral respiratory tract infections, climatological and social conditions and bacterial properties. The formation of protective antibodies against homologous strains was induced by nasopharyngeal carriage of *N. meningitidis*, but this also produced cross-reacting antibodies to heterologous strains of pathogenic meningococci [31]. Approximately 10% of the population harbors meningococci in the nasopharynx during endemic periods. Nine out of 10 strains isolated from carriers are, however, nonpathogenic *Neisseria lactamica* or nonpathogenic *N. meningitidis*, as they are not associated with the clones isolated from patients with meningococcal disease [32]. The carriage rate in children younger than four years was below 3%. This rate increases with age to a maximum of 24–37% at 15–24 years, and decreases to below 10% in older age groups [32–35]. The carriage rate of meningococci is higher in lower socioeconomic classes, probably because of crowding, and under conditions where people from different regions are brought

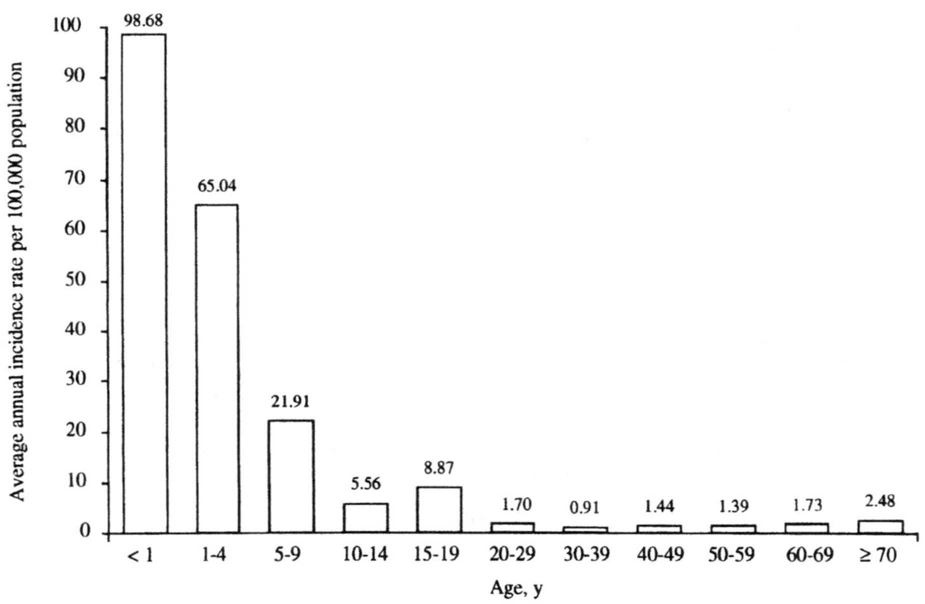

FIGURE 2. Meningococcal disease in Barcelona (1987–1992): Average annual incidence rate by age group (Cases detected by active surveillance).

together, for example military recruits, prisoners, boarding-school students, or pilgrims [31, 36–38]. Virulent clones have a higher transmission rate, with invasive disease often occurring within the first week after acquisition [39, 40], whereas some people may carry pathogenic meningococci for many months or years without falling ill [41, 42]. A randomly sampled population study performed in an endemic period suggests that acquisition of the pathogenic *N. meningitidis* strains induced illness in only 1% of persons harboring these strains [34].

Certain strains of enteric bacteria, such as *Escherichia coli* 07:K1(L):NM and *Bacillus pumilus*, produce capsular polysaccharides that are immunologically identical to the capsular polysaccharides of *N. meningitidis* serogroups A, B and C, and contribute to the defense against meningococci by the induction of cross-reacting antibodies. This is another potential source of immunization against meningococcal disease [43, 44].

Recently, it was suggested that the polymorphism in the neutrophilic receptor for the Fc portion of the immunoglobulins IgG (FcγRIIA) may play a role in the development of meningococcal disease, since neutrophils from patients with low affinity allotypes are less efficient in removing meningococci from the bloodstream [45]. Patients with deficits of the terminal factors of the complement are also colonized more frequently with virulent meningococcal strains that, as serum meningococcidal capacity is diminished, may more frequently cause invasive disease [46].

Pathogenesis and Pathophysiology

The development of full-blown meningococcal disease necessarily involves three steps, although sometimes only two are necessary to cause clinically apparent disease (Figure 3). First, *N. meningitidis* must colonize the nasopharyngeal mucosa of the patient and must also survive and eventually multiply there. Second, the meningo-

TABLE 1. Principal factors predisposing to the acquisition of meningococcal disease

Host dependent factors
Absence of bactericidal antibodies against antigens of the invasive strain
Age (maximum incidence between 6 months and 5 years)
Congenital or acquired deficits of complement factors (C2, C3, inactivator of C3b, C5, C6, C7, C8, C9)
Properdin deficiency
Immunoglobulin deficiency
Anatomic or functional asplenia
FcγRIIA polymorphism
Neisseria meningitidis dependent factors
Presence of capsule
Certain serogroups and serotypes
Production and release of endotoxin
Ability to capture and use iron
Production of hyaluronidase
Production of specific IgA1 proteases
Environment dependent factors
Exposure to a pathogenic strain of *Neisseria meningitidis* contained in nasopharyngeal secretions of a healthy carrier or patient with meningococcal disease
Crowding (household, day-care centers, schools, barracks, closed communities)
Climatic factors (winter and spring, windy weather in Sub-Saharan Africa)
Travel to areas with a high incidence of meningococcal disease

coccus must be able to pass through that mucosa and reach the bloodstream and successfully evade the host defense mechanisms, basically complement-mediated lysis and phagocytosis of immunoglobulin-opsonized meningococci by neutrophils [47]. Finally, if *N. meningitidis* has managed to survive in the bloodstream, it may reach the blood-brain barrier, cross it only to obtain a sanctuary, the subarachnoid space, where it will have virtually no real limitation to multiply and eventually cause a severe surbarachnoidal inflammatory response [48]. All these steps are modulated in a definite manner by the dynamic interaction established between the microorganism properties, the host and environmental conditions, the main factors being listed in Table 1.

Colonization of the human nasopharynx is the first event in the development of human meningococcal disease. The human nasopharyngeal mucosa is the only natural reservoir of *N. meningitidis*. Transmission of meningococcus always occurs from one person to another, by direct contact or via droplets, and the newly infected person is at the greatest risk of developing meningococcal disease [42]. The survival of bacteria in these droplets would appear to be influenced by climatological conditions, such as temperature and humidity. Multiple factors have been identified as favoring meningococcal nasopharyngeal carriage, such as being in close contact with a patient with meningococcal disease, for example household members, healthcare workers, and day-care center workers [49, 50]. Physical damage of nasopharyngeal mucosa by active or passive smoking increases the risk of *N. meningitidis* carriage and meningococcal disease [51–54], as do stressful events and preceding or concomitant *Mycoplasma pneumoniae* or viral upper respiratory tract infections which either alter the integrity of the mucosal surface or influence local or systemic immunity [55–59]. Pili contribute to the attachment to nasopharyngeal mucosal cells [47]. The mechanisms for nasopharyngeal colonization and survival of *N. meningitidis* are not well understood, but since IgA and ciliary activity constitutes the cornerstone of mucosal defense, the meningococcus is able to diminish the ciliary activity and to produce an IgA protease [60].

Meningococcus can survive and proliferate in the bloodstream when intravascular killing is impaired, either because of specific virulence factors of the meningococcus itself or because of a naive or defective immune system of the host. The polysaccharide capsule is the most important bacterial virulence factor for survival of meningococcus in the bloodstream. This protects against complement-mediated bacteriolysis and phagocytosis by neutrophils, and hepatic

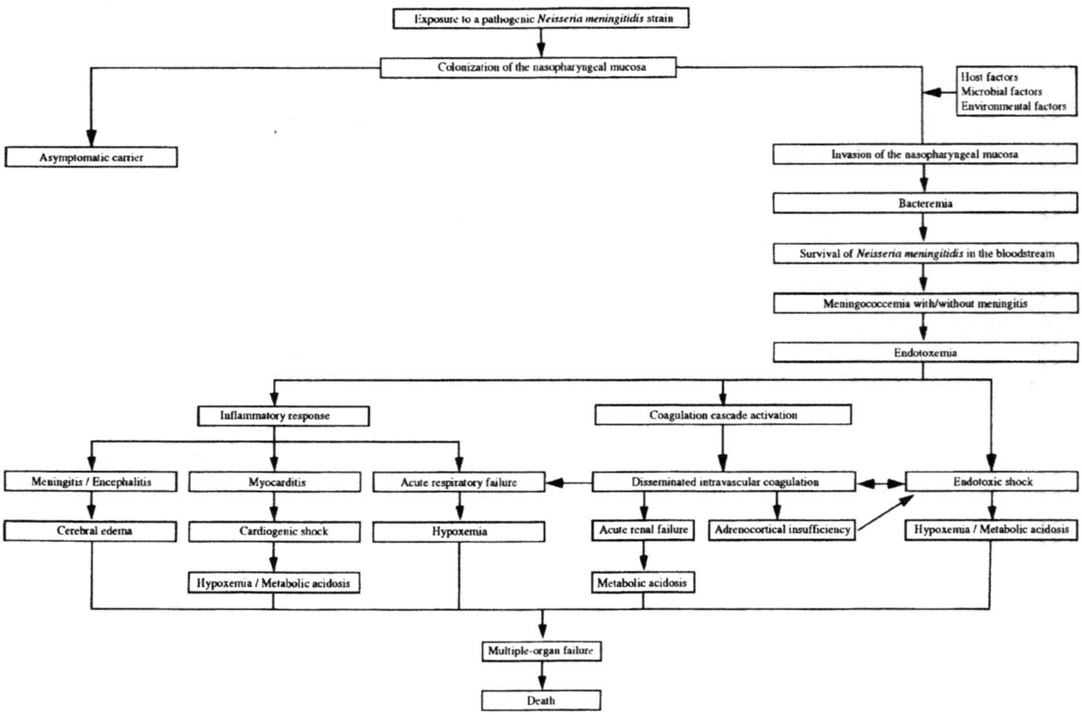

FIGURE 3. Algorithm of pathogenesis and pathophysiology of meningococcemia.

and spleen macrophages [61]. The capacity to acquire iron from human transferrin by using transferrin-binding proteins is another factor involved [62, 63].

Defense against meningococcus within the bloodstream is based on the presence of serum bactericidal antibodies against *N. meningitidis*, a functioning complement system, and its cornerstone is antibody-mediated lysis of meningococci via classical activation. The incidence of meningococcal disease in normal individuals is reciprocally related to the serum concentration of specific antibodies, with the highest incidence occurring from 6 to 24 months of age, when maternal antibodies have disappeared [28, 31, 36]. Specific antibodies are induced throughout life by the continuously repeated and intermittent carriage of meningococci and *N. lactamica* [64, 65]. As already mentioned, certain strains of enteric bacteria with capsular polysaccharides immunologically identical to certain capsular polysaccharides of *N. meningitidis* induce the production of cross-reacting antibodies [43, 44].

Effective removal of encapsulated bacteria requires phagocytosis of opsonized bacteria, a process that depends on efficient interaction between antibodies and Fc receptors and between complement and complement receptors [66]. The IgG receptors (FcγRs) are of crucial importance in directing the uptake and destruction of encapsulated bacteria, since FcγRs on phagocytes detect IgG-opsonized microorganisms [67, 68]. The naturally occurring polymorphism of the FcγRIIA may influence neutrophil phagocytic capacity, thus predisposing a patient to handling more or less efficiently the presence of meningococci within the bloodstream [69]. The presence of adequate concentrations of complement, especially terminal factors, is of

TABLE 2. Meningococcal disease in Barcelona (1987–1992):
Clinical manifestations by bacteriological form (cases detected by active surveillance)

	No. (%) of patients				
Clinical feature	Meningococcemia (n = 152)	Meningitis (n = 165)	Meningococcemia with meningitis (n = 150)	Meningococcal disease not microbiologically proved (n = 176)	All cases (n = 643)
Fever	148 (97.4)	165 (100)	148 (98.7)	176 (100)	637 (99.1)
Petechiae	112 (73.7)	94 (57.0)	121 (80.7)	176 (100)	503 (78.2)
Headache*	25 (16.4)	123 (74.5)	105 (70.0)	101 (57.4)	354 (55.1)
Nausea/vomiting	51 (33.6)	92 (55.8)	73 (48.7)	85 (48.3)	301 (46.8)
Meningeal signs	12 (7.9)	129 (78.2)	83 (55.3)	59 (33.5)	283 (44.0)
Pharyngeal erythema	46 (30.3)	70 (42.4)	58 (38.7)	65 (36.9)	239 (37.2)
Chills*	67 (44.1)	36 (21.8)	33 (22.0)	29 (16.5)	165 (25.7)
Abnormal level of consciousness (excluding coma)	11 (7.2)	55 (33.3)	49 (32.7)	40 (22.7)	155 (24.1)
Maculopapular rash	32 (21.1)	20 (12.1)	26 (17.3)	23 (13.1)	101 (15.7)
Ecchymosis	20 (13.2)	12 (7.3)	17 (11.3)	24 (13.6)	73 (11.4)
Myalgia*	22 (14.5)	9 (5.5)	15 (10.0)	21 (11.9)	67 (10.4)
Abdominal pain*	12 (7.9)	3 (1.8)	9 (6.0)	12 (6.8)	36 (5.6)
Coma	3 (2.0)	17 (10.3)	5 (3.3)	6 (3.4)	31 (4.8)
Arthralgia*	6 (3.9)	9 (5.5)	6 (4.0)	6 (3.4)	27 (4.2)
Hemorrhagic diathesis	9 (5.9)	3 (1.8)	8 (5.3)	5 (2.8)	25 (3.9)
Seizures	2 (1.3)	6 (3.6)	6 (4.0)	8 (4.5)	22 (3.4)
Cranial nerve palsies	1 (0.7)	10 (6.1)	3 (2.0)	1 (0.6)	15 (2.3)
Other focal neurologic signs	0 (0)	5 (3.0)	3 (2.0)	3 (1.7)	11 (1.7)

* Only patients aged ≥6 years were considered.
From Barquet N, Domingo P, Caylà JA, *et al.* Meningococcal disease in a large urban population (Barcelona, 1987–1992): Predictors of dismal prognosis. Arch Intern Med 159:2329, 1999.

paramount importance for killing meningococci, since they not only directly damage the bacterial membrane but also improve opsonization and phagocytosis [70]. Patients who have deficits of the terminal factors of the complement exemplify how important it is, and usually present recurrent episodes of meningococcal disease. The possibility of acquiring meningococcal disease increases by up to 6000-fold due to deficiency of one of the terminal complement factors [46]. Only a few cases can be explained by terminal complement factors or properdin deficiency, due to their rarity. Only five cases (1.0%) of 643 patients living in Barcelona diagnosed as having meningococcal disease during 1987–1992 had a complement deficit, this being C7 in three cases and C8 in two others [28].

Once *N. meningitidis* has been able to survive and eventually multiply within the bloodstream, it may reach the blood-brain barrier and cross it. However, the pathogenic events underlying the development of meningococcal meningitis are beyond the scope of this chapter and will be discussed in the chapter devoted to bacterial meningitis.

Common complications of meningococcemia are vascular collapse and shock and coagulation disorders ranging from laboratory abnormalities to disseminated intravascular coagulation (DIC) [71]. Both complications are primarily due to the effects of meningococcal lipooligosaacharide, which is a potent endotoxin [72]. There are common causal mechanisms for shock and DIC, two interrelated processes which reinforce each other. For example, microvascular thrombosis leads to hypoperfusion (i.e. shock) and shock induces endothelial damage and DIC [20]. Capillary leakage, inappropriate vascular tone, intravascular microthrombi, and myocardial dysfunction cause shock. DIC and myocardial depression further aggravate the state of shock. Its effects are mediated by TNF-α, IL-1 and IL-6 and by an extensive complement activation, and all these mediators may contribute to the multiple-organ failure and death occurring in the most severe cases [73, 74]. Cytokines also play a pivotal role in the activation and regulation of the coagulation cascade, which in its most severe form causes overwhelming DIC with the formation of microvascular thrombi in various organs [71].

It has recently been demonstrated that factors intrinsic to the host, such as genetic influences on cytokine production, may contribute to a severe or fatal outcome of meningococcal disease. Among them, death associated with meningococcal disease has been related to a TNF-α gene promoter polymorphism [75], to a low level of TNF production and a high level of IL-10 production *ex vivo* [76], and to a functional insertion/deletion (4G/5G) polymorphism in the promoter region of the plasminogen activator inhibitor (PAI)-1 gene resulting in high levels of PAI-1 in patients with severe meningococcal disease [77, 78]. These findings may constitute a genetic background that modulates the host response to meningococcal infection, and eventually its clinical manifestations and outcome.

Clinical Features and Forms of Meningococcemia

Meningococcal disease is a protean disease, i.e. its clinical manifestations can be quite varied, ranging from transient fever and bacteremia to fulminant disease with death ensuing within hours of the onset of clinically apparent disease [79]. Despite the fact that variations in the clinical manifestations of meningococcal disease can occur, the trained physician has little doubt when facing a case of full-blown meningococcemia, but diagnosis of sporadic cases requires a high index of suspicion and a careful search for clues of the disease. This is particularly true for patients of extreme ages, where subtle symptoms and sings may be the prodrome of overt disease.

Despite the variety of clinical presentations of meningococcal disease, fever and petechiae are usually present. Petechiae are present in 78.2% of patients, independently of the clinical form of the disease [28]. They usually appear as discrete lesions, 1–2 mm in diameter, most frequently on the trunk and lower portions of the body (Figures 4–7). However, in patients with scarce lesions, the mucous surfaces such as the conjunctiva may be the only site affected. Petechiae commonly cluster in areas where pressure may be applied to the skin by elastic underwear or stockings. The initial number and progression of petechiae is important and a simple means to monitor both the evolution of the disease and the effectiveness of therapy. A common practice is to circle areas with petechiae, count those within the circle, and document the number of petechial lesions present per a given unit of time. The counts should be performed hourly early in the disease or until the patient clinically stabilizes.

Petechial rash is not the only cutaneous manifestation of meningococcal disease, and a maculopapular eruption that can resemble a viral exanthem, particularly rubella, has also been described [80]. This rash is neither purpuric nor pruritic and is usually transient, generally not lasting more than two days, and most frequently disappears hours after the first observation. In cases of fulminant meningococcal disease, the skin lesions dominate the clinical appearance and may evidence coalescence of increasing petechiae, septic vasculitis, together with ecchymoses, purpura, and subcutaneous hematomata. Skin hemorrhages are the distinguishing feature par excellence of meningococcal disease and are usually the visual manifestations of DIC (Figures 8 and 9). These cutaneous signs frequently

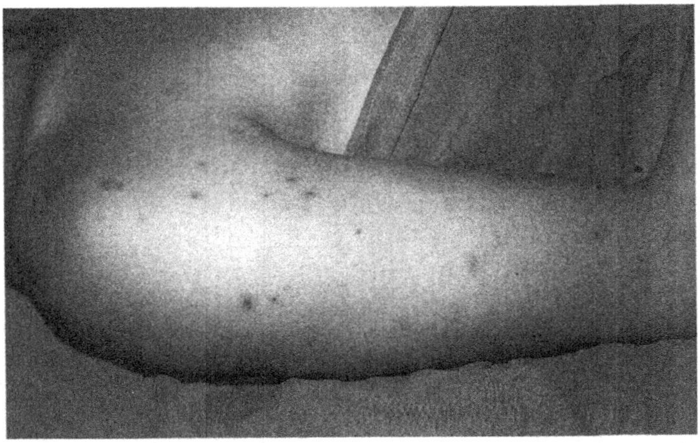

FIGURE 4. Petechiae in the arm of a patient with meningococcemia.

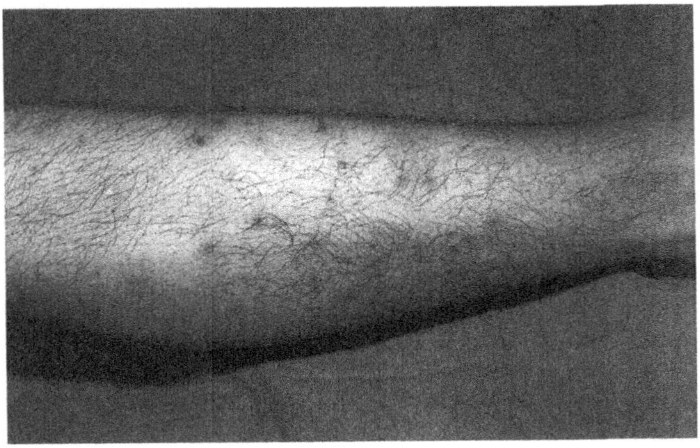

FIGURE 5. Petechiae in the leg of a patient with meningococcemia.

coexist with other signs of DIC, such as gastric or gingival bleeding, or oozing at the sites of venipuncture, lumbar puncture, arterial access or intravenous infusions. All of these are signs of ominous prognosis [28, 81] and are present characteristically in the fulminant form of meningococcemia, together with a profound endotoxic shock with hemorrhagic destruction of adrenal glands (Waterhouse-Friderichsen syndrome) or peripheral symmetric gangrene (*purpura fulminans*) (Figure 10). DIC is a generalized phenomenon which affects all organs, but the adrenals are especially vulnerable [82]. Adrenal hemorrhages can cause adrenal insufficiency [83]. However, the intracerebral vessels are spared during fluminant meningococcemia [20].

The fulminant form of meningococcal disease, defined as interval of symptoms to therapy lower than 7 hours and shock on hospital admission, affects 3.9–5.3% of patients [28, 81]. When present, shock dominates the clinical picture, with a poorly responsive patient, intense peripheral vasoconstriction and cyanotic and poorly perfused extremities. Blood analyses demonstrate metabolic acidosis and usually hypoxia. A very important prognostic sign is myocardial involvement that manifests itself by the presence of gallop rhythm, congestive cardiac failure with pulmonary edema and poor peripheral perfusion [84]. Some degree of myocarditis has been demonstrated in more than half of the patients who die of meningococcal disease [85, 86]. Another frequent complaint in meningococcemia is generalized muscle tenderness, sometimes with very intense pain, that can be an important differential sign [79].

Wolfe and Birbara have distinguished four clinical situations in meningococcal disease: bacteremia without sepsis, meningococcemia without meningitis, meningitis with or without meningococcemia, and the meningoencephalitic presentation [87]. The latter two clinical forms will be discussed in the chapter devoted to bacterial meningitis (see pages 421–434). Benign, occult or inapparent meningococcemia is caused by a low-degree bacteremia, ranging from 22 to 325 organisms per milliliter, from a primary upper respiratory source [88]. In fact, the patient or parent seeks medical attention because of an

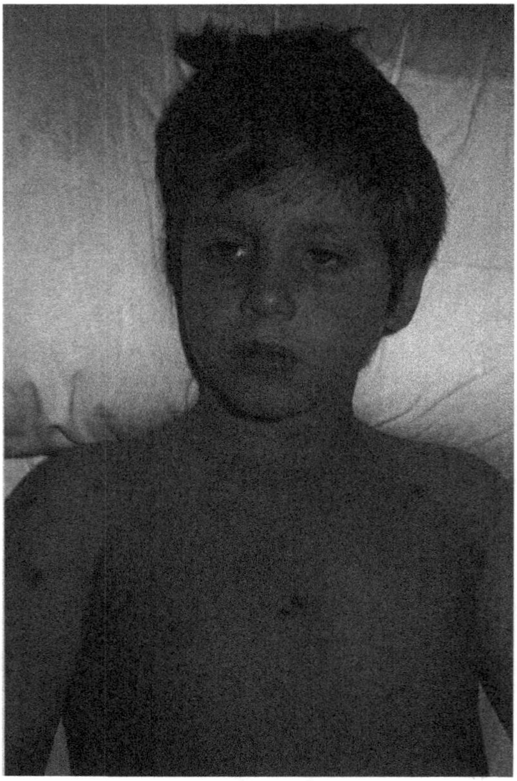

FIGURE 6. Purpuric lesions in a young child with meningococcemia.

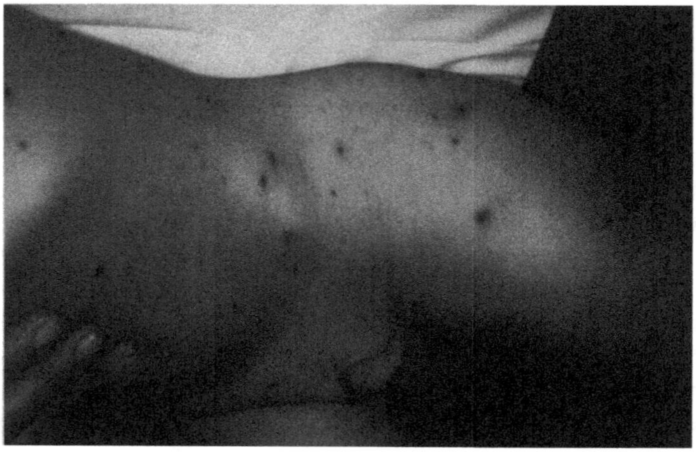

FIGURE 7. Septic vasculitis in a patient with meningococcemia.

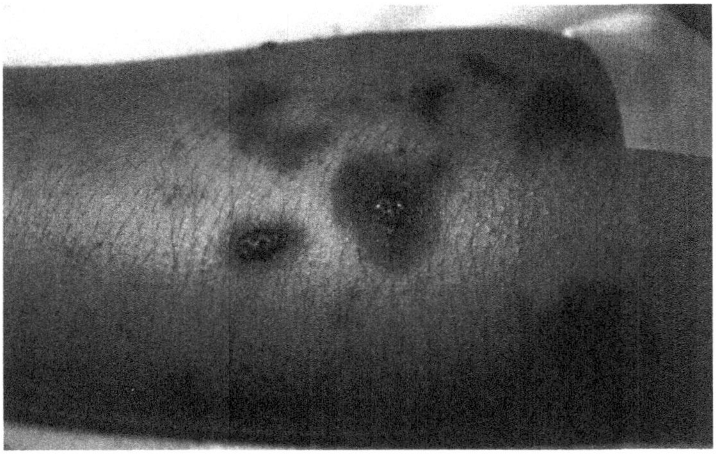

FIGURE 8. Subcutaneous ecchymosis in a patient with fulminant meningococcemia.

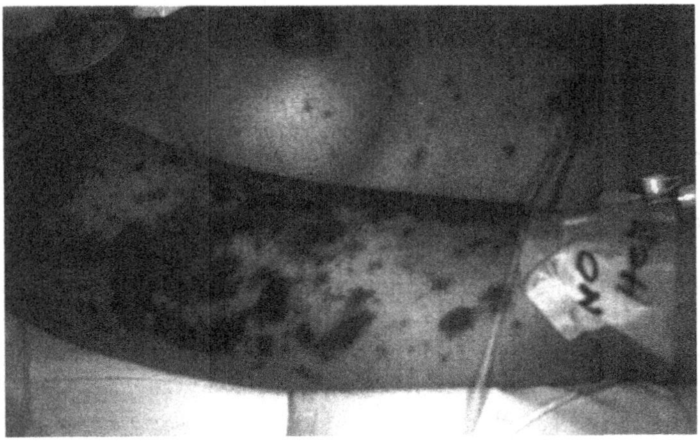

FIGURE 9. Extensive ecchymosis in a patient with fulminant meningococcemia and disseminated intravascular coagulation.

upper respiratory illness or rash of presumed viral origin [28]. After recovery, or more frequently after discharge from the hospital without specific antimicrobial therapy, the results of blood cultures are reported positive for *N. meningitidis*. This from of meningococcal disease accounts for 2% of the total number of cases [28]. When isolated meningococcemia or meningococcemia without meningitis is present, the patient looks septic, usually with a skin rash, generalized malaise, weakness, headache, and muscle tenderness. Frequently hypotension appears on admission or shortly thereafter. Isolated meningococcemia represent around 23.6% of the total cases of meningococcal disease [28]. When meningococcemia occurs in the setting of meningococcal meningitis, symptoms and signs attributable to meningitis usually dominate the clinical picture. Finally, variations of manifestations may occur, and the patient can progress from one to the other form during the course of the disease.

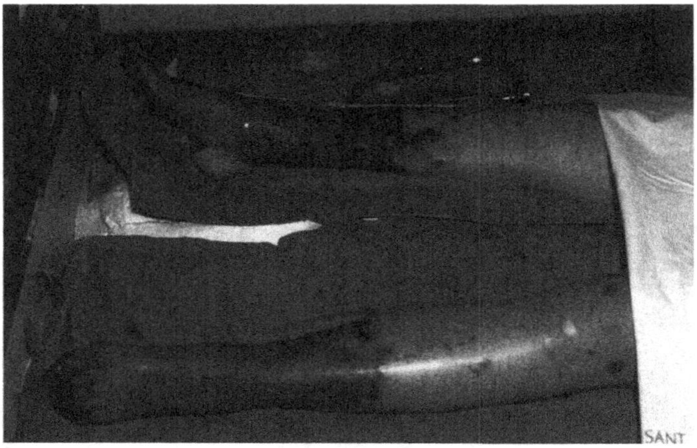

FIGURE 10. Symmetric peripheral gangrene in *purpura fulminans.*

A specific and infrequent form of meningococcal disease called chronic meningococcemia, that is characterized by low-grade fever, rash, and arthritis, is also known [89, 90]. From a clinical point of view, the cutaneous lesions are identical to those seen in chronic gonococcemia, and *N. meningitidis* is thought to be increasing as a cause of the arthritis-dermatitis syndrome [91]. In patients with repeated flares of meningococcemia, complement deficiencies must be ruled out [46]. Although a primary focus for meningococcemia is seldom found, a portal of entry can sometimes be identified. The most frequent are the conjunctiva, and the lung [92, 93].

Diagnosis

Early diagnosis and immediate recognition of deterioration are of crucial importance because meningococcal disease can be fatal within a few hours. The clinical diagnosis of meningococcal disease does not usually pose many problems for an experienced physician from an endemic area when faced with a characteristic case. However, in some cases, early diagnosis of meningococcemia is extremely difficult and requires a high degree of suspicion [94, 95].

The hallmarks for the clinical diagnosis of meningococcal disease are the presence of fever and petechiae, and they form the basis for the criteria of the Meningococcal Disease Surveillance Group to establish a clinical diagnosis of meningococcal disease [96]. Following its criteria, a patient can be diagnosed as having meningococcal disease when having an illness with fever and petechiae, diagnosed as meningococcal disease by the local physician, even if there is no blood or cerebrospinal fluid (CSF) isolate of *N. meningitidis*. In Western Europe there are only a few diseases that may resemble meningococcals disease. Among them, viral illnesses, bacteremia caused by *Haemophilus influenzae*, *Streptococcus pneumoniae* and other Gram-positive cocci, rickettsiosis, and autoimmune purpuras may cause a rash that can simulate meningococcal disease. In North America, rickettsiosis of the Rocky Mountain spotted fever group may pose a greater diagnostic dilemma. Furthermore, only 78% of the patients with meningococcal disease will present an identifiable rash, and in those cases in which there are no cutaneous signs, the clinical presentation is entirely indistinguishable from other bacteremic diseases, and these patients are more prone not to be identified when they first seek medical attention [28].

Twelve per cent of patients diagnosed as having meningococcal disease in Barcelona from

1987 to 1992 had been seen by a hospital physician but were sent home from the emergency service with erroneous diagnostic of upper respiratory tract infection or viral illness. Meningococcal disease was only diagnosed in a subsequent visit [28].

A definite diagnosis of meningococcal disease needs isolation and identification of *N. meningitidis* from a usually sterile body fluid such as blood, CSF, or rarely synovial, pleural or pericardial fluids. Obviously, the CSF and blood are the most fruitful sources of positive cultures. In our experience, blood cultures were positive in 47.0% of cases [28], whereas in the experience of others they were positive in 51.4% of the cases [97]. However, even in patients who do not have clinical meningitis, *N. meningitidis* can be recovered from a CSF culture, and CSF is otherwise normal in terms of protein and glucose contents and cellular count [98]. Another possible source of meningococci, although with a variable ability to isolate *N. meningitidis*, is the petechial skin or mucosal lesions. Some authors have reported isolation in 69.8% of petechial smears, but once again interpretation of these specimens may be difficult [97].

Throat swabs play a limited role in the diagnosis of meningococcal disease, since a third of young adults carry meningococci, and thus isolation of a meningococcus from a young adult with meningococcemia is uninformative. However, meningococci are rarely carried by infants and young children (1–4%), and therefore isolation of a well–capsulated meningococcus from such a patient with meningococcemia may be valid [99]. Rapid methods for microbiologic diagnosis, such as Gram stain, detection of meningococcal antigens by means of counterimmunoelectrophoresis, latex agglutination, and coagglutination, and the polymerase chain reaction, have been useful for the diagnosis of meningococcal meningitis, but their use in an environment of meningococcemia has yet to be determined.

A percentage of patients with meningococcal disease ranging from 35.2%–43.7% have received antibiotics prior to hospital admission [28, 81]. These patients, that can still be diagnosed as having meningococcal disease if they fulfill the criteria established by the Meningococcal Disease Surveillance Group [96], will have in a greater proportion no positive microbiologic data to support the diagnosis. Meningococcal disease without microbiologic proof represents 27.4% of the total number of patients with the disease [28]. In these patients, methods such as those that look for bacterial antigens or bacterial DNA may play a diagnostic role.

Management of Meningococcemia

Although significant advances in the treatment of meningococcal disease were made early in the twentieth century by means of serum therapy from immunized horses [100, 101], the introduction of sulfonamides by Schwentker *et al.* in 1937 [102], and penicillin in 1944 by Rosenberg and Arling [103] dramatically altered the previously ominous prognosis of meningococcal disease. However, sulfonamides play a very limited role in the treatment of meningococcal disease since meningococci became widely resistant to sulfonamides early in the 1960s [104]. Antibiotics are the cornerstone of treatment. It is necessary to begin antibiotic therapy as soon as possible, and this should never be delayed by diagnostic procedures. Therapy should be extended to include immediate fluid resuscitation, prompt beginning of mechanical ventilation, and transfer to a suitably equipped ICU in patients with poor prognostic signs or imminent shock [20]. The usual doses of the most common antibiotics used in the treatment of meningococcal disease are expressed in Table 3.

Penicillin has for decades been the treatment of choice for meningococcal disease. However, since the mid 1980s, there has been an increasing frequency of isolation of meningococcal strains with decreased susceptibility to penicillin, mainly from Spain [105], the United Kingdom [106], and South Africa [107]. In Spain, the prevalence of meningococcal strains

TABLE 3. Antibiotics used in the treatment and chemoprophylaxis of meningococcal disease

Meningococcemia treatment	
Non penicillin-allergic	Penicillin G Na
	Adults: 300,000 units/kg/day IV, up to 24 million units/day
	Ceftriaxone
	Adults: 100 mg/kg/day IV, up to 4 g/day
	Cefotaxime
	Adults: 200 mg/kg/day IV, up to 12 g/day
Penicillin-allergic	Chloramphenicol
	Adults: 100 mg/kg/day IV, up to 4 g/day
	Aztreonam
	Adults: 100–150 mg/kg/day IV, up to 12 g/day
Chemoprophylaxis	
	Rifampin
	Adults: 600 mg/12 h PO, for 2 days
	Children >1 month: 10 mg/kg/12 h PO, for 2 days
	Children <1 month: 5 mg/kg/12 h PO, for 2 days
	Ceftriaxone
	Adults: 250 mg IM, single dose
	Children <15 years: 125 mg IM, single dose
	Ciprofloxacin
	Adults: 500 mg PO, single dose
	Ofloxacin
	Adults: 400 mg PO, single dose
	Minocicline
	Adults: 100 mg/12 h PO, for 5 days
	Spiramycin
	Adults: 500 mg/6 h PO, for 5 days
	Children: 10 mg/kg/6 h PO, for 5 days

relatively resistant to penicillin rose from the mid 1980s to a maximum of 43.2% in 1990 and 70.0% in 1997 (Figure 11) [105]. Since then, these figures have stabilized at around 25% of strains. This reduced sensitivity is due to a reduced affinity to penicillin binding protein type 2 [105]. Penicillin resistance due to plasmid-related β-lactamase production occasionally occurs [108]. Although the present rate of partially resistant strains has potential implications for empiric therapy of bacterial meningitis, it probably should not affect penicillin-based therapeutic strategies of meningococcemia. Standard doses of penicillin (i.e., 250,000 units/kg/day) will provide an adequate serum level, that usually surpasses the MIC for partially resistant isolates by many times [109]. Thus, penicillin can still be used safely in the treatment of meningococcemia. The usual recommended dose of penicillin is 300,000 units/kg/day with an upper limit of 24 million units/day as two million units q2h.

Notwithstanding the fact that penicillin or chloramphenicol therapy may by successful, it does not eradicate the meningococcus from the nasopharynx [110], and thus patients treated with penicillin or chloramphenicol should be given rifampin chemoprophylaxis before discharge from the hospital to prevent reentry of the pathogenic *N. meningitidis* strain into the household or another group of which the patient forms part [111, 112]. It has, however, been shown that on discharge from hospital only 1% of patients were nasopharyngeal carriers of pathogenic meningococci [110, 113, 114]. With indiscriminate chemoprophylaxis it is possible

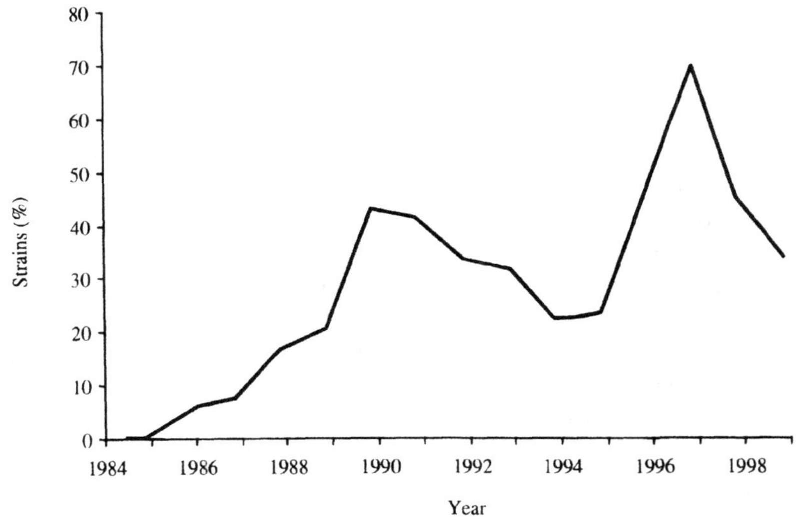

FIGURE 11. Prevalence of decreased susceptibility to penicillin *Neisseria meningitidis* strains isolated in Spain (1987–1994).

to sterilize the nasopharynx in the absence of pathogenic strains of meningococcus and to eliminate the nonpathogenic strains of *Neisseria* or of other nonpathogenic germs which compete with *N. meningitidis* for the colonization of the nasopharynx. Non-selective chemoprophylaxis prevents the protective immunological response by means of crossed reactivity and allows the colonization *de novo* of pathogenic *N. meningitidis* strains. It is therefore recommended to proceed with selective chemoprophylaxis which consists of carrying out a nasopharyngeal exudate culture, having obtained the sample by smear, and only carrying out chemoprophylaxis in the event of detecting the presence of pathogenic meningococcal strains.

Third-generation cephalosporins are increasingly used in the empirical treament of bacterial meningitis and meningococcal disease due to a better coverage of all possible etiologies of bacterial meningitis and because of the fear of resistance. Third-generation cephalosporins, including cefotaxime, ceftriaxone, ceftizoxime, and ceftazidime and the second-generation cefuroxime have been successfully used for the treatment of meningococcal meningitis [115–117]. For patients who are allergic to penicillin, aztreonam may be a safe alternative. Also, for patients allergic to penicillin, chloramphenicol at a dose of 100 mg/kg/day up to a maximum of 4 g/day administered intravenously may be an effective substitute for penicillin and in Third World countries it can be administered in its depot formulation by intramuscular route. The duration of antibiotic therapy will vary, but usually seven days is enough when the meningococcus is sensitive to the antibiotic used.

Recent studies in the United Kingdom have suggested that early administration of parenteral penicillin by general practitioners, as soon as the diagnosis was entertained, significantly improved the prognosis of patients pre-treated in this way [118–123]. Although not intended to demonstrate the ability of preadmission antibiotic therapy to modify the prognosis of meningococcal disease, in a recent study preadmission antibiotic therapy was an independent predictor of a better outcome in a large series of patients with meningococcal disease [81].

The most common and important manifestation requiring urgent intervention in meningococcal disease is vascular collapse and shock. This occurs in 12.1% of all the cases of meningococcal disease and is far more frequent in isolated meningococcemia than when there is concomitant meningitis [28]. For the first few hours, it is necessary to monitor patients closely as shock can develop after starting antibiotic therapy [124]. It should be taken into account that monitoring the systolic blood pressure in children is not sufficient to trace the development of shock. Low diastolic blood pressure, delayed capillary refill, cold extremities, and tachycardia are better indicators [20]. Good clinical surveillance and frequent laboratory monitoring are crucial. For example, on observing an increase in the number and size of skin hemorrhages and a decrease in the platelet count, it is easy to monitor the progression of DIC [20, 125].

Patients with fulminant form of meningococcal disease characteristically have a severe capillary leak syndrome together with myocardial dysfunction. Thus, supportive care should include optimizing preload, decreasing afterload, and improving myocardial contractility. All of this is best accomplished in the ICU setting. Intravenous fluid administration should be implemented, together with inotropic and vasopressive support with dobutamine or dopamine, tailored to the needs of each patient on the basis of clinical assessment and of monitoring of systemic arterial pressure and central venous pressure or pulmonary wedge pressure [126–129]. During the first 24 hours, administration of 8–10 liters of intravenous fluid may be necessary. The severity of shock has been correlated by various studies with serum levels of TNF-α, IL-1, IL-6, and lipo-oligosaccharide [73, 130, 131]. These findings and the encouraging results obtained in animal models have suggested that treatment with monoclonal antibodies against some of the cytokines or the endotoxin could be of use in humans [132–135]. However, the results of clinical trails in humans have been less promising and a number of them are still in progress [136, 137].

The use of glucocorticoids in the treatment of meningococcemia in patients with evidence of *purpura fulminans* and adrenal hemorrhagic necrosis (Waterhouse-Friderichsen syndrome) is still controversial [138, 139]. Several controlled studies of patients with shock have demonstrated no benefit of high-dose glucocorticoid treatment. However, in many acute care hospitals glucocorticoids belong to the standard treatment protocol of fulminant meningococcemia with extensive DIC and shock or suspicion of Waterhouse-Friderichsen syndrome [20]. Some patients with meningococcemia have a profound respiratory failure, and in this case and in those who have received high amounts of intravenous fluid and those in which profound shock has occurred, mechanical ventilation should be started immediately [140].

The problem of DIC is particularly ominous and its presence is an independent predictor of death [28, 81]. As shock and DIC are interrelated processes, the only successful treatment of DIC is the therapy against shock. The routine use of heparin has not improved the prognosis of DIC. Endovascular thrombosis, ischemia, and imminent autoamputation may, however, lead to additional treatment. Heparin therapy has been suggested for this purpose [141, 142]. Patients with impending peripheral gangrene (Figure 10) and severe coagulopathy should be treated with low-dose heparin (10 units/kg/hour) together with fresh frozen plasma with the aim of restoring depleted levels of antithrombin III, protein C, and protein S. Other proposed therapies in patients with severe meningococcemia have been recombinant aminoterminal fragment of human bactericidal/permeability-increasing protein, protein C concentrate and heparin and antithrombin III [141]. Other heroic measures such as extracorporeal membrane oxygenation [143], hemofiltration [142, 144] and plasma or whole-blood exchange with or without leukapheresis [145–148], have been tried in a few cases of fulminant and refractory meningococcemia with variable results. In order to restore perfusion to pregangrenous limbs, thrombolytic therapy offers the best hope, and there are

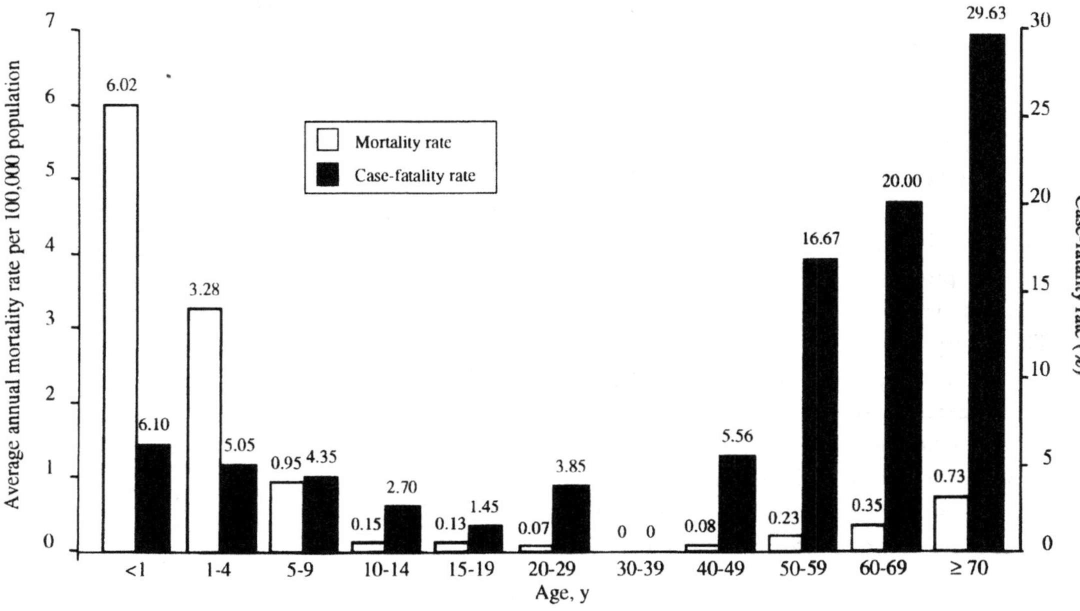

FIGURE 12. Meningococcal disease in Barcelona (1987–1992): Average annual mortality rate and case-fatality rate by age group (cases detected by active surveillance).

anecdotal reports of the beneficial effects of recombinant tissue plasminogen activator [128, 149, 150].

Metabolic acidosis as a result of poor tissue perfusion in shock may appear, and serum electrolytes and acid-base balance may be monitored closely and abnormalities corrected immediately. Correction is often hampered by acute renal failure, and thus continuous plasma filtration or dialysis may be necessary in anuria due to acute tubular necrosis or cortical necrosis associated with meningococcal septic shock [151]. Alkalinization is recommended in patients with severe rhabdomyolisis in order to prevent myoglobin-induced renal failure [20].

Outcome and Prognosis

Despite adequate antibiotic therapy and supportive care, meningococcal disease causes an overall mortality of 6–15% of patients [16, 28, 152, 153]. Still today meningococcal disease is the third cause of death in children, only surpassed by casual injuries and malignant diseases. In Barcelona, over six years, meningococcal disease caused the loss of 1842 potential years of life (average annual, 18 per 100,000 inhabitants) [28]. In this study performed in Barcelona by active surveillance systems from 1987 to 1992, the average annual mortality rate was 0.40 per 100,000 and among children under 10 years was 2.23 per 100,000 (Figure 12) [28]. Multiple-organ failure is the most frequent cause of death (65.0–76.5% of deaths), followed by cerebral edema (13.7–25.0%), and myocarditis (9.8–10.0%) [28, 81].

Meningococcemia is the clinical form of meningococcal disease with the highest case-fatality rate (11.2%), and with fulminant meningococcemia this is 43.8–44.0% of patients [28, 81]. There is rapid clinical deterioration, and approximately half of the patients who die will do so within 24 hours of the appearance of the first symptoms. A third of the patients with fatal meningococcal disease die within six hours of hospital admission and another third die between six and 18 hours [20, 154, 155]. Death at a later stage is still determined by the course in the early hours, as shown by the fact that the main cause of death after 24 hours is withdrawal of treatment because of poor neurological prognosis after prolonged cerebral hypoperfusion in the early hours [156].

The ability to define the outcome of meningococcal disease based on a number of indicators has been extensively studied [155, 157–167]. The Barcelona Meningococcal Disease Surveillance Group recently designed and validated a very simple scoring system that is based entirely on clinical parameters very easy to determine at the patient's bedside. Hemorrhagic diathesis was scored with two points, presence of focal neurologic sings with one point, age of 60 years or older with one point, and preadmission antibiotic therapy was scored as −1. The clinical scores of −1, 0, 1, 2 and 3 or more points were associated with a probability of death of 0%, 2.3%, 27.3%, 73.3%, and 100%, respectively (Table 4). This scoring system was predictive of death in 82.4% of the patients [81]. The probability of death in meningococcal disease related to the presence or absence of predictors of death is shown in Figure 13. Patients with the highest probability of dying were those with hemorrhagic diathesis, whereas those with no predictor of death and who had received preadmission adequate antibiotics had the best prognosis.

TABLE 4. Prognostic factors for patients with meningococcal disease: Bedside clinical parameters for prediction of outcome

Barcelona Meningococcal Disease Surveillance Group Score

Parameter	Points
Preadmission antibiotic therapy	−1
Age, ≥60 y	1
Focal neurologic signs	1
Hemorrhagic diathesis	2

Probability of death according to observed score

Prediction score	Case-fatality rate, %
−1	0
0	2.3
1	27.3
2	73.3
≥3	100

From Barquet N, Domingo P, Caylà JA, *et al.* Prognostic factors in meningococcal disease: Development of a bedside predictive model and scoring system. JAMA 278:491, 1997.

The rate of permanent and disabling sequelae in meningococcemia is 2.6–11% of patients [20, 28, 168]. When they occur they are usually severe, with limb, finger-toe or extremity amputation being the most prevalent. Approximately 15% of cases require extensive skin and peripheral limb necrosis requiring amputation or reconstructive skin surgery [169–171]. Independent predictors of sequelae in patients with meningococcal disease are age over 60 years, the presence of focal neurologic signs on admission to the hospital and the presence of hemorrhagic diathesis, whereas preadmission antibiotic therapy plays a protective role [28]. The clinical factors which independently allow the appearance of sequelae to be predicted are the same as those which allow death to be predicted.

Prevention

It has long been known that household members and day-care centers and school-children contacts of index patients with meningococcal disease have a 50–1000–fold-higher chance of acquiring invasive disease than do members of the general population [111, 172, 173]. Chemoprophylaxis can protect susceptible persons from acquiring meningococcal disease by eliminating meningococci colonization in close contacts. Chemoprophylaxis eradicates *N. meningitidis* from the nasopharynx and should be administered to intimate contacts and also to anyone who has had oral contact with the index case

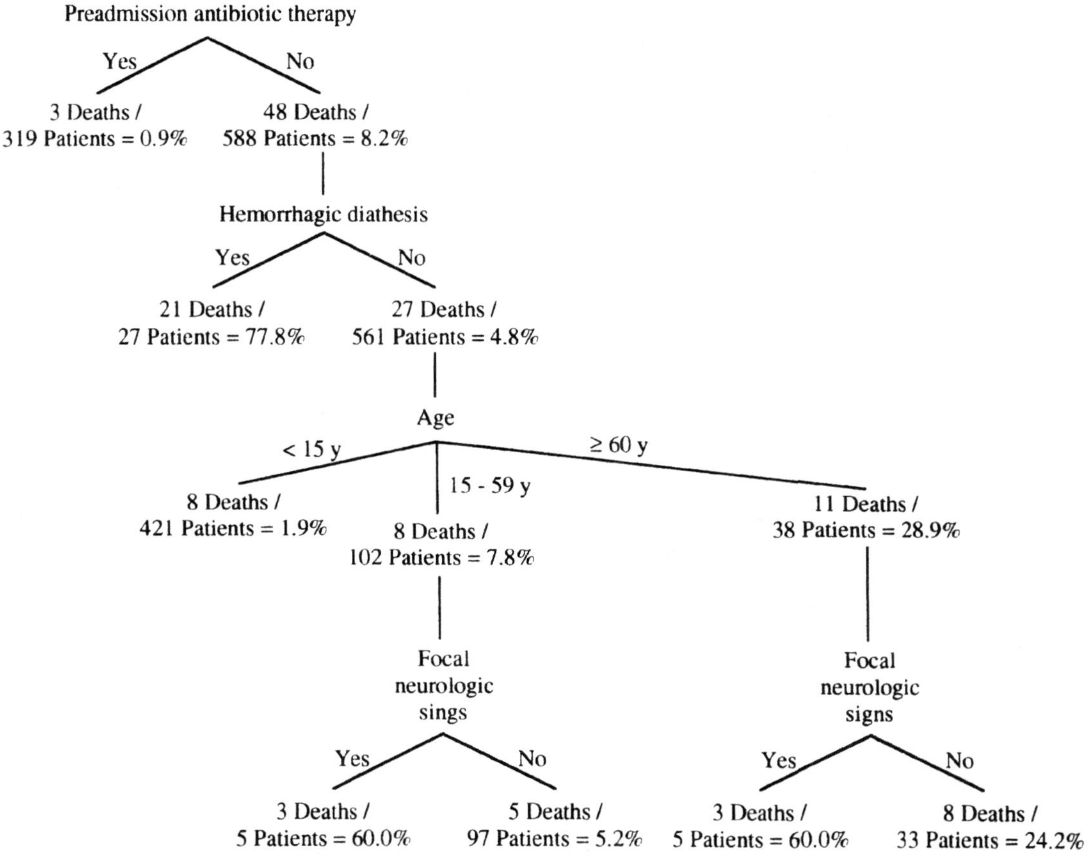

FIGURE 13. Algorithm of probability of death in meningococcal disease related to the presence or absence of predictors of death. The fraction expresses the number of deaths/the number of patients with condition, equal to the case-fatality rate.

(kissing, mouth-to-mouth resuscitation) [66, 174, 175]. Healthcare workers do not have an increased risk if the latter circumstances are excluded and should not be routinely offered chemoprophylaxis.

The antibiotics that are highly effective in eradicating meningococcus from the nasopharynx and the recommended chemoprophylaxis regime are listed in Table 3 [176–179]. Rifampin, which achieves high concentrations in nasopharyngeal and respiratory secretions, is one of the most effective antibiotics for eliminating meningococci from the nasopharynx. Rifampin is contraindicated in pregnant women and is generally well tolerated although it has various side effects, including orange urine, orange staining of contact lenses, stimulation of liver microsomal enzymes, and reduction in levels of other concurrent medications. Ciprofloxacin, ofloxacin, and minocicline are contraindicated in children and in pregnant woman. Ceftriaxone is probably the drug of choice for a pregnant contact [180].

Chemoprophylaxis should be instituted as soon as possible because the risk of secondary case is greatest during the first days after onset of disease in the index case. Chemoprophylaxis usually fail if given too late, to the inadequate person, because of meningococci resistance to the antibiotic administrated or due to incorrect dose or interval [181]. Physicians should not obtain nasopharyngeal cultures to determine whether or not to administer prophylaxis, this only delays prompt chemoprophylaxis. Selective chemoprophylaxis is only indicated in patients with meningococcal disease treated with penicillin or chloramphenicol.

Chemoprophylaxis is further limited as it does not prevent reintroduction of the pathogenic *N. meningitidis* strain from a carrier outside the group, and late secondary cases still therefore occur [182].

Immunization of contacts may be useful in order to prevent secondary cases as a supplement to chemoprophylaxis of household members, and day-care centers, school-children and another contacts of index cases of meningococcal disease caused by the serogroups carried by vaccine [183]. About 40% of secondary cases may occur five or more days after presentation of the index cases.

Due to the fact that half of secondary cases in household members develop within 24 hours in children under 15 years, the Norwegian health authorities advise treating these possible coprimary cases with phenoxymethyl-penicillin for one week [184–186]. The preventive treatment with penicillin has considerably reduced the number of coprimary fatalities in families [20].

Respiratory isolation of patients with meningococcal disease is recommended for the first 24 hours of admission to hospital. In all situations in which there is potential for secondary case, this risk must be explained to families and it is absolutely essential to educate contacts in relation to the need to seek immediate medical attention if they develop signs or symptoms of a febrile illness. No prophylactic strategy is 100 per cent effective, and ill contacts should therefore be evaluated with a high suspicion of meningococcal disease [180].

In view of the fact that the protection offered by vaccination is not immediate, and the limited value of chemoprophylaxis in the prevention of secondary cases, early diagnosis and prompt appropriate treatment are still the only ways to reduce morbidity and mortality [180].

Meningococcal disease only occurs in patients devoid of specific bactericidal or opsonizing antibodies. The best way to prevent meningococcal disease is therefore to use vaccination to induce these antibodies. Primary prevention is crucial for many reasons. For example, the presentation may be fulminant, with antibiotics being unable to influence the course of the disease. Antibiotic-resistant strains have now been discovered, and chemoprophylaxis of contacts is a difficult and often ineffective public health measure. Mass immunization is essential to help prevent both endemic and epidemic meningococcal disease world-wide [180].

The currently available A/C bivalent and A/C/Y/W135 tetravalent meningococcal unconjugate vaccines contain purified preparations of the specific capsular polysaccharide antigens of these two or four serogroups [187, 188]. These meningococcal unconjugated polysaccharide vaccines induce a T cell-independent immune response which is age-dependent, this being its main limitation: scarce immune response in children under 18 months old and, consequently, deficient protection in the age group at most risk of acquiring meningococcal disease; non-lasting protection, and a scarce antibody response to booster doses of serogroup C meningococcal vaccine [189, 190]. Administration of these vaccines does not therefore tend to be recommended for children under 18 months old. However, in people over this age they induce effective protection, having been extraordinarily useful to combat numerous epidemics and outbreaks of meningococcal disease caused by serogroups A and C [191–198].

The administration of meningococcal unconjugated polysaccharide vaccines (A/C or A/C/Y/W135) is indicated in the following situations: epidemics and outbreaks of meningococcal disease caused by the serogroups carried by vaccine; groups at high risk of acquiring meningococcal disease (individuals with functional or anatomic asplenia and persons with complement or properdin deficiencies); travelers who are visiting areas or countries with a high incidence of meningococcal disease; day-care center contacts, school children contacts and household members of an index case of meningococcal disease as an adjunct to antibiotic chemoprophylaxis; military training camps [199].

Polysaccharides are T cell-independent antigens and consequently induce an immune response through the direct presentation of the antigen and the activation of the B-cells without the intervention of the T-cells. In children under 18 months old this produces a response predominantly of IgM antibodies of little intensity and scarce duration and does not establish immune memory. The B-cells of this age group are in an insufficient stage of maturity to trigger an adequate immune response without the collaboration of the T-cells [200].

To obtain an effective response in children under 18 months old it is necessary to combine the capsular polysaccharides with a conveying protein, which grants them the characteristics of a T-cell-dependent antigen. The immune response then involves the stimulation of the T-cells which activate the B-cells by means of soluble factors. This allows an early production of long-lasting IgG antibodies, and the establishment of immune memory which is demonstrated by a marked strengthening effect after revaccination [199].

In order to overcome the lack of adequate immunogenicity of meningococcal unconjugated polysaccharide vaccines in infants, several C and A/C meningococcal protein-polysaccharide conjugate vaccines have been developed and are being evaluated in clinical trials. These vaccines have already demonstrated their ability to induce immunological memory and greater effectiveness in children under 18 months old, thus offering protection to the age group most in need of protection against meningococcal disease [201, 202]. The A/C meningococcal protein-polysaccharide conjugate vaccines are differentiated by the conveying protein (e.g. tetanic toxoid, bovine albumin, diphtheric toxoid CRM197), by the structure and length of the polysaccharide, by the method linking the protein to the polysaccharide which can be in a direct covalent manner or with an additional molecule and by the protein/polysaccharide ratio [199]. Research is currently being carried out into the value of these newly developed conjugated vaccines in mass vaccination.

The lack of activity against group B meningococci is the main disadvantage of the vaccines currently available in Western Europe. It has not been possible to develop serogroup B polysaccharide vaccines, because the specific capsular polysaccharide of serogroup B induces a weak immune response [200]. This polysaccharide is a 200-residue $\alpha(2 \rightarrow 8)$ homopolymer of *N*-acetilneuraminic acid and bears an extraordinary resemblance to the human neuronal cell adhesion molecule [203]. It is considered that this resemblance could be responsible for the scarce immunogenicity, due to a phenomenon of immunological tolerance. Given that the attempts to increase the tolerance for own antigens entails the risk of inducing autoimmunity, most research aimed at obtaining a vaccine against serogroup B concentrates on non-capsular antigens [199].

The disappointing immunogenic behavior of the specific capsular polysaccharide of serogroup B has not only been demonstrated in those vaccinated but also in patients surviving a recent episode of serogroup B meningococcal disease and in the nasopharyngeal carriers of strains of meningococcus of this serogroup. In all of them it is not possible to find plasmatic concentrations of antibodies aimed at the specific capsular polysaccharide of serogroup B.

A new approach is to use a conjugated chemically modified serogroup B polysaccharide capsule where the *N*-acetyl group has been replaced by the *N*-propionyl group [204]. Promising alternatives include the surface-exposed outer membrane proteins, iron regulating proteins and lipo-oligosaccharides. A B/C meningococcal vaccine, consisting of a mixture mainly of outer membrane proteins from serogroup B meningococci and capsular polysaccharide from serogroup C, was developed in Cuba. Different success rates were obtained from large-scale trials in Chile, Cuba and Brazil [205–209]. The vaccine effectiveness varied extraordinarily with age, being scarcely effective in children under four years old and ineffective under two years old.

A vaccine based on outer membrane proteins of a strain of serogroup B *N. meningitidis* was elaborated in Norway. The results of the clinical trial were so discouraging that it was concluded that the protection was insufficient to justify its inclusion in a systematic vaccination program [210]. A recent trial in the United Kingdom and the Netherlands with a Dutch outer membrane protein vaccine offered promising results [211, 212]. A nasal vaccine, consisting of outer membrane vesicles from serogroup B *N. meningitidis*, may induce systemic and local mucosal immune responses and offers protection against meningococcal disease in humans [213–215].

Current research into meningococcal vaccines is aimed at improving the immunogenicity of the capsular polysaccharides by conjugation with different types of proteins or using other components of the bacterial surface as antigens, such as outer membrane proteins, iron regulating proteins, lipo-oligosaccharides, pili, exotoxins, IgA proteases and nucleic acids [180]. The final objective is to obtain a polyvalent meningococcal vaccine, preferably for intranasal administration, which is highly effective and safe in all age groups, and which offers protection against all the serogroups of *N. meningitidis* which cause meningococcal disease.

References

1. Apicella MA. *Neisseria meningitidis*. In Mandell GL, Bennett JE, Dolin R (eds). Mandell, Douglas, and Bennett's Principles and Practice of Infectious Diseases. 5th edn, Vol. 2, Philadelphia: Churchill Livingstone, 2000: 2228.
2. Knapp JS, Rice RJ. *Neisseria* and *Branhamella*. In Murray PR, Baron EJ, Pfaller MA, Tenover FC, Yolken RH (eds). Manual of Clinical Microbiology. 6th edn, Washington, DC: American Society for Microbiology Press, 1995: 324.
3. Frasch CE, Zollinger WD, Poolman JT. Serotype antigens of *Neisseria meningitidis* and a proposed scheme for designation of serotypes. Rev Infect Dis 7:504, 1985.
4. Broud DD, Griffiss JM, Baker CJ. Heterogenity of serotypes of *Neisseria meningitidis* that cause endemic disease. J Infect Dis 140:465, 1979.
5. Mandrell RE, Zollinger WD. Lipopolysaccharide serotyping of *Neisseria meningitidis* by hemagglutination inhibition. Infect Immun 16:471, 1977.
6. Jennings HL, Johnson KG, Kenne L. The structure of the R-type oligosaccharide core obtained from some lipopolysaccharides of *Neisseria meningitidis*. Carbohydrate Res 121:233, 1983.
7. Gamian A, Beurret M, Michon F, *et al*. Structure of the L2 lipopolysaccharide core oligosaccharides of *Neisseria meningitidis*. J Biol Chem 267:922, 1992.
8. Scholten RJ, Kuipers B, Vankenburg A, Dankert J, Zollinger WD, Poolman JT. Lipo-oligosaccharide immunotyping of *Neisseria meningitidis* by a whole-cell ELISA with monoclonal antibodies. J Med Microbiol 41:236, 1994.
9. Stephens DS, Whitney AM, Rothbard J, Schoolnik GK. Pili of *Neisseria meningitidis*: analysis of structure and investigation of structural and antigenic relationship to gonococcal pili. J Exp Med 161:1539, 1985.
10. Caugant DA. Population genetics and molecular epidemiology of *Neisseria meningitidis*. APMIS 106:505, 1998.
11. Selander RK, Caugant DA, Ochman H, *et al*. Methods of multilocus enzyme electrophoresis for bacterial populations genetics and systematics. Appl Environ Microbiol 132:2855, 1986.
12. Fox AJ, Jones DM, Gray SJ, Caugant DA, Saunders NA. An epidemiologically valuable typing method for *Neisseria meningitidis* by analysis of restriction fragment length polymorphisms. J Med Microbiol 34:265, 1991.
13. Bjorvatn B, Hassan-King B, Greenwood B, Haimanot RT, Fekade D, Sperber G. DNA fingerprinting in the epidemiology of African serogroup A *Neisseria meningitidis*. Scand J Infect Dis 24:323, 1992.

14. Woods JP, Kersulyte D, Tolan RW Jr, Berg CM, Berg DE. Use of arbitrarily primed polymerase chain reaction analysis to type disease and carrier strains of *Neisseria meningitidis* isolated during a university outbreak. J Infect Dis 169: 1384, 1994.
15. Diaz PS. The epidemiology and control of invasive meningococcal disease. Pediatr Infect Dis J 18:633, 1999.
16. Peltola H. Meningococcal disease: still with us. Rev Infect Dis 5:71, 1983.
17. Achtman M. Global epidemiology of meningococcal disease. In Cartwright K (ed). Meningococcal disease. Chichester: John Wiley & Sons, 1995: 159.
18. Lapeyssonnie L. La méningite cerebro-spinale en Afrique. Bull World Health Organ 28 Suppl:1, 1963.
19. Moore PS. Meningococcal meningitis in subsaharan Africa: a model for epidemic process. Clin Infect Dis 14:515, 1992.
20. van Deuren M, Brandtzaeg P, van der Meer JW. Update on meningococcal disease with emphasis on pathogenesis and clinical management. Clin Microbiol Rev 13:144, 2000.
21. Moore PS, Reeves MW, Schwartz B, Gellin BG, Broome CV. Intercontinental spread of an epidemic group A *Neisseria meningitidis* strain. Lancet ii:260, 1989.
22. Zhu P, Hu X, Xu L. Typing *Neisseria meningitidis* by analysis of restriction fragment length polymorphisms in the gene encoding the class 1 outer membrane protein: application to assessment of epidemics throughout the last 4 decades in China. J Clin Microbiol 33:458, 1995.
23. Guibourdenche M, Høiby, Riou JY, Varaine F, Joguet C, Caugant DA. Epidemics of serogroup A *Neisseria meningitidis* of subgroup III in Africa, 1989–94. Epidemiol Infect 116:115, 1996.
24. McGee L, Koornhof HJ, Caugant DA. Epidemic spread of subgroup III of *Neisseria meningitidis* serogroup A to South Africa in 1996. Clin Infect Dis 27:1214, 1998.
25. Moore PS, Harrison LH, Telzak EE, Ajello GW, Broome CV. Group A meningococcal carriage in travelers returning from Saudi Arabia. JAMA 260:2686, 1988.
26. Stephens DS. Uncloacking the meningococcus: dynamics of carriage and disease. Lancet 353: 941, 1999.
27. Jones D. Epidemiology of meningococcal disease in Europe and the USA. In Cartwright K (ed). Meningococcal disease. Chichester: John Wiley & Sons, 1995: 147.
28. Barquet N, Domingo P, Caylà JA, *et al.* Meningococcal disease in a large urban population (Barcelona, 1987–1992): predictors of dismal prognosis. Arch Intern Med 159:2329, 1999.
29. Schwartz B, Moore PS, Broome CV. Global epidemiology of meningococcal disease. Clin Microbiol Rev 2 Suppl:S118, 1989.
30. Osler W. Special discussion on the epidemiology of cerebrospinal meningitis. Proc Roy Soc Med 8:41, 1915.
31. Goldschneider I, Gotschlich EC, Artenstein MS. Human immunity to the meningococcus: I. The role of humoral antibodies. J Exp Med 129:1307, 1969.
32. Bevanger L, Bergh K, Gisnås G, Caugant DA, Frøholm LO. Identification of nasopharyngeal carriage of an outbreak strain of *Neisseria meningitidis* by pulsed-field gel electrophoresis versus phenotypic methods. J Med Microbiol 47:993, 1998.
33. Cartwright KA, Stuart JM, Jones DM, Noah ND. The Stonehouse survey: nasopharyngeal carriage of meningococci and *Neisseria lactamica*. Epidemiol Infect 99:591, 1987.
34. Caugant DA, Høiby EA, Magnus P, *et al.* Asymptomatic carriage of *Neisseria meningitidis* in a randomly sampled population. J Clin Microbiol 32:323, 1994.
35. Caugant DA, Kristiansen BE, Frøholm LO, Bovre K, Selander RK. Clonal diversity of *Neisseria meningitidis* from a population of asymptomatic carriers. Infect Immun 56:2060, 1988.
36. Goldschneider I, Gotschlich EC, Artenstein MS. Human immunity to the meningococcus: II. Development of natural immunity. J Exp Med 129:1327, 1969.
37. Pether JV, Lightfood NF, Scott RJ, Morgan J, Steele-Perkins AP, Sheard SC. Carriage of *Neisseria meningitidis*: investigations in a military establishment. Epidemiol Infect 101:21, 1988.
38. Tappero JW, Reporter R, Wenger JD, *et al.* Meningococcal disease in Los Angeles County, California, and among men in the county jails. N Engl J Med 335:833, 1996.
39. Edwards EA, Devine LF, Sengbusch GH, Ward HW. Immunological investigations of meningococcal disease: III. Brevity of group C acquisition prior to disease occurrence. Scand J Infect Dis 9:105, 1977.
40. Marks MI, Frasch CE, Shapera RM. Meningococcal colonization and infection in children

and their household contacts. Am J Epidemiol 109:563, 1979.

41. Broome CV. The carrier state: *Neisseria meningitidis*. J Antimicrob Chemother 18 Suppl A:25, 1986.
42. Cartwright K. Meningococcal carriage and disease. In Cartwright K (ed). Meningococcal disease. Chichester: John Wiley & Sons, 1995: 115.
43. Kasper DL, Winkelhake JL, Zollinger WD, *et al.* Immunochemical similarity between polysaccharide antigens of *Escherichia coli* 07:K1(L):NM and group B *Neisseria meningitidis*. J Immunol 110:262, 1973.
44. Vann WF, Liu TY, Robbins JB. *Bacillus pumilus* polysaccharide cross-reactive with meningococcal group A polysaccharide. Infect Immun 13: 1654, 1976.
45. Platonov AE, Shipulin GA, Vershinina IV, Dankert J, van de Winkel JGJ, Kuijper EJ. Association of human Fc gamma RIIa (CD32) polymorphism with susceptibility to and severity of meningococcal disease. Clin Infect Dis 27:746, 1998.
46. Ross SC, Densen P. Complement deficiency states and infection: epidemiology, pathogenesis and consequences of neisserial and other infections in an immune deficiency. Medicine (Baltimore) 63:243, 1984.
47. DeVoe IW. The meningococcus and mechanisms of pathogenicity. Microbiol Rev 46:162, 1982.
48. Quagliarello V, Scheld WM. Bacterial meningitis: pathogenesis, pathophysiology, and progress. N Engl J Med 327:862, 1992.
49. Andersen J, Berthelsen L, Bech-Jensen B, Lind I. Dynamics of the meningococcal carrier state and characteristics of the carrier strains: a longitudinal study within three cohorts of military recruits. Epidemiol Infect 121:85, 1998.
50. Griffiss JMcL, Brandt BL, Jarvis GA. Natural immunity to *Neisseria meningitidis*. In Vedros NA (ed). Evolution of meningococcal disease. Vol. 2. Boca Raton: CRC Press, 1987: 99.
51. Haneberg B, Tønjum T, Rodahl K, Gedde Dahl TW. Factors preceding the onset of meningococcal disease, with special emphasis on passive smoking, stressful events, physical fitness and general symptoms of ill health. NIPH Ann 6:169, 1983.
52. Stuart JM, Cartwright KAV, Robinson PM, Noah ND. Effect of smoking on meningococcal carriage. Lancet ii:723, 1989.
53. Stanwell-Smith RE, Stuart JM, Hughes AO, Robinson P, Griffin MB, Cartwright K. Smoking, the environment and meningococcal disease: a case control study. Epidemiol Infect 112:315, 1994.
54. Fischer M, Hedberg K, Cardosi P, *et al.* Tobacco smoke as a risk factor for meningococcal disease. Pediatr Infect Dis J 16:979, 1997.
55. Levitt L, Bond JO, Hall IE, *et al.* Meningococcal and ECHO-9 meningitis: report of an outbreak. Neurology 20:45, 1970.
56. Young LS, LaForce FM, Head JJ, Feeley JC, Bennett JV. A simultaneous outbreak of meningococcal and influenza infections. N Engl J Med 287:5, 1972.
57. Moore PS, Hierholzer J, DeWitt W, *et al.* Respiratory viruses and mycoplasma as cofactors for epidemic group A meningococcal meningitis. JAMA 264:1271, 1990.
58. Cartwright KAV, Jones DM, Smith AJ, Stuart JM, Kaczmarski EB, Palmer SR. Influenza A and meningococcal disease. Lancet 338:554, 1991.
59. Raza MW, El Ahmer OR, Ogilvie MM, *et al.* Infection with respiratory syncytial virus enhances expression of native receptors for non-pilate *Neisseria meningitidis* on HEp-2 cells. FEMS Immunol Med Microbiol 23:115, 1999.
60. Plaut A. Microbial subversion of host defenses. In: Schaechter M, Medoff G, Schlessinger D (eds). Mechanisms on microbial diseases. Baltimore: Williams & Wilkins, 1989: 139.
61. Klein NJ, Ison CA, Peakman M, *et al.* The influence of capsulation and lipooligosaccharide structure on neutrophil adhesion molecule expression and endothelial injury by *Neisseria meningitidis*. J Infect Dis 173:172, 1996.
62. Schryvers AB, Gonzalez GC. Receptors for transferrin in pathogenic bacteria are specific for the host's protein. Can J Microbiol 36:145, 1990.
63. Pettersson A, Poolman JT, van der Ley P, Tommassen J. Response of *Neisseria meningitidis* to iron limitation. Antonie van Leeuwenhoek 71:129, 1997.
64. Gold R, Goldschneider I, Lepow ML, Draper TF, Randolph M. Carriage of *Neisseria meningitidis* and *Neisseria lactamica* in infants and children. J Infect Dis 137:112, 1978.
65. Jones GR, Christodoulides M, Brooks JL, Miller AR, Cartwright KA, Heckels JE. Dynamics of carriage of *Neisseria meningitidis* in a group of military recruits: subtype stability

and specifity of the immune response following colonization. J Infect Dis 178:451, 1998.
66. van de Winkel JGJ, Anderson CL. Biology of human immunoglobulin G Fc receptors. J Leukocyte Biol 49:511, 1991.
67. van de Winkel JGJ, Capel PJA. Human IgG Fc receptor heterogeneity molecular aspects and clinical implication. Immunol Today 14:215, 1993.
68. Gessner JE, Heiken H, Tamm A, Schmidt RE. The IgG Fc receptor family. Ann Hematol 76:231, 1998.
69. Salmon JE, Edberg JC, Brogie NL, Kimberly RP. Allelic polymorphisms of human Fcγ receptor IIA and Fcγ receptor IIIB: independent mechanisms for differences human phagocyte function. J Clin Invest 89:1274, 1992.
70. de Kleijn ED, Hazelzet JA, Kornelisse RF, de Groot R. Pathophysiology of meningococcal sepsis in children. Eur J Pediatr 157:869, 1998.
71. van Gorp ECM, Suharti C, ten Cate H, *et al.* Infectious diseases and coagulation disorders. J Infect Dis 180:176, 1999.
72. Brandtzaeg P, Kierulf P, Gaustad P, *et al.* Plasma endotoxin as a predictor of multiple organ failure and death in systemic meningococcal disease. J Infect Dis 159:195, 1989.
73. Girardin E, Grau GE, Dayr JM, *et al.* Tumor necrosis factor and interleukin-1 in the serum of children with severe infectious purpura. N Engl J Med 319:397, 1988.
74. Brandtzaeg P, Mollnes TE, Kierulf P. Complement activation and endotoxin levels in systemic meningococcal disease. J Infect Dis 160: 58, 1989.
75. Nadel S, Newport MJ, Booy R, Levin M. Variation in the tumor necrosis factor-α promoter region may be associated with death from meningococcal disease. J Infect Dis 174:878, 1996.
76. Westendorp RGJ, Langermans JAM, Huizinga TWJ, *et al.* Genetic influence on cytokine production and fatal meningococcal disease. Lancet 349:170, 1997.
77. Hermans PWM, Hibberd ML, Booy R, *et al.* 4G/5G promoter polymorphism in the plasminogen-activator-inhibitor-1 gene and outcome of meningococcal disease. Lancet 354:556, 1999.
78. Westendorp RGJ, Hottenga JJ, Slagboom PE. Variation in plasminogen-activator-inhibitor-1 gene and risk of meningococcal septic shock. Lancet 354:561, 1999.
79. Gold R. Clinical aspects of meningococcal disease. In Vedros NA (ed). Evolution of meningococcal disease. Vol. 2. Boca Raton: CRC Press, 1987: 69.
80. Kingston ME, Mackey D. Skin clues in the diagnosis of life-threatening infections. Rev Infect Dis 8:1, 1986.
81. Barquet N, Domingo P, Caylà JA, *et al.* Prognostic factors in meningococcal disease: development of a bedside predictive model and scoring system. JAMA 278:491, 1997.
82. Böhm N. Adrenal, cutaneous and myocardial lesions in fulminating endotoxinemia (Waterhouse-Friderichsen syndrome). Pathol Res Pract 174:92, 1982.
83. Hardman JM, Earle KM. Meningococcal infections: a review of 200 fatal cases. J Neuropathol Exp Neurol 26:119, 1967.
84. Levin S, Painter MB. The treatment of acute meningococcal infection in adults. Ann Intern Med 64:1049, 1966.
85. Gore I, Saphir Q. Myocarditis, a classification of 1402 cases. Am Heart J 34:827, 1947.
86. Hardman JM. Fatal meningococcal infections: the changing pathologic picture in the '60's. Milit Med 133:951, 1968.
87. Wolfe RE, Birbara CA. Meningococcal infections at an army training center. Am J Med 44:243, 1968.
88. Sullivan TD, LaScolea LJ. *Neisseria meningitidis* bacteremia in children: quantitation of bacteremia and spontaneous clinical recovery without antibiotic therapy. Pediatrics 80:63, 1987.
89. Frank ST, Gómez RM. Chronic meningococcemia. Milit Med 133:918, 1968.
90. Saslaw S. Chronic meningococcemia: report of a case. N Engl J Med 266:605, 1962.
91. Rompalo AM, Hood EW, Roberts PL, *et al.* The acute arthritis dermatitis syndrome: the changing importance of *Neisseria gonorrhoeae* and *Neisseria meningitidis*. Arch Intern Med 147:281, 1987.
92. Barquet N, Gasser I, Domingo P, Moraga FA, Macaya A, Elcuaz R. Primary meningococcal conjunctivitis: report of 21 patients and review. Rev Infect Dis 12:838, 1990.
93. Koppes GM, Ellenbogen C, Gebhart RJ. Group Y meningococcal disease in United States Air Force recruits. Am J Med 62:661, 1977.
94. Riordan FAI, Thomson APJ, Sills JA, Hart CA. Who spots the spots? Diagnosis and treatment of early meningococcal disease in children. BMJ 313:1255, 1996.

95. Granier S, Owen P, Pill R, Jacobson L. Recognising meningococcal disease in primary care: qualitative study of how general practitioners process clinical and contextual information. BMJ 316:276, 1998.
96. Meningococcal Disease Surveillance Group. Analysis of endemic meningococcal disease by serogroup and evaluation of chemoprophylaxis. J Infect Dis 134:201, 1976.
97. Hoyne AL, Brown RH. 727 meningococcic cases: an analysis. Ann Intern Med 28:248, 1948.
98. Domingo P, Mancebo J, Blanch L, Coll P, Net A, Nolla J. Bacterial meningitis with "normal" cerebrospinal fluid in adults: a report of five cases. Scand J Infect Dis 22:115, 1990.
99. Cartwright KAV. Early management of meningococcal disease. Infect Dis Clin North Am 13:661, 1999.
100. Jochmann G. Versuche zur serodiagnostik und serotherapie der epidemischen genickstarre. Dtsch Med Wochenschr 32:788, 1906.
101. Flexner S, Jobling JW. An analysis of four hundred cases of epidemic meningitis treated with the anti-meningitis serum. J Exp Med 10:690, 1908.
102. Schwentker FF, Gelman S, Long PH. The treatment of meningococcic meningitis with sulfanilamide: preliminary report. JAMA 108: 1407, 1937.
103. Rosenberg DH, Arling PA. Penicillin in the treatment of meningitis. JAMA 125:1011, 1944.
104. Scheld WM, Mandell GL. Sulfonamides and meningitis. JAMA 251:791, 1984.
105. Sáez-Nieto JA, Lujan R, Berrón S, *et al.* Epidemiology and molecular basis of penicillin-resistant *Neisseria meningitidis* in Spain: a 5-year history (1985–1989). Clin Infect Dis 14:394, 1992.
106. Sutcliffe EM, Jones DM, El-Sheikh S, Percival A. Penicillin-insensitive meningococci in the UK. Lancet i:657, 1988.
107. Botha P. Penicillin-resistant *Neisseria meningitidis* in Southern Africa. Lancet i:54, 1988.
108. Dillon JR, Paizé M, Yeung KH. Spread of penicillinase-producing and transfer plasmids from the gonococcus to *Neisseria meningitidis*. Lancet i:779, 1983.
109. Hieber JP, Nelson JD. A pharmacologic evaluation of penicillin in children with purulent meningitis. N Engl J Med 297:410, 1977.
110. Abramson JS, Spika JS. Persistence of *Neisseria meningitidis* in the upper respiratory tract after intravenous antibiotic therapy for systemic meningococcal disease. J Infect Dis 151:370, 1985.
111. Meningococcal Disease Surveillance Group. Meningococcal disease: secondary attack rate and chemoprophylaxis in the United States, 1974. JAMA 235:261, 1976.
112. Voss L, Lennon D. Epidemiology, management, and prevention of meningococcal infections. Curr Opin Pediatr 6:23, 1994.
113. Älvarez F, Aguilera A, García-Gago M. Effect of chemoprophylaxis on the meningococcal carrier state after infection. Pediatr Infect Dis J 10:700, 1991.
114. Weis N, Lind I. Pharyngeal carriage of *Neisseria meningitidis* before and after treatment of meningococcal disease. J Med Microbiol 41: 339, 1994.
115. Grubbauer HM, Dornbusch HJ, Weippli G, *et al.* Ceftriaxone monotherapy for bacterial meningitis in children. Chemotherapy 36:441, 1990.
116. Neu HC. Cephalosporins in the treatment of meningitis. Drugs 34(Suppl 2):135, 1987.
117. Shaad UB, Krucko J, Pfenninger J. An extended experience with cefuroxime therapy of childhood bacterial meningitis. Pediatr Infect Dis 3:410, 1984.
118. Begg N. Reducing mortality from meningococcal disease. BMJ 305:133, 1992.
119. Strang JR, Pugh EJ. Meningococcal infections: reducing the case fatality rate by giving penicillin before admission to hospital. BMJ 305: 141, 1992.
120. Cartwright K, Reilly S, White D, Stuart J. Early treatment with parenteral penicillin in meningococcal diseases. BMJ 305:143, 1992.
121. Palmer SR, Corson J, Hall R, *et al.* Meningococcal disease in Wales: clinical features, outcome and public health management. J Infect 25:321, 1992.
122. Woodward CM, Jessop EG, Wale MC. Early management of meningococcal disease. Commun Dis Rep Rev 5:R135, 1995.
123. Wilks D, Lever AMM. Reasons for delay in administration of antibiotics to patients with meningitis and meningococcaemia. J Infect 32:49, 1996.
124. Jacobs RF, Sowell MK, Moss MM, Fiser DH. Septic shock in children: bacterial etiologies and temporal relationships. Pediatr Infect Dis J 9:196, 1990.
125. van Deuren M, Neeleman C, van't Hek LGFM, van der Meer JWM. A normal platelet count at

admission in acute meningococcal disease does not exclude a fulminant course. Intensive Care Med 24:157, 1998.
126. Mercier JC, Beaufils F, Hartmann JF, Azema D. Hemodynamic patterns of meningococcal shock in children. Crit Care Med 16:27, 1988.
127. Kennedy NJ, Duncan AW. Acute meningococcaemia: recent advances in management (with particular reference to children). Anaesth Intensive Care 24:197, 1996.
128. Kirsch EA, Barton RP, Kitchen L, Giroir BP. Pathophysiology, treatment and outcome of meningococcemia: a review and recent experience. Pediatr Infect Dis J 15:967, 1996.
129. Hodgetts TJ, Brett A, Castle N. The early management of meningococcal disease. J Accid Emerg Med 15:72, 1998.
130. Waage A, Brandtzaeg P, Halstensen A, *et al.* The complex pattern of cytokines in serum from patients with meningococcal septic shock. J Exp Med 169:333, 1989.
131. Prins JM, Lauw FN, Derkx BH, *et al.* Endotoxin release and cytokine production in acute and chronic meningococcaemia. Clin Exp Immunol 114:215, 1998.
132. Nassif X, Mathison JC, Wolfson E, Koziol JA, Ulevitch RJ, So M. Tumour necrosis factor alpha antibody protects against lethal meningococcaemia. Mol Microbiol 6:591, 1992.
133. Wester JP, Breumelhof R, Geers AB. Monoclonal antibodies in the treatment of adult fulminant meningococcaemia. Eur J Med 1:372, 1992.
134. Villard J, Roux-Lombard P, Hugli A, Dayer JM. Could natural inhibitors of tumor necrosis factor-α modify the clinical course of fulminant meningococcemia? Crit Care Med 21:1396, 1993.
135. Hameter BM, Westra P, van der Zande FL, *et al.* Immunotherapy with human monoclonal antibody against endotoxin (HA-IA) in meningococcal sepsis/shock. Clin Intensive Care 4:116, 1993.
136. J5 Study Group. Treatment of severe infectious purpura in children with human plasma from donors immunized with *Escherichia coli* J5: a prospective double-blind study. J Infect Dis 165:695, 1992.
137. Derkx B, Wittes J, McCloskey R. Randomized placebo-controlled trial of HA-IA, a human monoclonal anti-endotoxin antibody, in children with meningococcal septic shock. Clin Infect Dis 28:770, 1999.
138. Riordan FA, Thomson AP, Ratcliffe JM, Sills JA, Diver MJ, Hart CA. Admission cortisol and adrenocorticotrophic hormone levels in children with meningococcal disease: evidence of adrenal insufficiency? Crit Care Med 27:2257, 1999.
139. Pollard AJ, Britto J, Nadel S, DeMunter C, Habibi P, Levin M. Emergency management of meningococcal disease. Arch Dis Child 80:290, 1999.
140. Wajchenberg BC, Leme CE, Tambascia M, *et al.* The adrenal response to exogenous adrenocorticotropin in patients with infections due to *Neisseria meningitidis*. J Infect Dis 138:387, 1978.
141. Corrigan JJ Jr, Jordan CM. Heparin therapy in septicemia with disseminated intravascular coagulation: effect on mortality and on correction of hemostatic defects. N Engl J Med 283:778, 1970.
142. Smith OP, White B, Vaoghan D, *et al.* Use of protein-C concentrate, heparin and haemodiafiltration in meningococcus-induced purpura fulminans. Lancet 350:1590, 1997.
143. Goldman AP, Kerr SJ, Butt W, *et al.* Extracorporeal support for intractable cardiorespiratory failure due to meningococcal disease. Lancet 349:466, 1997.
144. Kumar A, Kanagasundaram NS, Collyns TA, Davison AM. Plasma exchange and haemodiafiltration in fulminant meningococcal sepsis. Nephrol Dial Transplant 13:484, 1998.
145. Bjorvatn B, Bjertnaes L, Fadnes HO, *et al.* Meningococcal septicaemia treated with combined plasmapheresis and leucapheresis or with blood exchange. BMJ (Clin Res Ed) 288:439, 1984.
146. Drapkin MS, Wisch JS, Gelfand JA, Cannon JG, Dinarello CA. Plasmapheresis for fulminant meningococcemia. Pediatr Infect Dis J 8:399, 1989.
147. van Deuren M, Santman FW, van Dalen R, Sauerwein RW, Span LF, van der Meer JW. Plasma and whole blood exchange in meningococcal sepsis. Clin Infect Dis 15:424, 1992.
148. Churchwell KB, McManus ML, Kent P, *et al.* Intensive blood and plasma exchange for treatment of coagulopathy in meningococcemia. J Clin Apheresis 10:171, 1995.
149. Keeley SR, Matthews NT, Buist M. Tissue plasminogen activator for gangrene in fulminant meningococcaemia. Lancet 337:1359, 1991.
150. Zenz W, Muntean W. New therapies for severe meningococcal disease. Lancet 351:528, 1998.

151. Marotto MS, Marotto PC, Sztajnbok J, Seguro AC. Outcome of acute renal failure in meningococcemia. Renal Failure 19:807, 1997.
152. Havens PL, Garland JS, Brook MM, Dewitz BA, Stremski ES, Troshynski TJ. Trends in mortality in children hospitalized with meningococcal infections, 1957 to 1987. Pediatr Infect Dis J 8:8, 1989.
153. Hart CA, Rogers TRF. Meningococcal disease. J Med Microbiol 39:3, 1993.
154. Cahalane SF, Waters M. Fulminant meningococcal septicaemia: a hospital experience. Lancet ii:120, 1975.
155. Emparanza JI, Aldamiz-Echevarria L, Perez-Yarza EG, *et al.* Prognostic score in acute meningococcemia. Crit Care Med 16:168, 1988.
156. Mok Q, Butt W. The outcome of children admitted to intensive care with meningococcal septicaemia. Intensive Care Med 22:259, 1996.
157. Stiehm ER, Damrosch DS. Factors in the prognosis of meningococcal infection. J Pediatr 68: 457, 1966.
158. Niklasson PM, Lundbergh P, Strandell T. Prognostic factors in meningococcal disease. Scand J Infect Dis 3:17, 1971.
159. Kahn A, Blum D. Factors for poor prognosis in fulminating meningococcemia: conclusions from observations of 67 childhood cases. Clin Pediatr (Phila) 17:680, 1978.
160. Vik-Mo H, Lote K, Nordøy A. Disseminated intravascular coagulation in patients with meningococcal infection: laboratory diagnosis and prognostic factors. Scand J Infect Dis 10:187, 1978.
161. Lewis LS. Prognostic factors in acute meningococcemia. Arch Dis Child 54:44, 1979.
162. Gårdlund B. Prognostic evaluation in meningococcal disease. Intensive Care Med 12:302, 1986.
163. Sinclair JF, Skeoch CH, Hallworth D. Prognosis of meningococcal septicaemia. Lancet ii:38, 1987.
164. Gedde-Dahl TW, Bjark P, Høiby EA, Høst JH, Bruun JN. Severity of meningococcal disease: assessment by factors and scores and implications for patient management. Rev Infect Dis 12:973, 1990.
165. Giraud T, Dhainaut JF, Schremmer B, *et al.* Adult overwhelming meningococcal purpura: a study of 35 cases, 1977–1989. Arch Intern Med 151:310, 1991.
166. Thomson APJ, Sills JA, Hart CA. Validation of the Glasgow Meningococcal Septicemia Prognostic Score: a 10-year retrospective survey. Crit Care Med 19:26, 1991.
167. Busund R, Starume B, Revhaug A. Fatal course in severe meningococcemia: clinical predictors and effect of transfusion therapy. Crit Care Med 21:1699, 1993.
168. Edwards MS, Baker CJ. Complications and sequelae of meningococcal infections in children. J Pediatr 99:540, 1981.
169. Genoff MC, Hoffer MM, Achauer B, Formosa P. Extremity amputations in meningococcemia-induced purpura fulminans. Plast Reconstr Surg 89:878, 1992.
170. Harris NJ, Gosh M. Skin and extremity loss in meningococcal septicaemia treated in a burn unit. Burns 20:471, 1994.
171. Huang S, Clarkle JA. Severe skin loss after meningococcal septicaemia: complications and treatment. Acta Pediatr 86:1263, 1997.
172. De Wals P, Hertoghe L, Borlée-Grimée I, *et al.* Meningococcal disease in Belgium: secondary attack rate among household, day-care nursery and pre-elementary school contacts. J Infect 3(Suppl 1):53, 1981.
173. Cooke RPD, Riordan T, Jones DM, Painter MJ. Secondary cases of meningococcal infection among close family and household contacts in England and Wales, 1984–7. BMJ 298:555, 1989.
174. Schwartz B. Chemoprophylaxis for bacterial infections: principle of and application to meningococcal infections. Rev Infect Dis 13(Suppl 2):S170, 1991.
175. Jones DM. Control of meningococcal disease: chemoprophylaxis for some carriers and some contact groups. BMJ 298:542, 1989.
176. Pugsley MP, Dworzack DL, Horowitz EA, Cuevas TA, Sanders WE, Sanders CC. Efficacy of ciprofloxacin in the treatment of nasopharyngeal carriers of *Neisseria meningitidis*. J Infect Dis 156:211, 1987.
177. Schwartz B, Al-Tobaigi A, Al-Ruwais A, *et al.* Comparative efficacy of ceftriaxone and rifampicin in eradicating pharyngeal carriage of group A *Neisseria meningitidis*. Lancet ii:1239, 1988.
178. Gilja OH, Halstensen A, Didranes A, Mylvaganan H, Aksnes A, Høiby EA. Use of single-dose ofloxacin to eradicate tonsillopharyngeal carriage of *Neisseria meningitidis*. Antimicrob Agents Chemother 37:2024, 1993.
179. Cuevas LE, Kazembe P, Mughogho GK, *et al.* Eradication of nasopharyngeal carriage of *Neisseria meningitidis* in children and adults in rural

Africa: a comparison of ciprofloxacin and rifampin. J Infect Dis 171:728, 1995.

180. Anderson MS, Glodé MP, Smith AL. Meningococcal disease. In Feigin RD, Cherry JD (eds). Textbook of pediatric infectious diseases. 4th edn, Vol. 1. Philadelphia: WB Saunders 1998: 1143.

181. Foster G, Panigrahi H, Walker M. Failure of chemoprophylaxis to prevent meningococcal disease. BMJ (Clin Res Ed) 292:886, 1986.

182. Stuart JM, Cartwright KA, Robinson PM, Noah ND. Does eradication of meningococcal carriage in household contacts prevent secondary cases of meningococcal disease? BMJ 298:569, 1989.

183. Greenwood BM, Hassan-King M, Whittle HC. Prevention of secondary cases of meningococcal disease in household contacts by vaccination. BMJ 1:1317, 1978.

184. Høiby EA, Moe PJ, Lystad A, Frøholm LO, Bøvre K. Phenoxymethyl-penicilin treatment of household contacts of patients with meningococcal disease. Antonie van Leeuwenhoek 52:255, 1986.

185. Gedde-Dahl TW, Høiby EA, Brandtzaeg P, Eskerud JR, Bøvre K. Some arguments on early hospital admission and treatment of suspected meningococcal disease cases. NIPH Ann 13:45, 1990.

186. Kristiansen BE, Knapskog AB. Secondary prevention of meningococcal disease: high risk contacts should be given chemoprophylaxis and preventive treatment with penicilin. BMJ 312: 591, 1996.

187. Gotschlich EC, Goldschneider I, Artenstein MS. Human immunity to the meningococcus. IV. Immunogenicity of group A and group C meningococcal polysaccharides in human volunteers. J Exp Med 129:1367, 1969.

188. Hankins WA, Gwaltney JM Jr, Hendley JO, Farquhar JD, Samuelson JS. Clinical and serological evaluation of a meningococcal polysaccharide vaccine groups A, C, Y, and W135 (41306). Proc Soc Exp Biol Med 169:54, 1982.

189. Peltola H, Mäkelä HP, Käyhty H, *et al.* Clinical efficacy of meningococcus group A capsular polysaccharide vaccine in children three months to five years of age. N Engl J Med 297:686, 1977.

190. Ceesay SJ, Allen SJ, Menon A, *et al.* Decline in meningococcal antibody levels in African children 5 years after vaccination and the lack of an effect of booster immunization. J Infect Dis 167:1212, 1993.

191. Peltola H. Group A meningococcal polysaccharide vaccine and course of the group A meningococcal epidemic in Finland. Scand J Infect Dis 10:41, 1978.

192. Greenwood BM, Wali SS. Control of meningococcal infection in the African meningitis belt by selective vaccination. Lancet i:729, 1980.

193. Mohammed I, Zaruba K. Control of epidemic meningococcal infection by mass vaccination. Lancet i:80, 1981.

194. Binkin N, Band J. Epidemic of meningococcal meningitis in Bamako, Mali: epidemiological features and analysis of vaccine efficacy. Lancet ii:315, 1982.

195. Cochi SL, Markowitz LE, Joshi DD, *et al.* Control of epidemic group A meningococcal meningitis in Nepal. Int J Epidemiol 16:91, 1987.

196. Masterton RG, Youngs ER, Wardle JC, Croft KF, Jones DM. Control of an outbreak of group C meningococcal meningitis with a polysaccharide vaccine. J Infect 17:177, 1988.

197. Lennon D, Gellin B, Hood D, Voss L, Heffernan H, Thakur S. Successful intervention in a group A meningococcal outbreak in Auckland, New Zealand. Pediatr Infect Dis J 11:617, 1992.

198. Rosenstein N, Levine O, Taylor JP, *et al.* Efficacy of meningococcal vaccine and barriers to vaccination. JAMA 279:435, 1998.

199. Lepow ML, Perkins BA, Hughes PA, Poolman JT. Meningococcal vaccines. In Plotkin SA, Orenstein WA (eds). Vaccines. 3rd edn, Philadelphia: WB Saunders, 1999: 711.

200. Frasch CE. Vaccines for prevention of meningococcal disease. Clin Microbiol Rev 2(Suppl): S134, 1989.

201. Poolman JT. Development of a meningococcal vaccine. Infect Agents Dis 4:13, 1995.

202. Granoff DM, Forrest B, Rappuoli R. Meningococcal polysaccharide-protein conjugate vaccines. Int J Infect Dis 1:152, 1997.

203. Finne J, Leinonen M, Mäkelä PH. Antigenic similarities between brain components and bacteria causing meningitis: implications for vaccine development and pathogenesis. Lancet ii:355, 1983.

204. Jennings HJ. N-propionylated group B meningococcal polysaccharide glycoconjugate vaccine against group B meningococcal meningitis. Int J Infect Dis 1:158, 1997.

205. Sierra CVG, Campa HC, Valcárcel NW. Vaccine against group B *Neisseria meningitidis*:

protection trial and mass vaccination results in Cuba. NIPH Ann 14:195, 1991.

206. Zollinger WD, Boslego J, Moran E, *et al.* Meningococcal serogroup B vaccine protection trial and follow-up studies in Chile. NIPH Ann 14:211, 1991.

207. De Moraes JC, Perkins BA, Camargo MCC, *et al.* Protective efficacy of a serogroup B meningococcal vaccine in Sao Paulo, Brazil. Lancet 340:1074, 1992.

208. Milagres LG, Ramos SR, Sacchi CT, *et al.* Immune response of Brazilian children to a *Neisseria meningitidis* serogroup B outer membrane protein vaccine: comparison with efficacy. Infect Immun 62:4419, 1994.

209. Boslego J, García J, Cruz C, *et al.* Efficacy safety, and immunogenicity of a meningococcal group B (15:P1.3) outer membrane protein vaccine in Iquique, Chile. Vaccine 13:821, 1995.

210. Bjune G, Høiby EA, Grønnesby JK, *et al.* Effect of outer membrane vesicle vaccine against group B meningococcal disease in Norway. Lancet 388:1093, 1991.

211. Herbert MA, Heath PT, Mayon-White RT. Meningococcal vaccines for the United Kingdom. Commun Dis Rep CDR Rev 5:R130, 1995.

212. Cartwright K, Morris R, Rumke H, *et al.* Immunogenicity and reactogenicity in UK infants of a novel meningococcal vesicle vaccine containing multiple class 1 (PorA) outer membrane proteins. Vaccine 17:2612, 1999.

213. Haneberg B, Dalseg R, Oftung F, *et al.* Towards a nasal vaccine against meningococcal disease, and prospects for its use as a mucosal adjuvant. Dev Biol Stand 92:127, 1998.

214. Haneberg B, Dalseg R, Wedege E, *et al.* Intranasal administration of a meningococcal outer membrane vesicle vaccine induces persistent local mucosal antibodies and serum antibodies with strong bactericidal activity in humans. Infect Immun 66:1334, 1998.

215. Oftung F, Naess LM. Wetzler LM, *et al.* Antigen-specific T-cell responses in humans after intranasal immunization with a meningococcal serogroup B outer membrane vesicle vaccine. Infect Immun 67:921, 1999.

29. BRAIN ABSCESS

Linda M. Mundy and Susan J. Bersoff-Matcha

Introduction and Historical Perspective

Brain abscess is a focal, intracerebral infection that begins as a localized area of cerebritis and develops into a collection of pus surrounded by a well-vascularized capsule [1]. Prior to the late 1800s, brain abscess was a near fatal condition. Most cases were diagnosed post-mortem. The initial success in the treatment of brain abscess was surgical drainage or removal. This success was further enhanced during and after World War II when antibiotic therapy with penicillin and chloramphenicol became available.

Over the past two decades, there has been continued reduction in morbidity and mortality associated with brain abscess due to advances in diagnostic and treatment strategies. Neuroimaging studies, stereotactic brain biopsies, and aspiration techniques have contributed tremendously to the identification of lesion(s) size, number, location, potential approaches and evaluation over time. New antimicrobial therapies have simplified empiric- and pathogen-directed regimens. Interestingly, the epidemiology of this condition seems to have changed over the past two decades with the decreasing incidence of otogenic brain abscess and rising incident rates of brain abscess among immunocompromised host populations.

Pathophysiology and Microbiology

PATHOPHYSIOLOGY

The brain is rather resistant to bacterial and fungal infection, given the frequency of overt and occult bacteremia. This protection against seeding during bloodstream infection may be due to the abundant blood supply and relatively impermeable blood-brain barrier formed by the capillary-endothelial tight junctions. Through an experimental animal model, the natural history of brain abscess formation can be categorized into four distinct, chronological stages: early cerebritis (days one to three), late cerebritis (days four to nine), early capsule stage (days 10 to 14), and late capsule stage (>14 days) [2, 3].

Source

a. Contiguous focus of infection. Organisms invade the brain parenchyma usually as a consequence of a contiguous infection of nonneural tissues such as the middle ear, mastoids, paranasal sinuses, or soft tissues of the face, orbit, or scalp.
b. Hematogenous dissemination. Bloodstream infection serves as a source of inoculum. Patients with congenital cyanotic heart disease in whom venous blood is shunted into the systemic circulation are especially prone to brain abscess formation via this mechanism.
c. Traumatic inoculation. Direct inoculation of bacteria into the brain following penetrating brain injury is common, yet unlikely to result in brain abscess formation.
d. Post-craniotomy infections. Such infections are complications of post-surgical care.
e. Other. Congenital lesions, including dermal sinuses and various forms of ruptured encephaloceles may provide direct access for microorganisms to brain tissue. Ultimately, 20–30% of cases are cryptic and have no identified route of development.

MICROBIOLOGY

Although most abscesses are caused by a single pathogen, mixed infections occur in up to one third of cases and are especially common with otogenic infections. Typical intracranial brain abscess sites, likely pathogens and predisposing conditions are summarized in Table 1.

a. Immunocompetent hosts: Most infections in immunocompetent hosts are bacterial, often polymicrobial, with a combination of aerobic and anaerobic organisms. These occur in both adult and pediatric populations. In brain abscess associated with sinusitis, *Staphylococcus aureus*, aerobic streptococci, *Haemophilus influenzae*, and anaerobes are the most common isolates. In brain abscess associated with otogenic sources, anaerobic bacteria are the most frequent pathogens. In patients with congenital heart disease, streptococci are common. In post-craniotomy brain abscess (subdural empyema and intraparenchymal abscess), *S aureus* and *Staphylococcus epidermidis* are most common. In post-trauma cases, *S aureus* is the most frequent pathogen.
b. Immunosuppressed hosts: Patients with malignancy, HIV/AIDS, intravenous drug use, trauma, pregnancy, alcoholism, immunosuppression and diabetes mellitus are more vulnerable for brain abscess than fully immunocompetent hosts. Among those with human immunodeficiency virus type-1

TABLE 1. Typical intracranial locations and pathogens of brain abscess associated with identified predisposing conditions

Predisposing conditions	Intracranial location	Usual pathogen(s)	Initial empiric therapy[a]
Paranasal sinusitis or otitis	Frontal lobe	Aerobic streptococci, anaerobes, *S aureus*, *Haemophilus influenzae*	Amoxicillin-sulbactam or third generation cephalosporin and metronidazole
Otogenic infection	Temporal lobe or cerebellum	Mixed infections; *Fusobacterium* spp., *Actinomyces* spp.	Third generation cephalosporin and metronidazole
Hematogenous dissemination	MCA distribution	*S aureus*, *Enterobacteriaceae*	Third generation cephalosporin
Penetrating trauma	Site of injury	Streptococci, staphylococci	Third generation cephalosporin
HIV-1	Caudate nucleus	*Toxoplasma gondii*	Pyrimethamine, sulfadiazine, and folinic acid
Non-HIV immunosuppression	Varies	*Candida albicans* and *Aspergillus* spp.	Amphotericin B
Diabetes mellitus	Varies	*Mucor* or *Rhizopus*	Amphotericin B
Pyogenic lung infection	MCA distribution	Anaerobes	Penicillin G and clindamycin
Neonates/infants	MCA distribution	*Proteus* spp. or *Citrobacter* spp.	Third generation cephalosporin
Post-craniotomy	Post-surgical site	Staphylococci, streptococci	Penicillin G
Cryptogenic[b]	Varies	Varies	Broad-spectrum

MCA = middle cerebral artery.
HIV-1 = human immunodeficiency virus, type-1.
[a] Empiric therapy: initial therapy until pathogen identified.
[b] 20–30% of all brain abscess cases.

(HIV-1), pathogens associated with brain abscess include bacteria, atypical bacteria, fungi and parasites; *Toxoplasmosis gondii* is the most frequent etiology for brain abscess with enhancing lesions noted on neuroimaging studies. In non-HIV immunosuppressed hosts, fungi such as *Candida albicans* and *Aspergillus* spp. are much more common. Diabetic patients are vulnerable to the Zygomycetes infections of *Mucor* and *Rhizopus*.

Clinical Manifestations

The classic triad of symptoms for patients with brain abscess is fever, headache and focal neurologic deficit, yet less than half of patients present with all three symptoms [4]. Instead, the symptoms patients experience depend more on their underlying condition, the size and location of the abscess and the organisms causing the infection. Many of the clinical manifestations of brain abscess are nonspecific, which can lead to a delay in diagnosis, although, most patients (>75%) have symptoms for less than two weeks at the time the diagnosis is made [4, 5]. Headache, characterized by a dull, poorly localized ache occurs in 72–92% of patients and is the most common presenting symptom in those patients who are able to report a history of present illness [1, 4-6]. Fever >100°F is seen in only 40–60% of adults and 80% of children; thus the absence of fever is not a reliable way to rule out the diagnosis [1, 5, 6]. The presence of fever is not necessarily more likely in those patients with worse initial mental status or with multiple abscesses [4, 5]. In one study, patients without fever tended to be older, have temporal lobe lesions and have a higher mortality [4].

Nausea and vomiting occur in about 50% of patients, probably due to increased intracranial pressure. Other central nervous system (CNS) symptoms such as papilledema, lethargy and stupor occur in 10–66% of patients; these symptoms also indicate increased intracranial pressure [1, 4, 6]. Patients with significant altered mental status tend to have a poorer prognosis [5]. Focal neurological deficits such as hemiparesis (the most common focal neurological deficit in patients with brain abscess), ataxia, or aphasia may occur in one-third to one-half of patients, and their presence depends on the location of the abscess. Nuchal rigidity also occurs in up to 50% of patients, and when it occurs with abrupt onset, may indicate intraventricular rupture of the abscess [1, 4, 6]. This is a serious complication associated with a very high mortality rate of over 80% [1, 5]. Seizures have been the presenting symptom in 35% of patients and occur in 25–50% of cases during initial hospitalization [4, 5].

Children

Children account for up to 25% of patients who develop brain abscess, often as a complication of chronic otitis media and/or mastoiditis. When frontal lobe abscess occurs in children, it is most commonly seen in male adolescents as a complication of frontal sinusitis. These patients usually present with headache, fever and occasionally altered mental status. However, clinical findings for this condition are often subtle and routine head CT scans may initially be negative, thus a high index of suspicion is necessary. As with brain abscess in adults, both the brain abscess and sinusitis should be managed surgically and with appropriate antibiotics. In neonates, brain abscesses sometimes occur as a rare complication of meningitis from group B streptococci or *Escherichia coli* [1]. Other facultative Gram-negative organisms such as *Serratia marcescens*, *Proteus* spp., *Citrobacter* spp. and *Enterobacter* spp. are rare causes of meningitis in this age group. However, when such pathogens are cultured from the CSF, a brain abscess is present in >75% of cases [1]. Brain abscesses from these organisms are also associated with a very high mortality rate. Those who survive usually have significant long-term neurologic sequelae [1]. As with any patient with brain abscess, infants and children should be managed aggressively with both surgical drainage and antimicrobial therapy.

Congenital cyanotic heart disease, particularly tetralogy of Fallot and transposition of the great vessels (and any other condition resulting in a significant right-to-left shunt), is an important predisposing factor for brain abscess in as many as 50% of children [1]. The peak incidence of brain abscess in children with this risk factor is between four and seven years age and is rare in children under two years [7]. Brain abscess associated with congenital cyanotic heart disease may also occur in adults. Patients who have procedures to correct the right-to-left shunt significantly reduce their risk of brain abscess, while those patients who have palliative procedures that do not completely correct the shunt do not diminish their risk [1]. Thus, the earlier and more completely the cyanotic heart disease is corrected the lower the risk of brain abscess. The mortality from brain abscess associated with cyanotic congenital heart disease is high (30–40%) and as with brain abscess associated with other causes, requires both aggressive surgical and antimicrobial therapy [7].

Immunocompromised Hosts

Immunocompromised hosts, including those with diabetes, as well as those receiving corticosteroids or other immunosuppressive therapies may develop brain abscess due to a variety of etiologic agents, including fungi, nocardia and tuberculosis. The clinical presentation of brain abscess in these patients differs from those with pyogenic brain abscesses; they are less likely to develop headache or meningismus (presumably from a poor inflammatory response), and are more likely to present with fever, focal neurologic deficits and seizures [1]. Since the variety of etiologic agents that could potentially cause a brain abscess in these patients is so broad, choosing empiric therapy is difficult. Thus, in such cases, early surgical intervention is recommended so that cultures can be obtained and the correct antimicrobial agent(s) can be administered. The most common cause of a brain mass in patients with acquired immunodeficiency syndrome (AIDS) is toxoplasmosis. However, patients with AIDS may develop brain abscess from bacterial pathogens as well. AIDS patients with radiographic evidence of space-occupying CNS lesions should be started on empiric therapy for toxoplasmosis with pyrimethamine (for adults, a loading dose of 200 mg followed by 75–100 mg per day), sulfadiazine (1–1.5 g orally every six hours), and folinic acid (10 mg po qd) which helps prevent the bone marrow suppression that can occur with pyrimethamine. If the patient deteriorates or fails to show clinical improvement after two weeks of treatment, a brain biopsy or aspiration via neurosurgical or CT-guided techniques is recommended [8]. Patients with AIDS are also more susceptible to brain abscesses due to *Salmonella* spp., *L. monocytogenes*, *Nocardia* spp., tuberculosis, and the endemic mycoses (coccidioidomycosis, blastomycosis and histoplasmosis).

Diagnosis

The differential diagnosis for the clinical presentation consistent with brain abscess includes brain abscess, metastatic tumor, subdural abscess, sinus thrombosis, meningitis, mycotic aneurysm and encephalitis. In metastatic tumors, contrast studies are more likely to have irregular, diffuse borders on enhancement neuroimaging studies. In conjunction with the history and physical examination, supportive data include:

1. Laboratory data. Laboratory findings are of minimal assistance in the diagnosis or follow-up of patients with brain abscess. As many as 40% of patients have normal white blood cell counts with only 10% of patients having leukocytosis that exceeds 20,000/mm^3. Higher leukocyte counts suggest a concurrent meningitis or systemic infection. The erythrocyte sedimentation rate, although not specific, is elevated in 90% of cases. The mean erythrocyte sedimentation rate in patients with brain abscess is 45–55 mm/hr, but in many patients this,

too is normal [1]. C-reactive protein is also elevated. Hyponatremia may occur and in most cases indicates the syndrome of inappropriate antidiuretic hormone secretion. Blood cultures are most often negative, but two sets should be drawn from febrile patients, because when positive, can help direct antimicrobial therapy. Lumbar puncture is not recommended for patients with brain abscess due to the risk of herniation. When performed, CSF findings are nonspecific among patients with brain abscess; 25% of patients' CSF reveal hypoglycorrhachia, 67–81% show elevated protein, and 60–70% show a mononuclear pleocytosis [4]. In many cases, CSF findings are normal, and in only 10% of cases are cultures obtained from the CSF positive. The CSF Gram's stain and cultures are usually negative. Thus, because CSF does not provide useful clinical information and patients are at risk for potential "mass effect", lumbar puncture should not be routinely performed even after neuroimaging studies have been reviewed for open cisterns and evidence of potential or existing midline intracranial shift [1, 4]. The most reliable way to make a microbiological diagnosis is to culture specimens obtained during neurosurgery or CT-guided aspiration. With appropriate handling of specimens (i.e., careful attention to anaerobic transport techniques and prompt plating of culture material) aspirate or intraoperative culture yield can approximate 100% [5, 6]. In many cases, however, antimicrobial therapy has been initiated prior to surgery, and in those patients, cultures may be negative. While the incidence of negative cultures is greater for patients who have already begun antibiotics, material obtained during surgery should still be sent for Gram's stain and culture since Gram's stain findings may be helpful in guiding selection of antimicrobial agents.

2. Initial neuroimaging studies. The most important and expeditious part of the initial work-up for suspected brain abscess is a neuroimaging study with contrast, unless contraindicated. This can begin with either a head CT scan or brain magnetic radioimaging (MRI). The selection of head CT versus brain MRI may be guided by the suspected source or nidus of infection. Head CT will enhance evaluation of bone invasion and is a quicker procedure for unstable patients. Brain MRI is best if there is involvement of a paranasal sinus or suspicion of venous sinus thrombosis. The majority of brain abscesses are ring enhancing, usually with a thinner medial wall. Intense edema is often present. Gas within the ring enhancing lesion is highly suggestive of brain abscess. If noncontrast MRI is used, a rounded appearing lesion with edema is usually visualized. The T_1-weighted image reveals hypointensity at the central necrotic portion surrounded by less hypointensity which represents cerebritis and edema. The T_2-weighted images show increased or variable signal centrally surrounded by decreased signal intensity and then increased intensity (edema). After contrast the brain MRI reveals ring enhancement. If there is a brain abscess complicated by rupture of the abscess into the ventricle, there may be enhancement of the ependymal surfaces.
3. Follow-up neuroimaging studies. If nonsurgical management is selected for treatment, close clinical and radiographic follow-up is necessary. Serial head CT scanning is the usual neuroimaging modality for this purpose.
   a. Radionucleotide studies. Other imaging modalities such as indium 111-labeled leukocyte scans offer little to the initial or on-going evaluation of brain abscesses. The role of single-photon emission computed tomography (SPECT) and positron emission tomography (PET) remains to be determined.
   b. Cerebral Angiography. This modality can reveal that the lesion(s) are acellular in the central bulk.
   c. Repeat head CT or brain MRI. Each of these should reveal resolution over time (Figure 1).
4. Biopsy/Aspiration. CT- or MRI-guided stereotactic brain biopsy or aspirate of the brain abscess can be both diagnostic and therapeutic. Cultures and subsequent antibiograms can guide pathogen-directed therapy. In patients with HIV and brain mass lesions,

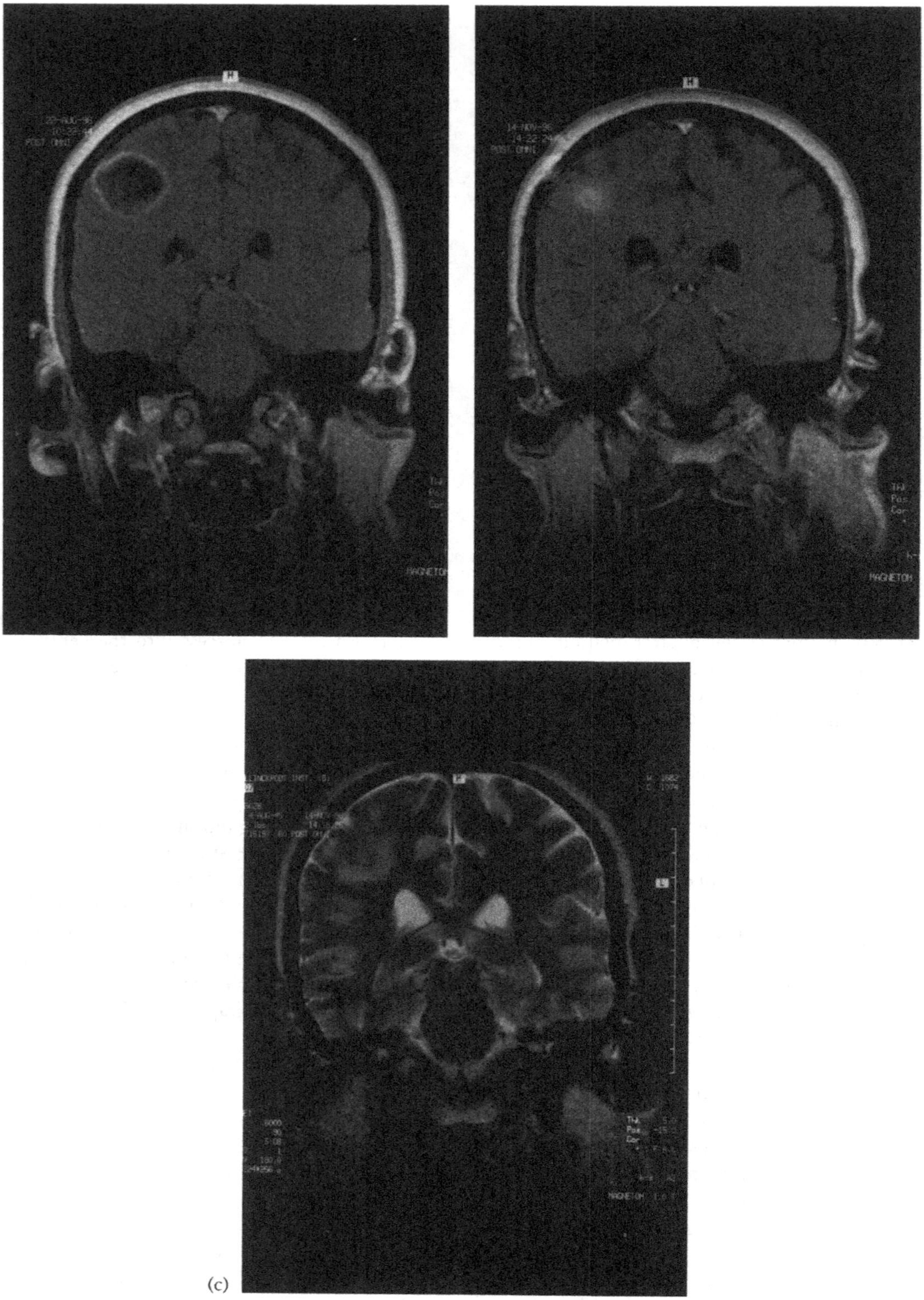

(a) (b) (c)

FIGURE 1. Serial intracranial imaging studies of host with brain abscess. At initial clinical presentation, brain MRI T-weighted imaging revealed 4.5 cm ring-enhancing lesion (Figure 1a). Figures 1b and 1c reveal pre- and post-gadolinium enhanced brain MRI resolution of the cavitary lesion 84 days after initial presentation.

stereotactic brain biopsy had a high diagnostic yield of 96% in 25 patients [9].

Therapy

Proper management of a patient with a brain abscess includes both antimicrobial therapy and a surgical drainage procedure during which abscess material can be obtained for Gram's stain and culture. Since brain abscesses are uncommon, there have been no randomized controlled trials to compare different therapies. Yet, based on the location of the abscess and previously reported experiences, some recommendations regarding therapy can be made. Brain abscesses are frequently polymicrobial and the organisms isolated depend to some extent, on the source, location and predisposing condition of the patient. However, the most common agents isolated in patients from large clinical series, are microaerophilic streptococci (particularly *Streptococcus milleri* and other streptococci) and anaerobic bacteria [4, 10, 11]. Other organisms such as *S aureus* and the Enterobacteriaceae have also been seen. Thus, empiric antibiotic coverage should include antimicrobials with activity against all these organisms until material from the abscess can be obtained for culture and organism specific antimicrobial therapy can be administered.

Surgery

Although there have been case reports documenting resolution of brain abscesses using antimicrobial therapy alone [12], in most cases, both medical and surgical intervention is recommended. The two most commonly performed procedures are open craniotomy and needle aspiration. Prior to the widespread availability of intracranial radiographic imagery studies, open craniotomy under general anesthesia was the only available procedure for brain abscess drainage. Now, head CT and brain MRI scans have made it possible to more definitively localize abscesses. In addition, needle aspiration under CT guidance is less invasive and has made brain abscess drainage possible with local anesthesia. Open craniotomy is now reserved for patients with multiloculated abscesses, multiple abscesses, abscesses that fail to resolve with needle aspiration and abscesses caused by resistant pathogens. While the two procedures have not been compared in a controlled clinical trial, retrospective analysis indicates that neither procedure has emerged as being superior in terms of outcome [5]. However, closed-needed aspiration is less invasive, most patients now initially undergo the stereotactic aspiration procedure, followed by the more invasive open procedure if deemed necessary. Interestingly, patients who do undergo open craniotomy have not been shown to have a higher incidence of seizures than those who have undergone needle aspiration [1].

Antimicrobial Agents

When choosing appropriate antimicrobial therapy for brain abscesses, several issues must be considered. First, the antimicrobial agent must have activity against the likely pathogen(s). Second, consideration must also be given as to whether the agent will penetrate the abscess cavity. While many studies have been carried out to determine antimicrobial penetration into the CSF, the data regarding antimicrobial penetration into brain abscess cavities is much more limited. It has been shown that the factors that predict whether an antibiotic will penetrate the CSF do not necessarily also predict penetration into a brain abscess cavity [13].

Chloramphenicol has many attractive attributes that made it one of the standard therapies for brain abscess for many years. It has a broad antimicrobial spectrum, good CNS penetration, and it has been shown to have good penetration into brain abscess cavities [4, 14]. However, because of its side effect profile, lack of available oral formulation, and because positive cultures from abscess fluid persist in many cases despite adequate drug concentrations, it has fallen out of favor as a first line therapy [4].

In spite of relatively poor CSF penetration, high-dose penicillin G (>24 million units daily in adults) has been found to reach therapeutic concentrations within brain abscess pus [15]. One study, however, found that after a 1-hour *in vitro* incubation within brain abscess pus, in some cases, greater than 90% of the drug was inactivated [16]. There is limited and conflicting data regarding the penetration of the semi-synthetic penicillins (methicillin, oxacillin and nafcillin) into abscess fluid. One study showed that methicillin was detectable in brain abscess pus after standard dosing, but nafcillin was not [14]. However, there is no data to suggest that these drugs should not be used to treat brain abscess when the organisms are susceptible. In patients with *staphylococci* who are allergic to penicillin, or in cases when the organism is resistant to methicillin, vancomycin should be used [17].

First generation cephalosporins do not have good CNS penetration and should therefore not be used to treat patients with brain abscess. On the other hand, third generation cephalosporins have excellent CSF penetration and many of the drugs are active against most of the organisms that cause both meningitis and brain abscess. While cefotaxime, ceftizoxime, ceftriaxone and ceftazidime all have good CSF penetration, activity within a brain abscess cavity cannot be inferred. Cefotaxime has been shown to penetrate into brain abscess cavities at therapeutic levels, and it is active against many of the bacteria that cause brain abscess [18]. When used for this purpose, cefotaxime should be given at high dose (3g iv q 8), in combination with metronidazole. This regimen has been shown to be an effective combination for the treatment of brain abscess [18, 19]. Ceftazidime has been shown in one study to have good penetration into brain abscess cavities, with high enough levels for bactericidal activity against most pathogens including streptococci [20]. There is limited data for ceftriaxone and ceftizoxime, but they have been used successfully in the treatment of brain abscess in small numbers of patients [1].

Metronidazole has gained popularity over chloramphenicol as one of the standard drugs in the treatment of brain abscess for several reasons. Metronidazole has been shown to have excellent and reproducible penetration into brain abscess pus and it is bactericidal against *Bacteroides fragilis*, whereas chloramphenicol is bacteriostatic [21]. Metronidazole, however, is useful only for treating strict anaerobes, and therefore must be used in combination with another agent that has activity against both aerotolerant anaerobes and microaerophilic streptococci, since these organisms are resistant to metronidazole [22]. Some patients, particularly those with hepatic failure, may experience side effects from metronidazole such as CNS toxicity, manifested by seizures, increased somnolence, and/or peripheral neuropathy. In many cases it may be difficult to distinguish whether these symptoms are due to drug side effects or to clinical deterioration.

Imipenem has a broad antimicrobial spectrum and has been used successfully in the treatment of brain abscess [23, 24]. However, because this drug has been known to induce seizures [25], it is usually reserved for CNS infections due to resistant pathogens [1].

Meropenem is a newer carbapenem with a similar antimicrobial spectrum to imipenem, but is associated with fewer CNS side effects. In addition to having good CNS penetration, the quinolones have excellent activity against Gram-negative facultative anaerobes (including the Enterobacteriaceae and *Pseudomonas* spp.). However, quinolones have been shown to lower the seizure threshold.

The definitive duration of antimicrobial therapy for brain abscess is unknown. In clinical series, most authors advocate that a 6–8 week course of intravenous antibiotics be directed at the pathogen(s) cultured from abscess pus postdrainage. Thus, if adequate surgical drainage is achieved, 6–8 weeks of intravenous therapy is likely to be sufficient. Other investigators believe that intravenous courses as short as three weeks may be adequate [18]. In most cases, however, decisions regarding duration should be individualized and based on the patient's response to therapy (both clinically and radiographically), the susceptibilities of the organism(s) to the chosen antimicrobial agent and the adequacy of surgical drainage. It is unclear whether oral antibiotics upon completion of an intravenous course is necessary; however, an additional 2–3 month course of oral antibiotics (given upon completion of the 6–8 weeks of intravenous therapy) has been suggested in order to prevent relapse [1]. As part of routine follow-up, patients should have both clinical examinations and radiographic (CT or MRI) scans on a monthly or bimonthly basis, in order to document resolution of the abscess.

Adjunctive Agents

The question of whether corticosteroids are useful as adjunctive therapy in patients with brain abscess has not been evaluated by controlled clinical trials. Studies using corticosteroids in animal models of brain abscess have had conflicting results [1]. A short course of high-dose corticosteroid therapy (given po or iv at 100 mg q six hours which is rapidly tapered over 5–7 days) for patients with increased intracranial pressure and/or impending herniation may be beneficial [1]. However, studies indicate that prolonged use of corticosteroids should probably not be used since they have been shown in some cases to decrease penetration of antibiotics into the abscess cavity or interfere with microbial clearance [1]. In spite of these findings, clinical series with relatively large numbers of patients have shown no significant difference in outcome in those patients who received corticosteroids over those patients who did not [1, 4, 10]. While corticosteroids may be beneficial in certain circumstances, their use should be determined on a case-by-case basis.

It has been recommended that anticonvulsant medications be given to patients, even with no previous history of seizures, as prophylaxis during treatment of brain abscess and continuing for at least three months post-surgery [1]. After three months, the decision regarding whether to continue the anticonvulsants should be based on the results of a neurological evaluation. It is recommended that a few months after completion of antimicrobial therapy that patients undergo an electroencephalogram. If the result is normal, discontinuation of anticonvulsant therapy can be considered [1]. If the electroencephalogram is abnormal, the medication should probably be continued [1].

Outcomes and Sequelae

The outcome of untreated bacterial abscess is usually death. In general, morbidity and mortality vary with location, degree of encapsulation, site or original infection, presence of complications and number of abscesses. In the literature, mortality has ranged from 35–55% with the highest rate occurring among lesions associated with pulmonary infections [26]. In a more recent study from Switzerland, the overall mortality rate was only 4% [27]. This lower rate of mortality was attributed to CT-guided stereotactic aspiration and early treatment.

Some complications of brain abscess result in worse outcomes, perhaps the most ominous of which is rupture of the brain abscess into the ventricular space. Patients present with sudden worsening of a preexisting headache accompanied by meningismus. This complication is usually fatal. If death is not immediate, neurosurgical intervention is warranted.

In a study by Seydoux and Francioli, sequelae of brain abscesses occurred in 44% of patients [5]. The only factor that influenced reduction in sequelae was the clinical presentation at admission. The sequelae of brain abscess include recurrence of brain abscess, new brain abscess formation, residual focal neurologic deficits and recurrent seizures. For recommendations on seizures prophylaxis and treatment see above Treatment section.

Summary

Major advances in diagnostic and therapeutic strategies have enhanced the management of brain abscess over the past two decades. Coordinated, strategic care between neuroradiologists, neurosurgeons and infectious disease specialists is recommended to optimize tailored short- and long-term patient care.

References

1. Mathisen GE, Johnson JP. Brain abscess. CID 25:763, 1997.
2. Britt RH, Enzmann DR. Clinical stages of human brain abscesses on serial CT scans after contrast infusion. J Neurosurgery 59:972, 1983.
3. Britt RH, Enzmann DR, Yeager AS. Neuropathological and computerized tomographic findings in experimental brain abscess. J Neurosurgery 55:590, 1981.
4. Chun CH, Johnson JD, Hofstetter M, Raff MJ. Brain abscess – a study of 45 consecutive cases. Medicine (Baltimore) 65:415, 1986.
5. Seydoux C, Francioli P. Bacterial brain abscesses: factors influencing mortality and sequelae. CID 15:394, 1992.
6. Mathiesen GE, Meyer RD, George WL, Citron DM, Finegold SM. Brain abscess and cerebritis. Rev Infect Dis 6(suppl 1):S101, 1984.
7. Kagawa M, Takeshita M, Yato S, Kitamura K. Brain abscess in congenital cyanotic heart disease. J Neurosurg 58:913, 1983.
8. Sande MA, Gilbert DN, Moellering RC. The Sanford Guide to HIV/AIDS Therapy. Eighth edn. Antimicrobial Therapy, Inc, 1999.
9. Hornef MW, Iten A, Maeder P, Villemure J, Regli L. Brain biopsy in patients with acquired immunodeficiency syndrome. Arch Intern Med 159:2590, 1999.
10. De Louvois J, Gortvai P, Hurley R. Bacteriology of abscesses of the central nervous system: a multicentre prospective study. Br Med J 2:981, 1977.
11. Lakshmi V, Rao RR, Dinakar I. Bacteriology of brain abscess – observations on 50 cases. J Med Microbiol 38:187, 1993.
12. Barsoum AH, Lewis HC, Cannillo KL. Nonoperative treatment of multiple brain abscesses. Surg Neurol 16:283, 1981.
13. Kramer PW, Griffith RS, Campbell RL. Antibiotic penetration of the brain: a comparative study. J Neurosurgery 31:295, 1969.
14. Black P, Graybill JR, Charache P. Penetration of brain abscess by systemically administered antibiotics. J Neurosurg 38:705, 1973.
15. De Louvois J, Gortvai P, Hurley R. Antibiotic treatment of abscesses of the central nervous system. Br Med J 2:985, 1977.
16. Picardi JL, Lewis HP, Tan JSeal. Clindamycin concentrations in the central nervous system of primates before and after head trauma. J Neurosurg 43:717, 1975.
17. Ogg G, Lynn WA, Peters M, Curati W, McLaughlin JE, Shaunak S. Cerebral nocardia abscesses in a patient with AIDS: correlation of magnetic resonance and white cell scanning images with neuropathological findings. Case Reports 311:3, 1997.
18. Sjolin J, Lilja A, Eriksson N, Arneborn P, Cars O. Treatment of brain abscess with cefotaxime and metronidazole: propsective study on 15 consecutive patients. CID 17:857, 1993.
19. Gomez J, Poza M, Martinez M, Martinez-Lage J, Hernandez JL, Valdes M. Use of cefotaxime and metronidazole for treating cerebral abscesses. CID [letter] 21:708, 1995.
20. Green HT, O'donoghue MAT, Shaw MDM, Dowling C. Penetration of ceftazidime into intracranial abscess. J Antimicrob Chemother 24:431, 1989.
21. Ingham HR, Selkon JB, Roxby CM. Bacteriological study of otogenic cerebral abscess: Chemotherapeutic role of metronidazole. Br Med J 2:991, 1977.
22. Ingham HR, Selkon JB. Metronidazole and brain abscess. Lancet, [letter] 2:613, 1982.
23. Asensi V, Carton JA, Maradona JA, Asensi JM, Perez Feal. Therapy of brain abscess with imipenem – a safe therapeutic choice. J Antimicrob Chemother 37:200, 1996.
24. Asensi V, Carton JA, Maradona JA, Asensi JM, Perez F, *et al*. Imipenem therapy of brain abscesses. Eur J Clin Microbiol Infect Dis 15:653, 1996.

25. Wong VK, Wright HT Jr, Ross LA, Mason WH, Inderlied CB, Kim KS. Imipenem/cilastin treatment of bacterial meningitis in children. Pediatr Infect Dis 10:122, 1991.
26. Loeser E Jr, Scheinberg L. Brain abscesses: A review of ninety-nine cases. Neurology 7:601, 1957.
27. Hasdemir MG, Ebeling U. CT-guided stereotactic aspiration and treatment of brain abscesses. Acta Neurochir 125:58, 1999.

30. ENCEPHALITIS

R. Jordá-Marcos

Introduction

Encephalitis refers to an inflammation of the cerebral parenchyma that can be caused by various nosologic agents, whether they are infectious or not. The viral encephalitis is a common disease that affects mainly children under 15 years of age, and represents the most frequent cause of disseminated lesions in the brain tissue.

Its incidence varies depending on age, ranging between 1 and 16.7 cases per 100,000 children per year [1]. Its mortality ranges from 0% of some seasonal encephalitis (mumps), to 70% of *herpes simplex* virus (HSV) encephalitis without treatment. Clinical symptoms include fever, headache and a decreased level of consciousness that can range from simple disorientation to a deep coma with seizures and motor focalities. According to our experience, acute infectious encephalitis corresponds to 9% of the total central nervous system (CNS) infections seen in the intensive care unit (ICU) at our hospital [2]. The viruses that most frequently cause encephalitis are shown in Table 1.

Apart from the infections caused by virus, other infectious agents can lead to cerebral inflammatory lesions such as *Mycoplasma pneumoniae*, *Rickettsios's*, *Spirochet Leptospir* tuberculosis, *Cryptococcus neoformans* or *Toxoplasma gondii*, that in most cases will occur as subacute or chronic diseases through the years (Table 2).

Another important group of illnesses are those that involve the brain vessels (vasculitis, cerebral hemorrhage) outside the area of infection, that can evolve into a diffuse cerebral lesion.

In this chapter we refer almost exclusively to the encephalitis caused by infectious agents, specifically the one caused by viruses, whose acute and, on some occasions, cataclysmic presentation qualifies them for admission in the ICU.

Etiology and Pathology

The term "infectious encephalitis" refers to a disseminated or a focal inflammation of the brain tissue. The pathogen enters the CNS basically through two pathways: the hematogenous and the neuronal.

- *The hematogenous pathway* is more frequently used by viruses and it takes place during a viremia that subsequently opens the way to cerebral invasion. In the USA the arbovirus encephalitis enters the blood stream through a mosquito bite. In Western Europe there is a prevalence of seasonal infectious diseases, related to non-polio enterovirus, parotiditis, respiratory virus and rubella [3, 4] whose entrance, despite being also through the blood stream, and a previous virus replication in another organ such as lungs or intestine. And then, viremia and cerebral invasion occur.
- *The neuronal pathway* is mainly used by two groups of virus: rabies and herpes. The rabies virus is transmitted by infected saliva that enters the healthy body usually from the bite of an infected animal. The virus travels from the wound to the brain through the motor and the sensitive nerves. Regarding the neuronal pathway, different studies carried out

TABLE 1. More frequent viruses that cause acute encephalomyelitis

Direct Infection	Postinfection
Eastern equine	Rubella
Western equine	Mumps
St. Louis	Measles
Venezuelan equine	
WeMurray Valley	Herpesvirus
Nile	Varicella-zoster virus
Japanese	Epstein-Barr virus
Dengue	
Tick-borne complex Measles	
LaCrosse	
Rift Valley	
Sindbi	
California	
Mumps	
Measles	
Poliovirus	
Coxsackieviruses	
Echovirus	
Hepatitis A virus	
Colorado tick fever	
Rabies	
Human immunodeficiency	
Herpes simplex virus types 1 and 2	
Varicela-zoster virus	
Herpes B virus	
Epstein-Barr virus	
Cytomegalolovirus	
Human herpesvirus 6	
Adenovirus	

TABLE 2. Nonviral infections that cause encephalomyelitis

Rocky Mountain spotted fever	Tuberculosis
Typhus	*Crypococcus* sp
Ehrlichia canis	*Histoplasma* sp
Q fever	*Naegleria* sp
Mycoplasma	*Acanthamoeba* sp
Brucellosis	*Toxoplasma gondii*
Subacute bacterial endocarditis	*Plasmodium falciparum*
Listeria	Trypanosomiasis
Syphilis (meningovascular)	Amebiasis
Lyme disease	
Leptospirosis	
Nocardia	
Actinomycosis	

on animals have shown that the entrance of the infectious agent can be through the olfactory nerves or the branches of the trigeminal nerve [5, 6]. Once the infection is established in the brain tissue, the viral replication takes place in the cortex and also in the neuroglia, including the epithelial cells of the blood vessels. As a result of this cellular lesion, lysis takes place resulting in a tissular necrosis and an inflammatory reaction [5, 7]. This invasive process can be gradual so that on occasions it occurs as lymphocytic meningitis, with a low mortality rate, or it becomes diffuse encephalitis with hemorrhage which has a worse prognosis. The evidence of this invasive phenomenon is that the agent that causes most of the lymphocytic meningitis also causes encephalitis, and in this clinical context they show a better outcome.

In addition, there are other mechanisms that would increase brain edema. While in bacterial infectious processes, the involvement of inflammatory mediators such as IL-1, IL-6, IL-8 and TNF are related to the occurrence of brain edema, this mechanism does not seem to be the main one in encephalitis, where the levels of cytokines are similar to the control group [8]. There are also other mechanisms that seem to be involved. A decrease of oxygen extraction has been noted, when controlling the dynamic consumption of cerebral oxygen, which indicates vascular hyperemia [9]. Highly hyperemic zones in basal frontotemporal zones have been observed when analyzing, by SPEC, the lesions caused by HSV. Therefore it seems that the vasogenic component is an important factor in the occurrence of secondary edema in encephalitis.

The injured area of the brain shows a variable distribution, from disseminated to focal lesions more or less dispersed, that will influence the clinical picture of the infection. Although some pathogens have a preference for certain cerebral areas, (HSV in temporal and frontal lobes, rabies virus in Purkinje's corpuscles, *Varicella Zoster* virus in motor zones), in most cases the sites vary. Modifications of the usual areas of infection may

TABLE 3. More frequent etiology of encephalitis in ICU

HSV	6 (46%)
VZV	1 (7%)
Borrellia	1 (7%)
Influenza B virus	1 (7%)
Unknown	4 (28%)
Total	13

HSV: *Herpes Simplex Virus*.
VZV: *Varicela-Zoster Virus*.
ARF: Acute Respiratory Failure.

TABLE 4. Encephalitis adverse events

Seizures	9 (69%)
ARF	9 (69%)
Ischemic lesion	5 (38%)
Focal lesion	5 (38%)
Shock	1 (7%)
Diabetes insipidus	1 (7%)
Brain abscess	1 (7%)

ARF: Acute Respiratory Failure.

occur, as recently observed with enterovirus 71 that from being a predominant dermatological infection involved the central nervous sistem in 35% of the cases [10].

Herpes Simplex Virus (HSV)

In spain HSV causes 46% of the encephalitis that require ICU admission (Table 3) [2]. The importance of HSV type 1 encephalitis lies in its frequent occurrence (first cause of non-seasonal encephalitis) and in the possibility of an early treatment with acyclovir, which represents a rise in the survival rate. Basically there are two types of infectious HSV:

- Type 1 responsible for most of herpes simplex illnes (HSI) in adults, and
- Type 2 responsible for HSI in newborns less than three weeks of age, although it is also responsible for approximately 6% of infections in older children [11].

Other types of herpes virus are less likely to cause encephalitis [12]. Investigations have shown that the entrance of HSV into the brain is through the olfactory tract and the branches of the trigeminal nerve until infiltrate the basal areas of the temporal and frontal lobes [5, 13]. It is unknown when this entrance occurs since the infection can appear in the course of a primary infection or can start from an infected sensorial ganglion in a retrograde way. Thus, the transmission of viral particles takes place without peripheral neuritis [3]. Labial herpes is present only in 6–10% of patients who are already seropositive for HSV at the onset of the symptoms [11].

The lesion caused by HSV-1 is typically a disseminated hemorrhagic lesion that mainly affects the basal areas of the anterior cerebral lobes (temporal and frontal) causing an acute reactive edema that may lead to a displacement and uncal herniation. It differs from type 2 because the lesion is diffuse and evolves into an encephalomalacia without hemorrhagic events [2, 14, 15].

Recent experimental studies have shown that brain damage is not only a result of direct lesions produced by viruses but also by other factors, which explains the therapeutic failure in some cases. In mouses has been noted that acyclovir decreases the immune expression of the nitric oxide synthetase in the early stages but not after six months [16].

SYMPTOMS

The symptoms of herpes simplex encephalitis (HSE) may be unspecific with some days of fever, headache, vomiting and coma. Table 4 shows the most frequent clinical events that lead to admission into the ICU. However, there may be unique signs of infection in the front-temporal lobes, which leads to a prodrome with hallucinations, and personality changes including delirium, and the occurrence of neurological focalities such as aphasia or anosmia. We can also observe non-specific signs such as seizures or hemiparesis [17]. Focal seizures are more frequent in patients younger than 18 years of age, while confusion and memory disorders occur in patients older than 18 years of age. Therefore, this disease may occur at any time of the year and at any age, although 50% of the cases are patients over 20 years of age [18]. Despite the radical change in the survival expectancies with the use of acyclovir, HSE is a severe infection. In 42 patients with a positive HSE diagnosis, and receiving an appropriate treatment, 97% of the survivors had some type of neurological sequelae, and among them, 12% had severe disorders. The mortality rate was 12% [19]. The severity, the duration, and the level of unconsciousness are decisive clinical factors in the evolution of HSE [18]. The development in newborns is completely different depending on the type of infection (HSV-1 or HSV-2), the seizures being when caused by HSV-2 more frequent, and in 77% of the cases, the neurological damage persists after three years [15].

DIAGNOSIS

Sometimes it is not easy to diagnose HSE. Only in 45% of the patients with clinically suspected HSE will it be possible to confirm the diagnosis. In 33% no diagnosis will be made, and the remainder of cases correspond to encephalitis caused by other viruses, non-viral infectious encephalitis, and non-infectious encephalitis [20].

An initial evaluation of the cerebrospinal fluid (CSF) is required to determine the clinical symptoms. CSF will be drawn by lumbar puncture. The cells are usually leukocytes below $500/mm^3$, and rarely above $3000/mm^3$, most of them being lymphocytes. Red blood cells related to the cerebral hemorrhagic lesion can be detected and, depending on the amount, the CSF could be classified as "clear" or "hematic fluid" [17]. Proteins are elevated although never as high as in bacterial meningitis, and the glucose is normal although it could be under 50% of the serum levels [21].

For many years, a reliable diagnosis of HSE has been carried out through a cerebral biopsy. The eosinophilic nuclear inclusion bodies in neurons and glia cells were pathognomonic. Nowadays, the cerebral biopsy is made in those patients with an inadequate response to acyclovir treatment. The development of new techniques of expression of the viral replication has reversed the performance terms, so today these techniques are the first ones that must be carried out for the etiologic diagnosis [22]. Detection of viral DNA through PCR techniques has a sensibility rate between 96 and 100% and a specificity range between 95–100% [23, 24]. Its use has allowed to rationalize acyclovir administration since empiric treatment can be withdrawn in those patients with a negative PCR for HSV, and with a stable clinical evolution [25]. It is interesting to note that the sensitivity and specificity of the procedure is maintained even when there are other underlying basal illnesses, such as HIV infection [26].

Recent studies based on the detection of viral copies in CSF would add a new prognostic value to this measurement, since patients with more than 100 copies show a higher degree of CT lesions and a worse prognosis [27]. However, some authors have demonstrated that the progressive disappearance of viral DNA in CSF is not correlated with treatment effectiveness, since DNA disappears and clinical and MRI disorders persist [28]. Viral DNA detection is a very specific and sensitive technique, and it is also very fast, so it has taken the place of other inmunofluorescent techniques such as the detection of viral antigenic levels in the wall of lymphocytes obtained from CSF. Although it is a fast technique and its use was praised at the beginning of this decade, it is expensive, and has low sensitivity due to not always being possible to obtain enough lymphocytes to get an adequate response [29]. Another feasible microbiologic method is the viral culture, although today it is not advisable as a routine practice, it can be useful in those cases where the etiologic diagnosis is uncertain [30].

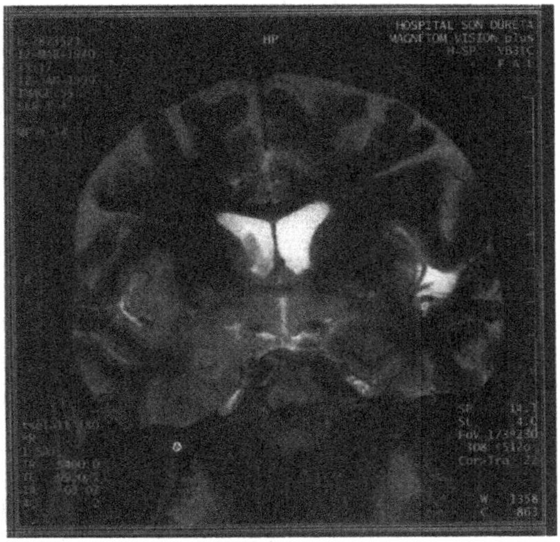

FIGURE 1. In the Axial T1 projection the arrow shows an abnormal increased level of the signal intensity to the level of mamilars bodies and of both temporary lobes, with hemorragic phenomenons in the left one.

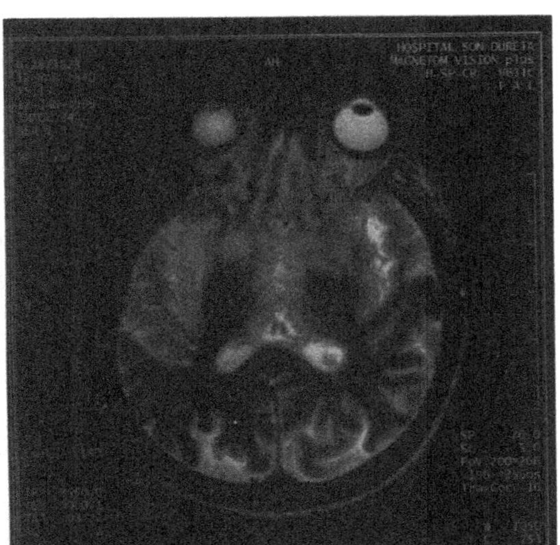

FIGURE 1. In the Axial T1 projection the arrow shows an abnormal increased level of the signal intensity to the level of mamilars bodies and of both temporary lobes, with hemorragic phenomenons in the left one.

Traditionally the electroencephalogram (EEG) is another diagnosis technique for HSE. Representative alterations are seen in 65% of the cases, consisting of lateral epileptiform waves in the temporal areas mixed with slow waves in latencies of two or three seconds. EEG evolution is not correlated with the patient's clinical evolution, because EEG alterations could go back to normal while the neurological symptoms persist [31].

Nowadays we can determine *in vivo* any lesion caused by the herpes infection. Both the computerized axial tomography (CT) and magnetic resonance imaging (MRI) can show the location of the lesions, but also their evolution and final sequelae, being a relationship between these and the pathology [11, 32–34]. MRI is a more sensitive, specific and a faster technique in detecting brain lesions. Low signal areas with surrounding edema can be observed in T1 before the occurrence of hemorrhagic lesions (Figure 1). The use of gadolinium increases the evidence of the inflammation areas (Figure 2). However, radiological images are not the base for HSE diagnosis, although they can discern other different processes [13], and are mandatory before making a cerebral biopsy since it enables enhancement of the effectiveness of the biopsy to 100%.

TREATMENT

Acyclovir is the first line drug for treatment of HSE. The administration of 10 mg/Kg q8 h I.V. has decreased the mortality rate from 70% to 28% [35]. Acyclovir inhibits the viral DNA polymerase by blocking the DNA synthesis. It is mainly excreted through the kidney so precautions need to be taken when administered to patients with renal failure. In general, it is a well tolerated drug, with very few side effects, the most important adverse events being nephrotoxicity and neurotoxicity.

Nephrotoxicity increase with the use of other nephrotoxic drugs (cyclosporine, aminoglycosides) and when there is renal failure, while neurotoxicity can show various clinical symptoms that could be taken as HSE symptoms. This toxicity is present in 1–4% of treatments being hallucinations, anxiousness and a decreased level of consciousness the most frequent symptoms. Other less frequent symptoms are tremors, myoclonus or seizures. As a general rule, the onset of symptoms usually occurs on the second day of the therapy, and they disappear after the drug is withdrawn [36]. The duration of the treatment can be between 14 and 21 days, depending on the severity of the clinical symptoms and the time of recovery. A relapse rate in 5–8% of cases has been seen. Under this circumstance the treatment with acyclovir will be rechallenged at a dose of 15 mg/kg q8 h over 21 days [3]. The combination with other drugs has not improved the clinical outcomes obtained with monotherapy. Only in a subgroup of children with severe CT images, the administration of β-interferon improved the mortality and the morbidity rates [37].

Other Herpes Virus

Other types of herpes virus can lead to encephalitis, especially in patients with an altered immune system. Cytomegalovirus (CMV) encephalitis in patients with AIDS or severely immunosupressed (i.e. transplanted patients) is the most common virus [38, 39]. In transplanted patients, it may appear as a diffuse meningoencephalitis, with a quick onset, quick evolution and usually a fatal outcome. The encephalitis in patients with AIDS can develop as focal or disseminated, with a subacute onset included within the AIDS dementia complex, although its role is still unclear. CMV identification is documented by observation of typical inclusion bodies in the neurons or by the presence of CMV antigens in the CSF. Currently, there are various highly effective techniques to identify CMV such as indirect inmunofluorescence, radioimmunoassay, the latex reaction or an ELISA test. Infection will be evident by detecting antigens that were not previously there, or by an increase in their title. The detection by PCR technique could distinguish an infected patient from a patient with antigens [38]. There is a specific treatment for CMV infection, ganciclovir at a dose of 5 mg/Kg q12 h over 14–21 days. Other effective drugs are foscarnet and cidofovir [40]. Currently, combination of drugs, live foscarnet plus ganciclovir, is under investigation in order to increase treatment effectiveness [38].

Varicella-Zoster encephalitis (VZ) or Epstein Barr encephalitis are rare. VZ encephalitis is present in less than 1% of population with encephalitis. Its evolution is usually better than the CMV encephalitis although AIDS patients with VZ encephalitis could have a leucoencephalitis, usually fatal, whose main symptom is a hemispheric necro-hemorrhagic involvement of all the cerebral lobes, and it can be documented by MRI [41]. Acyclovir is active against this virus at the same doses recommended for HSE [42].

Rabies Virus

Rabies virus (RV) is a *lyssavirus* that belongs to the *rhabdoviridae* family. Its extensiveness is universal, affecting mammals of different species, including humans. The RV infects the brain producing encephalitis that will inexorably lead to the subject's death. Although the most frequent way of infection is from the bite of an infected animal, there are other infection pathways that include mucosa, aerosol and cornea transplantation. Domestic mammals, dogs and cats, are free from infection in developed countries thanks to vaccination campaigns; however, in developing countries they can represent 10% of the reservoir [43, 44]. The virus migrates to the brain through the motor or the sensitive nerves. The incubation period (period from exposure to rabies virus to onset of illness) ranges from three to 12 weeks, in which time the virus replicates and implants in the brain [45].

The pathological lesions caused by RV are typical, with intracytoplasmic inclusion bodies (Negri bodies) in neurons, distributed in different levels of the CNS, including the cerebral cortex and the spinal ganglions. Also, perivascular involvement is observed, with the presence of lymphocytes and polymorphonuclear cells [6].

SYMPTOMS

Despite the general belief that rabies comes from the bite of dogs, it is eight times more common coming from cat bites of cats [46]. Initial rabies symptoms in humans are vague with episodes of fever, headache and malaise (not feeling well). Paresthesias can be observed at the site of the wound, although in 78% of cases there is no evidence of the bite [47]. In the next stage, the disease is asymptomatic up to the third week, when neurogenic hypersensitivity develops with signs of hydrophobia and pharyngeal spasms with consciousness impairment that evolves into to coma. In this stage, the disease is irreversible and the subject dies [6, 47].

The diagnosis of rabies is made by antigen detection using the fluorescent antibody test in the brain of the infected animal. This technique can also be applied to samples obtained from the inoculation area. Patient's serum, CSF and sputum samples must be taken for antigen detection. The PCR technique can be used in the salivary samples, where high concentrations of the virus can be found.

TREATMENT

The only treatment for rabies is prevention, as there are no antiviral drugs available against RV. The CDC recommends to control RV infection are shown in Table 5. The preventive vaccination and serologic control for antibodies titer are only advisable in those workers with daily manipulation of samples with high concentration of the virus, that can be infected by various pathways, and for those people in high risk occupations (veterinarians, sheerers, diagnosis laboratory workers) who work in enzootic areas of RV. The bite of an animal does not require immediate vaccination. Assuming that up to 65% of cats and 28% of dogs are not vaccinated [46], they will be placed under a 10 day quarantine. If the animal does not show any sign of rabies then it will not be necessary to carry out any procedure. If there is any sign of the disease, the animal will be put down for an immediate diagnosis of the infection and a passive immunization by rabies immune globulin (RIG) will start, as shown tables [48].

Arbovirus Encephalitis

The arboviruses that cause encephalitis in humans are distributed among several families: *Togaviridae* (Eastern equine encephalitis, Western equine encephalitis and Venezuelan equine encephalitis), *Flavviridiae* (St. Louis encephalitis, Japanese encephalitis, Dengue encephalitis, Murray Valley encephalitis, West Nile encephalitis and Tick-borne encephalitis), *Buyaviridiae* (LaCrosse encephalitis, Jamestown Canyon encephalitis and California encephalitis) and *Reoviridae* (Colorado, Sindbi) [49, 50]. All of them are zoonotic infections, with the virus being reproduced in birds or mammals and always transmitted by an arthropod. This fact is of vital importance to understand the spread of the disease, since the time of maximum outbreak is summer, when the transmission vector hatches. The infection in humans does not contribute to the spread of the virus. The biggest influence area corresponds to the USA, being the Sindbi virus and West Nile encephalitis more frequent in Europe, mainly in Center, East and Mediterranean countries [51]. In Japan and Southeast Asia, Japanese encephalitis clearly dominates. However, travelers make possible the spread of the infection from their epizootic zones [52].

The lesions in the brain structure involve the gray and the white matter, including the brain stem. Cortical lesions, menigeal enhancement, and periventricular white-matter changes were less common [53–55]. There is evidence of apoptosis in the swollen glial cells [54].

SYMPTOMS

Most of the time the illness is asymptomatic or it is present as a discomfort, without encephalic involvement. Encephalic symptoms are

TABLE 5. Recommendations of the CDC for the prevention and treatment of rabies [48]

Category of risk	Exhibition level	Control	Treatment	Comments
Preexposure	*Continuous*: Workers on continuous manipulation of the virus.	Serology every six months.	Vaccination if An titers are <1:5*	
	Frequent: Workers with episodic exposure regardless whether they know it or not. Epidemic areas.	Serology every two years.	Vaccination if An titers are <1:5*	
	Infrequent: Workers manipulating animals in areas with low frequency of rabies.	No measure required	No serology or vaccination required.	
	Rare: general population in areas of low frequency	No measure required	No serology or vaccination required.	
Postexposure (lesion produced by a non-vaccinated animal)	*Without previous vaccination*		Wound	Thorough cleaning with water and soap. Flush with a viral agent (povidone solution)
			RIG (Rabies immunoglobulin)	20 IU/kg. To be completely administered around the wound. Do not use the same syringe for RIG and the vaccine.
			Vaccines	HDCV, RVA, or PCEC at a dose of 1.0 ml, IM in deltoids on days 0, 3, 7, 14 and 28.
	Previous vaccination		Wound	Same as previous.
			RIG	It must not be administered.
			Vaccines	HDCV, RVA, or PCEC 1.0 ml, IM in deltoids & on days 0 and 3.

* RFFIT: Rapid Fluorescent Focus Inhibition Test. HDCV: human diploid cell vaccine. RVA: rabies vaccine absorbed. PCEC: purified chick embryo cell vaccine, & do not administer in the glutei, the number of antibodies reached is smaller.

TABLE 6. Non-infectious diseases that may cause encephalitis

Whipple's disease	Carcinoma
Behçet's disease	Lymphoma in HIV
Cat-scratch disease	Drug reactions
Vasculitis	

unspecific. After an incubation period between seven and 14 days, there will be fever, headache, nausea, vomiting and drowsiness. Subsequently convulsions, coma and focal lesions such as hemiparesis and cranial nerve involvement will occur.

For its correct identification we must keep in mind that the outbreak of infection in the animal reservoir usually happens before the infection in humans. The distribution area in which the infection takes place, patient's age and the animal reservoir will give us a clinical idea of the infectious virus. Thus, the Eastern and Western equine virus and the LaCrosse and West Nile infections are more frequent in children, whereas in adults Venezuelan equine, Western equine, St. Louis and Nile virus are isolated. People over 50 years of age are more likely to be infected by the last three viruses mentioned [3, 56].

Clinical outcome of the disease is variable, with the Eastern equine encephalitis having the highest mortality rate, that could reach 36%, with 35% of sequelae in survivors [53]. The most frequent arbovirus encephalitis in Europe is the encephalitis caused by a tick sting. It usually occurs as a meningoencephalitis, with a better prognosis. Mortality rate is below 2% [57]. Japanese encephalitis prevails in South-eastern Asia, including Japan, and has a mortality rate of 12%, with 60% of sequelae, being more than 40% severe [58].

DIAGNOSIS

The diagnosis of arbovirus encephalitis has been carried out so far through detection of immunoglobulines G and M by immunofluorescent assay. It requires an increase of the titration up to four times the baseline value, in the convalescence period between one and three weeks after the onset of the symptoms. Currently there are two methods that have improved the diagnosis:

- The detection on CSF serum, of IgG or IgM by ELISA or arthropod. In early stages, IgM is more specific, whereas IgG will be more reactive in later stages.
- The development of the PCR technique has allowed an early diagnosis of the encephalitis caused by the sting of arthropods, with higher sensitivity and specificity [57].

MRI is the radiological technique that has the highest sensitivity when revealing lesions. The distribution of the lesions could be disseminated, which corresponds to the anatomopathological lesions, and they may be found in the gray matter, basal nucleus, thalamus, cerebral stem, or white matter [55].

TREATMENT

As there is no specific antiviral treatment for this kind of lesion, the therapy must be based on prevention eliminating the natural reservoirs, the insects and the use of developed vaccines. So far, there are vaccines for Japanese encephalitis, tick encephalitis, and Eastern, Western and Venezuelan encephalitis. The choice of the vaccine depends on the spread area of the arboviruses. The vaccination of people who travel to endemic areas during summer is strongly recommended. Likewise it is advisable not to be outdoors during twilight hours, to wear trousers and long shirts, and to use mosquito repellent in these areas.

Besides the prophylactic measures, an effective method to control brain edema has not been found yet. The use of high doses of corticosteroids has been ineffective in decreasing the mortality rate in the Japanese encephalitis [59].

Enterovirus

The *Enterovirus* family is the leading cause of seasonal meningoencephalitis. Under this denomination poliovirus, echovirus, Coxsackieviruses, hepatitis A and viruses that causes intestinal infections are included. The initial symptoms are vague with fever, arthromyalgies and headache. Previous gastrointestinal dysfunction, such as nausea/vomiting may have occurred [6]. In the *enterovirus* 71 infection, myoclonia and ataxia may occur [10], while Coxsackie infection can cause polyserositis, herpangina, rash, and occasionally neurological focalities such as seizures in children [60].

Although the usual outcome is good (towards a complete recovery), mortality has been noted between 3–9% of cases [61].

The diagnosis is made by specific virus antibody detection in CSF and serum samples. The virus can also be isolated in the oropharynx or faeces [30]. EEG, CT and MRI do not help in the diagnosis although they are probably adequate in the follow-up of those cases with an unfavorable resolution.

There is no effective antiviral treatment for enteroviral encephalitis, with supportive treatment being the unique option [62].

Postinfectious Encephalitis

Postinfectious or postvaccine encephalitis refers to the cerebral damage, with an autoimmune etiology that occurs between 1–3 weeks after the onset of the viral infection or after the vaccination. The populations at high risk are older children and young adults. The viruses most frequently involved are chickenpox, measles and respiratory viruses. The vaccines most frequently involved are those for rubella, measles, smallpox, and mumps [63].

The pathologic changes of postinfectious and postvaccine encephalomyelitis are characterized by perivascular infiltration of mononuclear inflammatory cells and perivenous demyelination [63].

The use of high dose corticosteroids (prednisone 60 mg/day) is effective in the treatment of most postinfectious encephalitis, where the occurrence of death or permanent lesions is not unusual, especially in encephalitis caused by measles [45].

Toxoplasma gondii encephalitis

Toxoplasma gondii (TG) is an intracellular parasite that affect the CNS and it is common in AIDS patients with advanced disease, being isolated in 17% of these patients. The symptoms develop progressively, in days or weeks, being exceptional sudden onsets.

Symptoms range from lethargy and apathy to coma, from incoordination and ataxia to hemiparesis, from memory loss to severe dementia and from local to major motor seizures [64]. The variability of the symptoms is due to the type of lesion caused by the parasite in the brain. In 77% of the cases, lesions are multiple [65], involving white and gray matter of both cerebral hemispheres, although brain stem involvement is not unusual [66].

DIAGNOSIS

The diagnosis of TG encephalitis is based on compatible symptoms, serological criteria and radiological images. The CSF parameters are not different from other viral encephalitis. Hyperproteinorrhachia with a low cellular level, as well as normo or hypoglycorrachia may occur. The serum detection of IgG and IgM levels by ELISA is enough to make a diagnosis of acute infection, although their titration is variable, and sometimes it does not allow distinction from a post-exposition. The IgE is only positive in 33% of the cases [67]. The detection of the parasite's DNA in CSF by PCR has improved the diagnosis, with a 100% specificity and a 33% sensitivity, that increases to 50% if it is made within the first week of infection, not being altered by the administration of theropy [68, 69].

The radiological lesions obtained by CT and MRI shown characteristically hypodense bilateral lesions, revealing an aura after the administration of the contrast medium. They are usually in the cortex-medulla junction although they might show in the brain stem. MRI is more sensitive than CT. However, these techniques, by themselves, are not diagnostic assays as the results are not specific for *T. gondii* [70, 71].

TREATMENT

TG encephalitis in AIDS patients must be treated by using two drugs. The most recommended combination is pyrimethamine (75–100 mg/day with a load dose of 200 mg) plus sulfadiazine 1–1.5 gr q6 h, and a supplement of folinic acid (10–20 mg).

Pirimethamine and clindamycin (600 to 1200 mg q6 h) administration has proved to be as effective as the former combination [65, 72]. However, none of the two combinations is free of adverse events, mainly rash and hematologic disorders [65], that leads to a discontinuation of the treatment. Therefore, alternative treatments are being tested, such as cotrimoxazol [73].

Tuberculosis Encephalitis

Tuberculosis is an endemic and world-wide disease that has experienced an unusual growth thanks to AIDS. Usually, the immunocompetent patient suffers tuberculosis as a subacute meningoencephalitis, with several days of evolution, although AIDS patients may suffer it more acutely, with fever, headache, nausea and vomiting as the most frequent symptoms. Usually there is an involvement of cranial nerves [74]. The CSF shows a low number of cells, mainly lymphocytic, with glycorrhachia <40 mg/dl, and normal or slightly elevated number of proteins. Zhiel staining of the CSF may help for early diagnosis of the infection as it can be positive in 80% of the cases when there are three serial lumbar punctures performed [39]. The sensitivity to detect *M. tuberculosis* by PCR is 48%, with a 100% specificity [75], which makes this technique the most suitable for the diagnosis. The presence of tuberculomas in basal regions of the CNS shown by CT or MRI reinforces the diagnosis.

The mortality rate of patients admitted in the ICU with brain tuberculosis after four months is over 64%, being a delay of more than three days in the start of a treatment and an APACHE II score >11, of death independent prognosis factors [76].

Treatment must involve a minimum of three drugs (isoniazide 5 mg/kg, rifampin 10 mg/kg, and pyrazinamide 15–30 mg/kg), being strongly recommended the administration of a fourth tuberculosis drug (ethambutol 15–25 mg/kg, or streptomycin 15 mg/kg IM) in patients with AIDS. The use of dexametasone (0.2–0.4 mg/kg q8 h) decreases the number of adverse events and sequelae [77].

Non-Infectious Encephalitis

Thirty per cent of the encephalitis are not caused by a virus [3]. Among these, more than 50% of the cases are diagnosed as non-infectious encephalitis, usually being diseases with a diffuse vascular involvement. The usual symptoms of these lesions are subacute or chronic, which allows a suitable diagnosis and treatment. Only in those patients with AIDS who do not receive any treatment, tumoral lesions, specially brain lymphoma, may represents an acute problem of differential diagnosis in front of infectious processes [68]. In these cases, the incidence of neoplasia is higher than the infection allocated in the area, a situation that was found in 46% of the studied population, whereas *T. gondii* involvement is 15% [68].

Supportive Management

The management and control of some patients with acute encephalitis in ICUs may be warranted, not only to control the encephalitis which response is not correlated to the treatment (probably because the brain edema that coexists with the lesion is high) but also because there is an increased number of viral encephalitis without a suitable treatment. Therefore, controlling brain damage will help the patient to survive. This control involves (Table 7):

- Maintenance of the airway and adequate ventilation
- Control of brain edema
- Occurrence of any adverse event

TABLE 7. Suportive management

1. *Airway management*:
   - Isolation of the airway road if GCS < eight points with intubation oro/nasotraqueal
   - Control of ventilation by means of sedation (midazolam), and muscular relaxation if necessary
   - To assure an adequate oxygenation (Sat.O2 > 95%)
   - To prevent atelectasias using levels of PEEP 4–7 cm H_2O
2. *Control of cerebral edema*:
   - To monitor cerebral activity (ICP, $SjvO_2$, cranial doppler, EEG)
   - To maintain CPP > 60 mm Hg
   - Semirecumbent body possition > 30 degrees
   - To maintain hyperventilaxion ($paCO_2$ 34–37 mm Hg)
   - IV bolus of manitol 20% or glycerol, 0.5 to 1 g/kg, if ICP > 20 cm H_2O
   - IV bolus of tiopental of 2–3 mg/kg. If ICP decreases, establish perfusion of 0.5–3 microg/kg/h. It is advisable to control the cerebral activity by means of continous EEG
   - To avoid hyperglicemia, hypernatremia
   - Maintained body temperature < 38° by means of physical or pharmacological measures (paracetamol)
   - Dexamethasone 4 mg iv. q4 h Doubtful effectiveness
3. *Control complications*:
   - Treat convulsions with intravenous phenytoin load (20 mg/kg) followed by 3–5 mg maintenance/kg/day
   - Treat insipid diabetes with desmopressin 1–3 mg, intermittent
   - Control strict electrolytes in the event of inadequate secretion of ADH
   - Exquisite care of all the exogenous devices to diminish the incidence of nosocomial infection

CPP: Cerebral perfusion pressure. ICP: Intracranial pressure. $SjvO_2$: Jugular venous oxygen saturation.
GCS: Glasgow coma score.

The decrease in the level of consciousness of these patients will involve loss of the intake reflexes with, loss of swallowing and tusigen reflexes, that will be accompanied by abnormalities in the tongue movements with a likely airway obstruction. This problem can usually be noted in patients whose Glasgow Coma Score is equal or below eight [78]. Then, the airway must be opened using oropharyngeal or nasopharyngeal cannulas. This also allows tusigen stimulatiodrainage and secretions. The deep impairment of the level of consciousness and the specific brain lesions, are accompanied by severe impairment in the patient's ventilation in form of bradipnea, Cheyne-Stokes breathing or hyperventilation crisis. This implies an acute respiratory failure that leads to orotracheal or nasotracheal intubation and the use of ventilatory. Support the use of sedatives and muscle relaxants will depend on the difficulty to achieve the patient's adequate respiratory parameters. Use of sedatives may interfere with the neurological status of the patient. Ventilation control should be strict in the acute stages of the disease.

As an expression of brain damage in 69% of encephalitis, there is an increase in intracranial pressure ICP values above 15 mmHg [79]. However, ICP value is not to be assessed except as an indicator of the cerebral perfusion pressure (CPP) [80] which is the value that will really determine brain suffering. CPP values below 60 mmHg means the occurrence of secondary cerebral damage. Patients with sustained ICP values above 20 mmHg have a higher mortality rate than those with lower values [81]. Besides, GGS level is not correlated with PIC levels. There are no adequately evidences to determine the most suitable treatment for these patients. A simple measure is to keep patient's head at around 30°, since it facilitates the venous return. It may be reasonable using hyperventilation since hyperemia has been observed. The maintenance of low values of CO_2 around 34–37 mmHg produces a vasoconstrictor effect in the brain that would improve the vascular dynamics. Nevertheless, it must be kept in mind that the maintenance of this situation could lead to an undesirable cerebral ischemia [45]. Based on data from craneoencephalic trauma patients, it could be useful to place a catheter in the bulb of the jugular vein to control oxygen consumption. Oxygen saturation over 65% would indicate a hyperemic cerebral flow, despite treatment [82]. Another measure to control ICP is the use of osmotic diuretics, manitol 20% or glycerol 20%. In both cases the dose is 0.5–1 g/Kg in bolus. Glycerol is more frequently used in children and its effect is longer than manitol, although slow. In addition, the infusion rate can not be faster than 3.3 mOsm per minute [83]. If the previous measures are not effective an option is thiopental (0.5–3 mg/kg/mn, I.V.) to maintain the patient in barbiturate coma. The consequence of this decision will be to lose control on the patient's neurological status. The use of corticosteroids (dexametasone 4 mg q4 h) has been recommended by some authors as one of the effective treatments to control brain edema, since it has an anti-inflammatory effect in the vasogenic and neurogenic edema. However, it does not seem to be effective in all cases since in Japanese encephalitis with torpid resolution neither the mortality nor the sequelae decrease after three months. In selected groups of patients, some physicians praise the use of cranial decompression that could lead to an hemicraniectomy [84].

The occurrence of adverse events is the third situation that requires strict control. The most important is the occurrence of seizures. From a clinical point of view they are the expression of the patient's cerebral involvement, but they also represent an added factor that will worsen the patient's prognosis, since during their appearance the mechanisms that control brain edema will be altered, and the number of events will be significantly increased. The administration of benzodiazepines (lorazepam 0.05–0.1 mg/Kg, diazepam 0.2–0.5 mg/Kg or midazolam 0.05–2 mg/Kg) iv could be enough to control the event [85], provided that we keep in mind that their administration should be slow to avoid the occurrence of respiratory depression and hypotension. Subsequently, it is advisable to use phenitoin to prevent the occurrence of new seizures (load dose 20 mg/Kg, perfusion rate not higher than 50 mg/min; followed by a 3–5 mg/Kg/day maintenance dose). If the control is not effective and seizures continue, another treatment strategy should be used to control the event within 60 minutes to prevent ischaemic cerebral lesions due to seizures appear. Pentobarbital administration with a load dose of 12 mg/Kg, with a maximum perfusion rate of 50 mg/min, followed by a 10 mg/Kg in continuous perfusion until seizure suppression should be prescribed [85]. Hemodyramic control is indispensable since Pentothal has depressor effect of the myocardial function and the control of CCP should be maintained, using vasopressor amines (norepinephrine).

Since nosocomial infection is one of the most frequent events in neurologic patients, infection control measures to avoid their appearance should be reinforced. Patients with neurological disorders whose GCS is between six and eight, and have a nosocomial infection, have a significantly higher mortality versus those without infection [86]. The most frequent nosocomial infections are pulmonary infections, mainly caused by primary endogenous agents (*S. aureus*, *H. influenzae* or *S. pneumoniae*) that enter the lung after colonizing the pharying, either during intubation or through the orotracheal tube. Various systems have been suggeded for infection control, but the effectiveness is partial [87].

References

1. Koskiniem M, Rantonen J, Lehtokoski-Lehtimiemi E, *et al.* Epidemiology of encephalitis in children: a 20 year-survey. Ann Neurol 29:492, 1991.
2. Jordà Marcos R. Infección del SNC: Datos globales de un estudio multicentrico en la UCI. In Jordà Marcos R (ed). Infección del Sistema Nervioso Central en la Unidad de Cuidados Intensivos. Madrid: EMISA, 1996: 1.

3. Whitley RJ. Viral encephalitis. N Engl J Med 323:242, 1990.
4. Kennedy C, Robinson R, Valman H, *et al.* A major role for virus in acute chilhood encephalopaty. Lancet 3:989, 1986.
5. Lynas C, Hill TJ, Maitland NJ, *et al.* Latent infection with the MS strain of herpes simplex virus type 2 in the mouse following intracerebral inoculation. J Neurol Sci 120:107, 1993.
6. Griffin DE. Encephalitis, Myelitis and Neuritis. In Mandell GL, Bennet JE, Doblin R (eds). Principles and Practice of Infectious Diseases. New York: Churchill Livingstone, 1995: 874.
7. Bergstrom T, Alestig K, Svennerholm B, *et al.* Neurovirulence of herpes simplex virus types 1 and 2 isolates in diseases of the central nervous system. Eur J Clin Microbiol Infect Dis 9:751, 1990.
8. Tsai ML, Chen WC, Wang YC, *et al.* Cerebrospinal fluid interleukin-6, interleukin-8, and tumor necrosis factor-alpha in children with central nervous system infections. Acta Paediatr Sin 39:16, 1996.
9. Goetting MG, Haddad ML. Cerebral oxygen extraction during severe viral encephalitis. Henry Ford Hosp Med J 40:127, 1992.
10. Wang SM, Liu CC, Tseng HW, *et al.* Clinical spectrum of enterovirus 71 infection in children in southern Taiwan, with an emphasis on neurological complications. Clin Infect Dis 29:184, 1999.
11. Sköldenberg B. Herpes simplex encephalitis. Scand J Infect Dis Suppl 100:8, 1996.
12. Kolski H, Ford Jones EL, Richardson S, *et al.* Etiology of acute childhood encephalitis at The Hospital for Sick Children, Toronto, 1994–1995. Clin Infect Dis 26:398, 1998.
13. Miller RF, Lucas SB, Hall Craggs MA, *et al.* Comparison of magnetic resonance imaging with neuropathological findings in the diagnosis of HIV and CMV associated CNS disease in AIDS. J Neurol Neurosurg Psychiatry 62:346, 1997.
14. Whitley RJ. Herpes simplex virus infections of the central nervous system. Encephalitis and neonatal herpes. Drugs 42:406, 1991.
15. Corey L, Whitley RJ, Stone EF, *et al.* Difference between herpes simplex virus type 1 and type 2 neonatal encephalitis in neurological outcome. Lancet 1:1, 1988.
16. Haas J, Meyding LU, Fäth A, *et al.* Acyclovir treatment of experimentally induced herpes simplex virus encephalitis: monitoring the changes in immunologic NO synthase expression and viral load within brain tissue of SJL mice. Neurosci Lett 264:129, 1999.
17. Whitley RJ, Soong SJ, Linneman C. Herpes simplex encephalitis: Clinical assessment. JAMA 247:317, 1982.
18. Marton R, Gotlieb ST, Klein C, *et al.* Acute herpes simplex encephalitis: clinical assessment and prognostic data. Acta Neurol Scand 93:149, 1996.
19. McGrath N, Anderson NE, Croxson MC, *et al.* Herpes simplex encephalitis treated with acyclovir: diagnosis and long term outcome. J Neurol Neurosurg Psychiatry 63:321, 1997.
20. Whitley RJ, Cobbs CG, Alford CA Jr, *et al.* Diseases that mimic herpes simplex encephalitis. Diagnosis, presentation, and outcome. NIAD Collaborative Antiviral Study Group. JAMA 262:234, 1989.
21. Ratzan KR. Viral meningitis. Med Clin North Am 69:399, 1985.
22. Domingues RB, Tsanaclis AM, Pannuti CS, *et al.* Evaluation of the range of clinical presentations of herpes simplex encephalitis by using polymerase chain reaction assay of cerebrospinal fluid samples. Clin Infect Dis 25:86, 1997.
23. Aurelius E, Johansson B, Skoldenberg B, *et al.* Rapid diagnosis of herpes simplex encephalitis by nested polymerase chain reaction assay of cerebrospinal fluid. Lancet 337:189, 1991.
24. Guffond T, Dewilde A, Lobert PE, *et al.* Significance and clinical relevance of the detection of herpes simplex virus DNA by the polymerase chain reaction in cerebrospinal fluid from patients with presumed encephalitis. Clin Infect Dis 18:744, 1994.
25. Tebas P, Nease RF, Storch GA. Use of the polymerase chain reaction in the diagnosis of herpes simplex encephalitis: a decision analysis model. Am J Med 105:287, 1998.
26. Cinque P, Vago L, Marenzi R, *et al.* Herpes simplex virus infections of the central nervous system in human immunodeficiency virus-infected patients: clinical management by polymerase chain reaction assay of cerebrospinal fluid. Clin Infect Dis 27:303, 1998.
27. Domingues RB, Lakeman FD, Mayo MS, *et al.* Application of competitive PCR to cerebrospinal fluid samples from patients with *herpes simplex* encephalitis. J Clin Microbiol 36:2229, 1998.
28. Wildemann B, Ehrhart K, Storch HB, *et al.*

Quantitation of *herpes simplex* virus type 1 DNA in cells of cerebrospinal fluid of patients with herpes simplex virus encephalitis. Neurology 48:1341, 1997.
29. Grandien M, Olding-Stenkvist E. Rapid diagnosis of viral infections in the central nervous system. Scand J Infect Dis 16:1, 1984.
30. Reina J. Diagnóstico microbiológico de las infecciones del SNC. In Jordà Marcos R (ed). Infección del Sistema Nervioso Central en la Unidad de Cuidados Intensivos. Madrid: EMISA, 1996: 41.
31. Misra UK, Kalita J. Neurophysiological studies in *herpes simplex* encephalitis. Electromyogr Clin Neurophysiol 38:177, 1998.
32. Sze G, Zimmerman RD. The magnetic resonance imaging of infections and inflammatory diseases. Radiol Clin North Am 26:839, 1988.
33. Schmidbauer M, Podreka I, Wimberger D, *et al.* SPECT and MR imaging in *herpes simplex* encephalitis. J Comput Assist Tomogr 15:811, 1991.
34. Meyding LU, Lamadé W, Kehm R, *et al. Herpes simplex* virus encephalitis: cranial magnetic resonance imaging and neuropathology in a mouse model. Neurosci Lett 248:13, 1998.
35. Whitley RJ, Alford CA, Hirsch MS. Vidarabina versus acyclovir therapy in *herpes simplex* encephalitis. N Engl J Med 314:144, 1986.
36. Rashiq S, Briewa L, Mooney M, *et al.* Distinguishing acyclovir neurotoxicity from encephalomyelitis. J Intern Med 234:507, 1993.
37. Wintergerst U, Belohradsky BH. Acyclovir monotherapy versus acyclovir plus beta-interferon in focal viral encephalitis in children. Infection 20:207, 1992.
38. Cinque P, Cleator GM, Weber T, *et al.* Diagnosis and clinical management of neurological disorders caused by cytomegalovirus in AIDS patients. J Neurovirol 4:120, 1984.
39. Kita M, Laskowitz DT, Kolson DL. Central Nervous System Infections. In Miller DH, Raps EC (eds). Critical Care Neurology. Boston: Butterworth Heinemann, 1999: 279.
40. Anders HJ, Goebel FD. Neurological manifestations of cytomegalovirus infection in the acquired immunodeficiency syndrome. AIDS 10:151, 1999.
41. Aygun N, Finelli DA, Rodgers MS, *et al.* Multifocal varicella-zoster virus leukoencephalitis in a patient with AIDS: MR findings. Am J Neuroradiol 19:1897, 1998.
42. Otero J, Ribera E, Gavaldà J, *et al.* Response to acyclovir in two cases of herpes zoster leukoencephalitis and review of the literature. Eur J Clin Microbiol Infect Dis 17:286, 1998.
43. Human rabies–Montana and Washington, 1997. MMWR 46:770, 1997.
44. Human rabies–Virginia, 1998. MMWR 48:95, 1999.
45. Paczynski RP, Clifford DB. Encephalitis. In Webb AR, Shapiro MJ, Singer M, *et al.* (eds). Oxford Textbook of Critical Care. Oxford: Oxford University Press, 1999: 482.
46. Hensley JA. Potential rabies exposures in a Virginia county. Public Health Rep 113:258, 1998.
47. Noah DL, Drenzek CL, Smith JS, *et al.* Epidemiology of human rabies in the United States, 1980 to 1996. Ann Intern Med 128:922, 1998.
48. Human-Rabies prevention – United States, 1999. Recommendations of the Advisory Committee of Immunization Practices (ACIP). MMWR 48:1, 1999.
49. Calisher CH. Medically important arboviruses of the United States and Canada. Clin Microbiol Rev 7:89, 1994.
50. Ansari MZ, Shope RE. Epidemiology of arboviral infections. Public Health Rev 22:1, 1994.
51. Lundström JO. Mosquito-borne viruses in Western Europe: a review. J Vector Ecol 24:1, 1999.
52. Schwarz TF, Jäger G, Gilch S, *et al.* Travel-related vector-borne virus infections in Germany. Arch Virol Suppl 11:57, 1996.
53. Deresiewicz RL, Thaler SJ, Hsu L, *et al.* Clinical and neuroradiographic manifestations of eastern equine encephalitis. N Engl J Med 336:1867, 1997.
54. Garen PD, Tsai TF, Powers JM. Human eastern equine encephalitis: immunohistochemistry and ultrastructure. Mod Pathol 12:646, 1999.
55. Shoji H, Kida H, Hino H, *et al.* Magnetic resonance imaging findings in Japanese encephalitis. White matter lesions. J Neuroimaging 4:206, 1994.
56. Ho DD, Hirsch MS. Acute viral encephalitis. Med Clin North Am 69:415, 1985.
57. Tomazic J, Poljak M, Popovic P, *et al.* Tick-borne encephalitis: possibly a fatal disease in its acute stage. PCR amplificatioin of TBE RNA from postmortem brain tissue. Infection 25:41, 1997.

58. Misra UK, Kalita J, Srivastava M. Prognosis of Japanese encephalitis: a multivariate analysis. J Neurol Sci 161:143, 1998.
59. Hoke CH Jr, Vaughn DW, Nisalak A, *et al.* Effect of high-dose dexamethasone on the outcome of acute encephalitis due to Japanese encephalitis virus. J Infect Dis 165:631, 1992.
60. Modlin JF, Dagan R, Berlin LE, *et al.* Focal encephalitis with enterovirus infections. Pediatrics 88:841, 1991.
61. Koskiniemi M, Vaheri A. Effect of measles, mumps, rubella vaccination on pattern of encephalitis in children. Lancet 1:31, 1989.
62. Muir P, van Loon AM. Enterovirus infections of the central nervous system. Intervirology 40:153, 1997.
63. Davis LE. Postinfectious encephalitis. In Mohr JP (ed). Manual of clinical problems in neurology. Boston: Little, Brown and Company, 1989: 222.
64. Renold C, Sugar A, Chave JP, *et al.* Toxoplasma encephalitis in patients with the acquired immunodeficiency syndrome. Medicine (Baltimore) 71:224, 1992.
65. Danneman B, McCutchan JA, Israelski D, *et al.* Treatment of toxoplasmic encephalitis inpatients with AIDS. A randomized trial comparing pyrimethamine plus clindamycin to pyrimethamine plus sulfadiazime. The California collaborative treatment group. Ann Intern Med 116:33, 1992.
66. Elder GA, John LS. Neurologic disorders associated with AIDS retroviral infection. Rev Infect Dis 10:286, 1988.
67. Wong SY, Hajdu MP, Ramirez R, *et al.* Role of specific immunoglobulin E in diagnosis of acute toxoplasma infection and toxoplasmosis. J Clin Microbiol 31:2952, 1993.
68. Roberts TC, Storch GA. Multiplex PCR for diagnosis of AIDS-related central nervous system lymphoma and toxoplasmosis. J Clin Microbiol 35:268, 1997.
69. Cingolani A, De Luca A, Ammassari A, *et al.* PCR detection of *Toxoplasma gondii* DNA in CSF for the differential diagnosis of AIDS-related focal brain lesions. J Med Microbiol 45:472, 1996.
70. Davidson HD, Steiner RE. Magnetic resonance imaging in infections of the central nervous system. Am J Neuroradiol 6:499, 1985.
71. Luft BJ, Remington JS. Toxoplasmic encephalitis in AIDS. Clin Infect Dis 15:211, 1992.
72. Luft BJ, Hafner R, Korzun AH, *et al.* Toxoplasmic encephalitis in patients with the acquired immunodeficiency syndrome. N Engl J Med 329:995, 1993.
73. Canessa A, Del BV, De Leo P, *et al.* Cotrimoxazole therapy of *Toxoplasma gondii* encephalitis in AIDS patients. Eur J Clin Microbiol Infect Dis 11:125, 1992.
74. Podzamczer D, Gudiol F, Bolas F, *et al.* Tratamiento de las infecciones más frecuentes en pacientes con infección por el virus de inmunodeficiencia humana. Enf Infec Microbiol Clin 8:161, 1990.
75. Kox LF, Kuijper S, Kolk AH. Early diagnosis of tuberculous meningitis by polymerase chain reaction. Neurology 45:2228, 1995.
76. Verdon R, Chevret S, Laissy JP, *et al.* Tuberculous meningitis in adults: review of 48 cases. Clin Infect Dis 22:982, 1996.
77. Kumarvelu S, Prasad K, Khosla A, *et al.* Randomized controlled trial of dexamethasone in tuberculous meningitis. Tuber Lung Dis 75:203, 1994.
78. Rello J, Ausina V, Castella J, *et al.* Nosocomial respiratory tract infections in multiple trauma patients; Influence of level of consciousness with implications for therapy. Chest 102:525, 1992.
79. Rebaud P, Berthier JC, Hartemann E, *et al.* Intracranial pressure in childhood central nervous system infections. Intensive Care Med 14:522, 1988.
80. Goitein KJ, Tamir I. Cerebral perfusion pressure in central nervous system infections of infancy and childhood. J Pediatr 103:40, 1983.
81. Barnett GH, Ropper AH, Romeo J. Intracranial pressure and outcome in adult encephalitis. J Neurosurg 68:585, 1988.
82. Stocchetti N, Rossi S, Buzzi F, *et al.* Intracranial hypertension in head injury: management and results. Intensive Care Med 25:371, 1999.
83. McDonald JT, Under DL. Intravenous glycerol and mannitol therapy in children with intracranial hypertension. Neurology 32:437, 1982.
84. Schwab S, Jünger E, Spranger M, *et al.* Craniectomy: an aggressive treatment approach in severe encephalitis. Neurology 48:412, 1997.
85. Payne TA, Bleck TP. Status epilepticus. In Diringer MN (ed). Update on Neurologic Critical Care. Philadelphia: W.B. Saunders Company, 1997: 17.

86. Bueno-Cavanillas A, Delgado-Rodriguez M, López-Luque A, *et al.* Influence of nosocomial infection on mortality rate in an intensive care unit. Crit Care Med 22:55, 1994.

87. Kollef MH. Ventilator-associated pneumonia. A multivariate analysis. JAMA 270:1965, 1993.

9781461356745V01